DIABETES AND EXERCISE

CONTEMPORARY DIABETES

ARISTIDIS VEVES, MD, DSc
SERIES EDITOR

The Diabetic Foot: *Second Edition,* edited by *Aristidis Veves,* MD, *John M. Giurini,* DPM, *and Frank W. LoGerfo,* MD, *2006*

The Diabetic Kidney, edited by *Pedro Cortes,* MD *and Carl Erik Mogensen,* MD, *2006*

Obesity and Diabetes, edited by *Christos S. Mantzoros,* MD, *2006*

Diabetic Retinopathy, edited by *Elia J. Duh,* MD, *2008*

Diabetes and Exercise: edited by *Judith G. Regensteiner,* PhD, *Jane E.B. Reusch,* MD, *Kerry J. Stewart,* EDD, *Aristidis Veves,* MD, DSC, *2009*

DIABETES AND EXERCISE

Edited by

Judith G. Regensteiner, PhD
Divisions of General Internal Medicine and Cardiology, Department of Medicine,
University of Colorado Denver, Aurora, CO, USA

Jane E.B. Reusch, MD
Division of Endocrinology, Metabolism and Diabetes, Department of Medicine,
University of Colorado Denver, Aurora, CO, USA

Kerry J. Stewart, EDD
Division of Cardiology, Department of Medicine, Johns Hopkins School of Medicine,
Baltimore, MD, USA

Aristidis Veves, MD, DSc
Joslin-Beth Israel Deaconess Foot Center, Microcirculation Laboratory,
Department of Surgery, Beth Israel Deaconess Medical Center, Harvard Medical School,
Boston, MA, USA

Humana Press

Editors

Judith G. Regensteiner, PhD
Divisions of General Internal Medicine
  and Cardiology
Department of Medicine
University of Colorado
Denver, Aurora, CO, USA

Kerry J. Stewart, EDD
Division of Cardiology
Department of Medicine
Johns Hopkins School of Medicine
Baltimore, MD, USA

Jane E.B. Reusch, MD
Division of Endocrinology
Metabolism and Diabetes
Department of Medicine
Aurora, CO, USA

Aristidis Veves, MD, DSc
Joslin-Beth Israel Deaconess Foot Center
Microcirculation Laboratory
Department of Surgery
Beth Israel Deaconess Medical Center
Harvard Medical School
Boston, MA, USA

ISBN: 978-1-58829-926-0   e-ISBN: 978-1-59745-260-1
DOI: 10.1007/978-1-59745-260-1

Library of Congress Control Number: 2008942273

Printed on acid-free paper

springer.com

To my husband, Ken, and my daughter, Allie, for their unfailing support. Also to my mother, Dorothy, my in-laws, Herb and Inge and to the memory of my father, Max Regensteiner.

Judith G. Regensteiner

To Jay, Maddie, and Leah, and in memory of Roy Brown.

Jane E.B. Reusch

To my wife, Cherie, and children, Jordan and Rebecca, for their support and encouragement with this project and for their patience over the years through many other academic journeys. Also, to the memory of my parents, who may have benefited 20 years ago if we knew then what we know today about preventing and treating diabetes and heart disease.

Kerry J. Stewart

To my wife, Maria, and son, George.

Aristidis Veves

Also, to the patients in our studies, for their willingness to volunteer in research experiments that produce the evidence that make books like this possible. Collectively, their efforts will help many others in their quest for better health.

Preface

Diabetes is a highly significant public health problem in the United States. Approximately 21 million children and adults (7% of the population) have diabetes, although only about 14.6 million have been diagnosed. The estimated number of persons with prediabetes is 54 million. The prevalence of diabetes is higher among persons of Hispanic, African American and Native American heritage than among persons of non-Hispanic white origins. Of persons with type 2 diabetes, two of three deaths are caused by cardiovascular disease, myocardial infarction, or stroke, which may in part be due to an increased prevalence of atherosclerosis risk factors such as hypertension and dyslipidemias. Prevalence of peripheral arterial disease is also greatly increased in persons with diabetes.

Type 1 and type 2 diabetes raise common and disparate issues when it comes to exercise, and these issues are discussed in *Diabetes and Exercise*. At present, more data are available about exercise in type 2 diabetes than type 1 diabetes. However, there is a regenerating interest more recently in type 1 diabetes and new studies should be forthcoming.

Though exercise is recognized by the American Diabetes Association and others as a cornerstone of diabetes treatment, most people with type 2 diabetes are not physically active. Persons with type 2 diabetes have reduced exercise capacity, including lower maximal oxygen consumption and impairments in the submaximal measures of cardiorespiratory exercise performance. These exercise abnormalities appear early and may be related to cardiac and hemodynamic abnormalities. Whatever the reason for decreased physical activity levels, being sedentary is linked to increased levels of morbidity and mortality, which are already high in diabetes. The purpose of *Diabetes and Exercise* is to give the researcher and practitioner in the area of diabetes, information that is both theoretical and clinically useful to further understanding of the importance for persons with diabetes to be physically active as part of the standard of care for treating this condition. In addition, exercise guidelines and precautions are provided to maximize the benefits of activity and to minimize risk in order to avoid adverse events.

We are proud of the quality of all of the chapters in this book, all written by experts in their respective areas and wish to recognize the substantial efforts of all of the authors. Section I sets the stage essentially for the rest of the book. Dr. Kenneth Cusi reviews the epidemiology of diabetes. Prevention of diabetes is discussed by Dr. Jonathan Shaw. Finally, the metabolic syndrome is examined by Dr. Christos Mantzoros. In this way, the reader can understand the magnitude of the problem posed by diabetes and understand the compelling rationale for the use of exercise and increased physical activity in persons with diabetes.

In Part II, the scientific evidence for the importance of exercise/physical activity is provided in five chapters. This mechanistic information makes it possible to understand the reasons why this type of treatment is especially important for people with diabetes and has specific benefits in these individuals. Thus, the concept of exercise as medicine has a strong scientific basis for prevention and treatment of diabetes. Dr. Irene Schauer's chapter provides a thorough discussion of the abnormalities of exercise performance in type 2 diabetes and the benefit of exercise training for persons with type 2 diabetes. Dr. Sherita Hill Golden reviews the cardiovascular consequences of type 2 diabetes. Dr. John Doupis examines endothelial dysfunction, inflammation, and exercise. Dr. Kerry Stewart's chapter covers exercise, adiposity, and regional fat distribution. Finally, Dr. Amy Huebschmann discusses diabetes mellitus and exercise physiology in the presence of diabetic co-morbidities. These chapters all provide a compelling rationale for exercise as a treatment in diabetes from a scientific standpoint.

Part III addresses practical issues that are essential in order to safely engage patients with diabetes in exercise-related research protocols and clinical programs. Dr. Dalynn Badenhop provides guidelines for prescription of exercise for patients with diabetes. Dr. Brent Van Dorsten considers the critical behavioral issues that must be addressed to sustain exercise adherence in patients accustomed to sedentary behavior. Dr. Nora Tomuta's chapter provides information on diabetes and nutrition since this aspect of care is the other main behavioral cornerstone of diabetes treatment. Finally, Dr. Barry Franklin examines the medical evaluation and assessment that should be undertaken before beginning a program of exercise for persons with diabetes, including the value and limitations of exercise stress testing.

In Part IV, additional key issues concerning diabetes and exercise are discussed. Dr. Susan Herzlinger Botein addresses the difficult problem of conditions and co-morbidities that may interfere with exercise. Dr. David Maahs discusses type 1 diabetes and exercise and finally Dr. Kristen Nadeau examines the growing problem of type 2 diabetes in youth and the role of exercise.

We are proud to have been joined in this effort by the some leading authorities in this area, all of whom have made important contributions in the area of diabetes and exercise and whose collaboration made this book possible.

It is my hope that the reader will find the information in this book to be insightful and clinically useful. Furthermore, I hope that it will at the very least provoke more and perhaps different thinking about the important role of exercise in preventing diabetes and managing its consequences.

Judith G. Regensteiner
Jane E.B. Reusch
Kerry J. Stewart
Aristidis Veves

Contents

Contributors

DALYNN T. BADENHOP, PhD, FACSM • *Division of Cardiovascular Medicine, Department of Medicine, University of Toledo College of Medicine, Toledo, OH, USA*

TIMOTHY BAUER, PhD • *Division of General Internal Medicine, Department of Medicine, University of Colorado Denver, Aurora, CO, USA*

SUSAN HERZLINGER BOTEIN, MD • *Division of Endocrinology, Diabetes and Metabolism, Joslin Diabetes Center, Harvard Medical School, Boston, MA, USA*

AOIFE M. BRENNAN, MD • *Division of Endocrinology, Diabetes and Metabolism, Beth Israel Deaconess Medical Center and Joslin Diabetes Center, Harvard Medical School, Boston, MA, USA*

KENNETH CUSI, MD • *Diabetes Division, Department of Medicine, The University of Texas Health Science Center at San Antonio, San Antonio, TX, USA*

NICHOLA DAVIS, MD, MS • *Division of General Internal Medicine, Department of Medicine, Albert Einstein College of Medicine, Montefiore Medical Center, Bronx, NY, USA*

JOHN DOUPIS, MD • *Department of Clinical Research, Joslin Diabetes Center, Harvard Medical School, Boston, MA, USA*

ROSANNA FIALLO-SCHARER, MD • *Division of Endocrinology, Department of Pediatrics, Barbara Davis Center for Childhood Diabetes, University of Colorado Denver, Aurora, CO, USA*

BARRY A. FRANKLIN, PhD • *Division of Cardiology, Cardiac Rehabilitation/Exercise Laboratories, William Beaumont Hospital, Royal Oak, MI, USA*

SHERITA HILL GOLDEN, MD, MHS • *Division of Endocrinology and Metabolism, Welch Center for Prevention, Epidemiology, and Clinical Research, Departments of Medicine and Epidemiology, Johns Hopkins University, Baltimore, MD, USA*

EDWARD S. HORTON, MD • *Clinical Research Center, Joslin Diabetes Center, Harvard Medical School, Boston, MA, USA*

AMY G. HUEBSCHMANN, MD • *Division of General Internal Medicine, Department of Medicine, University of Colorado Denver, Aurora, CO, USA*

CARMEN ISASI, MD, PhD • *Division of Health Behavior and Nutrition, Department of Epidemiology and Population Health, Albert Einstein College of Medicine, Bronx-Lebanon Hospital Center, Bronx, NY, USA*

DAVID MAAHS, MD, MA • *Division of Endocrinology, Department of Pediatrics, Barbara Davis Center for Childhood Diabetes, University of Colorado Denver, Aurora, CO, USA*

CHRISTOS S. MANTZOROS , MD, DSc • *Division of Endocrinology, Diabetes and Metabolism, Department of Internal Medicine, Beth Israel Deaconess Medical Center, Harvard Medical School, Boston, MA, USA*

PETER A. MCCULLOUGH, MD, MPH • *Division of Nutrition and Preventive Medicine, Department of Medicine, William Beaumont Hospital, Royal Oak, MI, USA*

WENDY M. MILLER, MD • *Division of Nutrition and Preventive Medicine, Department of Medicine, William Beaumont Hospital, Royal Oak, MI, USA*

KRISTEN NADEAU, MD • *Division of Endocrinology, Department of Pediatrics, University of Colorado Denver, Aurora, CO, USA*

KATHERINE NORI, MD • *Division of Nutrition and Preventive Medicine, Department of Medicine, William Beaumont Hospital, Royal Oak, MI, USA*

JUDITH G. REGENSTEINER, PhD • *Divisions of General Internal Medicine and Cardiology, Center for Women's Health Research, Department of Medicine, University of Colorado Denver, Aurora, CO, USA*

JANE E.B. REUSCH, MD • *Division of Endocrinology, Metabolism and Diabetes, Department of Medicine, University of Colorado Denver, Aurora, CO, USA*

IRENE SCHAUER, MD • *Division of Endocrinology, Metabolism and Diabetes, Department of Medicine, University of Colorado Denver, Aurora, CO, USA*

JORDAN C. SCHRAMM, BA • *Microcirculation Laboratory, Beth Israel Deaconess Medical Center, Harvard Medical School, Boston, MA, USA*

JONATHAN E. SHAW, MD, MRCP (UK), FRACP • *Department of Epidemiology and Clinical Diabetes, Baker IDI Heart and Diabetes Institute and Monash University, Melbourne, Australia*

RICHARD W. SIMPSON, DM, FRCP (UK), FRACP • *Department of Medicine, Monash University, Box Hill Hospital, Melbourne, Australia*

KERRY J. STEWART, EDD, FAACVPR, FACSM, FSGC • *Division of Cardiology, Department of Medicine, Johns Hopkins School of Medicine, Baltimore, MD, USA*

LAURA SWEENEY, MD • *Department of Internal Medicine, Beth Israel Deaconess Medical Center, Harvard Medical School, Boston, MA, USA*

CRAIG E. TAPLIN, MD • *Division of Pediatric Endocrinology, Department of Pediatrics, University of Colorado Denver, Aurora, CO, USA*

NORA TOMUTA, MD • *General Clinical Research Center, Albert Einstein College of Medicine, Bronx, NY, USA*

VLAD TOMUTA, MD • *Department of Medicine, Albert Einstein College of Medicine, Bronx Lebanon Hospital Center, Bronx, NY, USA*

BRENT VAN DORSTEN, PhD • *Department of Physical Medicine and Rehabilitation, University of Colorado Denver, Aurora, CO, USA*

ARISTIDIS VEVES, MD, DSc • *Joslin-Beth Israel Deaconess Foot Center, Microcirculation Laboratory, Department of Surgery, Beth Israel Deaconess Medical Center, Harvard Medical School, Boston, MA, USA*

PETER WATSON, PhD • *Division of Endocrinology, Metabolism and Diabetes, Department of Medicine, University of Colorado Denver, Aurora, CO, USA*

JUDITH WYLIE-ROSETT, EDD, RD • *Division of Health Behavior and Nutrition, Department of Epidemiology and Population Health, Albert Einstein College of Medicine, Montefiore Medical Center, Bronx, NY, USA*

PHIL ZEITLER, MD, PhD • *Division of Endocrinology, Department of Pediatrics, University of Colorado Denver, Aurora, CO, USA*

I   EPIDEMIOLOGY AND PREVENTION

1

The Epidemic of Type 2 Diabetes Mellitus: Its Links to Obesity, Insulin Resistance, and Lipotoxicity

Kenneth Cusi

Contents

Abstract

The epidemic of type 2 diabetes (T2DM) is a public health problem that threatens to spiral out of control in the twenty-first century. Early intervention can greatly mitigate the serious socioeconomic impact of the disease, driven largely by disabling microvascular complications and cardiovascular disease. Obesity is at the core of the epidemic of T2DM, affecting 2/3 of adults and reaching alarming rates in children in modern society. Our understanding of adipose tissue has evolved drastically in the past decade being now viewed as a dynamic "endocrine organ" responsible for the development or worsening of insulin resistance and "lipotoxicity" in obese individuals. "Lipotoxicity" describes the damage that occurs when chronic energy supply exceeds metabolic needs and lipid accumulates in tissues that would not normally store large amounts of lipid. In this setting, lipid is redirected into harmful pathways of nonoxidative metabolism, with accumulation of toxic metabolites that activate inflammatory pathways and eventually lead to apoptosis. It affects organs responsible for maintaining normal energy homeostasis, such as the liver, skeletal muscle, and pancreatic beta-cells, but also the vascular bed. The ability of fatty acids to disrupt insulin signaling and how the mitochondria adapts to chronic lipid overload are essential steps in understanding FFA-induced insulin resistance and lipotoxicity across different tissues. Interventions that may prevent lipotoxicity in different target tissues, but in particular

From: *Contemporary Diabetes: Diabetes and Exercise*
Edited by: J. G. Regensteiner et al. (eds.), DOI: 10.1007/978-1-59745-260-1_1
© Humana Press, a part of Springer Science+Business Media, LLC 2009

pancreatic beta-cell lipotoxicity, such as exercise, weight loss, and/or pharmacological therapies such as thiazolidinediones, hold the key to prevent diabetes in subjects genetically predisposed to T2DM and tackle the looming epidemic of the coming century.

Key words: Type 2 diabetes mellitus; Obesity; Insulin resistance; Lipotoxicity; Free fatty acids; β-cell function; Fatty liver.

INTRODUCTION

In recent years, physicians and society at large have experienced the burden of obesity and type 2 diabetes mellitus (T2DM) as never before. The "diabetes epidemic" is a relatively new phenomenon of the last 2 decades that poses a unique challenge to health care providers. This review will first highlight the magnitude of the diabetes epidemic and its relationship to obesity and the metabolic syndrome (MS) to then examine the role of dysfunctional adipose tissue and "lipotoxicity" in promoting insulin resistance, β-cell failure and, eventually, T2DM. We will also briefly review how lifestyle intervention may reverse the deleterious metabolic effects of ectopic fat deposition in target organs (i.e., muscle, liver, pancreatic β-cells), providing the rationale for strategies to halt the epidemic of T2DM that threatens to spiral out of control in the twenty-first century.

THE EPIDEMIC OF TYPE 2 DIABETES MELLITUS

Magnitude of the Problem of T2DM in the Twenty-First Century

It has now become evident that T2DM is reaching epidemic proportions in the United States and worldwide. Although experts debate on the many reasons, all agree that increasingly sedentary lifestyles coupled with excessive caloric intake (in particular of caloric-rich foods high in carbohydrates and saturated fats) have led to an explosion in the prevalence of obesity and T2DM. This had devastating effects in the young and elder segments of modern societies, and in ethnic groups genetically predisposed to type 2 diabetes mellitus (T2DM) such as Hispanics, African-Americans, native Americans, and South Asians. Diabetes mellitus affects over 8% of the US population between ages 20 and 74. This amounts to 21 million Americans having diabetes (~90% T2DM) and 2,500 new diagnosis of diabetes every day *(1)*.

DIABETES AND CARDIOVASCULAR DISEASE

Despite the many medical advances done in recent years in the diagnosis and treatment of T2DM, for the most part, the diagnosis of diabetes continues to be done late, with about one in three individuals with diabetes (or an estimated 6 million subjects) believed to be undiagnosed in the United States. This has led us to estimate that there is a "diagnosis gap" of about 7 years between the development of asymptomatic hyperglycemia and clinical diagnosis *(2)*. A major problem of a delayed diagnosis of diabetes is the silent but relentless progression of diabetes complications, and particularly among them, of cardiovascular disease. It is likely that this diagnostic delay accounts for the observation that 50% of diabetics already have some manifestation of cardiovascular disease (CVD) at the time of diagnosis *(3)*. When cardiovascular (CV) burden is assessed by advanced imaging techniques, such as by measuring carotid intima-media thickness (CIMT) or arterial wall calcification, there is extensive "preclinical" plaque burden in otherwise "asymptomatic" patients with T2DM *(4)*. The risk of CVD developing in the years preceding the development of frank hyperglycemia is best exemplified in a long-term prospective study in which the relative risk of CVD was 2.8-fold higher in subjects with a normal fasting plasma glucose at baseline that developed T2DM during follow-up, compared with the control group that never developed T2DM *(5)*, although the highest CV risk belonged to those with diabetes at baseline (fivefold higher).

Diabetics are known to have CV death rates that are three to fourfold higher in the presence of similar traditional factors such as elevated blood pressure, dyslipidemia, and smoking compared with matched nondiabetic individuals *(6)*. This is consistent with the clinical observation that patients with diabetes fare much worse once they have coronary artery disease (CHD). CV events account for 75% of hospital admissions of subjects with diabetes *(4)*. Mortality from acute coronary syndromes before hospital arrival is twofold higher when compared with individuals without diabetes and is estimated that one-third die within the first month of hospital stay *(7, 8)*. It is also well established that revascularization interventions have higher initial failure rates and restenosis in subjects with diabetes *(9)* and a twofold higher mortality rate when examined either at 1 month, at 1 year, or after 5 years of follow-up *(4, 7, 8)*. The median life expectancy is believed to be up to 8 years lower for diabetic compared with nondiabetic adults aged 55–64 years and the age-adjusted mortality rate 50% higher for diabetic men compared diabetic women *(10)*. Although the rate of CV mortality has declined in the general population *(11)*, individuals with T2DM continue to have a much higher rate of morbidity and mortality compared with subjects without diabetes *(12, 13)*. This appears to be particularly true among ethnic minorities in the Unites States, although many of the ethnic differences reported in the incidence of CVD in patients with diabetes are predominantly a function of differences in education, socioeconomic status, and use of preventive and therapeutic health care resources *(14)*. This imposes the imperative to reverse health care disparities and promote initiatives for the early diagnosis and treatment of CVD among those in greater need.

THE EPIDEMIC OF TYPE 2 DIABETES: IS THE WORSE STILL TO COME?

Several recent alarming projections suggest that the epidemic of T2DM will become even worse in the near future. Wild et al. *(15)* estimated that the worldwide prevalence of diabetes would nearly double by 2030 affecting 366 million people. These figures are also in accordance with those from the International Diabetes Federation (IDF) that predict that 333 million people will suffer from diabetes by 2025 *(16)*. Diabetes represents a major problem for developing countries, being estimated that just China and India combined will be home to 24% of all subjects with diabetes worldwide by 2050 *(17, 18)*.

In the United States, future diabetes prevalence rates are already alarming and always characterized by constant revisions "upwards" to accommodate for the continuous rise in the prevalence of obesity. Initially, the World Health Organization (WHO) using data from the National Health and Nutrition Education Survey (NHANES) II (1976–1980), estimated that there would be 21.9 million people with diabetes in the United States by 2025 *(19)*. However, follow-up estimates by the WHO's 2000 report from the Global Burden of Disease study using NHANES III data (1988 and 1994), estimated 30.3 million people with diabetes in the United States by 2030 (a prevalence of 11.2%, a significant increase from the earlier 8.9% in NHANES II) *(15)*. Similarly, in an earlier report by the National Health Interview Survey (NHIS) using physician-diagnosed diabetes from face-to-face interviews from 1980–1998 data, estimated that 19.9 million people would have diabetes in the United States in 2025 *(1)*. However, the updated figures by the same group based on NHIS 1984–2004 data estimate that 36.4 million people will have diabetes in the United States in 2030 *(20)*. This is in striking consistency with findings from a study recently reported by Mainous and colleagues *(21)*, who created models from the NHANES II mortality survey (1976–1992), the NHANES III (1988–1994) and the NHANES 1999–2002 (Fig. 1). They applied a multivariable diabetes risk score for diabetes prevalence based on data from the NHANES III database that was later fitted to data from the NHANES 1999–2002 survey as a validity check of the accuracy of the model's estimates. They projected the number of individuals with diabetes in 10-year increments into the future. The authors estimated that the diabetes burden will be of 25.4 million (11.5%) by 2011 and will grow up to 32.6 million (13.5%) by 2021. By 2031, the authors estimated 14.5% of the entire US adult population (or 37.7 million people), with an overwhelming 20.2% of adults of Hispanic origin in the United States having diabetes.

The rapidly increasing number of individuals with diabetes and the severe atherosclerotic burden and microvascular complications that the disease imposes suggest that health care resources will be stretched to the limit in the near future, unless a collective and aggressive effort is done to reverse this trend. The cost of diabetes care is increasing out of control in the United States, exceeding $100 billion each year. Prevention of diabetes complications cannot be underestimated, as $3 out of $4 is spent on hospital admissions *(4, 17)*. While pharmacological interventions to treat hyperglycemia and the associated CV risk factors associated with diabetes have made major advances in recent times, lifestyle intervention strategies to reverse the metabolic abnormalities imposed by obesity and sedentary behaviors will be essential for long-term success. Large clinical trials have proven that lifestyle intervention effectively delays the onset of T2DM *(22)*. The increasing consensus in the field is that establishing early interventions may delay the onset of frank hyperglycemia, help preserve pancreatic β-cell function and potentially reduce CVD in high-risk populations *(23–26)*. Chronic hyperglycemia per se appears to be associated with a 15–18% increased risk of CVD in diabetes, as highlighted in a recent meta-analysis of 1,688 patients with type 1 diabetes mellitus (T1DM) and 7,435 patients with T2DM (pooled data from three and ten studies, respectively). It is important for practitioners to recognize that a comprehensive intervention, including control of hyperglycemia and of associated CV risk factors, has been proven to reduce complications in T1DM and T2DM *(27, 28)*. Aggressive management of hyperglycemia and associated CV risk factors is of critical importance because once plaque burden is established in patients with T2DM, CVD remains relatively high despite our best efforts *(4, 12, 13, 17)*.

Role of Obesity and Physical Inactivity to the Epidemic of T2DM

SOCIOECONOMIC IMPACT OF THE OBESITY EPIDEMIC

The normal body mass index (BMI) is considered to be between 18.5 and 25 kg/m^2 *(29)*. An individual is considered to be overweight if his BMI is between 25 and 29.9 kg/m^2, and obese if >30 kg/m^2.

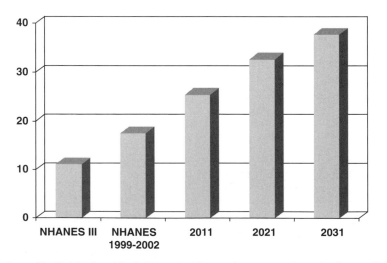

Fig. 1. Projected number of individuals with diabetes in 10-year increments into the future. It is estimated that the diabetes burden will be of 25.4 million (11.5%) by 2011, 32.6 million (13.5%) by 2021, and 37.7 million people (14.5% of the entire US adult population) by 2031. About 20.2% of adults of Hispanic origin in the United States will have diabetes. Adapted from Mainous et al. *(21)*.

Obesity has been further classified into stage I (BMI ranging from 30.0 to 34.9 kg/m²), stage II (BMI from 35.0 to 39.9 kg/m²), and stage III (if ≥40.0 kg/m² or morbid obesity). The most accepted direct measures of body fat include underwater weighing, bioimpedance, and dual energy X-ray absorptiometry. However, these tests are not widely available and not suitable for routine clinical practice, reason why BMI is the preferred alternative. However, one must point out that BMI is a simple and inexpensive way to quantify body fat, but that ethnicity, age, gender, cardiorespiratoy fitness, and body fat distribution are important factors that may modify considerably the health risks associated with obesity. For example, females and older adults have a higher proportion of adiposity for any given BMI compared to younger subjects, in particular males *(30)*. Meta-analysis examining the impact of ethnicity has concluded that estimates of body fat using BMI overestimate in African-Americans the percentage of body fat relative to that of Caucasians *(31)*.

While between 1960 and 2002 the average height has increased by 1.0–1.5 in. in the general adult population, weight has increased by ~25 lbs in both genders in the same period (or 14.8% in men and 17.2% in women) *(32)*. Both reduced levels of physical activity *(33)* and increased caloric intake *(34)* appear to account for this. Recent information from the 2002 Behavioral Risk Factor Surveillance Survey (BRFSS), an annual survey conducted by the Centers for Disease Control (CDC), has estimated that 59.2% of Americans are either overweight or obese *(29, 35)*. Obesity alone affects 60 million of adult Americans. Data from the most recent National Center for Health statistics using NHANES data report almost two out of three Americans as being overweight or obese (65.2%). Both sources coincide in that the "epidemic" of obesity is increasing at an alarming rate, particularly in Hispanics and African-Americans women and in socially disadvantaged groups, particularly those with the poorest levels of education and lowest income *(35, 36)*. In this regard, the social network appears to play a key role in the development of obesity as reported in a longitudinal follow-up between 1971 and 2003 from the Framingham Heart Study, in which the chances of a person becoming obese increased between 37% and 57% if he or she had a spouse, sibling, or friend who became obese in a given interval *(37)*. The United States leads the world as the country with more overweight and obese subjects at 64.5%, followed closely by Mexico, Australia, and the United Kingdom, with estimates that 60% of the increased incidence of diabetes can be attributed just to weight gain *(36)*. We live in the paradox of a world in which more people are overweight and obese than those undernourished (about one billion compared to 850 million, respectively) *(17)*. Health care expenditures also increase significantly once the BMI ≥30 kg/m² *(35, 36)*. In the United States, medical care expenses for obesity-associated conditions were estimated to be $117 billion or near 10% of the total health care costs.

Excess adiposity is also believed to be the driving force behind the development of early CVD and increased overall mortality observed in obese individuals in population-based studies *(33, 35, 38–47)*. Obesity is associated with a reduced life span, with 100,000–400,000 excess deaths per year, depending on the models used to assess the impact of obesity *(38, 47, 48)*. Mortality increases sharply as the BMI exceeds 30 kg/m² *(12, 33, 35, 38, 46, 47, 49, 50)*. It has been recently suggested that poor cardiorespiratory fitness may be more important than adiposity itself in older adults, being independent of overall or abdominal obesity, highlighting the importance of functional capacity beyond simple measures of adiposity such as BMI *(51)*. Moreover, it has been estimated that soon low levels of physical activity and poor dietary habits will overtake tobacco as the leading cause of death in the United States *(52)*. In the Framingham Heart Study, middle-aged overweight subjects had an average 7-year reduction in life expectancy *(38)*.

Recently, two large studies have assessed how obesity early in life may predict future CHD and overall life expectancy. Baker et al. *(53)* reported that in a large cohort of 276,835 Danish schoolchildren ages 7 through 13, there was a linear association between increasing BMI and risk of CHD, so that per each 1-unit increase in BMI at age 13 there was a 15% higher risk of CHD in adulthood.

Consistent with the deleterious effects of obesity, van Dam et al. *(39)* recently reported that increased adiposity at age 18 in women is associated with increased mortality later in life. The authors assessed body weight in 102,400 women from the Nurses' Health Study II and followed them for 12 years. They found that there was a 1.6-fold and 2.8 increase in mortality rates among overweight and obese women, respectively, compared to women with a BMI between 18.5 and 21.9 kg/m² at age 18. Obesity is also associated with significant functional impairment *(50, 54)*, another factor that predisposes to a more sedentary lifestyle and contributes to reduced CV fitness and a higher risk of CVD.

OBESITY AND BODY FAT DISTRIBUTION

Another important aspect of adiposity is the distribution of body fat. The waist circumference has been adopted as the practical way to measure central adiposity, but the accurate measurement of visceral fat calls for the use of imaging techniques such a magnetic resonance imaging (MRI) or computed tomography (CT). By these techniques, abdominal fat is typically measured with a single cut at the L4–5 vertebral bodies, although estimation of the total visceral fat volume is a more accurate approach *(55)*. High carbohydrate diets are known to promote hepatic very low-density lipoprotein (VLDL) oversecretion. In women, body fat deposition is primarily peripheral in the gluteo-femoral subcutaneous region. Adipose tissue expands in this area and the lower abdomen in overweight and obese women ("pear-shape" fat distribution). A key observation was that obese women with a predominantly upper-body fat distribution had much greater rates of lipolysis and free fatty acid (FFA) turnover than those with lower body obesity *(56)*. In contrast to women, fat takes more frequently a more central distribution in overweight and obese men ("apple-shape"). As with women with a more central fat distribution, this has been associated with insulin resistance, more visceral fat accumulation, higher triglycerides, and lower high-density lipoprotein-cholesterol (HDL-C) levels *(57)*. Subjects with "apple-shaped" fat distribution have a higher risk of CVD possibly related to the important metabolic differences between visceral and subcutaneous adipose tissue. This has made central obesity a criterion of significant value for the diagnosis of the MS (see discussion below).

Abdominal obesity is also associated with a greater risk of developing T2DM *(58)*. The Paris Prospective Study was the first large prospective study to confirm the close relationship between adipose tissue insulin resistance (i.e., elevated plasma FFA concentration) and the deterioration of glucose tolerance over time *(59)*. Visceral fat is believed to be more prone to lipolysis in response to counterregulatory hormones and more resistant to the antilipolytic effect of insulin *(57, 60)*. Moreover, it has been speculated that because it drains directly into the portal vein, FFA derived from the visceral bed would have a more direct impact on liver metabolism than fat from peripheral (subcutaneous) lipolysis. In any case, the role of visceral fat to overall CV risk remains highly controversial *(57, 61–63)*. For example, in a recent cross-sectional study across 21 research centers in Europe, simultaneously measuring insulin sensitivity by the gold-standard in euglycemic insulin clamp technique and the clustering of risk factors associated with the MS, it was not possible to isolate different measures of adiposity (BMI, fat mass, or fat distribution) as more prominent than the others as causative factors for insulin resistance or related CV risk factors *(63)*. We have found a closer correlation between visceral and liver fat accumulation than when compared with BMI or subcutaneous fat *(55, 64)*. However, while the "portal hypothesis" is appealing to the development of hepatic insulin resistance by visceral adipose tissue, the finding that in healthy obese individuals the contribution of visceral fat to the overall FFA pool increases only modestly (from 10% to only 25% compared to lean subjects) *(65)*, suggests that expansion of subcutaneous fat adipose tissue also plays an important role in the development of hepatic insulin resistance. Moreover, as FFA from visceral fat contributes only with 5% or less to the peripheral plasma FFA pool *(65)*, it is unlikely to be a primary responsible for peripheral (muscle) insulin resistance, again highlighting the damaging effect of overall adiposity (visceral and subcutaneous) as sources of FFA for subsequent ectopic (i.e., muscle, liver, β-cells) fat deposition. It is also possible that the deleterious role of visceral fat is mediated not so much by FFA but primarily by the release a number of adipocytokines [tumor necrosis factor-α (TNF-α), leptin, interleukins (IL), etc.] that have been shown to promote insulin resistance *(66, 67)*, offering a unifying explanation for how a rather modest amount of adipose tissue (i.e., 10–15% of total body fat) may hold the potential to impair hepatic and peripheral (muscle) insulin action.

OBESITY AND THE INSULIN RESISTANCE (METABOLIC) SYNDROME

In recent years, there has been great interest in the concept of a clustering of risk factors for CVD occurring in a given individual to a greater degree than expected by chance. This clustering, commonly referred to as the "metabolic syndrome," has clinical manifestations frequently observed in obesity and is believed to be associated with underlying insulin resistance in the majority, but not all, of individuals. In its original conception, "syndrome X" *(68)* or the "insulin resistance syndrome" *(69)* provided a framework to understand the relationship or association between insulin resistance, multiple metabolic abnormalities, and the development of T2DM. Interest in this "metabolic" clustering of risk factors evolved into an aggregation of risk factors (obesity, elevated TG (triglycerides) and low HDL-C, hypertension, insulin resistance and abnormal fasting or 2-h plasma glucose levels, and others) used primarily to predict in a given individual the risk of CVD.

Many studies have shown that the clustering of risk factors identifies subjects more likely to develop CVD *(33, 49, 57, 70–77)*. In a landmark study by Lakka et al. *(78)*, they prospectively followed 1,209 middle-aged Finnish men without CVD at baseline and showed that after 11.4 years of follow-up, those with the MS [defined using either National Cholesterol Education Program (NCEP) or WHO criteria] were 2.9-times more likely to die of CHD and had 1.9-fold higher CVD mortality rates. More recently, the San Antonio Heart Study examined the relationship between gender, the MS (NCEP definition) and diabetes in their ability to predict CHD mortality over 15.5 years of follow-up in 4,996 men and women *(71)*. Relative to women with neither diabetes nor MS, women with both had a 14-fold increased risk of CHD mortality whereas men had only a fourfold increased risk, respectively, gender being a strong modifier of the joint effect of diabetes and MS on CHD mortality. Still, three aspects are under considerable debate regarding the MS: (1) whether the association of multiple risk factors in the MS adds to CVD prediction more than the sum of its individual components; (2) which is the precise role of insulin resistance in its pathogenesis, and (3) which parameters/risk factors would best serve as predictors of CV disease (or T2DM) and what are their optimal cutoffs *(79–81)*. Regarding the first issue, it is unlikely that epidemiological studies alone using multiple regression analysis and other approaches will give us a definitive answer as to whether the whole (i.e., MS) will be more predictive than the sum of the parts (i.e., individual risk factors). This is because the mutual interaction of these metabolic abnormalities (i.e., the "embedded" impact of obesity and/or insulin resistance on atherogenic dyslipidemia, hypertension, or the plasma glucose concentration, among other factors) will likely make impossible that any statistical analysis will be able to dissect and quantify the relative contribution of these closely intertwined CV risk factors to overall CVD.

As for the role of insulin resistance in the pathogenesis of the MS, while controversial, it offers so far the best unifying hypothesis based on a large amount of basic and clinical data, with many prospective studies indicating that insulin resistance is an independent risk factor that strongly predicts future CV morbidity and mortality *(44, 49, 57, 66, 73, 82–84)*. Crude measurements of insulin resistance in some studies (i.e., such as a fasting plasma insulin level or the HOMA model, that is primarily a measure hepatic HOMA (homeostasis model assessment)) HOMA insulin resistance (but not of muscle or adipose tissue insulin sensitivity) may erroneously conclude that insulin resistance does not play a role. Alternatively, the effect of insulin resistance may already be accounted for by its impact on driving hepatic VLDL production (increasing plasma triglycerides) and promoting a high HDL-C turnover (lowering HDL) *(85, 86)*. Insulin resistance may also be promoting pancreatic β-cell failure and progressive hyperglycemia in individuals genetically predisposed to T2DM, so that when these variables are included in multiple regression analysis, the fasting insulin is no longer an "independent" risk factor to predict risk of CVD or T2DM. The role of insulin resistance has also been questioned on the grounds that not all patients with insulin resistance develop the MS, and also that not all patients with the MS are insulin-resistant. However, this reasoning is quite naive as to expect that every subject with insulin resistance will develop the MS, because disease always depends on a permissive factor (i.e., insulin resistance in the case of the MS) plus the diminished reserve to a given insult by the target organ (i.e., the vascular bed in atherosclerosis, the liver in nonalcoholic fatty liver disease (NAFLD), the ovary in polycystic ovary syndrome (PCOS), and the pancreatic β-cell in T2DM). In other words, insulin resistance create a fertile soil for end-organ damage and the genetic make-up determines the susceptibility to this permissive environment, in the same way that nobody questions today the roles of hypertension and dyslipidemia to the development of CVD, although many CV events will never develop even in the presence of this well-established risk factors.

Some of the confusion among the role of the MS arises on the emphasis placed on its different components/risk factors and variable cut-offs adopted by different organizations: the NCEP, the IDF, the Group for the Study of Insulin Resistance (EGIR), the American Association of Clinical Endocrinologists (AACE), and the WHO [elegantly reviewed by Meigs *(84)*]. These include obesity and/or a measure of waist circumference, fasting glucose [and some a measure of insulin resistance (EGIR) (WHO) or 2-h glucose (WHO)], triglycerides/HDL-C and elevated blood pressure. While obesity is important in all definitions, depending on the emphasis put on other risk factors, they appear to be defining slightly different populations. For example, the definition most widely held by clinicians is the NCEP ATP III 2005, which combines any of three out of five risk factors to meet the criteria. The criteria and cut-offs of the NCEP are fasting plasma glucose ≥100 mg/dL, central obesity (≥35 in in women and ≥40 in in men), low plasma HDL-C (≤40 mg/dL in males and ≤50 mg/dL in women); plasma triglycerides ≥150 mg/dL, and blood pressure ≥130 or ≥80 mmHg (or pharmacological treatment of any of these risk factors). This is a rather "lipid-centric" definition as most meet the MS criteria from having obesity and —one to two of the lipid criteria. It is limited also by not taking into account the weight of the different factors or by using measurements of insulin resistance, although its simplicity has made it a valuable tool for primary care physicians and for use in large epidemiological studies. Other definitions acknowledge directly or indirectly the importance of insulin resistance and the likelihood that it may have an important pathogenic role. The IDF requires abnormal waist-circumference as the driving criteria, emphasizing the role of abdominal/central obesity as a surrogate for insulin resistance. The EGIR and WHO definitions aim at identifying those with insulin resistance for its diagnosis, measured by the gold-standard euglycemic insulin clamp technique [or at least a fasting insulin in the top 25% (EGIR)], although these measurements are not costly and difficult to obtain by clinicians. In an attempt to assist physicians in clinical practice, AACE includes as criteria several conditions strongly associated with insulin resistance, such as NAFLD, polycystic ovary disease, and acanthosis nigricans. This has very practical implications and serves to increase awareness among doctors and patients on the importance of conditions with apparent no relation to the development of T2DM and CVD.

Future prospective studies will allow to "fine tune" the currently used MS criteria. From a practical perspective, many practitioners give value to the MS criteria by assisting them in searching for clusters of CV risk factors in patients who are overweight, or have either CVD or T2DM. It also helps them at the time of choosing a pharmacological agent to treat a given CV risk factor. For example, one may avoid treating one CV risk factor with an agent that may have deleterious effects on other risk factors, if alternative treatments are available. For example, beta blockers may increase the plasma cholesterol and plasma glucose levels and have been associated with increased incidence of T2DM in epidemiological and intervention studies *(4)*; use of an angiotensin converting enzyme inhibitors (ACEI) or angiotensin receptor blockers (ARB) may be preferable in the setting of uncomplicated hypertension and diabetes as both have no deleterious effects on glucose or lipid metabolism and have been reported to reduce the incidence of T2DM, with added benefits on preservation of renal function which is already at greater risk of damage in the setting of obesity, MS or T2DM.

THE CHALLENGE OF PREDICTING THE DEVELOPMENT OF T2DM

While the MS is a tool to predict CV risk, in the wake of the diabetes epidemic there has been significant interest about its ability to also predict T2DM, with several studies in Caucasians *(73, 75, 87)* and ethnic minorities *(74, 88)* confirming its value in this regard. This is important because if we can find the optimal way to identify early-on subjects that will develop T2DM later in life, aggressive lifestyle and/or pharmacological interventions before the development of hyperglycemia are likely to be very cost-effective (discussed at the end of the chapter).

A recent meta-analysis showed that the presence of MS increases the likelihood of developing T2DM by two to fourfold *(49)*. However, it is less sensitive than direct tests aimed at identifying subjects at risk of developing T2DM *(88)*. In testing a predictive tool for a disease, rather than estimating the relative risk, it is standard to use the area under the receiver–operator-characteristic curve (ROC) to determine the accuracy of a test to discriminate individuals that will develop a disease from those that will not. The ROC is always a balance between the ability of the test to correctly identify subjects (true positive rate) from its error in doing so (false positive), depending on the sensitivity and specificity set by the different parameters in the model. The gold-standard to predict T2DM has traditionally been the oral glucose tolerance test (OGTT), but it is somewhat inconvenient for widespread clinical use. Given the epidemic of T2DM, studies that have examined the value of the MS criteria to predict T2DM have concluded that it provides a reasonable prediction of future T2DM with a ROC between 0.75 and 0.82 *(76, 89–91)*. Of note, a ROC of 0.5 is considered simple chance discrimination while a perfect screening test would have an ROC of 1.0. However, the use of impaired fasting glucose (IFG) plays a key role in driving the predictive value of the different MS criteria, so that when required as one of the screening criteria for the prediction of T2DM, it greatly enhances the predictive value of the MS and it diminishes significantly when excluded *(73)*. However, models tailored to predict T2DM (that do not necessarily need to incorporate an OGTT in their model) are more accurate than the MS with ROCs of 0.84–0.85, such as the San Antonio Diabetes Prediction Model (SAPDM) *(76, 89)* and the Framingham Offspring Study database in middle-aged Caucasians *(92)*. Recently, the use of the 1-h OGTT, or factoring-in insulin resistance to insulin secretion during an OGTT, provided a slightly better prediction for T2DM compared to the SAPDM (ROC 0.86 vs. 0.80) or 2-h OGTT (ROC 0.79, both $p < 0.001$), but with the caveat of requiring invasive testing (OGTT) for the diagnosis of T2DM *(91)*.

One can expect in the future that the MS will have improved accuracy to predict T2DM if ethnicity (minorities being more prone to T2DM) and a family history (FH) of T2DM (a strong predictor of insulin resistance and diminished pancreatic β-cell reserve) are taken into consideration. For example, African-Americans tend to have higher blood pressure, lower triglycerides, and higher HDL-C (in contrast to higher triglycerides in Japanese) while insulin resistance and T2DM are more common in Mexican–Americans and American–Indians *(14)*. In high-risk populations (minorities, those with a FH of T2DM or gestational diabetes, obese patients with features of the MS), it may be cost-effective to use a minimally invasive and simple test such as an OGTT to establish an early diagnosis and consider intervention *(23)*. It is still quite a tragedy that diabetes continues to be diagnosed late and that still today about one-third of patients with T2DM are unaware of having the condition.

Pediatric Obesity and T2DM: An Inevitable Consequence of Living in an Age of Abundance?

Perhaps one of the greatest public health concerns of recent years has been the dismal increase in the prevalence of overweight and obese children and teenagers. Pediatric obesity is defined as a BMI greater than the 95th percentile while being overweight is defined as a BMI greater than the 85th percentile, adjusted for age and gender. While BMI is not the optimal way to quantify excessive adipose tissue, its simplicity has imposed it as a valuable surrogate test. However, one should keep in mind that there can be a significant variability when compared with direct measurements of body fat *(30, 93–95)*. In any case, the prevalence of obesity in children is believed to be 14% *(32, 35)*, representing about a threefold increase among children across all ages between 6 and 19 years. The CDC recently reported that the mean weight of 10-year-old boys and girls in 2002 increased by ~11 lbs (from 74.2 to 85 lb and 77.4 to 88 lbs, respectively) compared to data from 1963 to 1970. More recently, Li et al. *(96)* compared the mean waist circumference and waist–height ratio of boys and girls in four different age groups using NHANES data from 1988 to 1994 through 1999–2004. Using the 90th percentile values of waist circumference for gender and age, the prevalence of abdominal obesity increased by 65.4% (from 10.5% to 17.4%) and 69.4% (from 10.5% to 17.8%) for boys and girls, respectively. The implications of these statistics are serious because being obese during childhood is also a predictor of obesity as an adult *(35)*, with its serious health consequences. For example, an obese teenager has a 17-fold risk of being overweight when at ages 21–29.

Obesity in youth is also a strong predictor of future MS *(97)* and T2DM *(35, 98, 99)*. Obese children have a high prevalence of the MS, with a 50% chance if the BMI is greater than 40 kg/m^2. It is now estimated that in the pediatric population in the United States the number of new cases of diabetes having T2DM equals those of T1DM *(100)*. One recent study reported among 1,030 children ages 4–19, 20% already had the MS, which increased to 28% if elevated liver alanine aminotransferase was included in the analysis *(101)*. Elevated aminotransferases are also a predictor of CVD in large epidemiological studies *(102)*. In the study by Butte et al. *(101)*, obese Hispanic children were particularly affected. Of note, when the authors performed risk factor analysis and quantitative genetic analysis, they noted a marked heritability for traits of the MS and a clear clustering of CV risk factors among children affected, suggesting a complex web of genetic and environmental factors.

Obese children with the MS are also more prone to a number of additional medical conditions: NAFLD, sleep apnea, focal and segmental glomerulosclerosis, cranial hypertension, gallbladder disease, early maturation and obesity-related behavioral problems, poor school performance, and severe depression *(94, 97, 100, 101, 103–105)*. Hirsutism, PCOS, and infertility are also more common in girls with the MS *(106)*. In the long term, there is also an increased risk of osteoarthritis, CVD *(43, 45, 53, 107)*, and possibly of a variety of cancer types *(108)*. Debate on the long-term management is complicated by the multifactorial etiology of obesity in children (genetic, social, and economic forces at play) and lack of good data to set optimal guidelines.

Recently, the Expert Committee on the Assessment, Prevention and Treatment of Child and Adolescent Overweight and Obesity, a consortium of 15 health professional organizations including the American Medical Association (AMA), the Department of Health and Human Services' Health Resources and Services Administration (HRSA), and the CDC, proposed a number of measures to curve obesity in children *(109)*. As expected, treatment recommendations centered on a lifestyle modification approach with an emphasis on diet and exercise. They recognized as barriers parent denial of their child's weight problem (in as many as 40% of parents of overweight children), poor adherence to long-term goals, and inadequate third-party payer reimbursement for the team approach often needed for long-term success (physician, dietician, psychologist, exercise trainer, etc.). Many studies link obesity to physical inactivity *(33)* and overeating *(34)*, which in children is common during the many hours they spend in modern society watching TV or playing electronic games. This can be reversed with limiting the number of hours they spend watching television *(110)*. Unfortunately, there are few long-term weight loss studies in children, but modest success is possible *(99, 111, 112)*.

Other than for increase physical activity, few pharmacological alternatives are available for children: orlistat (Xenical®), which interferes with intestinal lipase function and enhances fecal fat loss, is approved for children ≥12 years of age, and sibutramine (Meridia®), working in the central nervous system, CNS, as a serotonin and norepinephrine reuptake inhibitor, for teenagers of age ≥16. Both have shown to be effective in achieving weight losses of ~8–10% in trials lasting 1–2 years *(113, 114)*, although potential for malabsorption with orlistat, and for tachycardia and hypertension with sibutramine, are of concern for long-term use in pediatric populations. There is limited short-term experience with bariatric surgery and no long-term studies to support its safety and efficacy in younger populations. It is recommended only for special cases, such as children with BMI ≥50 kg/m^2, or alternatively, with a BMI of 40 kg/m^2 if severe comorbidities are already present and after careful family counseling in the hands of experienced surgeons.

METABOLIC CONSEQUENCES OF OBESITY: WHY DOES IT PREDISPOSE TO T2DM?

Much work has been done in recent years to understand the links between physical inactivity, obesity, and the development of T2DM. Still no clear, unifying hypothesis has been able to encompass the complex web of metabolic and molecular defects that accompany T2DM. However, much has been learned on how dysfunctional adipose tissue in obesity impairs glucose homeostasis in humans, which can be separated conceptually in two major mechanisms: (a) dysfunctional fat viewed as an "endocrine organ," actively involved in releasing a number of cytokines that promote systemic inflammation that cause/promote muscle/liver insulin resistance, and (b) abnormal dysfunctional fat causing "lipotoxicity," where sick insulin-resistant adipocytes cause ectopic fat deposition in skeletal muscle, liver, and pancreatic β-cells, with devastating effects for glucose homeostasis.

Adipose Tissue as an "Endocrine Organ"

Obesity is the result of an increase in adipocyte size (fat storage) and number *(115, 116)*. Obesity can be interpreted based on our current understanding of fat biology as a pathological enlargement by fat cells and a failure to adequately proliferate and differentiate in response to excessive energy intake *(117–121)*. In addition to surplus energy, hypertrophic fat cells are challenged by chronic inflammation and perhaps insulin resistance itself, posing considerable stress to its various organelles. Among these, recently the role of the endoplasmic reticulum (ER) has been highlighted as a vital organelle that demonstrates significant signs of stress and dysfunction in obesity and insulin resistance *(121)*. Under normal conditions, the ER physiologically adapts to meet the demands related to protein and triglyceride synthesis in the differentiated fat cell, but when nutrients are in pathological excess, this overwhelms the ER activating the unfolded protein response (UPR) and triggering the development of insulin resistance through a host of mechanisms, including c-jun N-terminal kinase (JNK) activation, inflammation, and oxidative stress.

However, it was not until relatively recently that our perception of adipose tissue shifted from a rather "passive" fuel storage depot to a highly complex endocrine organ with an important role in causing systemic inflammation in obesity-related states. Because this topic has been the subjects of a number of recent in-depth reviews *(66, 83, 120–122)*, we will consider just briefly a few aspects of the link between abnormal fat cells and inflammation. Adipocytes develop from preadipocytes present in adipose tissue and their main mission has classically been restricted to the regulation of triglyceride storage and overall body energy metabolism by the secretion of hormones such as leptin. The observation by Hotaqmisligil et al. *(123)* and Feinstein et al. *(124)* that the fat-derived proinflammatory cytokine TNF-α could induce insulin resistance was a radical departure from the classical view of adipose tissue. While the role of TNF-α to induce insulin resistance in humans with T2DM remains controversial, nevertheless the realization that adipocytes were actively involved in the secretion of many inflammatory cytokines previously believed to be secreted only by macrophages – or simply unknown – opened a new horizon in the understanding of insulin resistance, obesity and T2DM [i.e., TNF-α, IL-6, resistin, monocyte chemoattractant protein-1 (MCP-1), plasminogen activator inhibitor-1 (PAI-1), visfatin, angiotensinogen, retinol-binding protein-4 (RBP-4), and serum amyloid A (SAA)]. In a general sense, adipocytokines such as TNF-α and IL-6 are viewed as mediating insulin resistance either through promoting serine phosphorylation of key insulin signaling steps (i.e., IRS-1 mediated by TNF-α or IL-6-induced IKKβ and JNK1 pathways) in liver and muscle or by infiltrating macrophages near adipose tissue cells that release cytokines and promote adipose tissue insulin resistance and the increased lipolysis that drives ectopic fat deposition in ectopic tissues. Another important observation was that 30–59% of the genes in adipocytes from obese subjects had a gene expression pattern closely related to macrophage biology *(125)*. Note that macrophages derive from a different cell lineage than adipocytes (bone marrow stem cells), but during nutritional excess triglyceride-loaded adipocytes produce a number of cytokines that are also typical of fat-loaded activated macrophages in the arterial plaque (foam cells) *(120)*. A high output of adipocytokines characterizes insulin-resistant fat cells, closing the loop by activating inflammatory pathways (i.e., NF-κβ) and inducing insulin resistance in target tissues. How obesity may alter gene expression and induce similarities among adipocytes and macrophages is unknown, but could be mediated by PPARγ activation *(115, 122, 125)*, an effect that has received extensive attention in recent times. This has been of particular interest in T2DM as PPARγ agonists have proven to have multiple beneficial effects on fat cell biology. Adipose tissue is infiltrated with macrophages, and its content of long-chain triacylglycerols (TAGs) and ceramides has been recently reported to be increased in subjects with increased hepatic fat content compared to equally obese subjects with normal liver fat content *(126)*. Lower plasma adiponectin levels in fatty liver disease (NAFLD), as well as in obesity and T2DM, may explain these differences and point toward dysfunctional adipocyte function in these pathological states *(127)*, being increased by PPARγ activation by thiazolidiendiones. Moreover, ob/ob mice overexpressing adiponectin are completely rescued from the diabetic phenotype at the expense of morbid obesity, offering an interesting paradox of how fat cells that can adapt successfully and store pathological amounts of fat while remaining insulin sensitive and free of diabetes *(128)*.

Adipose Tissue Insulin Resistance and "Lipotoxicity"

Type 2 diabetes is characterized by insulin resistance (at the level of skeletal muscle, adipose tissue, and liver) and by impaired β-cell function *(68, 129–134)*. Both genetic and acquired defects have been shown to play a role in affecting insulin action and insulin secretion. Among the acquired defects, obesity and glucotoxicity *(135–137)* have received special attention as both are believed to worsen insulin resistance and possibly contribute to the decline in β-cell function. Dissecting the role of genetic factors from those attributed to obesity and/or hyperglycemia itself has been particularly challenging. Equally difficult has been to define the sequence of events that results in the development of insulin resistance, and ultimately T2DM, in genetically predisposed subjects. For instance, it can be argued that adipose tissue insulin resistance may be the initiating event as it is present in nonobese normal glucose-tolerant subjects with a FH of type 2 diabetes long before the development of hyperglycemia. In such individuals, adipose tissue resistance to the action of insulin is characterized by increased rates of lipolysis with elevated plasma FFA levels despite chronic hyperinsulinemia and impaired suppression of plasma FFA by insulin, or just the latter with "normal" plasma FFA levels (although inadequately "normal" for the elevated plasma insulin concentration) *(138–142)*. This is also typical of obese nondiabetic *(143–145)* and in T2DM individuals *(68, 129–134, 146)*.

The term "lipotoxicity" was coined by Unger et al. *(147, 148)* to describe the deleterious effects of high fatty acid supply on β-cell function. Since then much work in the field has given the term lipotoxicity a broader sense and is currently applied more generally to the deleterious effects of fatty acids on tissues that would not normally be destined to store large amounts of fat. This places an extraordinary metabolic stress to these tissues. So when fat supply surpasses the metabolic needs of skeletal muscle, liver, and/or pancreatic β-cells, the offer of fatty acids in excess of their normal storage and oxidative capacity redirects lipid flux into harmful pathways of nonoxidative metabolism and intracellular accumulation of toxic metabolites renders tissues resistant to the action of insulin. Many studies have shown that hepatic and skeletal muscle insulin resistance can be readily induced in healthy individuals after short periods of lipid infusion that acutely raise plasma FFA levels *(68, 129–134, 146)*.

Liver and muscle insulin resistance are both central to the pathogenesis of T2DM. Hepatic insulin resistance per se may drive a chronic increase in insulin secretion aimed at refraining excessive rates of hepatic glucose production and prevent subsequent hyperglycemia. Hepatic insulin resistance is frequently associated with a fatty liver, diminished insulin clearance, and perpheral hyperinsulinemia. In such a scenario, hepatic insulin resistance could cause/contribute to muscle insulin resistance as mild chronic hyperinsulinemia per se (i.e., an approximately two- to threefold increase in plasma insulin concentration above normal, as seen in insulin-resistant states such as obesity or T2DM) may cause peripheral (muscle) insulin resistance just after 72 h in otherwise insulin-sensitive individuals *(149)*. Steatosis and hepatic insulin resistance are also characterized by an excessive secretion of proinflammatory cytokines [transforming growth factor-β (TGF-β), TNF-α, hsCRP, etc.] that also are known to promote peripheral insulin resistance and could "close the loop" of a self-perpetuating state of insulin resistance and systemic inflammation as described above for adipose tissue insulin resistance.

Finally, it is well established that there is an intrinsic defect in insulin action in skeletal muscle of patients with T2DM. Skeletal muscle insulin resistance has been well documented in muscle biopsy studies from lean normal glucose-tolerant and, otherwise, healthy subjects genetically predisposed to T2DM (without the confounding factor of obesity and elevated plasma FFA levels), long before the development of frank lipo- and/or gluco-toxicity observed in T2DM *(141, 142, 150)*. If skeletal muscle insulin resistance would be the initiating event in the cascade of events toward T2DM, one could put forward the hypothesis that skeletal muscle insulin resistance would lead to chronic hyperinsulinemia and place a sustained β-cell demand that could lead to T2DM in genetically susceptible individuals. Sustained systemic hyperinsulinemia is also known to promote hepatic steatosis, insulin resistance, and diminished hepatic insulin clearance, which combined would feed and perpetuate chronic hyperinsulinemia. It would also stimulate hepatic triglyceride secretion with potential to cause more lipotoxicity by delivering more lipid to insulin-sensitive tissues, such as muscle *(130)*, while potentially causing β-cell lipotoxicity *(147, 148)*, as well as promoting a MS phenotype by stimulating HDL-C turnover with increased clearance and lower plasma HDL-C levels *(86)*. Taken together, the above scenarios indicate that defects causing chronic hyperinsulinemia (either secondary to liver or muscle insulin resistance) can easily downregulate the insulin receptor and its downstream signaling steps and cause insulin resistance at the level of muscle, liver, and/or adipose tissue, again closing the loop for a state of self-sustaining insulin resistance and chronic inflammation as seen in obesity and T2DM.

In summary, genetic and acquired factors establish a tangled web of metabolic disturbances. Individual defects in each target tissue (muscle, liver, or adipose tissue) appear to be sufficient to trigger a self-perpetuating and down-spiraling cascade of events difficult to reverse. It is important to recognize that insulin resistance can be entirely acquired by fatty acid excess, as demonstrated in healthy lean insulin-sensitive individuals that develop muscle and hepatic insulin resistance within hours of a low-dose lipid infusion *(141, 142, 151)*. Therefore, we cannot miss the opportunity to apply this knowledge to the care of our patients; lifestyle interventions can reverse the acquired defects associated with sedentary behaviors that grip modern society (i.e., lipotoxicity from obesity), and delay the development of diabetes in subjects genetically predisposed to the disease as shown in clinical trials *(22, 23, 152)*, even as their intrinsic genetic abnormalities (i.e., insulin resistance, mitochondrial dysfunction, and aerobic capacity) appear to be more "fixed" and difficult to overcome compared to those without such a genetic background.

ROLE OF LIPOTOXICITY IN THE DEVELOPMENT OF SKELETAL MUSCLE INSULIN RESISTANCE

FFA-Induced Insulin Resistance: Early Studies

In 1963, Randle et al. *(153)* demonstrated that incubation of rat muscle with fatty acids diminished insulin-stimulated glucose uptake. They proposed a "glucose fatty-acid cycle" (better known later as the Randle cycle) that revolved around the notion that cardiac and skeletal (diaphragm) muscle could shift readily back and forth between carbohydrate and fat as sources of energy for oxidation, depending on substrate availability. In its original formulation of the Randle cycle, oxidation of fatty acids led to inhibition of the Krebs cycle and glucose oxidation, impairing glycolytic flux, and eventually leading to product inhibition of hexokinase function and glucose transport. More specifically, fat oxidation in muscle led to substrate accumulation of acetylCoA and citrate, which inhibited both pyruvate dehydrogenase (PDH) and phosphofructokinase (PFK), respectively. As a consequence of this inhibition, glucose-6-phosphate (G-6-P) would increase within the cell and inhibit hexokinase, which led to a reduction in glucose transport. A decrease in glucose transport would also impair glycogen synthesis.

As such, the theory was incredibly attractive to help explain defects in both pathways reported in T2DM. Early studies in healthy humans appeared to support this notion *(143, 154–159)*, as they demonstrated that a lipid infusion that increased plasma FFA, or just kept FFA constant during an infusion of insulin, inhibited glucose oxidation and/or impaired insulin-stimulated glucose uptake. Additional support came from observations in which lipid infusion increased approximately four- to fivefold muscle acetyl-CoA content and the acetyl CoA/freeCoA ratio *(160)* and inhibited muscle pyruvate dehydrogenase activity *(160, 161)*, as would be expected from elevated muscle acetyl-CoA levels.

However, in the early 1990s other mechanisms also appeared to play a role. For example, overnight hyperglycemia (plasma glucose clamped at ~180 mg/dL) prevented FFA-induced insulin resistance, an unexpected and rather puzzling finding if the glucose fatty-acid cycle was the basis for insulin resistance in T2DM *(162, 163)*. Additional studies suggested a direct effect of FFA on early steps of glucose metabolism (i.e., at the level of glucose transport and/or phosphorylation), and reported a discordance between the rapid FFA-induced reduction in glucose oxidation and the delay in the inhibition of insulin-stimulated glucose uptake *(164)*, as well as by inconsistencies in the temporal inhibition by FFAs of glucose uptake, glycogen synthesis, and glycolysis *(160, 163)*. Subsequent studies could not find the expected rise (based on the Randle hypothesis) in skeletal muscle G-6-P concentration at a time when lipid infusion had already decreased insulin-stimulated glucose uptake *(165–168)*.

Another important contradiction to the glucose fatty-acid cycle was the "metabolic inflexibility" observed in obese and T2DM subjects, in which they are unable to switch from fat to glucose oxidation to increase glucose uptake during insulin-stimulated conditions (fed state). In leg muscle of hyperglycemic T2DM subjects *(133, 162)* there was a substrate utilization "paradox" using leg (local) balance techniques that suggested that glucose oxidation was slightly increased in the fasting state (rather than decreased) and that the rate of fat oxidation during insulin stimulation was rather "fixed" with a lack of suppression to insulin, which would be the opposite of what would be expected by the glucose fatty-acid cycle hypothesis.

Taken together the above observations called for a broader view and clearly suggested that the glucose fatty-acid (Randle) cycle was inadequate to fully account for diminished insulin action by FFA. Likely, additional mechanisms were at play involving other than impaired glycolytic flux or accumulation of G-6-P regarding FFA-induced muscle insulin resistance in humans.

Impact of Lipotoxicity on Skeletal Muscle Insulin Signaling

EXCESS FFA INDUCES INSULIN RESISTANCE BY IMPAIRING INSULIN SIGNALING IN HEALTHY SUBJECTS

A series of studies have now suggested that FFA and triglyceride-derived metabolites from intramyocellular lipid accumulation directly disrupt early steps of insulin signaling (Fig. 2). Inhibition of insulin-stimulated muscle glucose transport has been reported by many laboratories both in vitro and in animal studies as fatty acid concentrations increase in the incubation medium or in plasma, respectively *(133, 169)*. Moreover, fatty acid lipotoxicity may be associated with mitochondrial deoxyribonucleic acid (DNA) fragmentation, caspase-3 cleavage, cytochrome-c release, and production of reactive oxygen species with subsequent apoptosis in L6 rat skeletal muscle *(170)*. In humans, FFA

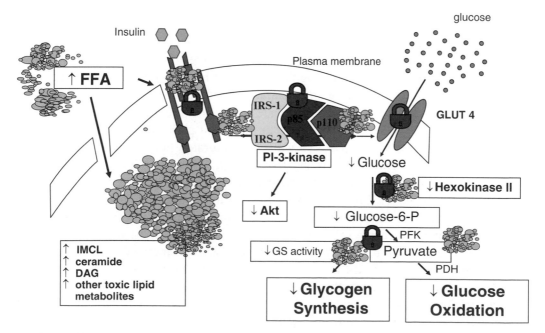

Fig. 2. Free fatty acids induce skeletal muscle insulin resistance in humans by inhibition of insulin signaling.

induce multiple defects in the insulin signaling cascade, at the level of glycogen synthesis, insulin-induced glucose transport and phosphorylation of the insulin receptor, insulin receptor substrate IRS-1, IRS-1–associated phosphatidylinositol (PI) 3-kinase activity, and of Akt *(142, 151, 166, 171–175)*, but this did not happen when lipid was infused to already insulin-resistant obese subjects *(175)*, suggesting that lipotoxicity may be already established in such individuals.

The role of FFA to cause insulin resistance and impair insulin signaling comes from a number of studies that show that an increase in fatty acid supply increases intramyocellular lipids (IMCL) and promotes the formation of a variety of fat-derived toxic metabolites, including fatty acyl-CoAs, ceramides, and diacylglycerol (DAG) with activation of the NF-κβ pathway. Boden et al. *(176)* and Bachmann et al. *(177)* quantified IMCL by 1H-MRS (magnetic resonance imaging and spectroscopy) in soleus and tibialis anterior muscles during lipid infusion studies and measured insulin sensitivity by means of the gold-standard euglycemic insulin clamp technique. Both groups showed that IMCL levels increased significantly within ~2 h of an intravenous lipid infusion, and continued to increase during the 4–6-h lipid infusion in parallel with a progressive reduction in insulin sensitivity throughout the lipid infusion period. Insulin sensitivity had a strong inverse correlation in these studies with the increase in IMCL, in both soleus and tibialis anterior muscles, suggesting an important role for triglyceride accumulation in the development of insulin resistance. These studies were consistent with the observation of increased IMCL in insulin-resistant nondiabetic subjects *(140, 178–182)* and in T2DM subjects *(182–184)*. It is now well established that lipid-derived metabolites [i.e, ceramide, DAG *(185)*, and long-chain acyl-CoA] activate cellular serine kinases and inhibit key insulin signaling molecules within muscle. Inflammatory pathways including both protein kinase C (PKC) activation of βII and δ isoforms in human skeletal muscle and Iκβ/NFκβ pathways have been clearly implicated in the FFA-induced impairment of IRS-1 tyrosine phosphorylation, and other downstream intracellular key signaling steps *(171, 186–188)*, being reversible by antiinflammatory agents, such as salicylates *(189)*. DAG is a powerful allosteric activator of PKC, a serine/threonine kinase with several isoforms, and increased serine phosphorylation of IRS-1 has been shown to inhibit IRS signaling *(129, 133, 134)*. Adams et al. *(187)* have showed that insulin sensitivity and stimulation of Akt phosphorylation by insulin is significantly impaired in obese nondiabetic subjects, being associated with a~twofold increase in muscle ceramide concentration. Moreover, ceramide content was significantly correlated with the plasma FFA concentration ($r = 0.51$, $p < 0.05$), providing another indication of the role of lipotoxicity in impairing insulin action in skeletal muscle.

More recently, there has been an increasing interest in toll-like receptor 4 (TLR4), the best characterized of the family of TLRs, as playing an essential role inflammation and insulin resistance in the setting of obesity, lipotoxicity, and T2DM. TLRs are important to the immune system by activating proinflammatory signaling pathways in response to microbial pathogens *(66, 190)*. TLR4 are activated by lipoplysaccharide (LPS) of bacterial walls and saturated fatty acids and play an important role in ligand recognition. IKK/Iκβ/NFκβ and JNK, which belong to the family of stress-activated protein kinases, are inflammatory pathways downstream of the TLR receptor and susceptible to activation by FFA. FFA activate TLR-driven signaling activating both inflammatory pathways and it is subject to intense research, as TLRs are believed to play an important role in the pathogenesis of FFA-induced insulin resistance. Recently Shi et al. *(191)* reported that in adipose tissue from insulin resistant high-fat-fed ob/ob and db/db mice, TLR gene expression was markedly increased compared to control normal animals and that TLR4 was required for FFA to generate the IKK/Iκβ/NFκβ-mediated inflammatory response. Furthermore, the investigators were able to demonstrate that the ability of FFA to activate the IKK/Iκβ/NFκβ pathway and induce an inflammatory response could be blocked in TLR4 null mice. Activation of these same pathways and protection from a high-fat diet-induced insulin resistance at the level of muscle, liver, and adipose tissue has also been reported in mice with a loss-of-function mutation in TLR4 *(192)*. Preliminary data from within our group indicates that TLR4 gene expression in vastus lateralis muscle from obese nondiabetic and T2DM subjects is increased, suggesting that TLR4 signaling is required for FFA-induced inflammation, and possibly insulin resistance (N. Musi, personal communication). Taken together, while much remains to be understood, it is now apparent that a decrease FFA cause insulin resistance largely by the accumulation of triglyceride and other lipid-derived metabolites with subsequent activation of intramyocellular inflammatory pathways that impair insulin signaling at different levels, rather than by substrate competition, as initially believed.

IMPAIRMENT OF MUSCLE INSULIN SIGNALING AND INSULIN SENSITIVITY BY FFA IS DOSE-DEPENDENT IN HUMANS: CLINICAL IMPLICATIONS

A limitation of most, but not all *(155, 160, 161, 164, 193)*, studies of humans examining the role of an increase in plasma FFA was the use of high-dose lipid infusion rates, which elevated plasma FFA usually ≥1,500 μmol/L. These levels are considerably higher than the usual FFA levels observed in obese and T2DM subjects. Fasting plasma FFA levels in healthy subjects range between ~300 and 400 μmol/L and increase to between ~800 and 1,100 μmol/L only under certain extreme conditions such as fasting for 2–3 days *(194, 195)*. As discussed earlier, in obese nondiabetic individuals *(145, 196, 197)* and in patients with T2DM *(198, 199)*, fasting and day-long plasma FFA levels are usually elevated (~600–700 μmol/L) because of resistance of adipose tissue to the antilipolytic effect of insulin, but plasma FFA usually rarely exceed ~1,000 μmol/L even in the presence of severe hypertriglyceridemia (with or without concomitant diabetes) *(86)* or poorly controlled diabetes *(200–202)*. Because few studies had used these lower lipid infusion doses *(155, 160, 161, 164, 193)*, one could argue against the clinical day-to-day relevance of FFA in human disease. These early studies did suggest that a small increase of plasma FFA levels in healthy subjects-induced insulin resistance, impaired glucose oxidation, and glycogen synthase activity *(160, 161)*, but no information was available on earlier steps of insulin signaling at plasma FFA elevations within the physiological range observed in T2DM. To better understand how FFA interacted with early molecular steps responsible for insulin action in muscle, we performed acute dose–response studies in healthy subjects at FFA spanning from plasma levels typically seen in obesity and T2DM (600–700 μmol/L), through the upper range of the physiological spectrum (~1,000–1,200 μmol/L) and on into the pharmacological range (~1,700 μmol/L) *(151)*. Of note, heparin was not coinfused to resemble as closely as possible physiological conditions, as it is uncertain whether a plasma FFA elevation achieved by dislodging lipoprotein lipase with heparin really resembles the physiologic delivery of FFA to tissues under normal living conditions. As observed in Fig. 3, FFA-induced insulin resistance in a dose-dependent manner, with most of the insulin resistance developing already with the low, physiological increase in plasma FFA concentrations (i.e., 695 μmol/L) observed in obesity and T2DM. Moreover, as observed in Fig. 4, there was a clear gradient of inhibition of all proximal insulin signaling steps ranging from the physiological to the pharmacological range.

This was the first demonstration in humans that plasma FFA inhibits insulin signal transduction in a dose-dependent manner. An important observation was that 70% of the maximal inhibition of insulin signaling was observed within just a few hours and at plasma FFA concentrations that were well within the physiological range (Fig. 3). Moreover, there was a close correlation between the plasma FFA concentration fasting and during the euglycemic insulin clamp and insulin sensitivity (Fig. 5). The clinical relevance of such a finding has far-reaching implications because it tells us that it takes only this small increase in plasma FFA to cause a broad inhibition of the signaling cascade, from the insulin receptor through Akt phosphorylation. This data also helps to understand how FFA can cause a significant impairment in skeletal muscle insulin action even in the presence of a mild expansion in

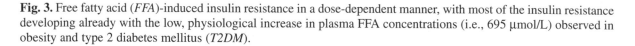

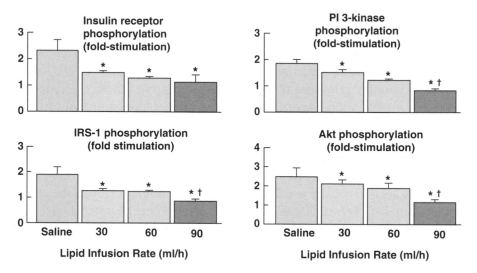

Fig. 3. Free fatty acid (*FFA*)-induced insulin resistance in a dose-dependent manner, with most of the insulin resistance developing already with the low, physiological increase in plasma FFA concentrations (i.e., 695 μmol/L) observed in obesity and type 2 diabetes mellitus (*T2DM*).

Fig. 4. Dose-dependent effect of an acute elevation in plasma free fatty acid (*FFA*) on insulin signaling in healthy nondiabetic subjects. Effect of saline vs. lipid (Liposyn III, a 20% triglyceride emulsion) infusion at 30, 60, and 90 mL/h on the percent reduction in insulin receptor (**a**) and IRS-1 tyrosine phosphorylation (**b**), PI 3-kinase activity associated with IRS-1 (**c**), and serine phosphorylation of Akt (**d**). $^{*}p < 0.01–0.05$, lipid vs. saline; $^{**}p < 0.05$, 90- vs. 30-mL/h lipid infusion rates.

adipose tissue mass, as seen in overweight individuals (BMI from 25 and 29.9 kg/m^2), and recognize why lipotoxicity is fully established in obese individuals (BMI ≥30 kg/m^2).

LESSONS ON LIPOTOXICITY FROM CHRONIC INCREASES IN PLASMA FFA LEVELS IN HEALTHY SUBJECTS GENETICALLY PREDISPOSED TO T2DM

Several laboratories have tried to separate intrinsic (genetic) defects in insulin action from those from acquired conditions such arising from adipose tissue insulin resistance in obesity or glucotoxicity of established T2DM. To this end, our group *(138, 141, 142, 150)* and others *(179, 203–210)* have

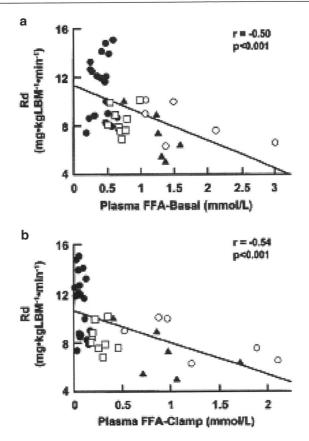

Fig. 5. Inverse correlation between total-body insulin-mediated glucose disposal and plasma free fatty acid (*FFA*) concentration during basal (fasting) conditions (**a**) and during the euglycemic insulin clamp (**b**). *Black circles*, saline infusion; *open circles*, lipid infusion at 90 mL/h; *black triangles*, lipid infusion at 60 mL/h; *open squares*, lipid infusion at 30 mL/h. *LBM* lean body mass.

studied *lean* healthy normal *glucose-tolerant* subjects genetically predisposed to T2DM (i.e., having both parents with T2DM or one parent and several siblings with T2DM). These family history positive (FH+) individuals are already insulin-resistant long before the development of β-cell failure (Fig. 6) and at high risk of T2DM as their pancreatic β-cells frequently cannot adapt with the chronic insulin secretory demand. This has been confirmed in longitudinal studies, with those at the highest risk of developing T2DM having a combination of both insulin resistance and low β-cell reserve *(211, 212)*. In vastus lateralis muscle biopsy studies, we have shown that FH+ subjects share the same early insulin signaling steps as seen later in life in patients with established T2DM *(142)* and suffered no further worsening after 4 days of increasing plasma FFA levels within the physiological range to levels typically seen in obesity and in T2DM (~600–700 µmol/L). In contrast, in subjects without a FH of T2DM, the same subtle increase in plasma FFA-reduced insulin sensitivity by ~25% and caused insulin-signaling defects in skeletal muscle similar to those seen in T2DM *(142)* (Fig. 6). Of note, in our study patients had "normal" plasma FFA concentration despite marked hyperinsulinemia (plasma insulin levels that were approximately twofold higher than lean insulin-sensitive controls), indicative of inadequate

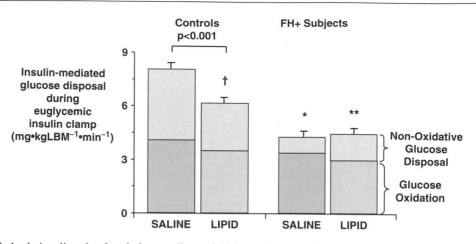

Fig. 6. Whole body insulin-stimulated glucose disposal (*R*d, total height of bars), glucose oxidation (closed part of bar) and nonoxidative glucose disposal (open part of bar) in healthy normal glucose-tolerant subjects without a family history of type 2 diabetes mellitus (*T2DM*) (controls) and in subjects with a strong family history of T2DM (FH + subjects 0 after 4 days of saline or low-dose lipid infusion. *LBM* lean body mass. *p < 0.01 vs. saline infusion; **p < 0.001 saline infusion in FH+ vs. controls; ***p < 0.01 lipid infusion in FH+ vs. controls. All data represented as means ±SEM.

FFA suppression by insulin, as has been reported by others (*140, 213*). Therefore, one cannot completely rule out a subtle degree of lipotoxicity. Whether this lack of additional deterioration in insulin signaling in FH+ subjects can be related to adipose tissue insulin resistance and early lipotoxicity, or to other (genetic) molecular mechanisms causing insulin resistance, remains to be determined. Taken together, lipotoxicity at the level of muscle could be a very early defect that may develop long before adulthood in FH+ individuals. Increased intramyocellular lipid content is already established in obese children (*213, 214*), but in the pediatric literature largely overweight adolescents have been examined, so that the contribution of genetic vs. acquired (obesity) factors remains cannot be dissected out. Studies of very early ages have not been done in lean FH+ children with the techniques employed at an older age due to their invasive nature, so the relative contribution very early lipotoxicity on top of genetic factors to the development of muscle insulin resistance in humans remains to be established.

Role of Mitochondrial Dysfunction in Muscle Insulin Resistance

Impaired muscle insulin action at an early stage in life could be the result from an intrinsic/genetic inability of muscle to increase its oxidative capacity upon demand, as reported in lean FH+ subjects and/or an acquired defect from excessive exogenous substrate (i.e., FFA) as in obesity and T2DM. Diminished lipid oxidative capacity has been reported by many laboratories in insulin-resistant lean FH+ and obese individuals, as well as in patients with T2DM (*133, 134, 184, 206, 215–218*). In Mexican-American FH+ subjects from San Antonio, Texas (*219*), and in Caucasian populations (*220*), it has been reported that there is a coordinate reduction of genes involved in oxidative metabolism in insulin-resistant diabetic and nondiabetic FH+ Mexican-Americans. Several studies have manipulated FFA availability to muscle and shown that a reduction of FFA availability prevents FFA-induced insulin resistance. Knockout mice with deletions in the fatty acid transport protein 1 (FATP1) or alterations in the activation of inflammatory pathways such as JNK, inhibitor of NF κB kinase β subunit (IKKβ), or PKCθ have all shown resistance to FFA-induced insulin resistance (*134*). Within our group, Richardson et al. *(221)* have reported that a 48-h increase in plasma FFA by means of a lipid infusion in healthy subjects in significantly reduced proliferator activated receptor-γ cofactor-1 (PGC-1) mRNA, along with messenger ribonucleic acids (mRNAs) for a number of nuclear encoded mitochondrial genes. Moreover, using microarray analysis, lipid infusion caused a significant overexpression of extracellular matrix genes and connective tissue growth factor. Quantitative reverse transcription PCR showed that the mRNA/protein expression of collagens and multiple extracellular matrix genes were also elevated after lipid infusion, in striking similarity to what has been observed in insulin-resistant subjects with a fatty liver in nonalcoholic steaothepatitis (as discussed below in the liver section of this chapter) *(222, 223)*, linking functional and structural abnormalities in different tissues by FFA oversupply. On the contrary, if plasma FFA levels are reduced by acipimox, an inhibitor of adipose tissue lipolysis, there is an enhancement of insulin action in FH+ subjects *(224)*, as well as in obese *(225)* and T2DM *(225, 226)* patients.

Recent studies have suggested that in insulin-resistant states, such as in FH+ and in T2DM subjects, there is an intrinsic mitochondrial substrate oxidation defect responsible for the accumulation of IMCL. In T2DM there are numerous functional and structural mitochondrial abnormalities when tissue from vastus lateralis muscle biopsies are examined *(216, 227, 228)*. Lean, insulin-resistant FH+ subjects have a reduced mitochondrial substrate oxidation capacity as measured by the incorporation of ^{13}C label into C_4 glutamate following [2-^{13}C] acetate infusion by MRS *(210)*. Consistent with these findings, Brehm et al. *(229)* have reported that when plasma FFA levels are maintained in the upper limit of the physiological range at 1,000 μmol/L during an hyperinsulinemic clamp (plasma insulin increased approximately tenfold), FFA-induced insulin resistance in skeletal muscle was associated with a 70% reduction in insulin-stimulated glucose transport/phosphorylation and a 24% reduction adenosine triphosphate (ATP) synthase flux compared to identical control (saline) studies. Recently, a lower mitochondrial content in muscle of diabetic subjects (rather than decreased function) has been proposed to play a role for the reduced mitochondrial oxidative capacity *(230)*. Taken together, these studies suggest that in genetically predisposed individuals the ability of the mitochondria to increase substrate oxidation may be limited by either a reduction in function and/or an overall mitochondrial content, making skeletal muscle particularly vulnerable to lipotoxicity, as observed in obesity and T2DM.

Can Weight Loss and/or Exercise Reverse Muscle Insulin Resistance?

It is unquestionable that cardiorespiratory fitness reduces the risk of CVD and that low rates of physical activity are associated with a greater risk of developing insulin resistance, obesity, MS, and T2DM *(51, 231–233)*. In the midst of an epidemic of obesity and diabetes, renewed interest has developed in understanding the molecular pathways by which exercise appears to reverse defects associated with insulin resistance [reviewed in-depth under *(234–236)*]. While the role of exercise will be reviewed in other chapters, a few points deserve attention. First, as discussed in the previous section, it is important to recognize that lipid accumulation in skeletal muscle and insulin resistance are not just the result of excessive fatty acid supply, but likely the combination of increased supply and a reduced capacity of muscle to use it as a fuel for energy needs. Because disruption in lipid metabolism/FFA flux appears to be causal in the development of insulin resistance, it follows that it should be possible to reverse FFA-induced insulin resistance with interventions that improve lipid homeostasis, such as aerobic endurance training. An increase in lipid oxidation plays an important role in the improvement observed in insulin sensitivity in skeletal muscle from high-fat-fed rodents *(237)* and in obese subjects following training *(238)*. Moderate-intensity physical activity (—four to five times per week for 30–40 min for 16 weeks), combined with weight loss, induces mitochondrial biogenesis, improved function, and morphologic changes (i.e., an increase in mitochondrial size) in previously sedentary obese subjects *(227, 239)*. These changes have also been reported in older sedentary individuals (>65 years of age) with rather modest amounts of training *(240)*. Exercise also enhances in a time- and intensity-dependent manner insulin signaling pathways at multiple levels in lean healthy subjects, including insulin receptor, IRS-1 and the PI 3-kinase association with IRS-1 phosphorylation *(241)*, HKII mRNA/activity *(242)*, GLUT-4 protein expression and glycogen synthase activity *(243)*, and AMPK activity and AS160 phosphorylation, although in skeletal muscle from obese and T2DM subjects the potential of exercise to stimulate the above steps is blunted *(188, 241, 242, 244)*. One mechanism by which regular exercise improves muscle insulin sensitivity involves inhibition of the inflammatory pathways discussed earlier, such as NF-κβ that interfere with insulin signaling in T2DM *(188)*.

While there is no doubt that aerobic exercise training is a potent and effective intervention strategy for individuals with insulin resistance, debate remains whether regular physical activity may improve insulin sensitivity independent of weight loss in T2DM, what is the minimum amount of exercise needed for health benefits and which exercise prescriptions may more successfully impact glycemic control and prevent CVD in patients with T2DM. The CV protection conferred by exercise includes antiinflammatory, hormonal, lipid, blood pressure, and multiple direct vascular effects beyond those related to improvements in muscle insulin sensitivity *(232, 233)*. To highlight an example of the adverse CV impact that disrupted fatty acid metabolism may have in humans, we have observed that just a mild increase in plasma FFA (to levels observed in T2DM) by means of a lipid infusion increases blood pressure *(245)* and induces endothelial dysfunction and systemic inflammation in lean healthy nondiabetic volunteers *(246)*. Exercise promotes an improvement in endothelial function and capillary recruitment in muscle, although this response is also reduced in patients with T2DM *(247)*. However, in a finding of value toward understanding the CV protective effects of exercise in diabetics, we demonstrated that just 8 weeks of moderate-intensity aerobic exercise training can improve endothelial dysfunction together with increased muscle insulin sensitivity in patients with T2DM *(248)*.

While regular exercise and weight loss combined appear to have the greatest impact on insulin resistance, reversal of lipotoxicity and CV risk *(51, 231–233)*, it is sometimes discouraging to patients that weight loss is minimal or none at all. However, it should be noted that training even without weight loss has been reported to improve insulin sensitivity *(22, 233, 249, 250)*, although not by all *(185)*. Whether aerobic training, resistance training, or both combined are best for subjects with diabetes is a matter of debate. A recent Canadian study performed across eight community-based facilities in 251 adults (age 39–70, mean = 54) addressed this issue. Subjects were asked to exercise with moderation three times a week for 22 weeks. The authors reported improved glycemic control with all three modalities (0.5%), although greater for combined aerobic and resistance training (an additional 0.5% reduction). These results are consistent with a large body of evidence about the metabolic benefits of moderate intensity exercise in terms of better glycemic control for patients with T2DM *(233)*. Regular physical activity is also important for the reduction of the risk of developing T2DM *(22, 152, 250)*. Recently, Sui et al. *(251)* confirmed this in an observational cohort of 6,249 women aged 20–79 years that were free of diabetes at baseline. During a 17-year follow-up, 143 cases of T2DM occurred. In multivariate analysis (including BMI), comparing the least fit third with the upper third of cardiorespiratory fitness there was a highly significant 39% reduction in the development of diabetes. From a practical perspective, a large body of evidence has led to recent "minimum recommendations" by the American College of Sports Medicine and the American Heart Association *(252, 253)* for physical activity. These recommend 30 min of moderate intensity (or 20 min of vigorous intensity) exercise 5 days per week for individuals between 18 and 65 years of age and to be adapted as possible to individual 65 and older or with chronic medical conditions as functional capacity allows. Fitness is a significant mortality predictor in older adults, independent of overall or abdominal adiposity and even after adjustment for smoking, baseline health, and either BMI, waist circumference, or percent body fat *(51)*. Clinicians should be aware of the importance of preserving functional capacity by recommending regular physical activity for overweight and obese insulin-resistant subjects, particularly in a high-risk category for developing T2DM (i.e., positive FH in a first-degree relative, ethnic minority, and history of gestational diabetes).

FFA AND THE LIVER

FFA and Hepatic Insulin Resistance

Insulin tightly regulates the rate of endogenous glucose production (EGP). Hepatic glucose production accounts for the majority (≥90%) of glucose output in the fasting state, except for a small proportion arising from renal gluconeogenesis *(254)*. The rate of EGP is important under fasting conditions to provide glucose for the metabolic needs of glucose-dependent tissues such as the brain and red blood cells. In lean insulin-sensitive healthy subjects, modest increases in the plasma insulin concentration (i.e., from 5 µU/mL to 40 µU/mL) rapidly inhibit EGP by 70–80% and nearly completely suppress EGP when they reach 50–100 µU/mL *(199, 255, 256)*. In contrast, in nondiabetic insulin-resistant subjects, such as obese individuals or lean subjects with a strong FH of T2DM, to maintain the rate of EGP within normal limits the fasting plasma insulin concentration needs to be two to threefold higher than in lean insulin-sensitive individuals. Fasting hyperglycemia has been shown in many studies to be closely correlated to the rate of EGP in T2DM, as insulin secretion cannot compensate adequately for hepatic insulin resistance and there is a progressive increase in the rate of EGP, particularly when the plasma glucose rises above 140–180 mg/dL *(199, 255–257)*. Glucogenolysis is particularly sensitive to small increases in the plasma insulin concentration, while inhibition of gluconeogenic flux requires higher levels of insulin *(258–261)*. In T2DM, overproduction of glucose by the liver is primarily due to resistance of hepatic gluconeogenesis to insulin action, while glycogeonlysis appears to preserve better its response to the inhibitory action of insulin *(258–260)*.

Insulin acts directly by binding to hepatic insulin receptors and thereby activating insulin signaling pathways in the liver. Insulin's indirect effects to regulate hepatic glucose production include reduction of pancreatic glucagon secretion *(262, 263)*, possible effects at the level of the hypothalamus *(264)*, and decreased substrate availability in the form of amino acids and FFA for gluceogenesis by inhibiting muscle protein catabolism and adipose tissue lipolysis, respectively *(265)*. Some have advocated that the indirect effects of insulin on peripheral tissues (mainly on adipose tissue) are keys to controlling hepatic glucose production *(266)*. However, recent evidence suggests that while FFA is important to glucose production by the liver, the direct effects of insulin on hepatocytes have primacy in the regulation of EGP *(267)*.

Plasma FFA levels play an important role in the relation to hepatic insulin sensitivity and glucose production in humans. In rodents, an increase in FFA supply causes insulin resistance and activates the proinflammatory nuclear factor-κB pathway *(268, 269)*, while perfusion of isolated rat livers with palmitate or oleate decreases insulin-receptor, IRS-1, PI 3-kinase, and Akt phosphorylation *(270)*. In dogs, elevated plasma FFA also stimulates hepatic glucose production and activates proinflammatory pathways that inhibit insulin signaling *(271)*. In lean healthy subjects, FFA have been reported to induce insulin resistance by stimulating both gluconeogenesis *(272)* and glycogenolysis *(261)*. In insulin-resistant states such as obesity and T2DM, adipose tissue is the primary source of fatty acids in insulin-resistant states *(273, 274)*, and elevated plasma FFA provide the liver with energy (ATP) and carbons to drive gluconeogenic pathways and de novo lipogenesis *(275)*. Increased plasma FFA also causes the dyslipidemia typically seen in insulin-resistant states, with increased rates of VLDL secretion, which in turn lower plasma HDL and lead to the formation of small dense LDL. Thus, adipose tissue insulin resistance with increased flux of FFA to the liver can lead to the full spectrum

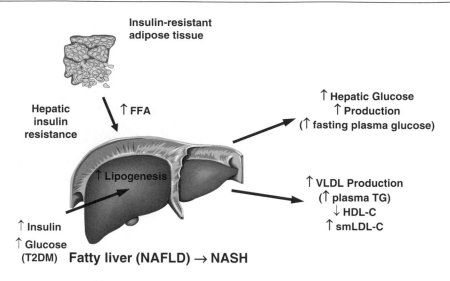

Fig. 7. Multiple abnormalities drive hepatic lipogenesis in insulin-resistant states. Excessive rates of lipolysis from adipose tissue increase plasma free fatty acids (*FFA*) and provide abundant substrate to the liver for triglyceride synthesis. Hyperinsulinemia activates SREBP1c and hyperglycemia ChREBP to stimulate hepatic steatosis. The clinical manifestations are common to patients with metabolic syndrome and type 2 diabetes mellitus (*T2DM*), increased fasting plasma glucose and atherogenic dyslipidemia.

of metabolic abnormalities that are so common clinically today, as summarized in Fig. 7. In our hands, a combined low-dose lipid and glucose infusion for 2 days can reproduce all the abnormalities seen in the MS in nondiabetic subjects genetically predisposed to T2DM: an increase in blood pressure, elevated triglycerides, and low HDL-C and systemic inflammation evidenced by an increase in hsCRP, ICAM (inter cell adhesion molecule)/VCAM (vascular cell adhesion molecule), etc. *(245)*. Moreover, 2–3 days of elevated plasma FFA in lean FH+ reduces insulin clearance and promotes chronic peripheral hyperinsulinemia, as has been reported in insulin-resistant states such as in obesity, PCOS, women with a history of gestational diabetes mellitus (GDM) and T2DM *(141)*. An acute (2–6 h) pharmacological (five to tenfold) elevation of plasma FFA levels *(82, 129, 132, 276)*, as well as low-dose chronic (48 h) lipid infusions *(141)*, induce hepatic insulin resistance, while reduction of plasma FFA by acipimox partially restore hepatic insulin sensitivity *(225)*. Taken together, these studies highlight the close relationship between increased FFA supply and hepatic insulin sensitivity. But perhaps where this interplay is best exemplified from a clinical standpoint is in the metabolic abnormalities observed in NAFLD.

Why do Obesity, T2DM, and NAFLD Cluster?
The Liver as the "Metabolic Sensor" of Lipotoxicity

NAFLD is a chronic liver condition frequently associated with T2DM and characterized by insulin resistance and hepatic fat accumulation. Liver fat may range from simple steatosis to severe steatohepatitis with necroinflammation and variable degrees of fibrosis (nonalcoholic steatohepatitis or NASH). About 40% of patients with NAFLD develop NASH *(277–279)*, with an early study reporting progression to fibrosis and/or cirrhosis in 15–20% of NASH *(280)*, although it is believed to be as high as 40% from data of more recent series *(281–284)*. Moreover, recent evidence suggests that the lifespan of patients with NAFLD is significantly shortened not only by a liver-related morbidity but also by a higher incidence of CVD *(285, 286)*.

As with obesity and T2DM, there is also considerable concern that NAFLD and NASH are reaching epidemic proportions *(287)*. However, the true magnitude of the disease is not appreciated by many clinicians because the majority (~70%) of patients affected have normal liver enzymes *(279, 288–290)*. It has been recently estimated that fatty liver disease affects ~1/3 of the adult population or ~80 million Americans, and as many as ~2/3 of obese subjects in the United States *(278, 279, 288)*. In a large population-based study (*n* = 2,287 subjects) performed in Dallas, Texas, in which liver fat was evaluated by means of the gold-standard MRS technique, 34% of the population had a fatty liver, being much more common in Hispanics (45%) compared to whites (33%) and African–Americans (22%) *(288)*. That adult Hispanic are affected more than Caucasians and African–Americans has been confirmed by others even after adjusting for major confounding variables *(94, 96, 99, 101, 291–294)*. Recent studies indicate that the prevalence of NAFLD is also rapidly increasing in children and adolescents, particularly in those of Hispanic ancestry *(94, 291, 293)*, being strongly associated with the triad of insulin resistance, increased visceral fat, and hypoadiponectinemia *(105)*.

While obese patients with the MS and T2DM are more prone to fatty liver and develop more severe disease (NASH), the reasons are unclear and most other aspects of the disease in T2DM remain poorly understood. It is tempting to speculate that the liver is like a "metabolic sensor" with the degree of steatosis being a reflection of the ability of the body to cope with a lipotoxic environment. There is an increasing awareness that insulin resistance, lipotoxicity, and T2DM are major risk factors for fatty liver disease, necroinflammation, and fibrosis. Still the information available on the natural history of the disease with paired biopsies is limited to a handful of small studies *(281–284)*. In these studies, involving from 22 to 103 patients with an average follow-up ranging from 3.2 *(283)* to 13.8 years *(284)*, fibrosis progressed over time in 32–41% of patients with NAFLD *(281–284)*. However, disease remained stable in 34–50% of patients and even improved in a minority. This has brought attention to try to dissect and understand better the prognostic factors that may lead to disease progression over time. Obesity *(281–284)* and T2DM *(281–284)* have been the two most prominent factors of poor prognosis, while elevated liver enzymes (ALT (aldnine aminotransferase) or AST (aspartate)/ALT ratio) have been of much less value to predict future disease, with levels frequently being normal even in cases of advanced disease. Some studies have compared subjects with NAFLD who had chronically elevated plasma ALT concentrations to individuals with persistently normal ALT levels and found that the prevalence of advanced fibrosis and cirrhosis was similar in both groups *(295, 296)*. Consistent with this, others have reported that in the setting of diabetes liver enzymes are poor predictors of disease activity *(297, 298)*. Complicating the issue is the accepted finding that AST tends to fall over time with the progression of fibrosis and development of cirrhosis *(283)*, making liver transaminases unreliable to identify patients at greater risk of advanced disease or to monitor therapy.

Many studies have reported that long-term prognosis in NAFLD varies widely depending upon the initial stage at diagnosis and the presence or not of obesity, MS, or T2DM. For example, the vast majority of patients with cryptogenic cirrhosis are obese or have T2DM *(299)*. Several studies have confirmed the strong impact of both factors, but in particular diabetes, to the progression of disease (e.g., fibrosis) *(280–284, 295–298, 300–305)*. Angulo et al. found that the combination of diabetes and obesity were predictors of advanced fibrosis in 66% of patients *(300)*. Hyperglycemia was identified as a key factor in disease progression in large early studies by Marceau et al. (*n* = 551) *(303)* and Luyckx et al. (*n* = 505) *(304)*. Dixon et al. *(302)* reported that 60% of patients with T2DM and NAFLD had biopsy-proven NASH, and that advanced fibrosis was present in 75% of those with diabetes and hypertension vs. 7% without either condition. Haukeland et al. *(305)* reported that the presence of diabetes or impaired glucose tolerance (IGT) increased by 3.8-fold the risk of fibrosis in patients with an unexplained elevation in LFT, diabetes being the only independent risk factor for NASH. Mofrad et al. *(295)* found that in patients with NAFLD and normal LFTs, 24% had severe fibrosis and >10% cirrhosis, concluding that normal plasma ALT levels does not guarantee freedom from underlying advanced fibrosis. Again, in this study diabetes was the only factor independently associated with increased risk of advanced fibrosis. Even if a low initial fibrosis stage is found, the presence of diabetes per se is a risk factor for progression *(283)*.

Given the poor prognosis that the combination of T2DM and NAFLD have, it is quite surprising that few studies have focused on screening patients with diabetes for NASH. A prospective study conducted by Gupte et al. *(306)* reported biopsy-proven NASH in 87% of diabetics, 22% having moderate to severe disease. In a retrospective analysis of 44 patients with T2DM worked-up for NAFLD, Younussi et al. also found that cirrhosis was more prevalent in diabetics vs. nondiabetics (25% vs. 10%, $p < 0.001$) *(301)*. More importantly, diabetics had increased not only liver-related mortality but also CV mortality was increased as well, consistent with recent epidemiological studies *(285, 286, 307)*. Moreover, by logistic regression analysis, the severity of histological features of NAFLD independently predicted carotid intima medial thickness or CIMT (a marker of atherosclerosis burden) ($p < 0.001$) after adjustment for all potential confounders *(307)*. In another study in 38 patients with NAFLD, in the absence of morbid obesity, hypertension, and diabetes, had altered left ventricular geometry and early features of left ventricular diastolic dysfunction *(308)*. While patients with T2DM are known to have increased CVD *(309)*, long-term studies have indicated that CVD is also the most common cause of death of patients with NAFLD, even after adjusting for classical CV risk factors *(284)*. NAFLD may increase CVD in T2DM by promoting a number of atherogenic risk factors, including chronic hyperinsulinemia (insulin resistance per se is known to be atherogenic) *(40, 310–312)*, by promoting atherogenic dyslipidemia (increased VLDL production, leading to a lowering HDL-C and small dense LDL-C) *(86, 313, 314)*, and by the induction of systemic inflammation *(64, 223, 315)*.

It has also been postulated that insulin resistance and/or its clinical correlate of the MS are the most reliable indicators of disease severity and future progression *(289, 316)*. In a study by Sorrentino et al. *(296)* in 80 patients with NAFLD but normal liver enzymes, 65% had NASH and 35% fibrosis, with the presence of the MS and long-standing history of obesity being the strongest predictors of disease, but not liver transaminase levels. Recently, Gholam et al. *(317)* reported in 97 obese individuals a 36% prevalence of NASH and 25% of fibrosis with hyperglycemia (A1c level), insulin resistance, and the MS, but not BMI, being strongly associated with NASH and fibrosis. Even modest increases in body weight and plasma triglycerides appear to support the role of insulin resistance in NAFLD, as suggested in an elegant study by Ratziu et al. *(318)* that found that a BMI $\geq$28 kg/m^2 and elevated triglycerides $\geq$145 mg/dL were both useful predictors of the severity of liver fibrosis. Even in nonobese, nondiabetic patients, the presence and severity of NAFLD can be strongly predicted on the basis of insulin resistance, central obesity, and elevated triglycerides *(319)*.

In summary, obese insulin-resistant T2DM patients are at the highest risk of fatty liver disease and progression to NASH and that NAFLD should be aggressively pursued in this population, although still today little is done to identify patients with the condition in routine clinical practice. The clustering of MS, T2DM, and NAFLD does not occur by chance, these conditions being tied together by the lipotoxicity brought about by adipose tissue insulin resistance. Lipotoxicity creates a permissive environment for NAFLD. However, despite the accepted role of excessive fat supply and inflammation to the pathogenesis of NAFLD, we cannot satisfactorily explain why some lean subjects develop NASH or some obese (or T2DM) individuals are spared from developing a fatty liver. Moreover, why fatty liver evolves into NASH in only ~30–40% of patients or cirrhosis in just ~10% is puzzling. It is possible that if more careful measures of insulin resistance and/or FFA metabolism are done we will be able to identify a profile of subjects prone to NAFLD and/or NASH, although it is likely that development of disease will depend on the adaptive flexibility of target tissues, primarily the liver, to adapt to the insult.

Is NASH a Mitochondrial Disease?

There is an increasing consensus that the inability of the mitochondria to adapt to insulin resistance and lipotoxicity play a key role in the development of fatty liver disease and NASH [reviewed in-depth by (223, 320–322)]. Adipose tissue insulin resistance, oversupply of FFA to the liver and the development of a state of local and systemic chronic inflammation are at center stage in the development of steatosis and liver damage in NAFLD. A key determinant for hepatic fat accumulation is the inability of the liver to adapt to the excessive FFA supply from dysfunctional, insulin-resistant adipose tissue. There may also be an altered composition of the fat that accumulates in fatty liver disease, with an increased content of TAG and DAG, and a shift toward a progressive increase in the TAG/DAG ratio, as patients progress from simple NAFLD to NASH (323). Adipose stores account for about ~60–70% of the FFA used for hepatic fat synthesis and for the secretion of VLDL in the setting of NAFLD and in obesity (273, 274). This excess FFA load places mitochondria within hepatocytes under severe functional stress, as their ability to increase fatty acid oxidation is limited in humans. An alternative adaptive mechanism by the liver in the setting of excessive FFA supply, chronic hyperinsulinemia, and hyperglycemia (all factors associated with increased hepatic triglyceride synthesis) is to increase the secretion of VLDL. This may be the way nature attempts to "unload" hepatic fat to prevent massive steatosis and may explain why so frequently high triglycerides and low HDL-C are seen in patients with MS, T2DM, and NAFLD. However, both mechanisms seem unable to prevent triglyceride accumulation in subjects that develop NAFLD. When mitochondrial adaptation is offset by chronic fat overload, it triggers the release of reactive oxygen species (ROS) with stimulation of Kupffer cells (local macrophages) and production of a myriad of cytokines that cause a chronic activation of multiple inflammatory pathways (i.e., JNK, NF-κβ) (223, 324). In rat liver, FFA have been reported to clearly induce hepatic/peripheral insulin resistance and activate the proinflammatory serine/threonine kinases and the NF-κβ pathway (268, 325), promote the accumulation of DAG and increase the expression of TNF-α and IL-1β (268), and impair insulin signaling (325), while both salycilate (325) and inhibition of hepatic lipid synthesis in high-fat-fed rats with antisense oligonucleotides prevents the development of steatosis (326–328).

Therefore, one may postulate several steps in the development of NASH. The "first step" in obese individuals is adipose tissue insulin resistance and the development of a lipotoxic environment. The "second step"" will depend on the ability of the liver to adapt to the fat load or not. Adaptation will depend on two main factors: the genetic background of the individual and the magnitude of the insult. The insult will commonly be varying degrees of adipose tissue expansion, insulin resistance, FFA flux to the liver ± chronic food overload, or additional factors such as genetically-determined insulin resistance (i.e., in lean subjects), hyperglycemia (i.e., in diabetes), concomitant conditions/medications associated with insulin resistance, and others. Genes will likely establish the metabolic flexibility of the liver to refrain from excessive lipogenesis, the oxidative capacity of mitochondrial hepatocytes to utilize fat, or to export triglycerides through VLDL secretion, all measures aimed at averting excessive accumulation of liver fat and the production of lipid-derived toxic metabolites and activation of inflammation. The "third step" will depend on the latter, that is, whether the hepatocytes will have enough metabolic flexibility to adapt with the "lipotoxic insult," or on the contrary, will collapse leading to the formation of reactive oxygen species and activation of inflammatory pathways. Failure will cause a chronic inflammatory and fibrotic response that might spiral out of control and lead progressively to end-stage liver disease. One may also consider if there is not also a "fourth step" from the cross-talk between stellate cells responsible for fibrogenesis and inflammatory pathways that may explain why severe fibrosis and cirrhosis develops just in a minority of patients who have chronic liver inflammation in NASH, an area that remains poorly understood.

Unfortunately, almost all the information available about NAFLD/NASH arises from animal models of the disease (largely rodents) with very limited information from human studies. An example of the shortcomings arising from animal data can be appreciated when examining the discrepant effects of fibrates and of rosiglitazone in mice compared to human studies. For example, fenofibrate markedly reduces hepatic steatosis and improves hepatic/muscle insulin sensitivity in mice models of fat-induced insulin resistance, obesity, and steatosis (329). In contrast, fenofibrate did not improve liver enzymes or hepatic/muscle insulin sensitivity when we treated obese nondiabetic subjects with the MS (330) or T2DM (331). In a similar way, while rosiglitazone has been reported to improve elevated liver transaminases and steatosis in humans (332, 333), studies in mice report that rosiglitazone increases hepatic transaminases and worsens necroinflammation and steatosis (334).

In NASH there is also altered insulin signaling and diminished activity of key energy regulators within the hepatocyte, such as AMP-activated protein kinase (AMPK), PGC-1α, PPAR-α, PPAR-γ, and others (321, 335). Adiponectin is also believed to play an important role in the pathogenesis of the fatty liver disease. Adiponectin plays a key role by regulating the activity of AMPK to inhibit lipogenesis (127, 223, 336–340) and also has systemic antiinflammatory effects (57, 127, 341, 342). Adiponectin gene expression is decreased in states of adipose tissue insulin resistance, such as in muscle (343) or adipose tissue of first-degree relatives of type 2 diabetic patients (344) or in obese patients with T2DM (345) or with NAFLD (346). Plasma adiponectin levels are also abnormally low as the result of dysfunctional adipose tissue in obese T2DM with NAFLD or NASH (64, 345–348). Hypoadiponectinemia and steatosis is already frequently seen in childhood obesity and strongly associated with insulin resistance and increased visceral fat (105). In this setting it becomes evident that beyond lifestyle intervention, effective pharmacological treatments will have to target adipose tissue metabolism and either increase plasma adiponectin concentration, ameliorate excessive adipose tissue lipolysis and FFA delivery to slow hepatic lipogenesis and deactivate inflammatory pathways.

Can Weight Loss and Exercise Improve NAFLD?

In general studies examining the effect of weight loss in fatty liver disease have been uncontrolled or of short duration, providing limited guidance for long-term management. Most have not used sophisticated measurements to assess insulin secretion or action, nor performed liver biopsies before and after to correlate weight loss with histological improvement, but have rather used surrogate markers such as liver transaminases or imaging. It is also unclear what kind of exercise would best improve hepatic insulin sensitivity and/or lead to the greatest loss of liver fat or histological improvement. It is also evident that until we better understand the mechanisms that lead to hepatic steatosis, inflammation, and fibrosis, exercise prescriptions (frequency, duration, what kind of exercise program, etc.) in NAFLD will not have a clear target and will remain rather empiric.

Beyond these limitations, there appears to be benefit from lifestyle modification involving increased physical activity and/or weight loss to reverse fatty liver disease, although the results have been variable (349–351). Intervention studies in patients with NAFLD illustrate the same kind of difficulties in achieving and maintaining weight loss that clinicians face in clinical practice. In a meta-analysis of 13 weight reduction studies spanning between the years 1967 through 2000, Wang et al. (349) found that most studies were typically small (only 3 had more than 50 patients while 9 had 25 or fewer subjects enrolled), uncontrolled (10 were case series), and frequently used a surrogate primary end point (i.e., liver aminotransferase levels instead of liver histology in 8 of the 13 trials). In the few studies that performed a liver biopsy before and after weight loss, only steatosis improved, but not necroinflammation or fibrosis. Moreover, improvement in aminotransferase levels did not necessarily translate into improved liver histologic scores, something well documented in a recent trial we performed in patients with NASH *(64)*.

The effect of exercise per se (independent of weight loss) in NAFLD has not been well studied. Most of the intervention studies in NAFLD have concentrated on the effect of weight loss alone, although a few studies have included exercise as part of the treatment program *(349, 352–356)*. Studies have been small (15–65 patients), of short duration (12–16 weeks) and largely used as the primary endpoint surrogate markers (i.e., AST/ALT and/or ultrasound). Only Ueno et al. performed liver biopsies before and after 3 months of diet and exercise and found a reduction in steatosis *(354)*. Moreover, none of these studies were designed to examine the effects of exercise per se from that of weight loss, but rather how both interventions were applied as part of an integrated lifestyle intervention. Recently, this issue was addressed by Tamura et al. *(357)* in 14 patients with T2DM exposed to a 2-week hypocaloric diet with or without moderate exercise (30-min exercise program – five to six times per week). Limitations of the study included the small sample size, short duration of the study, and unclear monitoring/compliance regarding the diet and activity program. Overall metabolic effects were small but insulin sensitivity slightly improved by exercise although such an exercise program had no significant impact on liver fat, being equally reduced in both groups by 27% *(357)*.

Recently, Huang et al. *(358)* reported a trend toward a histologic improvement but not a significant benefit after a year-long, intense nutritional counseling program in patients with nonalcoholic steatohepatitis. Those that lost more weight overall did better, but weight reduction was overall modest (−2.9 kg) in the two-thirds of patients who successfully completed the study. In a 6-month randomized controlled trial of weight loss plus pioglitazone or placebo, we only observed a mild reduction in inflammation in the diet-plus-placebo arm and a trend toward reduction in steatosis in the subjects. The results were overall similar in only those who lost a significant amount of weight were analyzed (unpublished). Nevertheless, weight reduction must be emphasized in NAFLD and NASH patients, with some studies reporting a significant reduction in liver steatosis as measured by MRS in small ($n = 7–10$), short-term low-fat calorie restriction studies lasting anywhere from 2 *(357, 359)* to 12 weeks *(360)* and involving nondiabetic obese *(357, 360)* or T2DM *(359)* patients with NAFLD.

Dietary composition may be another important but frequently overlooked aspect related to excessive hepatic fat deposition, as been suggested in single case reports *(361)* and small case series ($n = 5$) *(362)* in which low-carbohydrate diets were of particular benefit to rapidly reduce steatosis and elevated ALT in subjects with NAFLD. Recently, Ryan et al. *(363)* examined the effect of two hypocaloric diets containing either 60% carbohydrate/25% fat or 40% carbohydrate/45% fat (15% protein) for 16 weeks in 52 insulin-resistant obese subjects. While both diets resulted in significant decreases in weight, insulin resistance, and serum ALT concentrations, the low carbohydrate diet improved all three parameters significantly more than the high carbohydrate diet. Reduction of steatosis and of plasma triglycerides concentration by low carbohydrate diets is likely related to downregulation of hepatic sterol regulatoryelement-binding proteins (SREBP) activity by the amelioration of chronic hyperinsulinemia and by lowering the postprandial glucose load that stimulates hepatic ChREBP de novo lipogenesis *(335)*. However, long-term controlled trials using histologic findings as the primary endpoint remain very much needed. Of note, there was some concern from early studies *(304, 364)* that abrupt and/or massive weight loss with bariatric surgery could be detrimental in terms of paradoxically exacerbating liver inflammation and fibrosis. This concern has abated considerably as more recent bariatric surgery series report significant histological improvements, possibly associated with less malnutrition and procedure-related complications *(365)*. Furthermore, bariatric surgery is now backed by large, long-term follow-up studies showing a significant decrease in overall- and diabetes-related mortality by these procedures *(366, 367)*.

Weight loss remains the standard of care in NAFLD because no pharmacological therapy has conclusively proven to be effective in the long term. Pharmacological therapies with modest benefit have included pentoxifilline, orlistat, vitamin E, cytoprotective agents, ursodeoxycholic acid, and lipid-lowering agents *(368)*, while insulin sensitizers such as metformin *(369)* and thiazolidinediones yielded provocative results in small uncontrolled studies in NASH *(332, 370, 371)*. We recently demonstrated in a randomized, double-blind, placebo-controlled trial that pioglitazone treatment for 6 months in patients with T2DM and NASH significantly improved glycemic control, glucose tolerance, insulin sensitivity, and systemic inflammation *(64)*. This was associated with a 50% decrease in steatohepatitis ($p < 0.001$) and a 37% reduction of fibrosis within the pioglitazone-treated group (-37%, $p < 0.002$), although this fell short of statistical significance when compared with placebo ($p = 0.08$). Our results provided "proof-of-principle" that pioglitazone may be the first agent capable of altering the natural history of the disease. However, definitive proof requires establishing its safety and efficacy in a large long-term clinical trial.

PANCREATIC β-CELL LIPOTOXICITY AND THE DEVELOPMENT OF T2DM

There have been a number of in-depth reviews detailing the intricate interaction between FFA and glucose to tightly adapt insulin secretory needs under basal and postprandial conditions *(148, 276, 372–376)*. Here we will only highlight some aspects that help explain at the clinical level the role of β-cell lipotoxicity in the pathogenesis of T2DM and the link between both the epidemics of obesity and T2DM. Chronic hyperinsulinemia is an adaptation to insulin resistance that allows in the majority of individuals to maintain the 24-h plasma glucose levels within the normal range. Hyperglycemia develops when this compensation fails, although subtle defects in insulin secretion are present long before the development of frank hyperglycemia in lean healthy FH+ subjects with normal glucose tolerance *(141)*. As the fasting plasma glucose rises from normal to ~120 mg/dL, there is a gradual loss of first-phase insulin secretion (i.e., 0–10 min) in response to intravenous glucose *(129)*. Second-phase insulin secretion (i.e., insulin secretion produced after the initial 10 min) also decreases as glucose tolerance worsens in FH+ subjects prone to T2DM. This become quite evident in later stages of the disease, as subjects develop IFG or IGT *(91, 129, 276)*. For example, in data from the San Antonio Metabolism (SAM) study in 388 subjects with either NGT, IGT, or T2DM, β-cell dysfunction is already present long before the development of a 2-h plasma glucose of >140 mg/dL, which is the current definition of IGT. Moreover, in this cohort of otherwise healthy subjects, by the time the 2-h glucose was between 121 and 140 mg/dL (6.7–7.8 mmol/L) there was already a ~50% decline in insulin secretion, with more than a 90% deterioration when the 2-h plasma glucose reached above 200 mg/dL (11.1 mmol/L). Once hyperglycemia develops, β-cell function deteriorates rather rapidly over time *(377)*. Poor understanding of the underlying mechanisms causing this relentless decline in β-cell function over time has seriously limited the ability to implement rationale preventive interventions in subjects at high-risk of developing T2DM later in life. However, recent basic and clinical studies highlighting the importance of the glucose-fatty acid cross-talk that controls insulin secretion hold promise toward the prevention of T2DM by earlier interventions that may remove β-cell lipotoxicity (i.e., lifestyle interventions and/or thiazolidiendiones).

Role Fatty Acids in the Control of Insulin Secretion

In the fasting state, plasma FFA (not glucose) is the primary energy substrate for sustaining insulin secretion *(378)*. Following a meal, pancreatic β-cells switch from using FFA to glucose as the preferred energy source. This occurs as glucose enters the β-cell by high-capacity, low-affinity GLUT2 transporters and is rapidly phosphorylated to glucose-6-phosphate (G-6-P) by glucokinase that acts as the glucose sensor or "pacemaker" for insulin secretion *(379)*. Glucokinase is the rate-limiting step for insulin secretion as the capacity of GLUT2 to transport glucose inside the β-cell is much greater than the capacity of glucokinase to phosphorylate it. Most of the glucose is then converted through glycolysis to pyruvate (β-cells have limited capacity to generate glycogen or lactic acid from glucose), entering the mitochondria and generating ATP through the Krebs cycle as acetyl-CoA. This promotes the formation of citrate, which is transported to the cytoplasm inhibiting CPT-1, which is the transporter of fatty acids (as long-chain fatty acyl-CoA) into the mitochondria. This way, malonylCoA acts as the metabolic "switch" for insulin secretion from the fasting to the fed state: FFA goes from being oxidized as a fuel for basal insulin secretion in the fasting state, to being stored within the β-cell during the fed state for use in the next period of fasting. This rapid fuel switch requires intact mitochondrial function capable to adapt immediately to the changing metabolic state. It also seems that the composition of circulating fatty acids has a significant impact on the ability of fatty acids to promote glucose-stimulated insulin secretion, such that exposure to saturated fatty acids stimulates much more insulin secretion compared to unsaturated fats, although this remains to be confirmed in humans *(380–382)*. Therefore, it is important to recognize the importance of FFA (either exogenous or endogenous from lipolysis) to support normal insulin secretion and that a rapid increase of FFA may acutely potentiate glucose-stimulated secretion by increasing fatty acyl-CoA or complex lipids within the β-cell that act distally by modulating insulin exocytosis upon demand. Long chain acyl-CoA controls multiple functions within the β-cell, including function of ion channels, activation of PKC, nitric oxide-mediated apoptosis, protein acylation, transcription activity, and ceramide formation. The ability of the β-cell to switch between endogenous fatty acid synthesis and oxidation is critical to optimal function and molecular defects secondary to plasma FFA oversupply lead to the accumulation of reactive "toxic" lipids (i.e., ceramide and DAG) *(148, 276, 372–376)*. Therefore, a chronic increase of plasma FFA, meant to enhance basal and glucose-stimulated insulin secretion in obesity and in other insulin-resistant states, may lead in a minority of FH+ subjects to β-cell lipotoxicity and tip them over to diabetes, as they appear to have genetically-determined diminished β-cell adaptation to excess FFA supply, as discussed below.

Pancreatic β-Cell Lipotoxicity: Evidence from Studies in Subjects Genetically Predisposed to T2DM

The potential for fatty acids to cause β-cell lipotoxicity in vitro and in vivo, in many cases with subsequent apoptosis (depending on the cell line or animal model) has generated substantial interest as an explanation for the development of T2DM *(372–376)*. The concept of β-cell lipotoxicity was championed initially by Unger in a series of elegant experiments in islets of leptin-unresponsive Zucker diabetic (ZDF) rats *(147, 148)*. In brief, excess palmitoyl CoA would enter the ceramide pathway as it condenses with l-serine by the enzyme serine palmitoyl transferase (SPT). Ceramide induces inducible nitric oxide synthase (iNOS) and also promotes, through the activation of the NF-κβ pathway, the formation of ROS that lead to lipoapoptosis. It has been well demonstrated in vitro or in vivo that if ceramide production is prevented (i.e., by dietary restriction or AMPK activation by different means of agents such as AICAR, leptin, or thiazolidiendiones), β-cell lipotoxicity can be averted or greatly diminished in animals *(148)*.

As discussed above, acute fatty acids stimulate insulin secretion *(372–376)*, but chronic exposure to increased levels of fatty acids for ~24–48 h has been shown to impair β-cell function in vitro *(383)* and in vivo *(384, 385)*. It is now clear that oxidative stress plays an important role during chronic exposure to fatty acids and that it can be prevented in vitro and in vivo by coadministration of antioxidants such as *N*-acetylcysteine (NAC) or taurine *(386)*. In humans, an acute elevation in plasma FFA either has no effect *(387, 388)* or enhances *(389, 390)* glucose-induced insulin secretion, but the effect of a more prolonged increase in plasma FFA on glucose-stimulated insulin secretion has yielded variable results. In lean healthy subjects, a 24–48-h lipid infusion has been reported to increase *(391–393)*, not significantly change *(390)*, or decrease *(389)* insulin secretion. In obese insulin-resistant individuals, a 48-h lipid infusion has been reported to reduce insulin secretion by 20%, but plasma insulin concentration increased due to a ~50% reduction in insulin clearance *(394)*. In subjects with T2DM, who already have a marked impairment in β-cell function, an increase in plasma FFA concentration for 2 days by a lipid infusion did not further worsen insulin secretion *(394)*. These conflicting results may be explained, in part, by differences in study populations, plasma FFA levels achieved, variable duration of lipid infusion, or concomitant glucose infusion/hyperglycemia *(391)*.

Given the potential clinical implications about the role of FFA and lipotoxicity, we felt important to determine whether the lipotoxicity hypothesis could apply to healthy FH+ glucose-tolerant subjects genetically prone to T2DM, and whether the response to elevated plasma FFA would differ in FH+ subjects compared to those without any FH of T2DM (controls). To make it clinically relevant, we used a prolonged (72-h) but *physiological* increase in plasma FFA concentration (~600–700 μmol/L) as discussed earlier during studies examining insulin action in muscle. We studied 21 young healthy with (FH+, $n = 13$) and without (controls, $n = 8$) a FH of type 2 diabetes *(141)*. Of note, both groups were well matched and subjects were lean and with no clinical features of the MS, having normal glucose tolerance, blood pressure, and plasma lipid profile. They were admitted twice to the clinical research center and received, in random order, a lipid or saline infusion. On days 1 and 2, insulin secretion was measured as part of a metabolic profile following mixed meals and in response to a +125 mg/dL hyper-glycemic clamp (morning of day 3). Insulin action was examined on day 4 by the gold-standard eug-lycemic insulin clamp technique. Day-long plasma FFA concentrations with lipid infusion increased to levels seen frequently in obesity and T2DM (~600–700 μmol/L). A sustained elevation in plasma had strikingly opposite effects on insulin secretion between lean young healthy adults with or without a FH of T2DM. Day-long plasma C-peptide levels on days 1 and 2 increased with lipid infusion in controls but decreased significantly in the FH+ group (+28 compared to −30%, respectively, $p < 0.01$), as illus-trated in Fig. 8. During the hyperglycemic clamp (Fig. 9), lipid infusion enhanced the insulin secretion rates in controls but decreased β-cell function in the FH+ subjects: first-phase insulin secretion increased by 75% in controls compared to 60% reduction in FH+ subjects ($p < 0.001$), while second-phase insulin secretion increased by 25% compared to a 35% reduction in FH+ individuals ($p < 0.04$). Because insulin secretion adapts to the prevailing insulin resistance, we then adjusted the insulin secre-tion rate (ISR) for the degree of insulin resistance (as the inverse of the rate of insulin-stimulated glu-cose disposal or Rd) as measured during the euglycemic insulin clamp on day 4. We called this index ISR_{Rd} ($ISR_{Rd} = ISR/[1/Rd]$. By doing so, the inadequate β-cell response in the FH+ group became even more evident, as shown in Fig. 10. Although ISR_{Rd} was not different between the two groups before lipid infusion, in the FH+ subjects lipid infusion reduced significantly first- and second-phase ISR_{Rd} to 25 and 42% of that in control subjects, respectively (both $p < 0.001$). Lipid infusion in the FH+ group (but not in the controls) also caused severe hepatic insulin resistance with an increase in basal EGP, despite an elevation in fasting insulin levels, and also impaired suppression of EGP to insulin. However, peripheral (muscle) insulin resistance did not worsen by the mild elevation in plasma FFA.

From these set of studies we concluded that in subjects genetically predisposed to T2DM, a sustained physiological increase in plasma FFA impairs insulin secretion in response to mixed meals and to intra-venous glucose. This was the first documentation in humans that lipotoxicity may play a central role in the development of T2DM in genetically predisposed subjects. Moreover, it also served as "proof-of-concept" that β-cell lipotoxicity, but not a worsening of muscle insulin resistance, may be the most

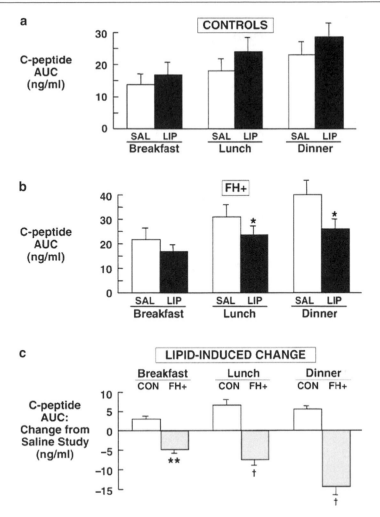

Fig. 8. Area under the curve (*AUC*) values for plasma C-peptide concentration (ng/mL) after breakfast (0800–1,200), lunch (1,200–1,800), and dinner (1,800–2,400) during the 48-h metabolic profile in control subjects (CON) (**a**) and in subjects with a strong family history of type 2 diabetes (FH) (**b**). *Open columns*, saline infusion; *closed (black) columns*, lipid infusion. (**c**) lipid-induced change. This panel summarizes the C-peptide area under the curve *change* induced by a 4-day lipid infusion compared with the respective salinestudy. *LIP* lipid infusion; *SAL* saline infusion. Data are means SE. *$p < 0.05$ vs. saline; **$p < 0.05$ vs. controlsubjects; ***$p < 0.01$ vs. control subjects. Adapted from Kashyap et al. *(141)*.

important feature determining the progression from normal glucose tolerance to overt hyperglycemia. If extended to the population at large, one may speculate that lipid-induced β-cell lipotoxicity may be the underlying mechanism for the observation that progression to T2DM is closely tied to the presence of obesity *(251, 395, 396)* and/or elevated plasma FFA *(59, 395, 397)*, although other factors are likely to contribute to β-cell failure over time in T2DM. While there is extensive literature that exposure to a chronic elevation of glucose causes β-cell damage and apoptosis in vitro and in vivo *(136, 373, 376)*, in human studies this has been harder to prove. In this regard, when a low-dose lipid, glucose, or both substrates were infused together (in separate admissions) for 48 h to lean healthy FH+ subjects, only FFA (but not hyperglycemia) induced β-cell dysfunction, suggesting the primacy of lipotoxicity over glucotoxicity in the "prediabetic stage" in subjects genetically predisposed to T2DM *(398)*.

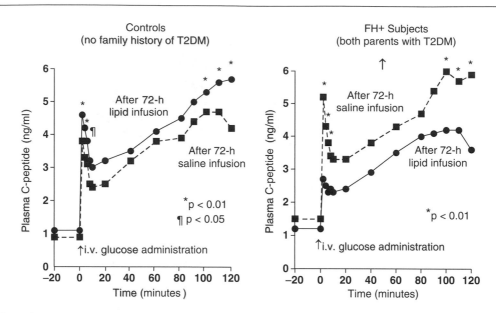

Fig. 9. Effect of a chronic physiologic elevation of plasma free fatty acids (*FFA*) by means of a low-dose lipid infusion on glucose-stimulated insulin secretion in subjects genetically predisposed to type 2 diabetes mellitus (*T2DM*) (i.e., both parents with T2DM). A sustained elevation in plasma had markedly opposite effects on insulin secretion between lean young healthy adults with or without a family history of T2DM. Adapted from Kashyap et al. *(141)*.

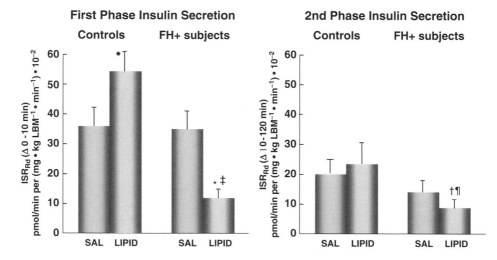

Fig. 10. Insulin secretion rates (*ISRs*) during the hyperglycemic clamp studies related to the prevailing severity of insulin resistance (ISR$_{Rd}$). (**a**) First phase ISR$_{Rd}$ 0–10. (**b**) Second-phase ISR$_{Rd}$ 10–120. Insulin resistance is the inverse of insulin-stimulated glucose disposal (*R*d), as determined during the euglycemic insulin clamps (1/*R*d). When comparing control vs. FH subjects, first-phase ISR$_{Rd}$ is similar during the saline studies; with lipid infusion, first-phase ISR$_{Rd}$ deteriorates in FH subjects, whereas it increases in control subjects. Second-phase ISR$_{Rd}$ is also reduced by lipid infusion in the FH + group but is unchanged in control subjects. $^*p < 0.01$ vs. saline; $^{**}p < 0.05$ vs. saline; $^{***}p < 0.001$ vs. control subjects; $\dagger p < 0.05$ vs. control subjects.

What Strategy to Use to Prevent T2DM in Subjects Genetically Predisposed to T2DM: Lifestyle Intervention, Pharmacological Therapy, or Both?

It is now clear that lifestyle interventions including dietary modification and regular physical activity delay the development of T2DM in genetically predisposed individuals [several excellent reviews are available *(22, 23, 152, 250, 396, 399)*]. Large prospective trials *(400–403)*, as well as a number of smaller ones [included in reviews by Norris et al. *(396)*, Gillies et al. *(22)* and Jeon et al. *(250)*], have confirmed this notion. In the Diabetes Prevention Program (DPP), the largest of the lifestyle intervention trials ($n = 3,234$ nondiabetic persons with elevated IFG and IGT), a lifestyle-modification program aimed at having patients reduce their weight by at least a 7% and perform at least 150 min of moderate intensity physical activity per week, led to a 58% reduction in the progression to T2DM over an average follow-up of 2.8 years as compared with the placebo group *(402)*. The mean weight loss at the end of the trial was rather modest (~3 kg) with a maximum weight loss of ~7 kg in the first year followed by a gradual regain thereafter. The weight loss achieved in the DPP appears to be an achievable goal for most patients, something that can be stimulated with simple measures such as the use of pedometers *(404)*. The DPP also showed that lifestyle intervention could be quite cost-effective, as to prevent one case of diabetes over a period of 3 years, only 6.9 persons would need to participate in such a program.

In addition to lifestyle-intervention, a number of drugs used to treat obesity *(405)* and T2DM, including acarbose *(406)*, metformin *(402, 407)* and thiazolidinediones *[(408–411)* and preliminary data from the ACT NOW trial using pioglitazone (Ralph De Fronzo, personal communication) *(412)]*, all have been successful to prevent the development of T2DM in high risk populations, despite very different mechanisms of action. This is puzzling as it suggests different/overlapping insults being implicated in β-cell dysfunction over time and calls for the need to better define the underlying causes. Of note, in the DPP most of the impact of metformin could be attributed to the induction of weight-loss *(413)*. For example, the 1.7-kg weight loss with metformin compared to the 0.3 kg gain with placebo alone explained 64% of the beneficial metformin effect on diabetes risk. Adjustment for weight, fasting insulin, proinsulin, and other metabolic factors combined explained 81% of the beneficial metformin effect, but it remained nominally significant ($p = 0.034$) *(413)*. On the basis of the important role of lipotoxicity in T2DM discussed so far in this chapter, the poorly understood and rather unspecific way that metformin appears to prevent the development of T2DM contrasts with the basic and clinical data on the impact of thiazolidinediones to restore dysfunctional adipose tissue back to health; in humans thiazolidinediones improve the expression of genes involved in lipid synthesis *(344, 346, 414)*, restore adipocyte sensitivity to insulin and prevent excessive release of FFA to ectopic tissues *(64, 331)* (and likely the β-cell *(148)*, although unproven in humans), increase the secretion of adiponectin – an effect with vast metabolic implications at the level of the liver *(64, 337, 340, 345, 415)*, muscle *(127)*, and vascular bed *(341, 342)* – and ameliorate the release of inflammatory adipokines from macrophages and adipose tissue linked to insulin resistance *(66, 126)* and atherogenesis *(416)*. In addition to the prevention of T2DM, early use of pioglitazone may reverse common metabolic complications of patients with IGT and T2DM, such as NAFLD *(64)* or PCOS *(417)*, and reduce subclinical inflammation *(418)* and atherosclerosis *(419)*. Pioglitazone has also been reported to reduce the risk of stroke and recurrent myocardial infarction in subjects with established CVD *(420–423)*, although for unclear reasons rosiglitazone paradoxically increases myocardial infarction in patients with T2DM *(424, 425)*. Clinical trials with thiazolidinediones also suggest that they are the most promising of the currently available pharmacological agents for the prevention of T2DM *(408–411)*.

In summary, until we understand better the mechanisms at play for β-cell preservation, treatment strategies will remain rather empiric for the prevention of T2DM in high-risk subjects. Nevertheless, prevention of obesity with amelioration of FFA-induced insulin resistance and β-cell lipotoxicity *(141)* appear as the most logical targets, at least in obese individuals genetically predisposed to diabetes. Perhaps in the future early screening for β-cell lipotoxicity by means of an acute intravenous lipid challenge *(426)*, or by other means, will offer a unique opportunity to identify those at the highest risk, but also with the greatest potential to benefit from early intervention. The benefit of early intervention has been recently suggested in a recent analysis of the DPP database, where higher insulin secretion and better insulin sensitivity at baseline were associated with a lower risk of progression to T2DM *(427)*. From a practical standpoint, we cannot remain passive as the epidemic of T2DM looms. While not systematically tested, it is not difficult to envision that a combined approach of early lifestyle and pharmacological intervention targeting those at the highest risk will be needed in the future to curve the epidemic of T2DM, likely the greatest public health problem of affluent societies of the twenty-first century.

REFERENCES

1. Boyle J, Honeycutt A, Narayan K, Hoerger T, Geiss L, Chen H, Thompson T: Projection of diabetes burden through 2050: impact of changing demography and disease prevalence in the U.S. *Diabetes Care* 24:1936–1940, 2001
2. Harris M, Klein R, Welborn TA et al.: Onset of NIDDM occurs at least 4–7 years before clinical diagnosis. *Diabetes Care* 15:815–819, 1992
3. Turner R, Cull C, Holman R: United Kingdom Prospective Diabetes Study 17: the effect of improved metabolic control on complications of NIDDM. *Ann Intern Med* 124:136–145, 1996
4. Cusi K: Cardiovascular risk management in type 2 diabetes: from clinical trials to clinical practice. *The Endocrinologist* 11:474–490, 2001
5. Hu F, Stampfer M, Haffner S, et al.: Elevated risk of cardiovascular disease prior to clinical diagnosis of type 2 diabetes. *Diabetes Care* 25:1129–1134, 2002
6. Stamler J, Vaccaro O, Neaton J, et al.: Diabetes, other risk factors, and the 12-year cardiovascular mortality for men screened in the Multiple Risk Factor Intervention Trial. *Diabetes Care* 16:434–444, 1993
7. Miettinen H, Lehto S, Salomaa V, et al.: Impact of diabetes on mortality after the first myocardial infarction. *Diabetes Care* 21:69–75, 1998
8. Tandl E, Schnell O: A new look at the heart in diabetes mellitus: from ailing to failing. *Diabetologia* 43:1455–1469, 2000
9. Elezi S, Kastrati A, Pache J, et al.: Diabetes mellitus and the clinical and angiographic outcome after coronary stent placement. *J Am Coll Cardiol* 32:1866–1873, 1998
10. Gu K, Cowie C, Harris M: Mortality in adults with and without diabetes in a national cohort of the U.S. population, 1971–1993. *Diabetes Care* 21:1138–1145, 1998
11. Ford E, Ajani U, Croft J, et al.: Explaining the decrease in U.S, deaths from coronary artery disease. *N Engl J Med* 356:2388–2398, 2007
12. Fox C, Coady S, Sorlie P, Levy D, Meigs J, D'Agostino RS, Wilson P, Savage P: Trends in cardiovascular complications of diabetes. *JAMA* 292:2495–2499, 2004
13. Fang J, Alderman M: Impact of the increasing burden of diabetes on acute myocardial infarction in New York city: 1999–2000. *Diabetes* 55:768–773, 2006
14. Kuller L, Lewis H: Ethnic differences in atherposclerosis, cardiovascular disease and lipid metabolism. *Curr Opin Lipidol* 15:109–113, 2004
15. Wild S, Roglic G, Green A, Sicree R, King H: Global prevalence of diabetes: estimates for the year 2000 and projections for 2030. *Diabetes Care* 27:1047–1053, 2004
17. Yach D, Stuckler S, Brownell D: Epidemiological and economic consequences of the global epidemics of obesity and diabetes. *Nat Med* 12:62–66, 2006
18. Wild SH, Forouhi NG: What is the scale of the future diabetes epidemic, and how certain are we about it? *Diabetologia* 50:903–905, 2007
19. King H, Aubert R, Herman W: Global burden of diabetes, 1995–2025: prevalence, numerical estimates, and projections. *Diabetes Care* 21:1414–1431, 1998
20. Narayan K, Boyle J, Geiss L, et al.: Impact of recent increase in incidence on future diabetes burden. *Diabetes Care* 29:2114–2116, 2006
21. Mainous A, Baker R, Koopman R, Saxena S, Diaz V, Everett C, Majeed A: Impact of the population at risk of diabetes on projections of diabetes burden in the United States: an epidemic on the way. *Diabetologia* 50:934–940, 2007

22. Gillies C, Abrams K, Lambert P, et al.: Pharmacological and lifestyle interventions to prevent or delay type 2 diabetes in people with impaired glucose tolerance: systematic review and meta-analysis. *BMJ* 334:299, 2007

23. Nathan D, Davidson M, DeFronzo R, Heine R, Henry R, Pratley R, Zinman B: Impaired fasting glucose and impaired glucose tolerance: implications for care. *Diabetes Care* 30:753–759, 2007

24. Tuomilehto J: Counterpoint: evidence-based prevention of type 2 diabetes: the power of lifestyle management. *Diabetes Care* 30:435–438, 2007

25. Alberti K, Zimmet P, Shaw J: International Diabetes Federation: a consensus on type 2 diabetes prevention. *Diabet Med* 24:451–463, 2007

26. Pi-Sunyer F: How effective are lifestyle changes in the prevention of type 2 diabetes mellitus? *Nutr Rev* 65:101–110, 2007

27. Hellman R, Regan J, Rosen H: Effect of intensive treatment of diabetes on the risk of death or renal failure in NIDDM and IDDM. *Diabetes Care* 20:258–264, 1997

28. Gaede P, Vedel P, Larsen N, Jensen GVH, Parving H-H, Pedersen O: Multifactorial intervention and cardiovascular disease in patients with type 2 diabetes. *N Engl J Med* 348:383–393, 2003

29. National Heart Lung and Blood Institute: Clinical guidelines on the identification, evaluation, and treatment of overweight and obesity in adults. The Evidence Report. National Intitutes of Health. *Obes Res* 6 (Suppl. 2):51S–209S, 1998

30. Gallagher D, Visser M, Sepulveda D, et al.: How useful is body mass index for comparison of body fatness accross age, sex, and ethnic groups? *Am J Epidemiol* 143:228–239, 1996

31. Deurenberg P, Yap M, van Staveren W: Body mass index and percent body fat: meta analysis among different ethnic groups. *Int J Obes Relat Metab Disord* 22:1164–1171, 1998

32. Bray G: Obesity: the disease. *J Med Chem* 49:4001–4007, 2006

33. Hamilton M, Hamilton D, Zderic T: Role of low energy expenditure and sitting in obesity, metabolic syndrome, type 2 diabetes, and cardiovascular disease. *Diabetes* 45:2655–2667, 2007

34. Jeffrey R, Harnack L: Evidence implicating eating as a primary driver for the obesity epidemic. *Diabetes* 56:2673–2676, 2007

35. Wyatt SB, Winters KP, Dubbert PM: Overweight and obesity: prevalence, consequences, and causes of a growing public health problem. *Am J Med Sci* 331:166–174, 2006

36. Runge C: Economic consequences of the obese. *Diabetes* 56:2668–2672, 2007

37. Christakis N, Fowler J: The spread of obesity in a large social network over 32 years. *N Engl J Med* 357:370–379, 2007

38. Peeters A, Barendregt J, Willekens F, et al.: Obesity in adulthood and its consequences for life expectancy: a life-table analysis. *Ann Intern Med* 138:1138–1145, 2003

39. van Dam RM, Willett WC, Manson JE, Hu FB: The relationship between overweight in adolescence and premature death in women. *Ann Intern Med* 145:91–97, 2006

40. Abbasi F, Brown B, Lamendola C, McLaughlin T, Reaven G: Relationship between obesity, insulin sensitivity and coronary artery disease risk. *J Am Coll Cardiol* 40:37–43, 2002

41. National Institutes of Health Consensus Development Conference Statement: health implications of obesity. *Ann Intern Med* 103:1073–1077, 1985

42. Pi-Sunyer F: Medical hazards of obesity. *Ann Intern Med* 119:655–660, 1993

43. Poirier P, Giles T, Bray G, Hong Y, Stern J: Obesity and cardiovascular disease: pathophysiology, evaluation, and effect of weight loss. *Arterioscler Thromb Vasc Biol* 26:968–976, 2006

44. Bray G, Bellanger T: Epidemiology, trends, and morbidities of obesity and the metabolic syndrome. *Endocrine* 29:109–117, 2006

45. Gunnell D, Frankel S, Nanchahal K, Peters T, Davey Smith G: Childhood obesity and adult cardiovascular mortality. *Am J Clin Nutr* 67:1111–1118, 1998

47. Flegal K, Graubard B, Williamson D, Gail M: Cause-specific excess deaths associated with underweight, overweight, and obesity. *JAMA* 298:2028–2037, 2007

48. Olshansky S, Passaro D, Hershow R, et al.: A potential decline in life expectancy in the United States in the 21st century. *N Engl J Med* 352:1138–1145, 2005

49. Ford E: Risks for all-cause mortality, cardiovascular disease, and diabetes associated with the metabolic syndrome: a summary of the evidence. *Diabetes Care* 28:1769–1778, 2005

50. Alley D, Chang V: The changing relationship of obesity and disability. *JAMA* 298:2020–2027, 2007

51. Sui X, LaMonte MJ, Laditka JN, Hardin JW, Chase N, Hooker SP, Blair SN: Cardiorespiratory fitness and adiposity as mortality predictors in older adults. *JAMA* 298:2507–2516, 2007

52. Mokdad A, Marks J, Stroup D, Gerberding J: Actual causes of death in the United States, 2000. *JAMA* 291:1238–1245, 2004

53. Baker J, Olsen L, Sorensen T: Childhood body-mass index and the risk of coronary heart disease in adulthood. *N Engl J Med* 357:2329–2337, 2007

54. Okoro C, Denny C, McGuire L, Balluz L, Goins R, Mokdad A: Disability among older American Indians and Alaska natives: disparities in prevalence, health-risk behaviors, obesity, and chronic conditions. *Ethn Dis* 17:686–692, 2007

55. Gastaldelli A, Cusi K, Pettiti M, Hardies J, Miyazaki Y, Berria R, Buzzigoli E, Sironi AM, Cersosimo E, Ferrannini E, DeFronzo RA: Relationship between hepatic/visceral fat and hepatic insulin resistance in nondiabetic and type 2 diabetic subjects. *Gastroenterology* 133:496–506, 2007

56. Jensen M, Haymond M, Rizza R, Cryer P, Miles J: Influence of body fat distribution on free fatty acid metabolism in obesity. *J Clin Invest* 83:1168–1172, 1989

57. Despres J: Cardiovascular disease under the influence of excess visceral fat. *Crit Pathways Cardiol* 6:51–59, 2007
58. Cassano P, Rosner B, Vokonas P, Weiss S: Obesity and body fat distribution in relation to the incidence of non-insulin-dependent diabetes mellitus. *Am J Epidemiol* 136:1474–1486, 1992
59. Charles M, Eschwege E, Thibult N, Claude J-R, Warnet J-M, Rosselin G, Girard J, Balkau B: The role of non-esterified fatty acids in the deterioration of glucose tolerance in Caucasian subjects: results of the Paris Prospective Study. *Diabetologia* 40:1101–1106, 1997
60. Ostman J, Arner P, Engfeldt P, Kager L: Regional differences in the control of lipolysis in human adipose tissue. *Metabolism* 29:1198–1205, 1979
61. Klein S: The case of visceral fat: argument for the defense. *J Clin Invest* 113:1530–1532, 2004
62. Miles J, Jensen M: Visceral adiposity is not causally related to insulin resistance. *Diabetes Care* 28:2326–2327, 2005
63. Ferrannini E, Balkau B, Coppack S, Dekker J, Mari A, Nolan J, Walker M, Natali A, Beck-Nielsen H, and the RISC Investigators: Insulin resistance, insulin response, and obesity as indicators of metabolic risk. *J Clin Endocrinol Metab* 92:2885–2892, 2007
64. Belfort R, Harrison SA, Brown K, Darland C, Finch J, Balas B, Gastaldelli A, Tio F, Hardies J, Pulcini J, Berria R, Ma J, Dwivedi S, Havranek R, Fincke C, DeFronzo R, Bannayan G, Schenker S, Cusi K: A placebo-controlled trial of pioglitazone in subjects with nonalcoholic steatohepatitis. *N Engl J Med* 355:2297–2307, 2006
65. Nielsen S, Guo Z, Johnson C, Hensrud D, Jensen M: Splanchnic lipolysis in human obesity. *J Clin Invest* 113:1582–1588, 2004
66. Shoelson S, Lee J, Goldfine A: Inflammation and insulin resistance. *J Clin Invest* 116:1793–1801, 2006
67. Fontana L, Eagon J, Trujillo M, Scherer P, Klein S: Visceral fat adipokine secretion is associatd with systemic inflammation in obese humans. *Diabetes* 56:1010–1013, 2007
68. Reaven G: Role of insulin resistance in human disease. *Diabetes* 37:1595–1607, 1988
69. DeFronzo RA, Ferrannini E: Insulin resistance. A multifaceted syndrome responsible for NIDDM, obesity, hypertension, dyslipidemia, and atherosclerotic cardiovascular disease. *Diabetes Care* 14:173–194, 1991
70. Ingelsson E, Sullivan LM, Murabito JM, Fox CS, Benjamin EJ, Polak JF, Meigs JB, Keyes MJ, O'Donnell CJ, Wang TJ, D'Agostino RB, Sr., Wolf PA, Vasan RS: Prevalence and prognostic impact of subclinical cardiovascular disease in individuals with the metabolic syndrome and diabetes. *Diabetes* 56:db07–0078, 2007
71. Hunt K, Williams K, Hazuda H, Stern M, Haffner S: The metabolic syndrome and the impact of diabetes on coronary heart disease mortality in women and men: the San Antonio Heart Study. *Ann Epidemiol. 2007 Jul 26*; [Epub ahead of print], 2007
72. Skilton MR: A comparison of the NCEP-ATPIII, IDF and AHA/NHLBI metabolic syndrome definitions with relation to early carotid atherosclerosis in subjects with hypercholesterolemia or at risk of CVD: evidence for sex-specific differences. *Atherosclerosis* 190:416–422, 2007
73. Wilson P, D'Agostino R, Parise H, Sullivan L, Meigs J: The metabolic syndrome as a precursor of cardiovascular disease and type 2 diabetes mellitus. *Circulation* 112:3066–3072, 2005
74. Resnick H, Jones K, Ruotolo G, Jain A, Henderson J, Lu W, Howard B, Study SH: Insulin resistance, the metabolic syndrome, and risk of incident cardiovascular disease in nondiabetic american indians: the Strong Heart Study. *Diabetes Care* 26:861–867, 2003
75. Klein B, Klein R, Lee K: Components of the metabolic syndrome and risk of cardiovascular disease and diabetes in Beaver Dam. *Diabetes Care* 25:1790–1794, 2002
76. Stern M, Williams K, González-Villalpando C, Hunt K, Haffner S: Does the metabolic syndrome improve identification of individuals at risk of type 2 diabetes and/or cardiovascular disease? *Diabetes Care* 27:2676–2681, 2004
77. Haffner SM: Relationship of metabolic risk factors and development of cardiovascular disease and diabetes. *Obesity* 14:121S–127S, 2006
78. Lakka H-M, Laaksonen D, Lakka T, Niskanen L, Kumpusalo E, Tuomilehto J, Salonen J: The metabolic syndrome and total and cardiovascular disease mortality in middle-aged men. *JAMA* 288:2709–2716, 2002
79. Kahn R, Buse J, Ferrannini E, Stern M: The metabolic syndrome: time for a critical appraisal. *Diabetes Care* 28:2289–2304, 2005
80. Eckel R, Grundy S, Zimmet P: The metabolic syndrome. *The Lancet* 365:1415–1428, 2005
81. Grundy S: Metabolic syndrome: connecting and reconciling cardiovascular and diabetes worlds. *J Am Coll Cardiol* 47:1093–1100, 2006
82. DeFronzo RA: Pathogenesis of type 2 diabetes: metabolic and molecular implications of identifying diabetes genes. *Diabetes Rev* 5:177–269, 1997
83. Dandona P, Aljada A, Chaudhuri A, Mohanty P, Garg R: Metabolic syndrome: a comprehensive perspective based on interactions between obesity, diabetes, and inflammation. *Circulation* 111:1448–1454, 2005
84. Meigs J: Metabolic syndrome and risk for type 2 diabetes. *Expert Rev Endocrin Metab* 1:57–66, 2006
85. Rashid S, Watanabe T, Sakaue T, Lewis G: Mechanisms of HDL lowering in insulin resistant, hypertriglyceridemic states: the combined effect of HDL triglyceride enrichment and elevated hepatic lipase activity. *Clin Biochem* 36:421–429, 2003
86. Ginsberg H, Zhang Y-L, Hernandez-Ono A: Regulation of plasma triglycerides in insulin resistance and diabetes. *Arch Med Res* 36:232–240, 2005
87. Laaksonen D, Lakka H, Niskanen L, Kaplan G, Salonen J, Lakka T: Metabolic syndrome and development of diabetes mellitus: application and validation of recently suggested definitions of the metabolic syndrome in a prospective cohort study. Am J Epidemiol 156:1070–1077, 2002

88. Lorenzo C, Okoloise M, Williams K, Stern M, Haffner S, Study SAH: The metabolic syndrome as predictor of type 2 diabetes: the San Antonio heart study. Diabetes Care 26:3153–3159, 2003

89. Stern M, Williams K, Haffner S: Identification of persons at high risk for type 2 diabetes mellitus: do we need the oral glucose tolerance test? Ann Intern Med 136:575–581, 2002

90. Schmidt M, Duncan B, Bang H, Pankow J, Ballantyne C, Golden S, Folsom A, Chambless L, the Atherosclerosis Risk in Communities Investigators: Identifying individuals at high risk for diabetes: The Atherosclerosis Risk in Communities study. Diabetes Care 28:2013–2018, 2005

91. Abdul-Ghani M, Williams K, DeFronzo R, Stern M: What is the best predictor of future type 2 diabetes? Diabetes Care 30:1544–1548, 2007

92. Wilson P, Meigs J, Sullivan L, Fox C, Nathan D, D'Agostino R: Prediction of incident diabetes mellitus in middle-aged adults. The Framingham Offspring Study. Arch Intern Med 167:1068–1074, 2007

93. Lazarus R, Baur L, Webb K, Blyth F: Body mass index in screening for adiposity in children and adolescents: systematic evalaution using receiver operating characteristic curves. Am J Clin Nutr 63:183–193, 1996

94. Schwimmer JB: Influence of gender, race, and ethnicity on suspected fatty liver in obese adolescents. Pediatrics 115:e561–e565, 2005

95. Westwood M, Fayter D, Hartley S, Rithalia A, Butler G, Glasziou P, Bland M, Nixon J, Stirk L, Rudolf M: Childhood obesity: should primary school children be routinely screened? A systematic review and discussion of the evidence. Arch Dis Child 92:416–422, 2007

96. Li C, Ford E, Mokdad A, Cook S: Recent trends in waist circumference and waist-height ratio among US children and adolescents. Pediatrics 118:1390–1398, 2006

97. Zimmet P, Alberti K, Kaufman F, Tajima N, Silink M, Arslanian S, Wong G, Bennett P, Shaw J, Caprio S, Group, ftIC: The metabolic syndrome in children and adolescents – an IDF consensus report. Pediatr Diabetes 8:299–306, 2007

98. Mokdad A, Ford E, Bowman B, Dietz W, Vinicor F, Bales V, Marks J: Prevalence of obesity, diabetes, and obesity-related health risk factors, 2001. JAMA 289:76–79, 2003

99. Caprio S, Genel M: Confronting the epidemic of childhood obesity. *Pediatrics* 115:494–495, 2005

100. Hellman R: Pediatric obesity: are we ready to pay the piper? *Rev Endocrinol* July/August:47–48, 2007

101. Butte N, Comuzzie A, Cole S, Mehta N, Cai G, Tejero M, Bastarrachea R, Smith E: Quantative genetic analysis of the metabolic syndrome in Hispanic children. *Pediatr Research* 58:1243–50, 2005

102. Targher G: Increased prevalence of cardiovascular disease in type 2 diabetic patients with non-alcoholic fatty liver disease. *Diabet Med* 23:403–409, 2006

103. de Piano A, Prado W, Caranti D, Siqueira K, Stella S, Lofrano M, Tock L, Cristofalo D, Lederman H, Tufik S, de Mello M, Damaso A: Metabolic and nutritional profile of obese adolescents with nonalcoholic fatty liver disease. *J Pediatr Gastroenterol Nutr* 44:446–452, 2007

104. Allen K, Byrne S, Blair E, Davis E: Why do some overweight children experience psychological problems? The role of weight and shape concern. *Int J Pediatr Obes* 1:239–247, 2006

105. Burgert TS, Taksali SE, Dziura J, Goodman TR, Yeckel CW, Papademetris X, Constable RT, Weiss R, Tamborlane WV, Savoye M, Seyal AA, Caprio S: Alanine aminotransferase levels and fatty liver in childhood obesity: associations with insulin resistance, adiponectin, and visceral Fat. *J Clin Endocrinol Metab* 91:4287–4294, 2006

106. Hassan A, Gordon C: Polycystic ovary syndrome update in adolescence. *Curr Opin Pediatr* 19:389–397, 2007

107. Nieto F, Szklo M, Comstock G: Childhood weight and growth rate as predictors of adult mortality. *Am J Epidemiol* 136:201–213, 1992

108. Calle E, Rodriguez C, Walker-Thurmond K, Thun M: Overweight, obesity, and mortality from cancer in a prospectively studied cohort of U.S. adults. *N Engl J Med* 348:1625–1638, 2003

110. Robinson T: Reducing children's television viewing to prevent obesity: a randomized controlled trial. *JAMA* 282:1561–1567, 1999

111. Collins C, Warren J, Neve M, McCoy P, Stokes B: Measuring effectiveness of dietetic interventions in child obesity: a systematic review of randomized trials. *Arch Pediatr Adolesc Med* 160:906–922, 2006

112. Savoye M, Shaw M, Dziura J, Tamborlane WV, Rose P, Guandalini C, Goldberg-Gell R, Burgert TS, Cali AMG, Weiss R, Caprio S: Effects of a weight management program on body composition and metabolic parameters in overweight children: a randomized controlled trial. *JAMA* 297:2697–2704, 2007

113. Rossner S, Sjostrom L, Noack R, Meinders A, Noseda G: Weight loss, weight mantenance, and improved cardiovascular risk factors after 2 years treatment with orlistat for obesity. European Orlistat Obesity Study Group. *Obes Res* 8:49–61, 2000

114. Berkowitz R, Fujioka K, Daniels S, et al. for the Sibutramine Adolescent Study Group: Effects of sibutramine treatment in obese adolescents. A randomized trial. *Ann Intern Med* 145:81–90, 2006

115. Bays H, Mandarino L, DeFronzo RA: Role of the adipocyte, free fatty acids, and ectopic fat in pathogenesis of type 2 diabetes mellitus: peroxisomal proliferator-activated receptor agonists provide a rational therapeutic approach. *J Clin Endocrinol Metab* 89:463–478, 2004

116. Bays H, Dujovne C: Adiposopathy is a more rational treatment target for metabolic disease than obesity alone. *Curr Sci* 8:144–156, 2006

117. Nadler S, Stoehr J, Schueler K, Tanimoto G, Yandell B, Attie A: The expression of adipogenic genes is decreased in obesity and diabetes mellitus. *PNAS* 97:11371–11376, 2000

118. Lazar M: How obesity causes diabetes: not a tall tale. *Science* 307:373–375, 2005

119. Dubois S, Heilbronn L, Smith S, Albu J, Kelley D, Ravussin E: Decreased expression of adipogenic genes in obese subjects with type 2 diabetes. *Obesity* 14:1543–1552, 2006

120. Qatanani M, Lazar M: Mechanisms of obesity-associated insulin resistance: many choices on the menu. *Genes Dev* 21:1443–1455, 2007

121. Gregor M, Hotamisligil G: Thematic review series: adipocyte biology. Adipocyte stress: the endoplasmic reticulum and metabolic disease. *J Lipid Res* 48:1905–1914, 2007

122. Spiegelman B, Enerbäck S: "The adipocyte: a multifunctional cell." *Cell Metabolism* 4:425–427, 2006

123. Hotamisligil G, Shargill N, Spiegelman B: Adipose expression of tumor necrosis factor-a: direct role in obesity-linked insulin resistance. *Science* 259:87–91, 1993

124. Feinstein R, Kanety H, Papa M, Lunenfeld B, Karasik A: Tumor necrosis factor-a suppresses insulin-induced tyrosine phophorylation of insulin receptor and its substrates. *J Biol Chem* 268:26055–26058, 1993

125. Lehrke M, Lazar M: Inflammed about obesity. *Nat Med* 10:126–127, 2004

126. Kolak M, Westerbacka J, Velagapudi VR, Wagsater D, Yetukuri L, Makkonen J, Rissanen A, Hakkinen A-M, Lindell M, Bergholm R, Hamsten A, Eriksson P, Fisher RM, Oresic M, Yki-Jarvinen H: Adipose tissue inflammation and increased ceramide content characterize subjects with high liver fat content independent of obesity. *Diabetes* 56:1960–1968, 2007

127. Kadowaki TYT: Adiponectin and adiponectin receptors. *Endocr Rev* 26:439–451, 2005

128. Kim J, van de Wall E, Laplante M, Azzara A, Trujillo M, Hofmann S, Schraw T, Durand J, Li H, Li G, Jelicks L, Mehler M, Hui D, Deshaies Y, Shulman G, Schwartz G, Scherer P: Obesity-associated improvements in metabolic profile through expansion of adipose tissue. *J Clin Invest* 117:2621–30, 2007

129. Cusi K, DeFronzo R: Non-insulin dependent diabetes mellitus. In *"The Endocrine Pancreas and Regulation of Metabolism"*, Handbook of Physiology, ed. *LS Jefferson and AD Cherrington, Oxford University Press Chap* 37:1115–1168, 2001

130. McGarry J: What if Minkowski had been ageusic? An alternative angle on diabetes. *Science* 258:766–770, 1992

131. DeFronzo RA: Lilly lecture 1987. The triumvirate: beta-cell, muscle, liver. A collusion responsible for NIDDM. *Diabetes* 37:667–687, 1988

132. Boden G: Role of fatty acids in the pathogenesis of insulin resistance and NIDDM. *Diabetes* 46:3–10, 1997

133. Kelley D, Mandarino L: Fuel selection in human skeletal muscle in insulin resistance. A reexamination. *Diabetes* 49:677–683, 2000

134. Morino K, Petersen K, Shulman G: Molecular mechanisms of insulin resistance in humans and their potential links with mitochondrial dysfunction. *Diabetes* 55:S9–S15, 2006

135. Unger R, Grundy S: Hyperglycemia as in inducer as well as a consequence of impaired islet cell function and insulin resistance: implications for the management of diabetes. *Diabetologia* 28:119–121, 1985

136. Rossetti L, Giaccari A, DeFronzo R: Glucose toxicity. *Diabetes Care* 13:610–630, 1990

137. Yki-Jarvinen Y, Makimattila S: Insulin resistance due to hyperglycaemia: an adaptation protecting insulin-sensitive tissues. *Diabetologia* 40:S141–S144, 1997

138. Gulli G, Ferrannini E, Stern M, Haffner S, DeFronzo R: The metabolic profile of NIDDM is fully established in glucose-tolerant offspring of two Mexican-American NIDDM parents. *Diabetes* 41:1575–1586, 1992

139. Vauhkonen INL, Vanninen E, Kainulainen S, Uusitupa M, Laakso M: Defects in insulin secretion and insulin action in non-insulin dependent diabetes mellitus are inherited. *J Clin Invest* 100:86–96, 1997

140. Virkamaki A, Korsheninnikova E, Seppala-Lindroos A, Vehkavaara S, Goto T, Halavaara J, Hakkinen A-M, Yki-Jarvinen H: Intramyocellular lipid is associated with resistance to in vivo insulin actions on glucose uptake, antilipolysis, and early insulin signaling pathways in human skeletal muscle. *Diabetes* 50:2337–2343, 2001

141. Kashyap S, Belfort R, Gastaldelli A, Pratipanawatr T, Berria R, Pratipanawatr W, Bajaj M, Mandarino L, DeFronzo R, Cusi K: A sustained increase in plasma free fatty acids impairs insulin secretion in nondiabetic subjects genetically predisposed to develop type 2 diabetes. *Diabetes* 52:2461–2474, 2003

142. Kashyap SR, Belfort R, Berria R, Suraamornkul S, Pratipranawatr T, Finlayson J, Barrentine A, Bajaj M, Mandarino L, DeFronzo R, Cusi K: Discordant effects of a chronic physiological increase in plasma FFA on insulin signaling in healthy subjects with or without a family history of type 2 diabetes. *Am J Physiol - Endocrinol Metab* 287:E537–E546, 2004

143. Felber J-P, Ferrannini E, Golay A, Meyer H, Theibaud D, Curchod B, Maeder E, Jequier E, DeFronzo R: Role of lipid oxidation in pathogenesis of insulin resistance of obesity and type II diabetes. *Diabetes* 36:1341–1350, 1987

144. Felber JP, Golay A, Jequier E, Curchod B, Temler E, DeFronzo RA, Ferrannini E: The metabolic consequences of long-term human obesity. *Int J Obes* 12:377–389, 1988

145. Bonadonna R, Groop L, Kraemer N, Ferrannini E, Del PS, DeFronzo R: Obesity and insulin resistance in humans: a dose-response study. *Metab Clin Exp* 39:452–459, 1990

146. Frayn K, Arner P, Yki-Järvinen H: Fatty acid metabolism in adipose tissue, muscle and liver in health and disease. *Essays Biochem* 42:89–103, 2006

147. Unger R: Lipotoxicity in the pathogenesis of obesity-dependent NIDDM. Genetic and clinical implications. *Diabetes* 44:861–870, 1995

148. Unger R, Zhou Y: Lipotoxicity of b-cells in obesity and in other causes of fatty acid spillover. *Diabetes* 50 (Suppl. 1):S118–S121, 2001

149. Iozzo P, Pranawatapatr T, Pijl H, Vogt C, Kumar V, Pipek R, Matsuda M, Mandarino L, Cusi K, DeFronzo R: Physiological hyperinsulinemia impairs insulin-stimulated glycogen synthase activity and glycogen synthesis. *Am J Physiol Endocrinol Metab* 280:E712–E719, 2001

150. Pratipanawatr W, Pratipanawatr T, Cusi K, Berria R, Adams JM, Jenkinson CP, Maezono K, DeFronzo RA, Mandarino LJ: Skeletal muscle insulin resistance in normoglycemic subjects with a strong family history of type 2 diabetes is associated with decreased insulin-stimulated insulin receptor substrate-1 tyrosine phosphorylation. *Diabetes* 50:2572–2578, 2001

151. Belfort R, Mandarino L, Kashyap S, Wirfel K, Pratipanawatr T, Berria R, DeFronzo RA, Cusi K: Dose-response effect of elevated plasma free fatty acid on insulin signaling. *Diabetes* 54:1640–1648, 2005

152. Buchanan TA: (How) Can we prevent type 2 diabetes? *Diabetes* 56:1502–1507, 2007

153. Randle P, Garland P, Hales C, Newsholme E: The glucose fatty acid cycle. Its role in insulin sensitivity and the metabolic disturbances of diabetes mellitus. *Lancet* 1:785–789, 1963

154. Felber J, Vanotti A: Effects of fat infusions on glucose tolerance and insulin plasma levels. *Med Exp* 10:153–156, 1964

155. Thiebaud D, DeFronzo RA, Jacot E, Golay A, Acheson K, Maeder E, Jequier E, Felber JP: Effect of long chain triglyceride infusion on glucose metabolism in man. *Metab Clin Exp* 31:1128–1136, 1982

156. Bevilacqua S, Bonnadona R, Buzzigoli G, Boni C, Ciocaro D, Maccari F, Giorico M, Ferranini E: Acute elevation of free fatty acid levels leads to hepatic insulin resistance in obese subjects. *Metab Clin Exp* 37:502–506, 1987

157. Wolfe B, Klein M, Peters E, Schmidt B, Wolfe R: Effect of elevated free fatty acids on glucose oxidation in normal humans. *Metabolism* 36:323–329, 1988

158. Bonadonna R, Zych K, Boni C, Ferrannini E, DeFronzo R: Time dependence of the interaction between lipid and glucose in humans. *Am J Physiol* 257:E49–E56, 1989

159. Bevilacqua S, Buzzigoli G, Bonnadona R, Brandi S, Oleggini M, Boni C, Geloni M, Ferranini E: Operation of the Randle's cycle in patients with NIDDM. *Diabetes* 39:383–389, 1990

160. Boden G, Chen X, Ruiz J, White J, Rossetti L: Mechanisms of fatty acid-induced inhibition of glucose uptake. *J Clin Invest* 93:2438–2446, 1994

161. Kelley DE, Mokan M, Simoneau JA, Mandarino LJ: Interaction between glucose and free fatty acid metabolism in human skeletal muscle. *J Clin Invest* 92:91–98, 1993

162. Kelley D, Mandarino L: Hyperglycemia normalizes insulin-stimulated skeletal muscle glucose oxidation and storage in noninsulin-dependent diabetes mellitus. *J Clin Invest* 86:1999–2007, 1990

163. Boden G, Chen X: Effects of fat on glucose uptake and utilization in patients with non-insulin-dependent diabetes. *J Clin Invest* 96:1261–1268, 1995

164. Boden G, Jadali F, White J, Liang Y, Mozzoli M, Chen X, Colemen E, Smith C: Effects of fat on insulin-stimulated carbohydrate metabolism in normal men. *J Clin Invest* 88:960–966, 1991

165. Roden M, Price T, Perseghin G, Petersen K, Rothman D, Cline G, Shulman G: Mechanism of free fatty acid-induced insulin resistance in humans. *J Clin Invest* 97:2859–2865, 1996

166. Dresner A, Laurent D, Marcucci M, Griffin M, Dufour S, Cline G, Slezak L, Andersen D, Hundal R, Rothman D, Petersen K, Shulman G: Effects of free fatty acids on glucose transport and IRS-1 associated phophatidylinositol 3-kinase activity. *J Clin Invest* 103:253–259, 1999

167. Roden M, Krssak M, Stingl H, Gruber S, Hofer A, Furnsinn C, Moser E, Waldhausl W: Rapid impairment of skeletal muscle glucose transport/phosphorylation by free fatty acids in humans. *Diabetes* 48:358–364, 1998

168. Krebs M, Krssak M, Nowotny P, Weghuber D, Gruber S, Mlynarik V, Bischof M, Stingl H, Furnsinn C, Waldhausl W, Roden M: Free fatty acids inhibit the glucose-stimulated increase of intramuscular glucose-6-phosphate concentration in humans. *J Clin Endocrinol Metab* 86:2153–2160, 2001

169. Holland W, Knotts T, Chavez J, Wang J-L, Hoehn K, Summers S: Lipid mediators of insulin resistance. *Nutr Rev* 65:S39–S46, 2007

170. Rachek LSIM, LeDoux S, Wilson G: Palmitate induced mitochondrial deoxyribonucleic acid damage and apoptosis in L6 rat skeletal muscle cells. *Endocrinology* 148:293–299, 2006

171. Ellis B, Poynten A, Lowy A, Furler S, Chisholm D, Kraegen E, Cooney G: Long-chain acyl-CoA esters as indicators of lipid metabolism and insulin sensitivity in rat and human muscle. *Am J Physiol Endocrinol Metab* 279:E554–E560, 2000

172. Kruszynska YWD, Ofrecio J, Frias J, Macaraeg G, Olefsky J: Fatty acid-induced insulin resistance: decreased muscle PI3K activation but unchanged AKT phophorylation. *J Clin Endocrinol Metab* 87:226–234, 2002

173. Chavez J, Summers S: Characterizing the effects of saturated fatty acids on insulin signaling and ceramide and diacylglycerol accumulation in 3T3-L1 adipocytes and C2C12 myotubes. *Arch Biochem Biophys* 419:101–109, 2003

174. Chavez JA, Knotts TA, Wang L-P, Li G, Dobrowsky RT, Florant GL, Summers SA: A role for ceramide, but not diacylglycerol, in the antagonism of insulin signal transduction by saturated fatty acids. *J Biol Chem* 278:10297–10303, 2003

175. Storgaard H, Jensen C, Bjornholm M, Song X, Madsbad S, Zierath J, Vaag A: Dissociation between fat-induced in vivo insulin resistance and proximal insulin signaling in skeletal muscle in men at risk for type 2 diabetes. *J Clin Endocrinol Metab* 89:1301–1311, 2004

176. Boden G, Lebed B, Schatz M, Homko C, Lemieux S: Effects of acute changes of plasma free fatty acids on intramyocellular fat content and insulin resistance in healthy subjects. *Diabetes* 50:1612–1617, 2001

177. Bachmann OP, Dahl DB, Brechtel K, Machann J, Haap M, Maier T, Loviscach M, Stumvoll M, Claussen CD, Schick F, Haring HU, Jacob S: Effects of intravenous and dietary lipid challenge on intramyocellular lipid content and the relation with insulin sensitivity in humans. *Diabetes* 50:2579–2584, 2001

178. Pan D, Lillioja S, Kriketos A, Milner M, Baur L, Bogardus C, Jenkins A, Storlien L: Skeletal muscle triglyceride levels are inversely related to insulin action. *Diabetes* 46:983–988, 1997

179. Jacob S, Machann J, Rett K, Brechtel K, Volk A, Renn W, Maerker E, Matthaei S, Schick F, Claussen C, Haring H-U: Association of increased intramyocellular lipid content with insulin resistance in lean nondiabetic offspring of type 2 diabetic subjects. *Diabetes* 48:1113–1119, 1999

180. Schick F, Machann J, Brechtel K, Strempfer A, Klumpp B, Stein D: MRI of muscular fat. *Magn Reson Med* 47:720–727, 2002

181. Thamer C, Machann J, Bachmann O, Haap M, Dahl D, Wietek B, Tschritter O, Niess A, Brechtel K, Fritsche A, Claussen C, Jacob S, Schick F, Haring H-U, Stumvoll M: Intramyocellular lipids: anthropometric determinants and relationships with maximal aerobic capacity and insulin sensitivity. *J Clin Endocrinol Metab* 88:1785–1791, 2003

182. Machann J, Haring HU, Schick F, Stumvoll M: Intramyocellular lipids and insulin resistance. *Diabetes Obes Metab* 6:239–248, 2004

183. Anderwald C, Bernroider E, Krssak M, Stingl H, Brehm A, Bischof MG, Nowotny P, Roden M, Waldhausl W: Effects of insulin treatment in type 2 diabetic patients on intracellular lipid content in liver and skeletal muscle. *Diabetes* 51:3025–3032, 2002

184. Roden M: Muscle triglycerides and mitochondrial function: possible mechanisms for the development of type 2 diabetes. *Int J Obes* 29 (Suppl. 2):S111–S115, 2005

185. Ross R, Dagnone D, Jones PJ, Smith H, Paddags A: Reduction in obesity and related comorbid conditions after diet-induced weight loss or exercise-induced weight loss in men. A randomized, controlled trial. *Ann Intern Med* 133:92–103, 2000

186. Itani SI, Ruderman NB, Schmieder F, Boden G: Lipid-induced insulin resistance in human muscle is associated with changes in diacylglycerol, protein kinase C, and IKB-a. *Diabetes* 51:2005–2011, 2002

187. Adams JM, II, Pratipanawatr T, Berria R, Wang E, DeFronzo RA, Sullards MC, Mandarino LJ: Ceramide content is increased in skeletal muscle from obese insulin-resistant humans. *Diabetes* 53:25–31, 2004

188. Sriwijitkamol A, Christ-Roberts C, Berria R, Eagan P, Pratipanawatr T, DeFronzo RA, Mandarino LJ, Musi N: Reduced skeletal muscle inhibitor of kappa-B beta content is associated with insulin resistance in subjects with type 2 diabetes: reversal by exercise training. *Diabetes* 55:760–767, 2006

189. Hundal R, Petersen K, Mayerson A, Randhawa P, Inzucchi S, Shoelson S, Shulman G: Mechanism by which high-dose aspirin improves glucose metabolism in type 2 diabetes. *J Clin Invest* 109:1321–1326, 2002

190. Evans J, Goldfine I, Maddux B, Grodsky G: Oxidative stress and stress-activated signaling pathways: a unifying hypothesis of type 2 diabetes. *Endocr Rev* 23:599–622, 2002

191. Shi H, Kokoeva M, Inouye K, Tzameli I, Yin H, Flier J: TLR4 links innate immunity and fatty acid-induced insulin resistance. *J Clin Invest* 116:3015–3025, 2006

192. Tsukumo DML, Carvalho-Filho MA, Carvalheira JBC, Prada PO, Hirabara SM, Schenka AA, Araujo EP, Vassallo J, Curi R, Velloso LA, Saad MJA: Loss-of-function mutation in toll-like receptor 4 prevents diet-induced obesity and insulin resistance. *Diabetes* 56:1986–1998, 2007

193. Johnson A, Argyraki M, Thow J, Cooper G, Fulcher G, Taylor R: Effect of increased free fatty acid supply on glucose metabolism and skeletal muscle glycogen synthase activity in normal man. *Clin Sci* 82:219–226, 1992

194. Wolfe B, Peters E, Klein S, Holland O, Rosenblatt J, Gary H: Effect of short-term fasting on lipolytic responsiveness in normal and obese subjects. *Am J Physiol Endocrinol Metab* 252:E189–E196, 1987

195. Dobbins R, Chester M, Daniels M, McGarry J, Stein D: Circulating fatty acids are essential for efficient glucose-stimulated insulin secretion after prolonged fasting in humans. *Diabetes* 47:1613–1618, 1998

196. Groop LC, Saloranta C, Shank M, Bonadonna RC, Ferrannini E, DeFronzo RA: The role of free fatty acid metabolism in the pathogenesis of insulin resistance in obesity and noninsulin-dependent diabetes mellitus. *J Clin Endocrinol Metab* 72:96–107, 1991

197. Golay A, Munger R, Felber J-P: Obesity and NIDDM: the retrograde regulation concept. *Diabetes Rev* 5:69–82, 1997

198. Reaven G, Hollenbeck C, Jeng C-Y, Shung M, Chen Y-DI: Measurement of plasma glucose, free fatty acid, lactate, and insulin for 24 h in patients with NIDDM. *Diabetes* 37:1020–1024, 1988

199. Groop LC, Bonadonna RC, DelPrato S, Ratheiser K, Zyck K, Ferrannini E, DeFronzo RA: Glucose and free fatty acid metabolism in non-insulin-dependent diabetes mellitus. Evidence for multiple sites of insulin resistance. *J Clin Invest* 84:205–213, 1989

200. Cusi K, Conmstock J, Cunningham G: Safety and efficacy of normalizing fasting glucose with bedtime NPH insulin alone in NIDDM. *Diabetes Care* 18:843–851, 1995

201. Cusi K, Consoli A, DeFronzo R: Metabolic effects of metformin on glucose and lactate metabolism in NIDDM. *J Clin Endo Metab* 81:4059–4067, 1996

202. Pratipanawatr T, Cusi K, Ngo P, Pratipanawatr W, Mandarino LJ, DeFronzo RA: Normalization of plasma glucose concentration by insulin therapy improves insulin-stimulated glycogen synthesis in type 2 diabetes. *Diabetes* 51:462–468, 2002

203. Perseghin G, Ghosh S, Gerow K, Shulman G: Metabolic defects in lean nondiabetic offspring of NIDDM parents. A cross-sectional study. *Diabetes* 46:1001–1009, 1997

204. Nyholm B, Walker M, Gravholt C, Shearing P, Sturis J, Alberti K: Twenty-four-hour insulin secretion rates, circulating concentrations of fuel substrates and gut incretin hormones in healthy offspring of Type II (non-insulin-dependent) diabetic parents: evidence of several aberrations. *Diabetologia* 42:1314–1323, 1999

205. Nyholm B, Nielsen MF, Kristensen K, Nielsen S, Ostergard T, Pedersen SB, Christiansen T, Richelsen B, Jensen MD, Schmitz O: Evidence of increased visceral obesity and reduced physical fitness in healthy insulin-resistant first-degree relatives of type 2 diabetic patients. *Eur J Endocrinol* 150:207–214, 2004

206. Petersen KF, Dufour S, Befroy D, Garcia R, Shulman GI: Impaired mitochondrial activity in the insulin-resistant offspring of patients with type 2 diabetes. *N Engl J Med* 350:664–671, 2004

207. Ostergard T, Nyholm B, Hansen TK, Rasmussen LM, Ingerslev J, Sorensen KE, Botker HE, Saltin B, Schmitz O: Endothelial function and biochemical vascular markers in first-degree relatives of type 2 diabetic patients: the effect of exercise training. *Metabolism* 55:1508–1515, 2006

208. Ostergard T, Andersen JL, Nyholm B, Lund S, Nair KS, Saltin B, Schmitz O: Impact of exercise training on insulin sensitivity, physical fitness, and muscle oxidative capacity in first-degree relatives of type 2 diabetic patients. *Am J Physiol Endocrinol Metab* 290:E998–E1005, 2006

209. Heilbronn L, Gregersen S, Shirkhedkar D, Hu D, Campbell L: Impaired fat oxidation after a single high fat meal in insulin sensitive non-diabetic individuals with a family history of type 2 diabetes. *Diabetes* 56:2046–2053, 2007

210. Befroy DE, Petersen KF, Dufour S, Mason GF, de Graaf RA, Rothman DL, Shulman GI: Impaired mitochondrial substrate oxidation in muscle of insulin-resistant offspring of type 2 diabetic patients. *Diabetes* 56:1376–1381, 2007

211. Warram J, Krolewski A, Kahn C: Slow glucose removal rate and hyperinsulinemia precede the development of type 2 diabetes in offspring of diabetic parents. *Ann Intern Med* 113:909–915, 1990

212. Martin B, Warram J, Krolewski A, Soeldner J, Kahn C, Martin B, Bergman R: Role of glucose and insulin resistance in development of type 2 diabetes mellitus: results of a 25-year follow-up study. *Lancet* 340:925–929, 1992

213. Sinha R, Dufour S, Petersen KF, LeBon V, Enoksson S, Ma Y-Z, Savoye M, Rothman DL, Shulman GI, Caprio S: Assessment of skeletal muscle triglyceride content by 1H nuclear magnetic resonance spectroscopy in lean and obese adolescents: relationships to insulin sensitivity, total body fat, and central adiposity. *Diabetes* 51:1022–1027, 2002

214. Liska D, Dufour S, Zern T, Taksali S, Calí A, Dziura J, Shulman G, Pierpont B, Caprio S: Interethnic differences in muscle, liver and abdominal fat partitioning in obese adolescents. *PLoS ONE* Jun 27, 2(6):e569, 2007

215. Kelley DE, Mokan M, Mandarino LJ: Intracellular defects in glucose metabolism in obese patients with NIDDM. *Diabetes* 41:698–706, 1992

216. Kelley DE, He J, Menshikova EV, Ritov VB: Dysfunction of mitochondria in human skeletal muscle in type 2 diabetes. *Diabetes* 51:2944–2950, 2002

217. Lane N: Mitochondrial disease: Powerhouse of disease. *Nature* 440:600–602, 2006

218. Schrauwen-Hinderling V, Roden M, Kooi M, Hesselink MPS: Muscular mitochondrial dysfunction and type 2 diabetes mellitus. *Curr Opin Clin Nutr Metab Care* 10:698–703, 2007

219. Patti ME, Butte AJ, Crunkhorn S, Cusi K, Berria R, Kashyap S, Miyazaki Y, Kohane I, Costello M, Saccone R, Landaker EJ, Goldfine AB, Mun E, DeFronzo R, Finlayson J, Kahn CR, Mandarino LJ: Coordinated reduction of genes of oxidative metabolism in humans with insulin resistance and diabetes: Potential role of PGC1 and NRF1. *Proc Natl Acad Sci* 100:8466–8471, 2003

220. Mootha VK, Lindgren CM, Eriksson KF, Subramanian A, Sihag S, Lehar J, Puigserver P, Carlsson E, Ridderstråle M, Laurila E, Houstis N, Daly MJ, Patterson N, Mesirov JP, Golub TR, Tamayo P, Spiegelman B, Lander ES, Hirschhorn JN, Altshuler D, Groop LC: PGC-1alpha-responsive genes involved in oxidative phosphorylation are coordinately downregulated in human diabetes. *Nat Genet* 34:267–273, 2003

221. Richardson DK, Kashyap S, Bajaj M, Cusi K, Mandarino SJ, Finlayson J, DeFronzo RA, Jenkinson CP, Mandarino LJ: Lipid infusion decreases the expression of nuclear encoded mitochondrial genes and increases the expression of extra-cellular matrix genes in human skeletal muscle. *J Biol Chem* 280:10290–10297, 2005

222. Fromenty B, Robin M, Igoudjil A, Mansouri A, Pessayre D: The ins and outs of mitochondrial dysfunction in NASH. *Diabetes Metab* 30:121–138, 2004

223. Diehl AM, Li ZP, Lin HZ, Yang SQ: Cytokines and the pathogenesis of non-alcoholic steatohepatitis. *Gut* 54:303–306, 2005

224. Cusi K, Kashyap S, Belfort R, Bajaj M, Cersosimo E, Lee S: Effects on insulin secretion and action of short-term reduction of plasma free fatty acids with acipimox in non-diabetic subjects genetically predisposed to type 2 diabetes. *Am J Physiol Endocrinol Metab* 292:E1775–E1781, 2007

225. Santomauro A, Boden G, Silva M, Rocha D, Santos R, Ursich M, Strassmann P, Wajchenberg B: Overnight lowering of free fatty acids with acipimox improves insulin resistance and glucose tolerance in obese diabetic and nondiabetic subjects. *Diabetes* 48:1836–1841, 1999

226. Bajaj M, Suraamornkul S, Romanelli A, Cline GW, Mandarino LJ, Shulman GI, DeFronzo RA: Effect of a sustained reduction in plasma free fatty acid concentration on intramuscular long-chain fatty acyl-Co as and insulin action in type 2 diabetic patients. *Diabetes* 54:3148–3153, 2005

227. Toledo FGS, Menshikova EV, Ritov VB, Azuma K, Radikova Z, DeLany J, Kelley DE: Effects of physical activity and weight loss on skeletal muscle mitochondria and relationship with glucose control in type 2 diabetes. *Diabetes* 56:2142–2147, 2007

228. Mogensen M, Sahlin K, Fernstrom M, Glintborg D, Vind BF, Beck-Nielsen H, Hojlund K: Mitochondrial respiration is decreased in skeletal muscle of patients with type 2 diabetes. *Diabetes* 56:1592–1599, 2007

229. Brehm A, Krssak M, Schmid AI, Nowotny P, Waldhausl W, Roden M: Increased lipid availability impairs insulin-stimulated ATP synthesis in human skeletal muscle. *Diabetes* 55:136–140, 2006

230. Boushel R, Gnaiger E, Schjerling P, Skovbro M, Kraunsøe R, Dela F: Patients with type 2 diabetes have normal mito-chondrial function in skeletal muscle. *Diabetologia* 50:790–796, 2007

231. LaMonte M, Barlow C, Jurca R, Kampert J, Church T, Blair S: Cardiorespiratory fitness is inversely associated with the incidence of metabolic syndrome: a prospective study of men and women. *Circulation* 112:505–512, 2005

232. Braith R, Stewart K: Resistance exercise training: its role in the prevention of cardiovascular disease. *Contemp Rev Cardiovasc Med* 113:2642–2650, 2006

233. Gill JMR, Malkova D: Physical activity, fitness and cardiovascular disease risk in adults: interactions with insulin resis-tance and obesity. *Clin Sci* 110:409–425, 2006

234. Goodpaster B, Brown N: Skeletal muscle lipid and its association with insulin resistance: What is the role for exercise? *Exerc Sport Sci Rev:* 33:150–154, 2005

235. Hawley J, Hargreaves M, Zierath J: Signalling mechanisms in skeletal muscle: role in substrate selection and muscle adaptation. *Essays Biochem* 42:1–12, 2006

236. Coffey VGRD, Lancaster GI, Yeo WK, Febbraio MA, Yaspelkis BB III, Hawley JA: Effect of high-frequency resistance exercise on adaptive responses in skeletal muscle. *Med Sci Sports Exerc* 39:2135–2144, 2007

237. Yaspelkis BB III, Lessard SJ, Reeder DW, Limon JJ, Saito M, Rivas DA, Kvasha I, Hawley JA: Exercise reverses high-fat diet-induced impairments on compartmentalization and activation of components of the insulin-signaling cascade in skeletal muscle. *Am J Physiol Endocrinol Metab* 293:E941–E949, 2007

238. Goodpaster BH, Katsiaras A, Kelley DE: Enhanced fat oxidation through physical activity Is associated with improve-ments in insulin sensitivity in obesity. *Diabetes* 52:2191–2197, 2003

239. Menshikova EV, Ritov VB, Ferrell RE, Azuma K, Goodpaster BH, Kelley DE: Characteristics of skeletal muscle mito-chondrial biogenesis induced by moderate-intensity exercise and weight loss in obesity. *J Appl Physiol* 103:21–27, 2007

240. Menshikova EV, Ritov VB, Fairfull L, Ferrell RE, Kelley DE, Goodpaster BH: Effects of exercise on mitochondrial content and function in aging human skeletal muscle. *J Gerontol A Biol Sci Med Sci* 61:534–540, 2006

241. Cusi K, Maezono K, Osman A, Pendergrass M, Patti M, Pranawatapatr T, DeFronzo R, Kahn C, Mandarino L: Insulin resistance differentially affects the PI 3-kinase- and MAP kinase-mediated signaling in human muscle. *J Clin Invest* 105:311–320, 2000

242. Cusi KJ, Pratipanawatr T, Koval J, Printz R, Ardehali H, Granner DK, DeFronzo RA, Mandarino LJ: Exercise increases hexokinase II mRNA, but not activity in obesity and type 2 diabetes. *Metabolism* 50:602–606, 2001

243. Christ-Roberts CY, Pratipanawatr T, Pratipanawatr W, Berria R, Belfort R, Kashyap S, Mandarino LJ: Exercise training increases glycogen synthase activity and GLUT4 expression but not insulin signaling in overweight nondiabetic and type 2 diabetic subjects. *Metabolism* 53:1233–1242, 2004

244. Sriwijitkamol A, Coletta D, Estela W, Gabriela B, Sara M, John B, Eagan P Jenkinson C, Cersosimo E, DeFronzo R, Sakamoto K, Musi N: Effect of acute exercise on AMPK signaling in skeletal muscle of subjects with type 2 diabetes: a time-course and dose-response study. *Diabetes* 56:836–848, 2007

245. Tay C, Belfort R, Mathew M, Cusi K: A 2-day lipid or combined lipid-glucose infusion reproduce in healthy subjects the metabolic abnormalities seen in the metabolic syndrome. *Diabetes* 55 (Suppl. 1):A66, 2006

246. Kashyap S, Belfort R, Cersosimo E, Lee S, Cusi K: Chronic low-dose lipid infusion in healthy subjects induces markers of endothelial activation independent of its metabolic effects. *J Cardiometabolic Syndrome* 3:141–146, 2008

247. Rattigan S, Wheatley C, Richards S, Barrett E, Clark M: Exercise and insulin mediated capillary recruitment in muscle. *Exerc Sport Sci Rev* 32:43–48, 2004

248. De Filippis E, Cusi K, Ocampo G, Berria R, Buck S, Consoli A, Mandarino LJ: Exercise-induced improvement in vasodilatory function accompanies increased insulin sensitivity in obesity and type 2 diabetes mellitus. *J Clin Endocrinol Metab* 91:4903–4910, 2006

249. Duncan GE, Perri MG, Theriaque DW, Hutson AD, Eckel RH, Stacpoole PW: Exercise training, without weight loss, increases insulin sensitivity and postheparin plasma lipase activity in previously sedentary adults. *Diabetes Care* 26:557–562, 2003

250. Jeon CY, Lokken RP, Hu FB, van Dam RM: Physical activity of moderate intensity and risk of type 2 diabetes: a sys-tematic review. *Diabetes Care* 30:744–752, 2007

251. Sui X, Hooker SP, Lee IM, Church TS, Colabianchi N, Lee C-D, Blair SN: A prospective study of cardiorespiratory fitness and risk of type 2 diabetes in women. *Diabetes Care* 30:dc07–1870, 2007

252. Physical Activity and Public Health: Updated recommendation for adults from the American College of Sports Medicine and the American Heart Association. *Circulation* 116:1081–1093, 2007

253. Physical Activity and Public Health in Older Adults: recommendation from the American College of Sports Medicine and the American Heart Association. *Circulation* 116:1094–1105, 2007

254. Ekberg K, Landau B, Wajngot A, Chandramouli V, Efendic S, Brunengraber H, Wahren J: Contributions of kidney and liver to glucose production in the postabsorptive state and after 60 h of fasting. *Diabetes* 48:292–298, 1999

255. DeFronzo RA, Ferrannini E: Regulation of hepatic glucose metabolism in humans. *Diabetes Metab Rev* 3:415–459, 1987

256. Campbell PJ, Mandarino LJ, Gerich JE: Quantification of the relative impairment in actions of insulin on hepatic glucose production and peripheral glucose uptake in non-insulin-dependent diabetes mellitus. *Metab Clin Exp* 37:15–21, 1988

257. Lewis GF, Carpentier A, Vranic M, Giacca A: Resistance to insulin's acute direct hepatic effect in suppressing steady-state glucose production in individuals with type 2 diabetes. *Diabetes* 48:570–576, 1999

258. Gastaldelli A, Baldi S, Pettiti M, Toschi E, Camastra S, Natali A, Landau BR, Ferrannini E: Influence of obesity and type 2 diabetes on gluconeogenesis and glucose output in humans: a quantitative study. *Diabetes* 49:1367–1373, 2000

259. Edgerton DS, Cardin S, Emshwiller M, Neal D, Chandramouli V, Schumann WC, Landau BR, Rossetti L, Cherrington AD: Small increases in insulin inhibit hepatic glucose production solely caused by an effect on glycogen metabolism. *Diabetes* 50:1872–1882, 2001

260. Gastaldelli A, Toschi E, Pettiti M, Frascerra S, Quinones-Galvan A, Sironi AM, Natali A, Ferrannini E: Effect of physi-ological hyperinsulinemia on gluconeogenesis in nondiabetic subjects and in type 2 diabetic patients. *Diabetes* 50:1807–1812, 2001

261. Boden G, Cheung P, Stein TP, Kresge K, Mozzoli M: FFA cause hepatic insulin resistance by inhibiting insulin suppression of glycogenolysis. *Am J Physiol Endocrinol Metab* 283:E12–E19, 2002

262. Steiner K, Williams P, Lacy W, Cherrington A: Effects of insulin on glucagon-stimulated glucose production in the conscious dog. *Metabolism* 39:1325–1333, 1990

263. Ito KMH, Hirose H, Kido K, Koyama K, Kataoka K, Saruta T.: Exogenous insulin dose-dependently suppresses glucopenia-induced glucagon secretion from perfused rat pancreas. *Metabolism* 44:358–362, 1995

264. Obici S, Feng Z, Karkanias G, Baskin D, Rossetti L: Decreasing hypothalamic insulin receptors causes hyperphagia and insulin resistance in rats. *Nat Neurosci* 5:566, 2002

265. Sindelar DK, Chu CA, Rohlie M, Neal DW, Swift LL, Cherrington AD: The role of fatty acids in mediating the effects of peripheral insulin on hepatic glucose production in the conscious dog. *Diabetes* 46:187–196, 1997

266. Bergman RN: Non-esterified fatty acids and the liver: why is insulin secreted into the portal vein? *Diabetologia* 43:946–952, 2000

267. Edgerton DS, Lautz M, Scott M, Everett CA, Stettler KM, Neal DW, Chu CA, Cherrington AD: Insulin's direct effects on the liver dominate the control of hepatic glucose production. *J Clin Invest* 116:521–527, 2006

268. Boden G, She P, Mozzoli M: Free fatty acids produce insulin resistance and activate the proinflammatory nuclear factor-kB pathway in rat liver. *Diabetes* 54:3458–3465, 2005

269. Boden G: Fatty acid-induced inflammation and insulin resistance in skeletal muscle and liver. *Curr Diabetes Rep* 6:177–181, 2006

270. Anderwald C, Brunmair B, Stadlbauer K, Krebs M, Furnsinn C, Roden M: Effects of free fatty acids on carbohydrate metabolism and insulin signalling in perfused rat liver. *Eur J Clin Invest* 37:774–782, 2007

271. Moore MC, Satake S, Lautz M, Soleimanpour SA, Neal DW, Smith M, Cherrington AD: Nonesterified fatty acids and hepatic glucose metabolism in the conscious dog. *Diabetes* 53:32–40, 2004

272. Roden M, Stingl H, Chandramouli V, Schumann WC, Hofer A, Landau BR, Nowotny P, Waldhausl W, Shulman GI: Effects of free fatty acid elevation on postabsorptive endogenous glucose production and gluconeogenesis in humans. *Diabetes* 49:701–707, 2000

273. Donnelly KL, Smith CI, Schwarzenberg SJ, Jessurun J, Boldt MD, Parks EJ: Sources of fatty acids stored in liver and secreted via lipoproteins in patients with nonalcoholic fatty liver disease. *J Clin Invest* 115:1343–1351, 2005

274. Barrows BR, Parks EJ: Contributions of different fatty acid sources to very low-density lipoprotein-triacylglycerol in the fasted and fed states. *J Clin Endocrinol Metab* 91:1446–1452, 2006

275. Moore MC, Cherrington AD, Wasserman DH: Regulation of hepatic and peripheral glucose disposal. *Best Pract Res Clin Endocrinol Metab* 17:343–364, 2003

276. McGarry J: Banting lecture 2001: dysregulation of fatty acid metabolism in the etiology of type 2 diabetes. *Diabetes* 51:7–18, 2002

277. Sanyal AJ, Colin B, Carol S, Velimir AL, Richard KS, Richard TS: Similarities and differences in outcomes of cirrhosis due to nonalcoholic steatohepatitis and hepatitis C. *Hepatology* 43:682–689, 2006

278. Angulo P: GI epidemiology: nonalcoholic fatty liver disease. *Aliment Pharmacol Ther* 25:883–889, 2007

279. Wieckowska A, McCullough A, Feldstein A: Noninvasive diagnosis and monitoring of nonalcoholic steatohepatitis: present and future. *Hepatology* 46:582–589, 2007

280. Powell E, Cooksley W, Hanson R: The natural history of nonalcoholic steatohepatitis: a follow-up study of forty-two patients for up to 21 years. *Hepatology* 11:74–80, 1990

281. Harrison S, Torgerson S, Hayashi P: The natural history of nonalcoholic fatty liver disease: a clinical histopathological study. *Am J Gastroenterol* 98:2042–2047, 2003

282. Fassio E, Estela A, Nora DN, Graciela L, Cristina L: Natural history of nonalcoholic steatohepatitis: a longitudinal study of repeat liver biopsies. *Hepatology* 40:820–826, 2004

283. Adams LA: The natural history of nonalcoholic fatty liver disease: a population-based cohort study. *Gastroenterology* 129:113–121, 2005

284. Ekstedt M, Franzén L, Mathiesen U, Thorelius L, Holmqvist M, Bodemar G, Kechagias S: Long-term follow-up of patients with NAFLD and elevated liver enzymes. *Hepatology* 44:865–873, 2006

285. Targher G, Lorenzo B, Roberto P, Stefano R, Roberto T, Luciano Z: Prevalence of nonalcoholic fatty liver disease and its association with cardiovascular disease among type 2 diabetic patients. *Diabetes Care* 30:1212–1218, 2007

286. Hamaguchi M: Nonalcoholic fatty liver disease is a novel predictor of cardiovascular disease. *World J Gastroenterol* 13:1579–1584, 2007

287. Kowdley K, Caldwell S: Nonalcoholic steatohepatitis: a twenty-first century epidemic? *J Clin Gastroenterol* 40:S2–S4, 2006

288. Browning JD, Szczepaniak LS, Dobbins R, Nuremberg P, Horton JD, Cohen JC, Grundy SM, Hobbs HH: Prevalence of hepatic steatosis in an urban population in the United States: impact of ethnicity. *Hepatology* 40:1387–1395, 2004

289. Zelber-Sagi S: Prevalence of primary non-alcoholic fatty liver disease in a population-based study and its association with biochemical and anthropometric measures. *Liver Int* 26:856–863, 2006

290. Adams L, Talwalkar J: Diagnostic evaluation of nonalcoholic fatty liver disease. *J Clin Gastroenterol* 40:S34–S38, 2006

291. Patton HM: Pediatric nonalcoholic fatty liver disease: a critical appraisal of current data and implications for future research. *J Pediatr Gastroenterol Nutr* 43:413–427, 2006

292. Quiros-Tejeira RE, Rivera CA, Ziba TT, Mehta N, Smith CW, Butte NF: Risk for nonalcoholic fatty liver disease in Hispanic youth with BMI > or = 95th percentile. *J Pediatr Gastroenterol Nutr* 44:228–236, 2007

293. Roberts EA: Pediatric nonalcoholic fatty liver disease (NAFLD): a "growing" problem? J *Hepatology* 46:1133–1141, 2008

294. Aslander-van Vliet E, Smart C, Waldron S: Nutritional management in childhood and adolescent diabetes. *Pediatr Diabetes* 8:323–339, 2007

295. Mofrad P: Clinical and histologic spectrum of nonalcoholic fatty liver disease associated with normal ALT values. *Hepatology* 37:1286–1292, 2003

296. Sorrentino P: Silent non-alcoholic fatty liver disease-a clinical-histological study. *J Hepatol* 41:751–757, 2004

297. Amarapurkar D, Patel N: Clinical spectrum and natural history of non-alcoholic steatohepatitis with normal alanine aminotransferase values. *Trop Gastroenterol* 25:130–134, 2004

298. Kunde S, Larenzby A, Clements R, Abrams G: Spectrum of NAFLD and diagnostic implications of the proposed new normal range for serum ALT in obese women. *Hepatology* 42:650–656, 2005

299. Maheshwari A, Paul JT: Cryptogenic cirrhosis and NAFLD: are they related? *Am J Gastroenterol* 101:664–668, 2006

300. Angulo P, Keach J, Batts K, Lindor K: Independent predictors of liver fibrosis in patients with nonalcoholic steatohepatitis. *Hepatology* 30:1356–1362, 1999

301. Younossi ZM: Nonalcoholic fatty liver disease in patients with type 2 diabetes. *Clin Gastroenterol Hepatol* 2:262–265, 2004

302. Dixon J, Bhathal P, O'Brien P: Nonalcoholic fatty liver disease: predictors of nonalcoholic steatohepatitis and liver fibrosis in the severely obese. *Gastroenterology* 121:91–100, 2001

303. Marceau P, Biro S, Hould F: Liver pathology and the metabolic syndrome X in severe obesity. *J Clin Endocrinol Metab* 84:1513–1517, 1999

304. Luyckx FH, Desaive C, Thiry A, Dewe W, Scheen AJ, Gielsen JE, Lefevre PJ: Liver abnormalities in severely obese subjects: effects of drastic weight loss after gastroplasty. *Int J Obes Relat Metab Disord* 22:222–226, 1998

305. Haukeland JW: Abnormal glucose tolerance is a predictor of steatohepatitis and fibrosis in patients with non-alcoholic fatty liver disease. *Scand J Gastroenterol* 40:1469–1477, 2005

306. Gupte P: Non-alcoholic steatohepatitis in type 2 diabetes mellitus. *J Gastroenterol Hepatol* 19:854–858, 2004

307. Targher G: Relations between carotid artery wall thickness and liver histology in subjects with nonalcoholic fatty liver disease. *Diabetes Care* 29:1325–1330, 2006

308. Goland S, Goland S, Shimoni S, Zornitzki T, Knobler H, Azoulai O, Lutaty G: Cardiac abnormalities as a new manifestation of nonalcoholic fatty liver disease: echocardiographic and tissue Doppler imaging assessment. *J Clin Gastroenterol* 40: 949–955, 2006

309. Engelgau MM, Geiss LS, Saaddine JB, Boyle JP, Benjamin SM, Gregg EW: The evolving diabetes burden in the United States. *Ann Intern Med* 140:945–950, 2004

310. DeFronzo R, Ferrannini E: Insulin resistance: a multifaceted syndrome responsible for NIDDM, obesity, hypertension, dyslipidemia, and ASCVD. *Diabetes Care-Rev* 14:173–194, 1991

311. Ginsberg HN: Insulin resistance and cardiovascular disease. *JCI* 106:453–458, 2000

312. Seppala-Lindroos A, Vehkavaara S, Hakkinen A-M, Goto T, Westerbacka J, Sovijarvi A, Halavaara J, Yki-Jarvinen H: Fat accumulation in the liver is associated with defects in insulin suppression of glucose production and serum free fatty acids independent of obesity in normal men. *J Clin Endocrinol Metab* 87:3023–3028, 2002

313. Taghibiglou C, Carpentier A, Van Iderstine SC, Chen B, Rudy D, Aiton A, Lewis GF, Adeli K: Mechanisms of hepatic very low density lipoprotein overproduction in insulin resistance. *J Biol Chem* 275:8416–8425, 2000

314. Zambon A, Cusi K: The role of fenofibrate in clinical practice. *Diab Vasc Dis Res* 4 (Suppl. 3):S15–S20, 2007

315. Kotronen A, Westerbacka J, Bergholm R, Pietilainen K, Yki-Jarvinen H: Liver fat in the metabolic syndrome. *J Clin Endocrinol* 92:3490–3497, 2007

317. Gholam PM, Flancbaum L, Machan JT, Charney DA, Kotler DP: Nonalcoholic fatty liver disease in severely obese subjects. *Am J Gastroenterol* 102:399–408, 2007

318. Ratziu V: Liver fibrosis in overweight patients. *Gastroenterology* 118:1117–1123, 2000

319. Hamaguchi M: The metabolic syndrome as a predictor of nonalcoholic fatty liver disease. *Ann Intern Med* 143:722–728, 2005

320. Caldwell S, Chang Y, Nakamoto R, Krugner-Higby L: Mitochondria in nonalcoholic fatty liver disease. *Clin Liver Dis* 8:595–617, 2004

321. Pessayre D, Fromenty B: NASH: a mitochondrial disease. *J Hepatol* 42:928–940, 2005

322. Delarue J, Magnan C: Free fatty acids and insulin resistance. *Curr Opin Clin Nutr Metab Care* 10:142–148, 2007

323. Puri P, Baillie R, Wiest M, Mirshahi F, Choudhury J, Cheung O, Sargeant C, Contos M, Sanyal A: A lipidomic analysis of nonalcoholic fatty liver disease. *Hepatology* 46:1081–1090, 2007

324. Elsharkawy A, Mann D: Nuclear factor-kappa-B and the hepatic inflammation-fibrosis-cancer axis. *Hepatology* 46:590–597, 2007

325. Park E, Wong V, Guan X, Oprescu AI, Giacca A: Salicylate prevents hepatic insulin resistance caused by short-term elevation of free fatty acids in vivo. *J Endocrinol* 195:323–331, 2007

326. Savage DB, Choi CS, Samuel VT, Liu Z-X, Zhang D, Wang A, Zhang X-M, Cline GW, Yu XX, Geisler JG, Bhanot S, Monia BP, Shulman GI: Reversal of diet-induced hepatic steatosis and hepatic insulin resistance by antisense oligonucleotide inhibitors of acetyl-CoA carboxylases 1 and 2. *J Clin Invest* 116:817–824, 2006

327. Samuel VT, Liu Z-X, Wang A, Beddow SA, Geisler JG, Kahn M, Zhang X-m, Monia BP, Bhanot S, Shulman GI: Inhibition of protein kinase Ce prevents hepatic insulin resistance in nonalcoholic fatty liver disease. *J Clin Invest* 117:739–745, 2007

328. Choi CS, Savage DB, Kulkarni A, Yu XX, Liu Z-X, Morino K, Kim S, Distefano A, Samuel VT, Neschen S, Zhang D, Wang A, Zhang X-M, Kahn M, Cline GW, Pandey SK, Geisler JG, Bhanot S, Monia BP, Shulman GI: Suppression of diacylglycerol acyltransferase-2 (DGAT2), but not DGAT1, with antisense oligonucleotides reverses diet-induced hepatic steatosis and insulin resistance. *J Biol Chem* 282:22678–22688, 2007

329. Chakravarthy M, Pan Z, Zhu Y, Tordjman K, Schneider J, Coleman T, Turk J, Semenkovich C: "New" hepatic fat activates PPARalpha to maintain glucose, lipid, and cholesterol homeostasis.*Cell Metab* 1:309–322, 2005

330. Belfort R, Berria R, DeFronzo R, Cusi K: Effect of fenofibrate on glucose metabolism and insulin sensitivity in hypertriglyceridemic subjects with the metabolic syndrome. *Diabetes* 53 (Suppl. 1):A2183, 2004

331. Bajaj M, Suraamornkul S, Hardies J, Glass L, Musi N, Defronzo R: Effects of peroxisome proliferator-activated receptor (PPAR)-alpha and PPAR-gamma agonists on glucose and lipid metabolism in patients with type 2 diabetes mellitus. *Diabetologia* 50:1723–1731, 2007

332. Neuschwander-Tetri BA, Brunt EM, Kent R, Wehmeier D, Oliver B, Bacon R: Improved nonalcoholic steatohepatitis after 48 weeks of treatment with the PPAR-g ligand rosiglitazone. *Hepatology* 38:1008–1017, 2003

334. García-Ruiz I, Rodríguez-Juan C, Díaz-Sanjuán T, Martínez M, Muñoz-Yagüe T, Solís-Herruzo J: Effects of rosiglitazone on the liver histology and mitochondrial function in ob/ob mice. *Hepatology* 46:414–423, 2007

335. Browning JD, Horton JD: Molecular mediators of hepatic steatosis and liver injury. *J Clin Invest* 114:147–152, 2004

336. Heilbronn L, Smith S, Ravussin E: The insulin-sensitizing role of the fat derived hormone adiponectin. *Curr Pharm Des* 9:1411–1418, 2003

337. Xu A, Wang Y, Keshaw H, Xu LY, Lam KSL, Cooper GJS: The fat-derived hormone adiponectin alleviates alcoholic and nonalcoholic fatty liver diseases in mice. *J Clin Invest* 112:91–100, 2003

338. Hui J, Hodge A, Farrell G, Kench J, Kriketos A, George J: Beyond insulin resistance in NASH: TNF-alpha or adiponectin? *Hepatology* 40:46, 2004

339. Towler M, Hardie D: AMP-activated protein kinase in metabolic control and insulin signaling. *Circ Res* 100:328–341, 2007

340. Yang G, Li L, Tang Y, Boden G: Short-term pioglitazone treatment prevents free fatty acid-induced hepatic insulin resistance in normal rats: possible role of the resistin and adiponectin. *Biochem Biophys Res Commun* 339:1190–1196, 2006

341. Ouchi NKS, Arita Y, Maeda K, Kuriyama H, Okamoto Y, Hotta K, Nishida M, Takahashi M, Nakamura T, Yamashita S, Funahashi T, Matsuzawa Y: Novel modulator for endothelial adhesion molecules: adipocyte-derived plasma protein adiponectin. *Circulation* 100:2473–2476, 1999

342. Chen HMM, Funahashi T, Shimomura I, Quon M Adiponectin stimulates production of nitric oxide in vascular endothelial cells. *J Biol Chem* 278:45021–45026, 2003

343. Civitarese A, Jenkinson C, Richardson D, Bajaj M, Cusi K, Kashyap S, Berria R, Belfort R, DeFronzo R, Mandarino L, Ravussin E: Adiponectin receptors gene expression and insulin sensitivity in non-diabetic Mexican Americans with or without a family history of type 2 diabetes. *Diabetologia* 47:816, 2004

344. Lihn AS, Ostergard T, Nyholm B, Pedersen SB, Richelsen B, Schmitz O: Adiponectin expression in adipose tissue is reduced in first-degree relatives of type 2 diabetic patients. *Am J Physiol Endocrinol Metab* 284:E443–E448, 2003

345. Tiikkainen M, Hakkinen A-M, Korsheninnikova E, Nyman T, Makimattila S, Yki-Jarvinen H: Effects of rosiglitazone and metformin on liver fat content, hepatic insulin resistance, insulin clearance, and gene expression in adipose tissue in patients with type 2 diabetes. *Diabetes* 53:2169–2176, 2004

346. Baranova A, Gowder SJ, Schlauch K, Elariny H, Collantes R, Afendy A, Ong JP, Goodman Z, Chandhoke V, Younossi ZM: Gene expression of leptin, resistin, and adiponectin in the white adipose tissue of obese patients with non-alcoholic fatty liver disease and insulin resistance. *Obes Surg* 16:1118–1125, 2006

347. Bajaj M, Suraamornkul S, Piper P, Hardies LJ, Glass L, Cersosimo E, Pratipanawatr T, Miyazaki Y, DeFronzo RA: Decreased plasma adiponectin concentrations are closely related to hepatic fat content and hepatic insulin resistance in pioglitazone-treated type 2 diabetic patients. *J Clin Endocrinol Metab* 89:200–206, 2004

348. Lutchman G, Promrat K, Kleiner DE, Heller T, Ghany MG, Yanovski JA, Liang TJ, Hoofnagle JH: Changes in serum adipokine levels during pioglitazone treatment for nonalcoholic steatohepatitis: relationship to histological improvement. *Clin Gastroenterol Hepatol* 4:1048–1052, 2006

349. Wang RT, Koretz RL, Yee HF: Is weight reduction an effective therapy for nonalcoholic fatty liver? A systematic review. *Am J Med* 115:554–559, 2003

350. Zivkovic AM, German JB, Sanyal AJ: Comparative review of diets for the metabolic syndrome: implications for non-alcoholic fatty liver disease. *Am J Clin Nutr* 86:285–300, 2007

351. Harrison S, Day C: Benefits of lifestyle modification in NAFLD. *Gut* 56:1760–1769, 2007

352. Palmer M, Schaffner F: Effect of weight reduction on hepatic abnormalities in overweight subjects. *Gastroenterology* 99:1408–1413, 1990

353. Park H, Kim M, Shin E: Effect of weight control on hepatic abnormalities in obese patients with fatty liver. *J Korean Med Sci* 10:414–421, 1995

354. Ueno T, Sugawara H, Sujaku K, Hashimoto O, Tsuji R, Tamaki S, Torimura T, Inuzuka S, Sata M, Tanikawa K: Therapeutic effects of restricted diet and exercise in obese patients with fatty liver. *J Hepatol* 27:103–107, 1997

355. Kugelmas M, Hill D, Vivian B, Marsano L, McClain C: Cytokines and NASH: a pilot study of the effects of lifestyle modification and vitamin E. *Hepatology* 38:413, 2003

356. Baba CS, Alexander G, Kalyani B, Pandey R, Rastogi S, Pandey A, Choudhuri G: Effect of exercise and dietary modification on serum aminotransferase levels in patients with nonalcoholic steatohepatitis. *J Gastroenterol Hepatol* 21:191–198, 2006

357. Tamura Y, Tanaka Y, Sato F, et al.: Effects of diet and exercise on muscle and liver intracellular lipid contents and insulin sensitivity in type 2 diabetic patients. *J Clin Endo Metab* 90:3191–3196, 2005

358. Huang MA, Greenson JK, Chao C, Anderson L, Peterman D, Jacobson J, Emick D, Lok AS, Conjeevaram HS: One-year intense nutritional counseling results in histological improvement in patients with non-alcoholic steatohepatitis: a pilot study. *Am J Gastroenterol* 100:1072–1081, 2005

359. Westerbacka J, Lammi K, Hakkinen A-M, Rissanen A, Salminen I, Aro A, Yki-Jarvinen H: Dietary fat content modifies liver fat in overweight nondiabetic subjects. *J Clin Endocrinol Metab* 90:2804–2809, 2005

360. Petersen KF, Dufour S, Befroy D, Lehrke M, Hendler RE, Shulman GI: Reversal of nonalcoholic hepatic steatosis, hepatic insulin resistance, and hyperglycemia by moderate weight reduction in patients with type 2 diabetes. *Diabetes* 54:603–608, 2005

361. Browning J, Davis J, Saboorian M, Burgess S: A low-carbohydrate diet rapidly and dramatically reduces intrahepatic triglyceride content. *Hepatology* 44:487–488, 2006

362. Tendler D, Lin S, Yancy WS, Jr., Mavropoulos J, Sylvestre P, Rockey DC, Westman EC: The effect of a low-carbohydrate, ketogenic diet on nonalcoholic fatty liver disease: a pilot study. *Dig Dis Sci* 52:589–593, 2007

363. Ryan MC, Abbasi F, Lamendola C, Carter S, McLaughlin TL: Serum alanine aminotransferase levels decrease further with carbohydrate than fat restriction in insulin-resistant adults. *Diabetes Care* 30:1075–1080, 2007

364. Andersen T, Gluud C, Franzmann MB, Christoffersen P: Hepatic-effects of dietary weight-loss in morbidly obese subjects. *J Hepatol* 12:224–229, 1991

365. Shaffer E: Bariatric surgery. A promising solution for nonalcoholic steatohepatitis in the very obese. *J Clin Gastroenterol* 40:S44–S50, 2006

366. Sjostrom L, Narbro K, Sjostrom CD, Karason K, Larsson B, Wedel H, Lystig T, Sullivan M, Bouchard C, Carlsson B, Bengtsson C, Dahlgren S, Gummesson A, Jacobson P, Karlsson J, Lindroos A-K, Lonroth H, Naslund I, Olbers T, Stenlof K, Torgerson J, Agren G, Carlsson LMS: Effects of bariatric surgery on mortality in Swedish obese subjects. *N Engl J Med* 357:741–752, 2007

367. Adams TD, Gress RE, Smith SC, Halverson RC, Simper SC, Rosamond WD, LaMonte MJ, Stroup AM, Hunt SC: Long-term mortality after gastric bypass surgery. *N Engl J Med* 357:753–761, 2007

368. Bugianesi E, Marzocchi R, Villanova N, Marchesini G: Non-alcoholic fatty liver disease/non-alcoholic steatohepatitis (NAFLD/NASH): treatment. *Best Pract Res Clin Gastroenterol* 18:1105–1116, 2004

369. Bugianesi E, Gentilcore E, Manini R, Natale S, Vanni E, Villanova N: A randomized controlled trial of metformin versus vitamin E or prescriptive diet in nonalcoholic fatty liver disease. *Am J Gastroenterol* 100:1082–1090, 2005

370. Caldwell SH, Hespenheide EE, Redick JA, Iezzoni JC, Battle EH, Sheppard BL: A pilot study of a thiazolidinedione, troglitazone, in nonalcoholic steatohepatitis. *Am J Gastroenterol* 96:519–525, 2001

371. Promrat K, Lutchman G, Uwaifo GI, Freedman RJ, Soza A, Heller T: A pilot study of pioglitazone treatment for non-alcoholic steatohepatitis. *Hepatology* 39:188–196, 2004

372. Yaney G, Corkey B: Fatty acid metabolism and insulin secretion in pancreatic beta cells. *Diabetologia* 46:1297–1312, 2003

373. Robertson R, Harmon J, Tran P, Poitout V: b-cell glucose toxicity, lipotoxicity, and chronic oxidative stress in type 2 diabetes. *Diabetes* 53 (Suppl. 1):S119–S124, 2004

374. Wiederkehr A, Wollheim C: Minireview: Implication of mitochondria in insulin secretion and action. *Endocrinology* 147:2643–2649, 2006

375. Nolan CJ, Madiraju MSR, Delghingaro-Augusto V, Peyot M-L, Prentki M: Fatty acid signaling in the b-cell and insulin secretion. *Diabetes* 55 (Suppl. 2):S16–S23, 2006

376. Maedler K: Beta cells in type 2 diabetes – a crucial contribution to pathogenesis. *Diabetes, Obes Metab* 10:408–420, 2008

377. Kahn SE, Haffner SM, Heise MA, Herman WH, Holman RR, Jones NP, Kravitz BG, Lachin JM, O'Neill MC, Zinman B, Viberti G: Glycemic durability of rosiglitazone, metformin, or glyburide monotherapy. *N Engl J Med* 355:2427–2443, 2006

378. Malaisse WJ, Best L, Kawazu S, Malaisse-Lagae F, Sener A: The stimulus-secretion coupling of glucose-induced insulin release: fuel metabolism in islets deprived of exogenous nutrient. *Arch Biochem Biophys* 224:102–110, 1983

379. Matschinsky F: Banting Lecture 1995: a lesson in metabolic regulation inspired by the glucokinase glucose sensor paradigm. *Diabetes* 45:223–241, 1996

380. Stein D, Esser V, Stevenson B: Essentially of circulating fatty acids for glucose-stimulated insulin secretion in the fasted rat. *J Clin Invest* 97:2728–2735, 1996

381. Stein DT, Stevenson BE, Chester MW, Basit M, Daniels MB, Turley SD, McGarry JD: The insulinotropic potency of fatty acids is influenced profoundly by their chain length and degree of saturation. *J Clin Invest* 100:398–403, 1997

382. Dobbins RL, Szczepaniak LS, Myhill J, Tamura Y, Uchino H, Giacca A, McGarry JD: The composition of dietary fat directly influences glucose-stimulated insulin secretion in rats. *Diabetes* 51:1825–1833, 2002

383. Zhou Y, Grill V: Long term exposure of rat pancreatic islets to fatty acids inhibits glucose-induced insulin secretion and biosynthesis through a glucose fatty acid cycle. *J Clin Invest* 1994:870–876, 1994

384. Sako Y, Grill V: A 48-hour lipid infusion in the rat time-dependently inhibits glucose-induced insulin secretion and B cell oxidation through a process likely coupled to fatty acid oxidation. *Endocrinology* 127:1580–1589, 1990

385. Bollheimer L, Skelly R, Chester M, McGarry J, Rhodes C: Chronic exposure to free fatty acid reduces pancreatic beta cell insulin content by increasing basal insulin secretion that is not compensated for by a corresponding increase in proinsulin biosynthesis translation. *J Clin Invest* 101:1094–1101, 1998

386. Oprescu AI, Bikopoulos G, Naassan A, Allister EM, Tang C, Park E, Uchino H, Lewis GF, Fantus IG, Rozakis-Adcock M, Wheeler MB, Giacca A: Free fatty acid induced reduction in glucose-stimulated insulin secretion: evidence for a role of oxidative stress in vitro and in vivo. *Diabetes* 56:2927–2937, 2007

387. Amery CM, Round RA, Smith JM, Nattrass M: Elevation of plasma fatty acids by ten-hour intralipid infusion has no effect on basal or glucose-stimulated insulin secretion in normal man. *Metabolism* 49:450–454, 2000

388. Balent B, Goswami G, Goodloe G, Rogatsky E, Rauta O, Nezami R, Mints L, Angeletti RH, Stein DT: Acute elevation of NEFA causes hyperinsulinemia without effect on insulin secretion rate in healthy human subjects. *Ann NY Acad Sci* 967:535–543, 2002

389. Paolisso G, Gambardella A, Amato L, Tortoriello R, D'Amore A, Varricchio M: Opposite effects of short- and long-term fatty acid infusion on insulin secretion in healthy subjects. *Diabetologia* 38:1295–1299, 1995

390. Carpentier A, Mittelman SD, Bergman RN, Giacca A, Lewis GF: Acute enhancement of insulin secretion by FFA in humans is lost with prolonged FFA elevation. *Am J Physiol Endocrinol Metab* 276:E1055–E1066, 1999

391. Boden G, Chen X, Rosner J, Barton M: Effects of a 48-h fat infusion on insulin secretion and glucose utilization. *Diabetes* 44:1239–1242, 1995

392. Magnan C, Collins S, Berthault M-F, Kassis N, Vincent M, Gilbert M, Penicaud L, Ktorza A, Assimacopoulos-Jeannet F: Lipid infusion lowers sympathetic nervous activity and leads to increased β-cell responsiveness to glucose. *J Clin Invest* 103:413–419, 1999

393. Magnan C, Cruciani C, Clement L, Adnot P, Vincent M, Kergoat M, Girard A, Elghozi J-L, Velho G, Beressi N, Bresson J-L, Ktorza A: Glucose-induced insulin hypersecretion in lipid-infused healthy subjects is associated with a decrease in plasma norepinephrine concentration and urinary excretion. *J Clin Endocrinol Metab* 86:4901–4907, 2001

394. Carpentier A, Mittelman SD, Bergman RN, Giacca A, Lewis GF: Prolonged elevation of plasma free fatty acids impairs pancreatic beta-cell function in obese nondiabetic humans but not in individuals with type 2 diabetes. *Diabetes* 49:399–408, 2000

395. Edelstein SL, Knowler WC, Bain RP, Andres R, Barrett-Connor EL, Dowse GK, Haffner SM, Pettitt DJ, Sorkin JD, Muller DC, Collins VR, Hamman RF: Predictors of progression from impaired glucose tolerance to NIDDM: an analysis of six prospective studies. *Diabetes* 46:701–710, 1997

396. Norris SL, Zhang X, Avenell A, Gregg E, Bowman B, Schmid CH, Lau J: Long-term effectiveness of weight-loss interventions in adults with pre-diabetes: a review. *Am J Prev Med* 28:126–139, 2005

397. Paolisso G, Tataranni P, Foley J, Bogardus C, Howard B, Ravussin E: A high concentration of fasting plasma non-esterified fatty acids is a risk factor for the development of NIDDM. *Diabetologia* 38:1213–1217, 1995

398. Mathew M, Tay C, Belfort R, Gastaldelli A, Wang S, Cusi K: A 48-hour elevation in plasma FFA, but not hyperglyce-mia, Iimpairs insulin secretion in lean Mexican-American subjects genetically predisposed to type 2 diabetes. *Diabetes* 56 (s1):A674, 2007

399. Chiasson JL, Rabasa-Lhoret R: Prevention of type 2 diabetes: insulin resistance and beta-cell function. *Diabetes* 53 (Suppl. 3):S34–38, 2004

400. Pan X-R, Li G-W, Hu Y-H, et al.: Effects of diet and exercise in preventing NIDDM in people with impaired glucose tolerance. The Da Qing IGT and Diabetes Study. *Diabetes Care* 20:537–544, 1997

401. Tuomilehto J, Lindstrom J, Eriksson JG, Valle TT, Hamalainen H, Ilanne-Parikka P, Keinanen-Kiukaanniemi S, Laakso M, Louheranta A, Rastas M, Salminen V, Aunola S, Cepaitis Z, Moltchanov V, Hakumaki M, Mannelin M, Martikkala V, Sundvall J, Uusitupa M: the Finnish Diabetes Prevention Study G: prevention of type 2 diabetes mellitus by changes in lifestyle among subjects with impaired glucose tolerance. *N Engl J Med* 344:1343–1350, 2001

402. Group DPPR: Reduction in the incidence of type 2 diabetes with lifestyle intervention or metformin. *N Engl J Med* 346:393–403, 2002

403. Laaksonen DE, Lindstrom J, Lakka TA, Eriksson JG, Niskanen L, Wikstrom K, Aunola S, Keinanen-Kiukaanniemi S, Laakso M, Valle TT, Ilanne-Parikka P, Louheranta A, Hamalainen H, Rastas M, Salminen V, Cepaitis Z, Hakumaki M, Kaikkonen H, Harkonen P, Sundvall J, Tuomilehto J, Uusitupa M: physical activity in the prevention of type 2 diabetes: the Finnish Diabetes Prevention Study. *Diabetes* 54:158–165, 2005

404. Bravata DM, Smith-Spangler C, Sundaram V, Gienger AL, Lin N, Lewis R, Stave CD, Olkin I, Sirard JR: Using pedometers to increase physical activity and improve health: a systematic review. *JAMA* 298:2296–2304, 2007

405. Torgerson J, Hauptman J, Boldrin M, Sjostrom L: XENical in the prevention of diabetes in obese subjects (XENDOS) study: a randomized study of orlistat as an adjunct to lifestyle changes for the prevention of type 2 diabetes in obese patients. *Diabetes Care* 27:155–161, 2004

406. Chiasson J-L, Josse RG, Gomis R, Hanefeld M, Karasik A, Laakso M, Group. ftS-NTR: acarbose for prevention of type 2 diabetes mellitus: the STOP-NIDDM randomised trial. *Lancet* 359:2072–2077, 2002

407. The Diabetes Prevention Program Research Group: Effects of withdrawal from metformin on the development of diabetes in the Diabetes Prevention Program. *Diabetes Care* 26:977–980, 2003

408. Buchanan TA, Xiang AH, Peters RK, Kjos SL, Marroquin A, Goico J, Ochoa C, Tan S, Berkowitz K, Hodis HN, Azen SP: Preservation of pancreatic b-cell function and prevention of type 2 diabetes by pharmacological treatment of insulin resistance in high-risk Hispanic women. *Diabetes* 51:2796–2803, 2002

409. Group TDPPR: Prevention of type 2 diabetes with troglitazone in the Diabetes Prevention Program. *Diabetes* 54:1150–1156, 2005

410. Xiang AH, Peters RK, Kjos SL, Marroquin A, Goico J, Ochoa C, Kawakubo M, Buchanan TA: Effect of pioglitazone on pancreatic b-cell function and diabetes risk in Hispanic women with prior gestational diabetes. *Diabetes* 55: 517–522, 2006

411. The DREAM (Diabetes Reduction Assessment with Ramipril and Rosiglitazone Medication) Trial Investigators: Effect of rosiglitazone on the frequency of diabetes in patients with impaired glucose tolerance or impaired fasting glucose: a randomised controlled trial. *Lancet* 368:1096–1105, 2006

412. DeFronzo RA et al. ACTos NOW for the prevention of diabetes (ACTNOW) study. American diabetes Assoc. Meeting 2008.

413. Lachin J, Christophi C, Edelstein S, Ehrmann DA, Hamman R, Kahn S, Knowler W, Nathan D, on behalf of the DPP Research Group: Factors associated with diabetes onset during metformin versus placebo therapy in the Diabetes Prevention Program. *Diabetes* 56:1153–1159, 2007

414. Bogacka I, Xie H, Bray GA, Smith SR: The effect of pioglitazone on peroxisome proliferator-activated receptor-gamma target genes related to lipid storage in vivo. *Diabetes Care* 27:1660–1667, 2004

415. Targher G: Associations between plasma adiponectin concentrations and liver histology in patients with nonalcoholic fatty liver disease. *Clin Endocrinol* 64:679–683, 2006

416. Brown J, Plutzky J: Peroxisome proliferator activated receptors as transcriptional nodal points and therapeutic targets. *Circulation* 115:518–533, 2007

417. Brettenthaler N, De Geyter C, Huber PR, Keller U: Effect of the insulin sensitizer pioglitazone on insulin resistance, hyperandrogenism, and ovulatory dysfunction in women with polycystic ovary syndrome. *J Clin Endocrinol Metab* 89:3835–3840, 2004

418. Hanefeld M, Marx N, Pfutzner A, Baurecht W, Lubben G, Karagiannis E, Stier U, Forst T: Anti-inflammatory effects of pioglitazone and/or simvastatin in high cardiovascular risk patients with elevated high sensitivity C-reactive protein: the PIOSTAT study. *J Am Coll Cardiol* 49:290–297, 2007

420. Dormandy JA, Charbonnel B, Eckland DJA, Erdmann E, Massi-Benedetti M, Moules IK, Skene AM, Tan MH, Lefebvre PJ, Standl E, Murray GD, Wilcox RG, Wilhelmsen L, Betteridge J, Birkeland KR, Golay A, Heine RJ, Koranyi L, Laakso M, Moka ÄM: Secondary prevention of macrovascular events in patients with type 2 diabetes in the PROactive Study (PROspective pioglitAzone Clinical Trial In macroVascular Events): a randomised controlled trial Secondary

prevention of macrovascular events in patients with type 2 diabetes in the PROactive Study (PROspective pioglitAzone Clinical Trial in MacroVascular Events): a randomised controlled trial. *Lancet* 366:1279–1289, 2005

421. Wilcox R, Bousser M-G, Betteridge DJ, Schernthaner G, Pirags V, Kupfer S, Dormandy J, for the PI: Effects of pioglitazone in patients with type 2 diabetes with or without previous stroke: results from PROactive (PROspective PioglitAzone Clinical Trial in MacroVascular Events 04). *Stroke* 38:865–873, 2007

422. Erdmann E, Dormandy JA, Charbonnel B, Massi-Benedetti M, Moules IK: The effect of pioglitazone on recurrent myocardial infarction in 2,445 patients with type 2 diabetes and previous myocardial infarction: results from the PROactive (PROactive 05) Study. *J Am Coll Cardiol* 49:1772–1780, 2007

423. Lincoff AM, Wolski K, Nicholls SJ, Nissen SE: Pioglitazone and risk of cardiovascular events in patients with type 2 diabetes mellitus: a meta-analysis of randomized trials. *JAMA* 298:1180–1188, 2007

424. Nissen SE, Wolski K: Effect of rosiglitazone on the risk of myocardial infarction and death from cardiovascular causes. *N Engl J Med* 356:2457–2471, 2007

425. Singh S, Loke YK, Furberg CD: Long-term risk of cardiovascular events with rosiglitazone: a meta-analysis. *JAMA* 298:1189–1195, 2007

427. The Diabetes Prevention Program Research Group: Role of insulin secretion and sensitivity in the evolution of type 2 diabetes in the Diabetes Prevention Program: effects of lifestyle intervention and metformin. *Diabetes* 54:2404–2414, 2005

2 Prevention of Type 2 Diabetes

Jonathan E. Shaw and Richard W. Simpson

CONTENTS

ABSTRACT

The numbers of people with type 2 diabetes are rising rapidly around the world, making it imperative to develop and introduce methods of preventing the condition. A series of clinical trials over the last decade has shown conclusively that lifestyle interventions focusing on physical activity, diet, and weight loss can reduce the risk of developing type 2 diabetes by approximately 60%. Trials examining pharmaceutical interventions have shown that metformin, acarbose, and glitazones also reduce the risk of developing diabetes, but have shown no benefit of ACE inhibitors. Although uncertainty remains about the widespread use of pharmaceutical agents for diabetes prevention, programmes to implement lifestyle changes in those at high risk of developing type 2 diabetes now need to be put in place.

Key words: Type 2 diabetes; Lifestyle intervention; Physical activity; Diet.

From: *Contemporary Diabetes: Diabetes and Exercise*
Edited by: J. G. Regensteiner et al. (eds.), DOI: 10.1007/978-1-59745-260-1_2
© Humana Press, a part of Springer Science+Business Media, LLC 2009

INTRODUCTION

Over recent decades, type 2 diabetes has become a major public health threat. As its prevalence has risen, it has become an increasingly important cause of cardiovascular disease (CVD), renal failure, visual loss and lower limb amputation. In many developed countries, its rising prevalence threatens to reverse the declines in cardiovascular mortality witnessed over the last 40–50 years, whilst in developing countries diabetes is one of the key factors in the switch from communicable to non-communicable diseases.

The most recent data suggest that there are currently 246 million adults with diabetes worldwide (at least 90% of this is type 2 diabetes), and that this will rise to 380 million individuals by the year 2025 *(1)* (Fig. 1). Although some of the increase in numbers of individuals with type 2 diabetes is due to the ageing of the population, lifestyle change has also played a major role in increasing the risk of type 2 diabetes. At a population level, the link with lifestyle is demonstrated by the approximately fourfold higher prevalence of diabetes among South Asians living in urbanised settings in the UK *(2)*, Mauritius *(3)* and India *(4)*, compared with those living in rural India *(5)*. Longitudinal studies have demonstrated that reduced physical activity and certain dietary aspects are risk factors for the development of type 2 diabetes *(6–8)*, while O'Dea has shown that when Australian aboriginals (who are among the populations with the greatest risk for and prevalence of type 2 diabetes) revert from a westernized lifestyle to a traditional hunter-gatherer lifestyle, they rapidly show profound metabolic improvement *(9)*.

The accumulating observational evidence linking both physical activity and diet to type 2 diabetes led to the belief that it would be possible to prevent type 2 diabetes with lifestyle change and, potentially, with glucose-lowering drugs. The rising tide of type 2 diabetes and the personal, social and societal impact of diabetic complications has made it imperative that all avenues of diabetes prevention are explored, and the last few years have seen the results of a number of major trials of diabetes prevention published.

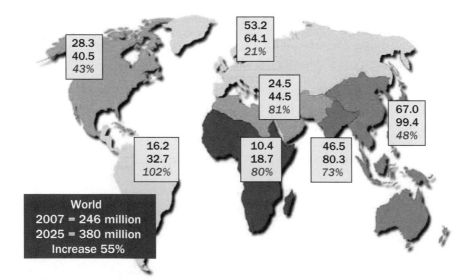

Fig. 1. The predicted global distribution and increase of diabetes: 2007–2025. The estimate is based on expected growth and ageing of the population *(1)*. The *upper* and *middle* figures represent the numbers of adults aged 20–79 (in millions) with diabetes for 2007 and 2025, respectively. The *lower* figures represent the percentage increase in numbers between 2007 and 2025.

This chapter will review the findings from the major diabetes prevention trials, with a focus mainly on those using lifestyle interventions, but will also describe the results of the pharmaceutical trials.

LIFESTYLE INTERVENTION STUDIES

A number of small, generally short-term, studies involving participants with various degrees of impaired glucose regulation were reported in the 1980s and 1990s *(10–12)*. Most of them had problems with design. Generally, however, these studies showed a benefit of healthy (or traditional) lifestyle on improving or delaying deterioration of glucose tolerance.

There have now been six large controlled and longer-term trials examining the effect of lifestyle changes on the progression from impaired glucose tolerance (IGT) to type 2 diabetes. The main lifestyle intervention targets were body weight, diet and physical activity. The intervention methods used to modify lifestyle varied between the studies as socio-cultural issues and the available facilities and personnel differed. Although there remained some methodological problems with the first two of these trials *(13, 14)*, the others were classical randomised controlled trials and provided a high level of evidence on the benefits of lifestyle change.

THE MALMÖ STUDY

This feasibility study examined the benefits of diet and exercise in 217 middle-aged men in MalmO with IGT *(13)*. The subjects chose whether they would be in the intervention or reference groups (in ratio 3:1). Thus, the subjects were not randomly assigned to the study groups and this diminishes the ability to generalise the results. The treatment group received detailed dietary advice and support within an exercise program while the other group received standard medical care according to requirements. Neither group received any form of anti-diabetic drug. Over a period of 5 years, the treated subjects significantly reduced and maintained weight loss (body mass index, BMI, fell 2.5% in the intervention group and rose 0.5% in the reference group). In addition, the estimated maximal oxygen uptake (a measure of physical fitness) increased by 10% in the intervention subjects, while it decreased by 5% in the control men. In the treated group 10.6% developed type 2 diabetes vs. 28.6% of the reference subjects. The relative risk reduction (RRR) in the incidence in the intervention group was 59% and the absolute risk reduction (ARR) was 17% points. Although the progression to diabetes in the reference group of Swedish men was lower than would be predicted from the observational studies (which may have been due to a relatively low BMI), this study demonstrated the feasibility of carrying out a diet and exercise program for 5 years among volunteers, and suggested that such a program might have significant benefits in the prevention of type 2 diabetes.

THE DA QING STUDY

The Da Qing IGT and Diabetes Study, published in 1997, involved a large population-based screening program to identify people with IGT *(14)*. The effect of exercise and diet in preventing the development of type 2 diabetes in 577 subjects with IGT was examined over 6 years in 33 hospital clinics across China. There were four intervention groups; diet alone, exercise alone, diet–exercise combined or no intervention. Randomisation into these groups was undertaken on a clinic rather than an individual basis. For dietary intervention, the participants were recommended a high-carbohydrate and low-fat diet and encouraged to reduce weight if BMI was ≥25 kg/m^2 aiming at 23 kg/m^2. Group sessions were organised weekly for the first month, monthly for 3 months and then three monthly. For the clinics assigned physical exercise, counselling sessions were arranged at a similar frequency. The participants were encouraged to increase their level of leisure-time physical activity by at least 1–2 'units'/day. One unit was defined as 30 min slow walking, 10 min slow running or 5 min swimming.

The annual risk of progressing to type 2 diabetes from IGT in this population was reduced from 15.7% in the control group to 8% in the three intervention groups. The cumulative 6-year incidence of type 2 diabetes in the three intervention groups was 41–46% compared with 68% in the control group. The reported changes in risk factor patterns were modest. There was an approximate 1 kg/m^2 reduction of BMI in subjects with baseline BMI >25 kg/m^2 with no change in BMI for the lean subjects. The estimated changes in habitual dietary nutrient intakes were small and non-significant between groups. Thus, it appears that neither weight change nor even diet were the major determinants of the outcome. Physical activity and possibly subtle qualitative changes in diet played a key role.

There is a major methodological limitation in this study as allocation to intervention group was based on clinic (cluster) rather than the individual subject randomisation. Individual data analysis must, therefore, be interpreted with caution. The study subjects were relatively lean (mean BMI 25.8 kg/m^2) compared with subjects with IGT from other ethnic groups, and the progression from IGT to diabetes was high (over 10% per year in the control group) compared with findings in observational studies. These issues make it difficult to generalise the conclusions. Furthermore, the similarity in outcomes for the three different intervention groups was somewhat surprising, as it suggested that there was no benefit in combining diet and exercise over pursuing either one individually. Thus, like the MalmO study, the Da Qing study was suggestive of the benefits of lifestyle intervention, but not conclusive.

THE FINNISH DIABETES PREVENTION STUDY

The Finnish Diabetes Prevention Study (FDPS) *(15)*, the first properly controlled trial on prevention of type 2 diabetes with lifestyle modification (diet and exercise) alone, enrolled 523 subjects with IGT from five clinics in Finland between 1993 and 1998. Subjects (age 40–64 years, BMI over 25 kg/m^2) were individually randomly allocated into the intervention and control groups with stratification according to centre, gender and severity of IGT.

In the intervention group, subjects received advice from a nutritionist seven times during the first year and then every 3 months. The intervention goals were reduction in weight of 5% or more, total fat intake to less than 30% of energy consumed, saturated fat intake to less than 10% of energy consumed, fibre intake of at least 15 g/1,000 kcal and moderate exercise of at least 30 min/day. The subjects were individually counselled to increase their level of endurance exercise (walking, jogging, swimming, aerobic ball games, skiing). Supervised and individually tailored resistance training sessions were also offered. There were seven personal counselling sessions in the first 12 months, with three-monthly sessions thereafter. The control group subjects were given general verbal and written advice about healthy lifestyle at the beginning of the study. An oral glucose tolerance test (OGTT) was performed annually but the study end-point of type 2 diabetes was based on a confirmatory second OGTT.

After a median follow-up of 3 years, 86 cases of diabetes had developed which was about half of the 160 cases predicted for the full period of the planned 6-year study. The cumulative incidence of diabetes after 4 years was 11% in the intervention group and 23% in the control group, a reduction of 58% (*P* < 0.001) in risk of diabetes in the intervention group. The reduction in the incidence of diabetes was directly associated with changes in lifestyle (Fig. 2); none of the people (either in the intervention or in the control group) who had reached all five lifestyle targets by the 1-year visit developed diabetes.

A further publication from this study has shown the status of participants 3 years after the end of the intervention *(16)*. Although the trial intervention was no longer being provided, a significant difference in the incidence of diabetes has persisted throughout this post-intervention follow-up

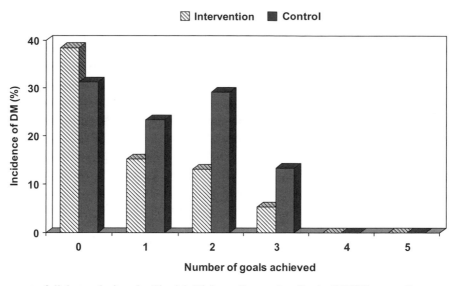

Fig. 2. Development of diabetes during the Finnish Diabetes Prevention Study (*FDPS*), according to number of intervention goals achieved *(15)*.

period, with the group originally in the lifestyle intervention arm still showing a 43% reduction in the incidence of diabetes over the lifetime of the trial. Even during the post-intervention period, the incidence of diabetes was 36% lower in the 'intervention' than the 'control' group. The mechanism of this profound 'hangover' effect remains uncertain, and some have suggested that the initial intervention produced a 'metabolic memory'. However, it seems likely that at least part of the explanation can be accounted for by the persistence of differences in lifestyle between the two groups beyond the end of the structured intervention and by the weight differences (or at least differences in fat mass) between the two groups during the intervention period. Indeed, the intervention group continued to achieve more of the lifestyle goals during the post-intervention phase than did the control group.

The study has also been analysed to determine which of the key goals was of most importance in producing the benefits *(16)*. When considered individually, achievement of each of the lifestyle goals, except the goal for saturated fat, was associated with a reduced incidence of diabetes. However, when considered together, only weight loss was significantly associated with benefits, indicating that most of the benefits of diet and exercise were mediated through weight loss. Thus, individuals who did not lose weight were unlikely to reduce their risk of developing diabetes, even if they reported that they were complying with the other lifestyle targets.

THE DIABETES PREVENTION PROGRAM

Recently, but prematurely completed, the Diabetes Prevention Program (DPP) (the data safety and monitoring board-advised closure) was a large multi-centre, randomised and placebo-controlled clinical trial carried out in the USA *(17)*. It involved an ethnically diverse population and was designed to investigate the effect of very aggressive lifestyle intervention (and metformin and troglitazone to be discussed below) in IGT patients. The study included 2,161 (in lifestyle and placebo arms) high-risk individuals with IGT and a fasting plasma glucose over 5.5 mmol/L. Special educators ('case managers' who were not regular health personnel) primarily carried out the lifestyle intervention in DPP. The lifestyle intervention involved a 16-session structured core curriculum within the first 24 weeks after randomisation, with sessions occurring approximately monthly for the remainder of the trial. The focus of the dietary intervention was initially on reducing total fat intake but later calorie balance was introduced with a goal to achieve and maintain a weight loss of at least 7%. A physical activity target was set of ~700-kcal/week expenditure (this equalled ~150 min of moderate physical activity, such as brisk walking, every week). Clinical centres also offered voluntary-supervised activity sessions.

In the DPP, of the participants assigned to intensive lifestyle intervention, 74% achieved the study goal of ≥150 min of activity per week at 24 weeks and at the 1-year visit the mean weight loss was 7 kg (about 7% of baseline weight). With intensive lifestyle intervention there was a 58% RRR in progression to type 2 diabetes compared with the placebo group. The lifestyle intervention was effective over a range of age, BMI and racial or ethnic subgroups.

In an analysis of those in the intensive lifestyle arm of the study (18), increased physical activity and reduced percent of fat in the diet predicted weight loss, but only weight loss was independently associated with a reduced incidence of diabetes. For every kilogram of weight loss, there was a 16% reduction in the risk of developing diabetes. Thus, like the FDPS, this study also showed that dietary and exercise goals are important in achieving weight loss, but unless weight loss is achieved, the risks of developing diabetes do not alter.

THE INDIAN DIABETES PREVENTION PROGRAME

The Indian Diabetes Prevention Programe (19) randomised 531 Asian Indian participants with IGT (79% men) into four groups – control, lifestyle modification, metformin and lifestyle plus metformin. The lifestyle intervention included both physical activity and dietary advice. Participants in the lifestyle groups were advised to walk briskly for at least 30 min daily, and those who were already achieving this goal at recruitment were encouraged to maintain their activity level. Dietary advice included avoidance of simple sugars and refined carbohydrates, fat intake not to exceed 20 g/day and an increase in fibre-rich food. Direct face-to-face counselling sessions were undertaken at baseline and every 6 months during the study, with telephone contact maintained monthly.

Over 3 years of follow-up, the cumulative incidence of diabetes was 55% in the control group, and was 39.3% in the lifestyle group. Thus, the RRR attributable to the lifestyle intervention was 28.5%, while the ARR was 15.7% points. There was no additive benefit of combining lifestyle with metformin – with the cumulative incidence of diabetes of 39.5% in this group being almost identical to that in the lifestyle alone group. Despite the more modest RRR than in some of the other studies, the high absolute conversion rate to diabetes meant that the number of individuals needed to treat over 3 years to prevent one case of diabetes was only 6.4 for the lifestyle intervention.

It is unclear exactly why the benefits of lifestyle intervention were smaller in this Indian population than in the US, Finnish and Chinese studies. However, there are a number of possible explanations. First, there were fewer face-to-face lifestyle counselling sessions in the Indian study, and this may have diminished the capacity to deliver an intensive lifestyle programe. Indeed, body weight hardly changed in the lifestyle group, and change in the body weight was not correlated with change in the plasma glucose. Second, the Indian population was described as being 'already physically active and were on a diet similar to that prescribed' at baseline. Thus, the lifestyle differences during the study (i.e. resulting from the intervention) between the lifestyle and control groups may not have been as great as in the other studies. Third, it is possible that ethnic differences in response to intervention may play a role, although the small number of Asians (4.4%) in the American DPP responded as well as other ethnic groups in that study. Finally, the Indian study population was younger and leaner (mean BMI 26 kg/m^2) than the American and Finnish populations.

JAPANESE DIABETES PREVENTION TRIAL

The Japanese diabetes prevention trial recruited 458 males with IGT (80% were government employees), and randomised them to a control or intensive lifestyle intervention in a 4:1 ratio *(20)*. The intervention was focused on reducing BMI to 22 kg/m². Dietary targets were individualised and targeted portion size, fat intake (advised to be <50 g daily), alcohol intake and limited eating out. A physical activity target of 30–40 min of moderate activity/day was set, and was being achieved by 15% of participants at baseline. The intervention was reinforced at study visits conducted every 2–3 months throughout the study.

Over the 4 years that the study ran for, the cumulative incidence of diabetes was 3.0% in the intervention group and 9.3% in the control group. Thus, the intervention resulted in a RRR of 67.4% and an ARR of 6.3% points. It was noteworthy that within the control group, the cumulative incidence of diabetes varied from 14.7% among those who gained at least 1.0 kg to only 4.3% in those who lost at least 1.0 kg. The intervention group had a mean weight loss of 2.18 kg. Whilst weight loss was a major mediator of the reduced incidence, it did not explain all the benefits observed.

The lifestyle prevention trials have now provided unequivocal evidence that type 2 diabetes can be prevented (or at least delayed) in subjects with IGT. The major findings of the six studies are summarised and compared in Table 1.

The similarity of the RRR of five of the six studies is striking over a range of BMI values (**Table 1**). The near identical RRR of Malmö, FDPS and DPP is remarkable. The higher ARR in the Da Qing study was a result of the higher risk of diabetes in that study population, while the lower ARR in the Japanese study reflects the lower risks of diabetes in that population. The lesser impact of an intensive lifestyle intervention in the Indian study most likely represents the lesser intensity of the delivery of the lifestyle intervention, with face-to-face appointments only occurring every 6 months.

SURGICAL OR DRUG-INDUCED WEIGHT LOSS

As yet there are no randomised-controlled trials of surgical treatment of obesity but in a group of severely overweight subjects with IGT undergoing gastric bypass surgery, the rate of conversion over 4–6 years to type 2 diabetes after an average weight loss of 22.5 kg was 0.15/100 persons/year. This was compared to a conversion rate of 4.72/100 persons/year in an un-operated group, a 30-fold reduction in risk with this intervention *(21)*. Likewise, in the Swedish Obese Subjects (SOS) Intervention Study *(22)*, gastric surgery in very obese subjects reduced the 2-year incidence of diabetes 30-fold in

Table 1
Summary of the Findings of the Six Lifestyle Intervention Studies in People with IGT

Study	Cohort size	Mean BMI (kg/m²)	Duration (years)	RRR (%)	ARR (%)	NNT
MalmO *(10)*	217	26.6	5	63	18	28
FDPS *(15)*	523	31.0	3	58	12	22
DPP *(17)*	2,161[a]	34.0	3	58	15	21
Da Qing *(14)*	259[a]	25.8	6	46	27	25
Indian *(19)*	269[a]	26.0	2.5	29	16	19
Japanese *(20)*	458	23.9	4	67	6	63

[a] Combined numbers for placebo and diet and exercise groups
FDPS Finnish Diabetes Prevention Study, *DPP* Diabetes Prevention Program, *IGT* impaired glucose tolerance, *BMI* body mass index, *RRR* relative risk reduction, *ARR* absolute risk reduction, *NNT* number needed to treat for 1 year to prevent one case of diabetes

grossly obese subjects (weight loss 28 kg) compared with control subjects who were receiving regular care (weight loss 0.5 kg). More recently, data on laparascopic gastric band surgery have been reported. Among 434 non-diabetic patients (BMI ≥ 35 kg/m²), followed up over 923 patient years after the procedure, none developed diabetes *(23)*. These results suggest that severe obesity can be treated surgically and lead to a marked reduction in the incidence of diabetes.

The Xendos [Xenical (orlistat) in the prevention of diabetes in obese subjects] *(24)* trial randomised 3,305 obese participants, aged 30–60 years of whom 21% had IGT to orlistat (which leads to weight loss by reducing intestinal fat absorption) or placebo. All participants received lifestyle advice (calorie-reduced diet and exercise counselling) initially two weekly for 6 months and thereafter monthly. Over 4 years, among those with IGT, orlistat reduced the incidence of diabetes by 45% (RRR 45%, ARR 10% points). Weight reduction was 6.9 kg in the orlistat group and 4.1 kg in the placebo group. Unfortunately, there was a high drop out rate over the 4-year treatment phase in both groups; 52% in orlistat and 34% in placebo.

Both the surgical and the orlistat studies in obese subjects indicate that probably weight control alone is an efficient way to prevent the development of type 2 diabetes.

PHARMACOLOGICAL INTERVENTION STUDIES

Prior to the last few years, there were nine, generally small and poorly designed, intervention studies using oral hypoglycemic agents published that examined patients over 1–10 years. All were commenced prior to 1979 when there was no agreement on the definition of pre-diabetic states and the subjects, according to recent diagnostic criteria, were probably a mixture of early type 2 diabetes and IGT. Seven studies investigated tolbutamide, and on an intention to treat analysis, four *(25–28)* reported improvement in glucose tolerance and/or reduced incidence of type 2 diabetes while three reported no benefit *(10, 29, 30)*. However, the Malmöhus study *(10)* reported a large non-compliance rate in the tolbutamide group and found prevention of progression when analysis was based on treatment compliance. This is an intriguing observation in view of the four earlier positive studies and awaits further study. Two intervention studies with phenformin did not show benefit *(31, 32)*. Finally, two studies examined glibenclamide with mixed results *(32, 33)* and one study employing World Health Organisation (WHO) criteria examined gliclazide and reported no benefit *(34)*. All these pharmacological studies, most containing fewer than 200 subjects in each of the intervention groups, would now be regarded as significantly underpowered.

Study to Prevent Noninsulin-Dependent Diabetes Mellitus Study

The Study to Prevent Noninsulin-Dependent Diabetes Mellitus (STOP–NIDDM) study *(35)*, a Canadian–European double-blind, placebo-controlled randomised trial evaluated whether acarbose (an α-glucosidase inhibitor) could prevent the development of diabetes in 1,429 high-risk subjects with IGT. After a mean of 3.3 years of follow up, but including an approximate 25% discontinuation rate on acarbose, there was a 25% reduction in progression to diabetes (based on a single OGTT) attributable to acarbose. The main results were based on an intention-to-treat analysis. The drug was effective in the different subgroups of age, gender and BMI. However, the benefit of treatment on prevention seemed to be reduced after only 3 months following cessation of active treatment.

Diabetes Prevention Program

The Diabetes Prevention Program (DPP) was initially set up to investigate individually the benefits of metformin, troglitazone (a PPARγ agonist), and diet and exercise. As a result of the increased risk of severe liver damage and in some instances fatal hepatic toxicity caused by troglitazone, this arm was discontinued after 2 years. The DPP found that metformin reduced the risk of progression to type 2 diabetes from IGT by 31% while still taking the drug. The reduction in progression was less (24.9%) when metformin was ceased, and allowed drug washout to occur before assessing glucose tolerance *(36)*. The benefit of metformin was not seen in subjects over the age of 60 years or in those with a BMI less than 30 kg/m² *(17)*.

Analysis of the troglitazone arm of the study over a mean of 0.9 years showed a 75% reduction in the incidence of diabetes, with most of the benefit being due to an improvement in insulin sensitivity *(37)*.

Troglitazone in the Prevention of Diabetes

Although the troglitazone arm of DPP was discontinued, a small 5-year double-blind study involving 250 Hispanic women living in Los Angeles with a history of gestational diabetes (~70% with IGT) were randomised to either troglitazone or placebo *(38)*. Women with a history of gestational diabetes mellitus (GDM) are at a high risk for developing type 2 diabetes. Over a median follow-up period of 31 months, there was a 56% reduction in the conversion of these patients to type 2 diabetes. The average annual incidence of diabetes was 5.4% in women randomised to troglitazone and 12.1% in the placebo group ($P < 0.01$). The group of women most responsive to intervention with troglitazone was those who 3 months after randomisation showed the greatest reduction in insulin resistance and fall in insulin secretion to an intravenous glucose tolerance test. There was also evidence that the protection conferred by troglitazone against developing type 2 diabetes persisted for about 8 months after treatment ceased.

Chinese Diabetes Prevention Study

In a small multi-centre study ($n = 321$) *(39)* subjects with IGT were divided into four groups: controls who received conventional education, diet and exercise, metformin and acarbose. As in the Da Qing study, allocation into groups was not random, but took place by geographical location. Over a 3-year period 34.9%, 24.6%, 12.4%, and 6.0% of each group, respectively, progressed to diabetes. This represents a RRR of 76.8% for metformin and 87.8% for acarbose compared with the control group. The mean BMI for the three groups was ~25 kg/m², which in relation to metformin is inconsistent with the DPP findings, which showed no benefit of metformin in those with a BMI <30 kg/m².

Diabetes Reduction Assessment with Ramipril and Rosiglitazone Medication Trial

The Diabetes Reduction Assessment with Ramipril and Rosiglitazone Medication (DREAM) trial is the largest of all the diabetes prevention studies, and the only one to include participants with both IGT and impaired fasting glucose (IFG). The 2 × 2 factorial design of the study allowed it to separately test whether the angiotensin converting enzyme (ACE) inhibitor, ramipril, and the PPARγ agonist, rosiglitazone, could prevent the development of diabetes. In addition to the smaller studies discussed above that showed the potential of PPARγ agonists in diabetes prevention, a significant body of evidence had suggested that ACE inhibitors might also play a role in the prevention of diabetes. In particular, the Heart Outcomes Prevention Evaluation (HOPE) study showed in post-hoc analyses that ramipril was associated with a 34% reduction in the incidence of diabetes *(40)*. HOPE, like a number of other cardiovascular studies showing similar results, was not designed to test the value of ACE inhibitors in diabetes prevention – hence, the need for a trial designed specifically to test this hypothesis. DREAM randomised 5,269 adults from 21 countries, and followed the participants for a median of 3 years. Ramipril was associated with a non-significant 9% reduction in the incidence of diabetes *(41)*, while rosiglitazone led to a highly significant 60% reduction in the development of diabetes *(42)*.

The benefits of rosiglitazone were seen in all the pre-specified sub-groups, but were greatest in those who were most overweight at baseline. Indeed, while the incidence of diabetes increased, as expected, with increasing adiposity in the placebo group, there was no such increase in the rosiglitazone group.

It is also important to note the side effects of rosiglitazone, which were similar to those reported in trials of the drug in people with established diabetes – weight gain, and a small, but significant, increase in risk of cardiac failure. Somewhat disappointingly, the DREAM trial failed to show even a trend towards cardiovascular benefit with either of the drugs, though it should be noted that DREAM was not designed to determine the effect on CVD, and the small number of CVD events occurring in the trial was consistent with the exclusion from the trial at baseline of anyone with a prior history of CVD. However, significant concern has subsequently developed over the safety of PPARγ agonists, with regard to CVD and to fractures. First, a meta-analysis indicated a higher risk of CVD in patients treated with rosiglitazone (ref), though an interim analysis of a large clinical trial focusing on CVD has not confirmed this (ref). Second, an excess of fractures (possibly osteoporotic) has been reported with both of the currently available PPARγ agonists (ref). Thus, the use of PPARγ agonists for diabetes prevention is not currently recommended.

DIABETES PREVENTION: REAL PREVENTION OR JUST DELAY IN ONSET?

Much debate over recent years has centred on whether any of the so-called diabetes prevention trials are actually reporting disease prevention or simply a delay in the time of disease onset. People have argued that the apparently impressive findings of the prevention of 60% of the expected cases of diabetes equates to no more than a delay in the onset of diabetes of a year or so. Within the confines of a 3-year clinical trial, a 1–2 year delay in disease development will have profound effects on the total number of people developing diabetes, but the average 50-year old, who might hope to live for another 25–30 years might be less impressed with an intervention that postpones his date of diabetes onset from his 60th to his 62nd birthday.

The term 'prevention' is often interpreted as meaning stopping diabetes from ever happening (although most dictionaries definitions include the meaning of hindering as well as stopping), and as such could only be shown in very long clinical trials. Of course, delaying the onset of diabetes until the individual dies of something else amounts to lifetime prevention for that individual.

Interventions that 'fix' a problem and genuinely prevent a disease from ever occurring are generally restricted to the arena of conditions such as infectious diseases, where vaccinations, or public health measures, such as providing clean water, have virtually eliminated a number of infections. However, for diseases such as type 2 diabetes, which appear to be strongly linked to age-related functional decline or degeneration in physiological systems, interventions that can be expected to 'fix' the problem seem much less likely. Specifically for type 2 diabetes, the age-related decline in beta cell function often leads to diabetes among the elderly even if they remain relatively lean.

Interestingly, although this debate could equally apply to other chronic diseases, such as CVD, it does not seem to have taken place. Thus, no one discusses whether lipid lowering with statins prevents or only delays myocardial infarction, though it is abundantly clear that a sizeable proportion of those successfully treated in the intervention arm of a statin trial will still suffer a vascular event at some time after the study ends. The results of such studies are usually reported in terms of the reduction of risk or reduction of incidence of the endpoint over the duration of the study. This would likely be a more useful way of presenting the diabetes prevention trials. The conclusion that over 3 years, a lifestyle intervention reduces the risk of developing diabetes or reduces the incidence of diabetes by 58% is a simple statement of the results, is in the same format as most other prevention studies, and describes the results of the trial without making any implications about lifetime risk. In retrospect, the use of the term 'prevention', though justifiably a high priority for researchers to achieve, has probably led to unrealistic beliefs about the long-term effects of interventions among the public and to a sterile debate between healthcare professionals about the meaning of delay and prevention. A focus on describing findings in terms of risk reduction and lowering of blood glucose would be much more constructive. The real debate could then address issues such as cost-effectiveness and the implementation of the trial results into clinical practice, which will ultimately be far more important in delivering effective interventions to populations.

POPULATION APPROACHES TO PREVENTION OF TYPE 2 DIABETES

The series of lifestyle intervention trials have shown beyond any shadow of a doubt that changes to diet and exercise patterns can markedly reduce the risk of developing diabetes. Furthermore, the findings have been applicable across a wide range of demographic groups. In addition, the results of drug trials show that there are also a number of effective pharmacological options. When attempting to translate these findings into benefits for the wider population, several questions need to be addressed. The first is to what extent the lifestyle interventions tested in the clinical trials could be effective outside a research setting. It needs to be remembered that clinical trials only recruit those volunteers who are already prepared to undertake the intervention – those who are not interested in making such changes are unlikely to volunteer, though may represent a significant proportion of the at-risk population. Furthermore, the funding and infrastructure available are far greater in a clinical trial than clinical practice or public health can offer even in the wealthiest of healthcare systems. Currently, we do not know whether the level of intervention available outside clinical trials would be effective, especially when delivered to individuals who would not have had the personal motivation to volunteer for a trial. No studies have compared different intensities of lifestyle intervention. However, the similarity of risk reduction observed in the DPP, the DPS and the Japanese study suggests that the lesser intensity of intervention applied by the two latter trials (study visits every 2–3 months) may provide as much benefit as the more intensive DPP (16 study visits in the first 6 months). The lesser risk reduction seen in the Indian study, with face-to-face study visits occurring only every 6 months, suggests that the optimal level of intervention involves more frequent lifestyle counselling, and probably requires approximately four to six face-to-face visits annually. The length and intensity of a program, the frequency of program visits and the use of self-monitoring have all been shown to be important for weight loss programs *(43)*, and, hence, are likely to be important in diabetes prevention. Studies examining different intensities of intervention, and studies designed to include all of the at-risk population (rather than just clinical trial enthusiasts) are now needed.

A second crucial issue in designing a population approach to diabetes prevention is determining the balance between targeting high-risk groups and targeting the general population. The potential impact of rolling out a high-risk approach (i.e. programs designed to reproduce clinical trial results in people with IGT) will always be limited. Reasons for this include the difficulty of identifying all those at high risk, and the fact that epidemiological studies show that over a 5-year period, ~20% of new cases of diabetes had normal glucose tolerance at baseline *(44)*. To maximise the population impact, this high-risk approach needs to be coupled with a lower intensity, but more broadly-based population-wide approach focused on weight loss, or at least on the prevention of weight gain. A small shift in the population means BMI would have profound effects on the numbers of individuals within the population developing type 2 diabetes.

The third important issue is the role of pharmacological therapy. None of the pharmacological (or lifestyle) trials reported so far have been designed to look at hard clinical end-points (such as CVD or microvascular complications). The first trial to do so will be the NAVIGATOR trial, examining the effects of valsartan and nateglinide in the prevention of diabetes and of CVD. Thus, while it is likely that lowering blood glucose in people with IGT will ultimately result in clinical benefits, this is unproven. Given the potential financial costs of treating the 10–15% of adults who have IFG and IGT, and the risk of side-effects over the many years of drug exposure that would be required, widespread use of drugs in the attempt to prevent type 2 diabetes cannot currently be justified. However, while lifestyle change appears to be a much better option (with far fewer side-effects, and an additional beneficial impact on cardiovascular risk factors other than glucose), there are those who are unable to make substantial changes (e.g. those in whom disease or old age limit their exercise capacity), some who fail to respond to an intensive lifestyle program, and some who might be judged to be at such high risk that a combined lifestyle and pharmacological approach might be appropriate from the outset. No consensus has emerged on the role of drugs, but the two groups that would seem the most important to consider for drug therapy are those who fail to lose weight in a lifestyle program, and those who are at highest risk (probably determined by blood glucose levels – the co-occurrence of IFG and IGT in the same individual is probably a useful definition of this high-risk group). Public funding or reimbursement of the costs of such pharmacological therapy is unlikely to be widely approved, given the currently available data, but after a full explanation of the risks, benefits and costs, it would not be unreasonable for an individual with IGT or IFG to choose to pay for drug treatment.

Finally, it is becoming increasingly apparent that in order to achieve meaningful lifestyle changes across a whole population, input from outside the health sector will be required. In order to alter the obesogenic environment that is now so prevalent, changes to food labelling and taxation, education, advertising, urban planning and transport will all need to be considered. In both Finland *(45)* and Mauritius *(46)*, changes at a governmental level including public health campaigns and changes in taxation and food supply were highly successful in lowering the mean population cholesterol level. Without similar societal action directed at weight control, it is unlikely that even the best organised health system can translate the findings of clinical trials into substantial population-wide reductions in diabetes incidence.

SUMMARY

It is now abundantly clear that the risk of developing type 2 diabetes can be substantially reduced by lifestyle change and by a number of glucose-lowering drugs. Lifestyle intervention directed at fat and calorie restriction, increased dietary fibre intake, and at achieving a minimum of 30 min of moderate exercise daily is the method of choice in reducing the incidence of type 2 diabetes. The focus should be on achieving weight loss and surgery and weight loss drugs may also be appropriate. However, weight loss is achieved, the greater the reduction in weight back to a healthy level, the greater the impact on reducing the risk of developing diabetes. While pharmacological therapy is clearly able to lower blood glucose in those with IGT and IFG, the lack of information on its impact on hard clinical outcomes makes it currently unsuitable for widespread use in those with IGT and IFG.

Health systems need to develop ways of identifying those at high risk of developing diabetes, and implementing intensive lifestyle programs. This needs to be supported by societal changes that facilitate the pursuit of healthy lifestyles for everyone.

REFERENCES

1. Sicree R, Shaw JE, Zimmet PZ: Diabetes and impaired glucose tolerance. In *Diabetes Atlas*, 3rd ed. Gan D, Ed. Brussels, International Diabetes Federation, 2006, 10–149.
2. Riste L, Khan F, Cruickshank K: High prevalence of type 2 diabetes in all ethnic groups, including Europeans, in a British inner city: relative poverty, history, inactivity, or 21st century Europe? *Diabetes Care* 24:1377–1383, 2001.

3. Soderberg S, Zimmet P, Tuomilehto J, de Courten M, Dowse GK, Chitson P, Gareeboo H, Alberti KG, Shaw JE: Increasing prevalence of type 2 diabetes mellitus in all ethnic groups in Mauritius. *Diabetes Med* 22:61–68, 2005.
4. Ramachandran A, Snehalatha C, Kapur A, Vijay V, Mohan V, Das AK, Rao PV, Yajnik CS, Prasannakumar KM, Nair JD: High prevalence of diabetes and impaired glucose tolerance in India: National Urban Diabetes Survey. *Diabetologia* 44: 1094–1101, 2001.
5. Sadikot SM, Nigam A, Das S, Bajaj S, Zargar AH, Prasannakumar KM, Sosale A, Munichoodappa C, Seshiah V, Singh SK, Jamal A, Sai K, Sadasivrao Y, Murthy SS, Hazra DK, Jain S, Mukherjee S, Bandyopadhay S, Sinha NK, Mishra R, Dora M, Jena B, Patra P, Goenka K: The burden of diabetes and impaired glucose tolerance in India using the WHO 1999 criteria: prevalence of diabetes in India study (PODIS). *Diabetes Res Clin Pract* 66:301–307, 2004.
6. Salme ron J, Hu FB, Manson JE, Stampfer MJ, Colditz GA, Rimm EB, Willett WC: Dietary fat intake and risk of type 2 diabetes in women. *Am J Clin Nutr* 73:1019–1026, 2001.
7. Salmerón J, Manson JE, Stampfer MJ, Colditz GA, Wing AL, Willet WC: Dietary fiber, glycemic load, and risk of non-insulin-dependent diabetes mellitus in women. *JAMA* 277:472–477, 1997.
8. Perry I, Wannamethee S, Walker M, Thomson AG, Whincup PH, Shaper AG: Prospective study of risk factors for development of non-insulin dependent diabetes in middle aged British men. *Br J Med* 310:560–564, 1995.
9. O'Dea K: Marked improvement in carbohydrate and lipid metabolism in diabetic Australian aborigines after temporary reversion to traditional lifestyle. *Diabetes* 33:596–603, 1984.
10. Sartor G, Scherstén B, Carlström S, Melander A, Nordén Å, Persson G: Ten-year follow-up of subjects with impaired glucose tolerance. Prevention of diabetes by tolbutamide and diet regulation. *Diabetes* 29:41–49, 1980.
11. Bourn D, Mann J, McSkimming B, Waldron M, Wishart J: Impaired glucose tolerance and NIDDM: does a lifestyle intervention have and effect? *Diabetes Care* 17:1311–1319, 1994.
12. Torjesen P, Birkeland K, Anderssen S, Hjermann I, Holme I, Urdal P: Lifestyle changes may reverse development of the insulin resistance syndrome. The Oslo diet and exercise study: a randomized trial. *Diabetes Care* 20:26–31, 1997.
13. Eriksson KF, Lindgarde F: Prevention of type 2 (non-insulin-dependent) diabetes mellitus by diet and physical exercise. The 6-year MalmO feasibility study. *Diabetologia* 34:891–898, 1991.
14. Pan X, Li G, Hu Y, Wang J, Yang W, An Z, Hu Z, Lin J, Xiao J, Cao H, Liu P, Jiang X, Wang J, Zheng H, Zhang H, Bennett P, Howard B: Effects of diet and exercise in preventing NIDDM in people with impaired glucose tolerance: the Da Qing IGT and diabetes study. *Diabetes Care* 20:537–544, 1997.
15. Tuomilehto J, Lindstrom J, Eriksson J, Valle T, Hamalainen H, Ilanne-Parikka P, Keinanen-Kiukaanniemi S, Laakso M, Louheranta A, Rastas M, Salminen V, Uusitupa M: Finnish Diabetes Prevention Study Group: Prevention of type 2 diabetes mellitus by changes in lifestyle among subjects with impaired glucose tolerance. *N Engl J Med* 344:1343–1350, 2001.
16. Lindstrom J, Ilanne-Parikka P, Peltonen M, Aunola S, Eriksson JG, Hemio K, Hamalainen H, Harkonen P, Keinanen-Kiukaanniemi S, Laakso M, Louheranta A, Mannelin M, Paturi M, Sundvall J, Valle TT, Uusitupa M, Tuomilehto J: Sustained reduction in the incidence of type 2 diabetes by lifestyle intervention: follow-up of the Finnish Diabetes Prevention Study. *Lancet* 368:1673–1679, 2006.
17. Knowler WC, Barrett-Connor E, Fowler SE, Hamman RF, Lachin JM, Walker EA, Nathan DM: Reduction in the incidence of type 2 diabetes with lifestyle intervention or metformin. *N Engl J Med* 346:393–403, 2002.
18. Hamman RF, Wing RR, Edelstein SL, Lachin JM, Bray GA, Delahanty L, Hoskin M, Kriska AM, Mayer-Davis EJ, Pi-Sunyer X, Regensteiner J, Venditti B, Wylie-Rosett J: Effect of weight loss with lifestyle intervention on risk of diabetes. *Diabetes Care* 29:2102–2107, 2006.
19. Ramachandran A, Snehalatha C, Mary S, Mukesh B, Bhaskar AD, Vijay V: The Indian Diabetes Prevention Programme shows that lifestyle modification and metformin prevent type 2 diabetes in Asian Indian subjects with impaired glucose tolerance (IDPP-1). *Diabetologia* 49:289–297, 2006.
20. Kosaka K, Noda M, Kuzuya T: Prevention of type 2 diabetes by lifestyle intervention: a Japanese trial in IGT males. *Diabetes Res Clin Pract* 67:152–162, 2005.
21. Long S, O'Brien K, MacDonald K, Leggett-Frazier N, Swanson M, Pories W, Caro J: Weight loss in severely obese subjects prevents the progression of impaired glucose tolerance to type II diabetes. A longitudinal intervention study. *Diabetes Care* 17:372–375, 1994.
22. Sjostrom CD, Lissner L, Wedel H, Sjostrom L: Reduction in incidence of diabetes, hypertension and lipid disturbances after intentional weight loss induced by bariatric surgery: the SOS Intervention Study. *Obes Res* 7:477–484, 1999.
23. Dixon JB, O'Brien PE: Health outcomes of severely obese type 2 diabetic subjects 1 year after laparoscopic adjustable gastric banding. *Diabetes Care* 25:358–363, 2002.
24. Torgerson JS, Hauptman J, Boldrin MN, Sjostrom L: XENical in the prevention of diabetes in obese subjects (XENDOS) study: a randomized study of orlistat as an adjunct to lifestyle changes for the prevention of type 2 diabetes in obese patients. *Diabetes Care* 27:155–161, 2004.
25. Fajans SS, Conn JW: Tolbutamide-induced improvement in carbohydrate tolerance of young people with mild diabetes mellitus. *Diabetes* 9:83–88, 1960.
26. Engelhardt HT, Vecchio TJ: The long-term effect of Tolbutamide on glucose tolerance in adult, asymptomatic, latent diabetics. *Metabolism* 14:885–890, 1965.
27. Belknap B, Bagdade J, Amaral J, Bierman E: Plasma lipids and mild glucose intolerance II: a double blind study of the effect of tolbutamide and placebo in mild adult diabetic outpatients. *Excepta Med Int Congr Ser* 149:171–176, 1967.

28. Paasikivi J, Wahlberg F: Preventive tolbutamide treatment and arterial disease in mild hyperglycaemia. *Diabetologia* 7:323–327, 1971.
29. Keen H, Jarrett R, McCartney P: The ten-year follow-up of the Bedford survey (1962–1972): glucose tolerance and diabetes. *Diabetologia* 22:73–78, 1982.
30. Camerini-Davalosra R: Treatment of chemical diabetes. *Exepta Med Int Congr Ser* 149:228–242, 1967.
31. Jarrett RJ, Keen H, Fuller JH, McCartney M: Treatment of borderline diabetes: controlled trial using carbohydrate restriction and phenformin. *Br Med J* 2:861–865, 1977.
32. Papoz L, Job D, Eschwege E, Aboulker JP, Cubeau J, Pequignot G, Rathery M, Rosselin G: Effect of oral hypoglycaemic drugs on glucose tolerance and insulin secretion in borderline diabetic patients. *Diabetologia* 15:373–380, 1978.
33. Ratzmann KP, Witt S, Schulz B: The effect of long-term glibenclamide treatment on glucose tolerance, insulin secretion and serum lipids in subjects with impaired glucose tolerance. *Diabete Metab* 9:87–93, 1983.
34. Cederholm J: Short-term treatment of glucose intolerance in middle-aged subjects by diet, exercise and sulfonylurea. *Ups J Med Sci* 90:229–242, 1985.
35. Chiasson JL, Josse RG, Gomis R, Hanefeld M, Karasik A, Laakso M: Acarbose for prevention of type 2 diabetes mellitus: the STOP-NIDDM randomised trial. *Lancet* 359:2072–2077, 2002.
36. Diabetes Prevention Program Research Group: Effects of withdrawal from metformin on the development of diabetes in the diabetes prevention program. *Diabetes Care* 26:977–980, 2003.
37. Knowler WC, Hamman RF, Edelstein SL, Barrett-Connor E, Ehrmann DA, Walker EA, Fowler SE, Nathan DM, Kahn SE: Prevention of type 2 diabetes with troglitazone in the Diabetes Prevention Program. *Diabetes* 54:1150–1156, 2005.
38. Buchanan TA, Xiang AH, Peters RK, Kjos SL, Marroquin A, Goico J, Ochoa C, Tan S, Berkowitz K, Hodis HN, Azen SP: Preservation of pancreatic beta-cell function and prevention of type 2 diabetes by pharmacological treatment of insulin resistance in high-risk hispanic women. *Diabetes* 51:2796–2803, 2002.
39. Wenying Y, Lixiang L, Jinwu Q, Zhiqing Y, Haicheng P, Guofeng H, Zaojun Y, Fan W, Guangwei L, Xiaoren P: The preventive effect of Acarbose and Metformin on the progression to diabetes mellitus in the IGT population: a 3-year multicenter prospective study. *Chin J Endocrinol Metab* 17:131–136, 2001.
40. Yusuf S, Gerstein H, Hoogwerf B, Pogue J, Bosch J, Wolffenbuttel BH, Zinman B: Ramipril and the development of diabetes. *JAMA* 286:1882–1885, 2001.
41. Bosch J, Yusuf S, Gerstein HC, Pogue J, Sheridan P, Dagenais G, Diaz R, Avezum A, Lanas F, Probstfield J, Fodor G, Holman RR: Effect of ramipril on the incidence of diabetes. *N Engl J Med* 355:1551–1562, 2006.
42. Gerstein HC, Yusuf S, Bosch J, Pogue J, Sheridan P, Dinccag N, Hanefeld M, Hoogwerf B, Laakso M, Mohan V, Shaw J, Zinman B, Holman RR: Effect of rosiglitazone on the frequency of diabetes in patients with impaired glucose tolerance or impaired fasting glucose: a randomised controlled trial. *Lancet* 368:1096–1105, 2006.
43. Wylie-Rosett J, Herman WH, Goldberg RB: Lifestyle intervention to prevent diabetes: intensive and cost effective. *Curr Opin Lipidol* 17:37–44, 2006.
44. Shaw J, Zimmet P, de Courten M, Dowse G, Chitson P, Gareeboo H, Hemraj F, Fareed D, Tuomilehto J, Alberti K: Impaired fasting glucose or impaired glucose tolerance. What best predicts future diabetes in Mauritius? *Diabetes Care* 22:399–402, 1999.
45. Vartiainen E, Jousilahti P, Alfthan G, Sundvall J, Pietinen P, Puska P: Cardiovascular risk factor changes in Finland, 1972–1997. *Int J Epidemiol* 29:49–56, 2000.
46. Uusitalo U, Feskens E, Tuomilehto J, Dowse G, Haw U, Fareed D, Hemraj F, Gareeboo H, Alberti K, Zimmet P: Fall in total cholesterol concentration over five years in association with changes in fatty acid composition of cooking oil in Mauritius: cross sectional survey. *BMJ* 313:1044–1046, 1996.
47. Home PD, Pocock SJ, Beck-Nielsen H, et al. Rosiglitazone Evaluated for Cardiac Outcomes and Regulation of Glycaemia in Diabetes (RECORD) Study: interim findings on cardovascular hospitalizations and deaths. *N Engl J Med* 357:28–38, 2007

3

The Metabolic Syndrome

*Aoife M. Brennan, Laura Sweeney,
and Christos S. Mantzoros*

CONTENTS

ABSTRACT

The metabolic syndrome refers to the clustering of metabolic abnormalities more frequently than would be expected by chance alone. These metabolic abnormalities are all risk factors for cardiovascular disease (CVD), and the epidemiological association between these multiple risk factors points to the possibility of a unifying underlying pathophysiology. Obesity, in particular visceral adiposity, insulin resistance, and some degree of abnormal glucose metabolism coupled with dyslipidemia and abnormal blood pressure are the hallmarks of the syndrome. Epidemiological data correlates the presence of the metabolic syndrome with a proinflammatory state and greater risk for diabetes and CVD. There is also emerging evidence that the syndrome is associated with an increased risk of several malignancies. Since obesity is an increasing global burden, it is expected that the number of individuals with the metabolic syndrome will increase worldwide. An internationally accepted definition of the syndrome would facilitate both clinical diagnosis and future research to accurately assess risk and to identify preventative and therapeutic strategies.

Key words: Obesity; Insulin resistance; Type 2 diabetes; Visceral obesity; Dyslipidemia; Cardiovascular disease; Hypertension; Proinflammatory state; Diagnosis; Epidemiology.

INTRODUCTION

The metabolic syndrome is the name given to the cluster of metabolic abnormalities associated with an increased risk of diabetes and cardiovascular disease (CVD). Several different definitions of the syndrome are in use. There has been recent controversy regarding the concept of a metabolic

From: *Contemporary Diabetes: Diabetes and Exercise*
Edited by: J. G. Regensteiner et al. (eds.), DOI: 10.1007/978-1-59745-260-1_3
© Humana Press, a part of Springer Science+Business Media, LLC 2009

syndrome, due largely to uncertainty regarding clinical utility in terms of predicting CVD and lack of evidence of an underlying pathophysiology, despite a vast research effort in this area *(1)*. Nonetheless, the concept of a metabolic syndrome is seen as helpful by many clinicians in emphasizing the importance and health implications of obesity, insulin resistance, and related traits. Herein, we will discuss the definition of the syndrome and present international prevalence figures. We will also discuss the features of the syndrome and associated abnormalities.

DEFINITION

In 1998, the World Health Organization (WHO) became the first organization to publish an internationally recognized definition of the metabolic syndrome *(2)* (Table 1). In 2001, the National Cholesterol Education Program's Adult Treatment Panel III (NCEP/ATP III) released its own definition adding central obesity to its list of criteria *(3)* (Table 1). While these two definitions agree on their basic components, they differ in what they identified as the major underlying abnormality. The WHO stated that insulin resistance is the driving force behind the disorder, while ATP III used central obesity as the defining factor.

In 2003, the American College of Endocrinology (ACCE/ACE) convened and published a position statement, which suggested that "The Metabolic Syndrome" should be termed "Insulin Resistance Syndrome"; thereby focusing on the underlying pathophysiology that was felt to underlie the cluster of related abnormalities *(4)*. The presence of multiple definitions made it increasingly difficult to compare prevalence and impact in different areas of the world. The International Diabetes Foundation (IDF) convened in 2005 to develop a new unifying worldwide definition building upon the WHO and ATP III definitions *(5)*. The new definition put forth by the IDF highlights both central obesity and insulin resistance as important causative factors. On the basis of this new definition, for a patient to be defined as having the metabolic syndrome/insulin-resistance syndrome, central obesity plus two or

Table 1
WHO and ATP III Definitions of the Metabolic Syndrome

1999 WHO definition of the metabolic syndrome

Glucose intolerance of diabetes and/or insulin resistance and two or more of the following:

    Raised arterial blood pressure ≥140/90 mmHg

    Raised plasma triglycerides 150 mg/dl (1.7 mmol/l) and/or low HDL lipoprotein cholesterol <35 mg/dl
        men (0.9 mmol/l), <39 mg/dl women (<1.0 mmol/l)

    Central obesity (males – waist to hip ratio >0.90; females – waist to hip ratio >0.85) and/or BMI >30 kg/m^2

    Microalbuminuria (urinary albumin excretion rate ≥20 μg/min or albumin:creatinine ratio 30 mg/g)

2001 NCEP ATP III definition of the metabolic syndrome

Three or more of the following risk factors

    Waist circumference >102 cm in men and >88 cm in women

    Triglycerides > 150 mg/dl (1.7 mmol/l)

    HDL-c <40 mg/dl (1.03 mmol/l) in men, <50 mg/dl (1.29 mmol/l) in women

    Blood pressure 130/85 mmHg

    Fasting plasma glucose 110 mg/dl

WHO World Health Organization, *ATP III* Adult Treatment Panel III, *NCEP* National Cholesterol Education Program, *BMI* body mass index, *HDL-c* high-density lipoprotein-cholesterol more of the following four factors must be present: (a) raised concentrations of triglycerides: 150 mg/dl (1.7 mmol/l) or specific treatment for this lipid abnormality, (b) reduced concentration of high-density lipoprotein-c (HDL-cholesterol): <40 mg/dl (1.03 mmol/l) in men and <50 mg/dl (1.29 mmol/l) in women or specific treatment for this lipid abnormality, (c) raised blood pressure: systolic blood pressure (SBP) ≥130 mmHg or diastolic blood pressure (DBP) ≥85 mmHg or treatment of previously diagnosed hypertension, and (d) raised fasting plasma glucose concentration ≥100 mg/dl (5.6 mmol/l) or previously diagnosed type 2 diabetes (5) (Table 2).

The IDF definition is the first to identify different cutoffs for waist circumference by ethnic groups, based on data from Asia that showed interethnic differences between various obesity indices and the risks of CVD (Table 3) (5). In addition, the IDF consensus group highlighted a number of other parameters that appear to be related to the metabolic syndrome but are not currently included in the definition criteria (Table 4) (5). The future study of these factors will hopefully allow for further modification of the definition and validation of the new clinical definition in various ethnic groups (5). At the present time, it is important to recognize that ongoing research continuously changes our understanding of this evolving syndrome.

Table 2
IDF Definitions of the Metabolic Syndrome

2005 IDF criteria

Central obesity (defined by waist circumference, see Table 3)
Plus any two of the following:
   Raised triglycerides >150 mg/dl (1.7 mmol/l)
   Reduced HDL cholesterol <40 mg/dl (1.03 mmol/l) in men; <50 mg/dl (1.29 mmol/l) in women
   Raised blood pressure systolic >130 mmHg or diastolic >85 mmHg (or previously treated hypertension)
   Raised fasting plasma glucose >100 mg/dl (5.6 mmol/l) or previous diagnosis of diabetes

IDF International Diabetes Foundation, *HDL* high-density lipoprotein

Table 3
Ethnic Specific Values for Waist Circumference

Ethnic group		*Waist circumference*
Europids	Male	≥94 cm
	Female	≥80 cm
South Asians	Male	≥90 cm
	Female	≥80 cm
Chinese	Male	≥90 cm
	Female	≥80 cm
Japanese	Male	≥85 cm
	Female	≥90 cm
Ethnic South/Central Americans	See South Asian recommendations until more specific data are available	
Sub-Saharan Africans	See European recommendations until more specific data are available	
Eastern Mediterranean	See European recommendations until more specific data are available	
Middle East	See European recommendations until more specific data are available	

Table 4
Additional Metabolic Criteria for Which the IDF Thinks Further Research Is Necessary

Possible new criteria	Areas of potential research
Abnormal fat distribution	Leptin, adiponectin, liver fat content
Atherogenic dyslipidemia	Apo B (or non-HDL-c), small LDL particles
Insulin resistance	Fasting insulin/proinsulin levels, HOMA-IR, insulin resistence, elevated free fatty acids, M value from clamp
Vascular dysregulation	Measurement of endothelial dysfunction, microalbuminuria
Proinflammatory state	Elevated high sensitivity c-reactive protein, elevated inflamma-tory cytokines, decrease in adiponectin levels
Prothrombotic state	Fibrinolytic factors, clotting factors
Hormonal factors	Pituitaryadrenal axis

These metabolic criteria may later be linked to the metabolic syndrome
Adapted from the International Diabetes Federation
IDF International Diabetes Foundation, *LDL* l ow-density lipoprotein, *HDL* high-density lipoprotein

EPIDEMIOLOGY/PREVALENCE

The metabolic syndrome and obesity/overweight are becoming increasingly common throughout the world, as shown by emerging prevalence data *(6, 7)*. Research in several countries, including Canada, Finland, New Zealand, the United Kingdom, the United States, and Western Samoa, has demonstrated large increases in prevalence *(8)*. Using the most recent national data available for adults in the USA and the definition of the metabolic syndrome proposed by the IDF, almost 40% of US adults are classified as having the metabolic syndrome *(9)*. This is significantly higher than the 34% of US adults that would be classified under the ATP III definition. The IDF criteria for defining central obesity appeared to account for much of this difference *(9)*, since these require central obesity (rather than obesity being one of five criteria as in the ATP III definition) and substantially lower the threshold for waist circumference.

Ethnicity is a powerful predictor of insulin resistance the metabolic syndrome *(10)*. Epidemiologic studies have shown that this syndrome occurs in a wide variety of ethnic groups including Caucasians, African-Americans, Mexican-Americans, Asian-Indians, and Chinese *(11–14)*, and manifestations of the metabolic syndrome are increased in essentially every group of non-Caucasian ancestry in which comparisons have been made *(4)*. With the lower thresholds of waist circumference, new estimates of prevalence are especially increased for Mexican-Americans and Asians, and the application of the IDF definition to estimate the prevalence of the metabolic syndrome will likely have a substantial effect on the estimates in Latin American countries as well *(9, 15, 16)*.

Using the ATP III definition, the InterASIA Collaborative Group recently found that, in China, the age-standardized prevalence of overweight was 26.9% in men and 31.1% in women and the age-standardized prevalence of metabolic syndrome was 9.8% in men and 17.8% in women *(7)*. One can assume that these figures would be even higher using the new IDF definition. In 2003, also using the ATP III definition, the Tehran Lipid and Glucose Study found that the age-standardized prevalence of the metabolic syndrome was 33.7%. The prevalence increased with age in both sexes but was more commonly seen in women than in men *(17)*. A study in 2006 by Harzallah et al. examining the meta-bolic syndrome in Arab men and women found that the prevalence was 45.5% using the new IDF criteria: 55.8% in women and 30.0% in men *(18)*. The prevalence rates of the metabolic syndrome according to the WHO and the NCEP ATPIII are similar, 28.4 and 24.3%, but both are strikingly lower than the rate using the new IDF criteria. Similar results were recently found in a study in Korea, where the prevalence of the metabolic syndrome was lower than that of the ATP III-defined metabolic syndrome *(19)*. Regardless of which definition is used, the reported prevalence tends to be higher in women than in men predominantly because of significant differences in central obesity and HDL-c and, to a lesser extent, hypertension *(18)*.

The prevalence of the metabolic syndrome has been shown to correlate positively with body mass index (BMI), hyperglycemia, and concentrations of C-reactive protein (CRP) *(9)*. Individuals with hypertension have more than twice the prevalence of the metabolic syndrome than those who are normotensive. In addition, individuals with hypercholesterolemia have a higher prevalence of the metabolic syndrome than individuals who have concentrations of total cholesterol <200 mg/dl. Also, women with PCOS *(20)*, or a history of gestational diabetes *(21)*, are likely to be insulin resistant and at increased risk to develop one or more of the clinical components of the metabolic syndrome. Insulin resistance has been shown to be a familial characteristic *(22)*, and a family history of type 2 diabetes, hypertension, or CVD increases the risk of insulin resistance and the risk of subsequently developing the metabolic syndrome.

Not unexpectedly, the metabolic syndrome is highly age dependent. Using data from the National Health and Nutrition Examination Study (NHANES III), the prevalence of the metabolic syndrome rose from 7% at age 20–29 to 44% for individuals of age 60–69 *(9)*. These data have been replicated in several ethnic groups *(9, 17, 23)*.

Importantly, reports over the past several decades have shown that the prevalence of obesity/overweight and type 2 diabetes is increasing in children *(23)*. In addition, the metabolic syndrome is far more common among children and adolescents than previously reported and its prevalence increases directly with the degree of obesity *(24)*. For each half-unit increase in the BMI there is an associated increase in the risk of the metabolic syndrome among overweight and obese youth *(24)*. In a sample of adolescents in the USA who were included in the third NHANES III, conducted between 1988 and 1994, the prevalence of the metabolic syndrome was 6.8% among overweight adolescents and 28.7% among obese adolescents *(25, 26)*. Further, it has been shown that insulin resistance in obese children is strongly associated with specific biomarkers of inflammation and potential predictors of adverse cardiovascular outcomes *(24)* including CRP and interleukin-6 (IL-6), the levels of which rise with increasing levels of obesity.

CLINICAL DIAGNOSIS

On the basis of the IDF definition, central obesity is required for a diagnosis of the metabolic syndrome. The IDF has recognized and emphasized ethnic differences in the correlation between abdominal obesity and other metabolic syndrome risk factors. For this reason, the criterion of abdominal obesity is specified by nationality or ethnicity based on the best available population estimates. For people of European origin (Europid), the IDF-specified thresholds for abdominal obesity are waist circumferences ≥94 cm in men and ≥80 cm in women. For Asian populations, except for Japanese subjects, thresholds are ≥90 cm in men and ≥80 cm in women; for Japanese, they are ≥85 cm for men and ≥90 cm for women (see Table 3). If the criterion of abdominal obesity is met, two of the following criteria are also required for the diagnosis of the metabolic syndrome: triglycerides >150 mg/dl, low HDL (men <40 mg/dl and women <50 mg/dl), elevated blood pressure (SBP > 130 or DBP > 85) or previously treated hypertension, or raised fasting plasma glucose >100 mg/dl (or previous diagnosis of diabetes) (see Table 2).

CLINICAL MANIFESTATION, ASSOCIATIONS, AND COMPLICATIONS OF THE METABOLIC SYNDROME

As mentioned earlier, the metabolic syndrome is the name given to a constellation of metabolic abnormalities, which cooccur more often than would be expected by chance. While insulin resistance may be the underlying mechanism, patients generally present with one or more of the following features:

Diabetes and Prediabetes

Abnormal glucose metabolism, associated with central obesity, was first described by Vague in 1947, and studies in many populations have shown a relationship between the presence of obesity, insulin resistance, and the subsequent development of type 2 diabetes *(27, 28)*. Research to understand the pathophysiology of this association and the resulting CVD is ongoing. Insulin resistance is thought to be the primary abnormality leading initially to postprandial hyperinsulinemia and then fasting hyperinsulinemia as the pancreatic beta cells secrete increasing amounts of insulin to overcome resistance at the tissue level. Only after pancreatic beta cell function cannot keep up with the increased demands for insulin production does hyperglycemia, impaired glucose tolerance (IGT), and diabetes develop. Recently, early defects in pancreatic beta cell function have been described, which challenge this traditional view *(29)*.

Increased circulating free fatty acid levels appear to play a central role in the development of insulin resistance. Insulin has an important role to inhibit lipolysis in adipose tissue and the increased circulating fatty acid levels observed in insulin-resistant states further impair insulin action in insulin-sensitive tissues such as muscle and liver *(30)*. Increased circulating free fatty acids may also contribute to insulin resistance at the level of the pancreatic beta cell, resulting in inappropriate insulin secretion for a given blood glucose *(31)*.

Insulin resistance results in impaired suppression of glucose production by the kidneys and liver together with reduced glucose uptake by muscle and adipose tissue leading to high blood glucose values. IGT and impaired fasting glucose (IFG) are defining abnormalities of the metabolic syndrome, and several studies have evaluated the sensitivity and specificity of the metabolic syndrome in predicting future development of diabetes. A study comparing the metabolic syndrome to the Diabetes Predicting Model and the Framingham Risk Score found that the metabolic syndrome had a sensitivity of approximately 65% in predicting development of diabetes over an average follow-up of 7 years *(32)*. Moreover, in subjects with preexisting diabetes, diagnosis of the metabolic syndrome has been shown to predict both the presence of micro- and macrovascular complications *(33)*.

Diabetes is frequently asymptomatic and many individuals are not diagnosed until complications appear. Common presenting symptoms of high blood glucose include excessive thirst, polyuria, visual disturbance, and unexplained weight loss. Although the effectiveness of screening in asymptomatic individuals has not been clearly demonstrated, consensus recommendations are in favor of screening for diabetes at 3-year intervals in individuals over 45 years of age or in those less than 45 who have risk factors for diabetes including other features of the metabolic syndrome *(34)*. The recommended screening test is a fasting plasma glucose but the 75 g, 2-h oral glucose tolerance test (OGTT) is also used in several parts of the world *(34)*. More frequent testing is required in individuals with multiple risk factors and in those with preexisting IFG and IGT. Screening using glycosylated hemoglobin is not currently recommended *(34)*.

Diagnosis of diabetes is based on one of the following three criteria:

• Polydipsia, polyuria, or unexplained weight loss and random plasma glucose >200 mg/dl (11.1 mmol/l)

- Fasting plasma glucose >126 mg/dl (7.0 mmol/l)
- Plasma glucose of >200 mg/dl (11.1 mmol/l) 2 h after 75 g of anhydrous glucose

Individuals who have a positive diagnostic test require comprehensive diabetes evaluation and referral to an appropriate multidisciplinary team (34).

IGT and IFG have been defined as prediabetes in recognition of the increased risk of developing overt diabetes in this population. 11.9 million Americans were estimated to have prediabetes in 2000 (35). The threshold for IFG was lowered by the American Diabetes Association in 2003 based on epidemiological evidence from several cohorts such that fasting plasma glucose values above 100 mg/dl (5.5 mmol/l) are now considered abnormal. This change has increased the prevalence of prediabetes further.

IGT is diagnosed on the basis of OGTT when fasting blood sugar is normal and the 2-h postload plasma glucose is 140–199 mg/dl (7.811.0 mmol/l). It has been suggested that, if fasting plasma glucose alone is used for screening, a proportion of these individuals will be missed (36). Based on cost, convenience, and ease of administration, however, fasting plasma glucose alone continues to be recommended for screening (34).

Cardiovascular Disease

Many prospective cohort studies have evaluated the risk of CVD in individuals with the metabolic syndrome. While these studies have been hampered by the lack of consensus regarding definition, all have shown increased risk of CVD in individuals with the syndrome, irrespective of the definition used (37–46). The risks of CVD appear to differ between races and ethnic groups and further study is required to define race-specific risk (46). In general, the relative hazard ratio for CVD outcomes in men and women with the metabolic syndrome ranges between 2 and 5 in most studies (43, 45–47).

Data from NHANES III study revealed that the presence of the syndrome is associated with a more than twofold increase in myocardial infarction and stroke in both men and women. Moreover, insulin resistance, low HDL-c, hypertension, and hypertriglyceridemia were all independently associated with risk of myocardial infarction (MI) and stroke (45). The absence of the metabolic syndrome in the NHANES cohort correlated with a low age-adjusted prevalence of coronary heart disease, that is, 8.7%. The prevalence of coronary heart disease in the presence of the metabolic syndrome was 13.9% and 19.2% for those without and with diabetes, respectively (44).

In addition to CVD, the metabolic syndrome also appears to be a significant risk factor for cardiovascular and total mortality, providing additional information to models including established risk factors for CVD (41, 42). The presence of the metabolic syndrome also predicted mortality in individuals without diabetes or CVD at baseline in one recent study (41). Moreover, there appears to be a dose response relationship between number of components of the metabolic syndrome present and cardiovascular morbidity and mortality, with risk being greatest in subjects with multiple components of the syndrome and in those who are smokers (42).

Obesity and Increased Waist/Hip Ratio

The increasing worldwide prevalence of obesity has contributed to the increased recognition and diagnosis of the metabolic syndrome. Although numerous studies have demonstrated a positive relationship between obesity and insulin resistance (48, 49), it must be emphasized that individuals with a BMI in the normal range may also have insulin resistance and the metabolic syndrome (50). In addition, BMI and insulin sensitivity do not have a simple linear relationship since body fat distribution appears to be an important determinant of insulin sensitivity (51). Waist circumference and waist to hip ratio are used in large observational studies to assess visceral adiposity, since the most accurate measurements of central adiposity, namely computerized tomography (CT) and magnetic resonance imaging (MRI) and, possibly, dual-energy X-ray absorptiometry scanning (DEXA) *(52, 53)*, cannot be utilized in large population studies. CT, MRI, and DEXA have enabled an examination of the relationship between visceral adiposity and insulin resistance in research studies but are not recommended for routine clinical use. In subjects who lose weight, improvement in insulin sensitivity is correlated with the reduction in visceral fat *(54)*, with visceral adipose tissue explaining 54% of the variance in insulin sensitivity between lean insulin-resistant, lean insulin-sensitive, and obese insulin-resistant subjects in one study *(55)*.

The relative importance of visceral adiposity has been linked to the release of free fatty acids directly into the splanchnic circulation, as opposed to the systemic circulation where fatty acids from subcutaneous fat are released. Release of free fatty acids into the splanchnic circulation leads to direct effects on hepatic metabolism and pancreatic function. An alternative explanation is the differential secretion of metabolically active hormones by subcutaneous and visceral adipose tissue. Several metabolically active hormones, such as leptin and adiponectin, are secreted preferentially by subcutaneous adipose tissue *(56)*. Adiponectin appears to have an important role in the pathogenesis of the metabolic syndrome, and its levels are reduced in subjects with visceral adiposity *(57)* and levels increase with weight loss and exercise. Adiponectin levels are inversely correlated with insulin resistance *(58, 59)* and have been shown to predict future development of diabetes and CVD and may also be linked with several obesity-associated malignancies. In addition, visceral adipose tissue secretes a number of proinflammatory cytokines, which may contribute to the increased CVD risk in this population.

Dyslipidemia

The classic lipid profile in individuals with the metabolic syndrome includes elevated triglycerides, reduced HDL, and elevated atherogenic low-density lipoprotein (LDL) (predominantly small dense particles) *(60)*. The association between dyslipidemia-increased visceral adiposity and insulin resistance has been confirmed by several studies including a study of middle-aged men and women who were either lean and insulin-sensitive or obese and insulin-resistant. Increasing visceral adiposity was associated with increased triglycerides, LDL-cholesterol, LDL particle size and apolipoprotein B, and decreased HDL-c *(61)*.

The process through which insulin resistance leads to these changes in lipid profile is incompletely understood as, under normal circumstances, insulin inhibits the secretion of very low-density lipoproteins (VLDL) into the circulation *(62)*. In the metabolic syndrome, increased delivery of free fatty acids to the liver and increased production of apo B-containing, triglyceride-rich VLDL occurs. The reduced HDL levels observed may be a result of increased clearance, a consequence of the high triglyceride levels and thus may be an indirect consequence of insulin resistance.

Small dense LDL particles result from the increased triglyceride content of the serum as unesterified and esterified cholesterol is depleted from the particles leaving predominantly LDL triglyceride *(63)*. Whether LDL particle size is an independent risk factor for CVD or merely reflects other changes in lipid profile associated with the metabolic syndrome is debated. There is evidence from animal and ex vivo studies suggesting that these small particles may be more atherogenic as they are more easily able to transit through endothelial basement membrane, are more toxic to the endothelium, and have increased susceptibility to oxidation *(64)*.

Fasting lipid profile should be obtained at least yearly in individuals with the metabolic syndrome. There is evidence that individuals with the metabolic syndrome may benefit from more aggressive lipid-lowering therapy *(65)*; however, cardiovascular risk assessment and international guidelines should be used as a basis for therapeutic decisions *(3)*.

Hypertension

The relationship between elevated blood pressure and risk for CVD is well known *(66)*. Hypertension is one of the key features of the metabolic syndrome and the association appears to be multifactorial with both obesity and insulin resistance contributing. In an analysis of the NHANES data on trends in hypertension, about 2%, or more than half, of the increase in the prevalence of hypertension could be attributed to increases in BMI in the population *(67)*.

Insulin resistance is thought to contribute to hypertension in the metabolic syndrome through an effect of insulin to increase renal sodium absorption and activation of the sympathetic nervous system *(68, 69)*. In contrast, the normal vasodilatory effects of insulin are lost in states of insulin resistance, and fatty acids may also contribute to vasoconstriction *(70)*. In spite of these proposed mechanisms, insulin resistance alone does not completely account for the increased prevalence of hypertension in the metabolic syndrome and further study in this area is warranted *(71)*.

Whatever the etiology, individuals with the metabolic syndrome should have close monitoring and aggressive management of hypertension. In individuals with type 2 diabetes, the goal of therapy is blood pressure <130/80 mmHg *(34)*. In persons with hypertension (blood pressure 140/90 mmHg), drug therapies are required according to Joint National Committee 7 recommendations *(72)*.

Proinflammatory State

Insulin resistance and obesity are recognized proinflammatory states and the increased proinflammatory cytokines in the circulation may be involved in the increased risk of CVD in this population. There is increased secretion of tumor necrosis factor-alpha (TNF-α) and IL-6 from adipose tissue and increased production of acute phase reactants, CRP and fibrinogen, by the liver *(73)*. These inflammatory mediators in turn impair insulin action in target tissues and contribute to insulin resistance *(73)*.

Measurement of CRP is the most practical way to assess the presence of an inflammatory state. CRP levels tend to be higher than normal in patients with the metabolic syndrome and although elevated CRP levels are an emerging risk factor for CVD *(74)*, the utility of routine measurement of CRP in practice remains unproven. The American Heart Association (AHA) and Centers for Disease Control and Prevention (CDC) have issued guidelines for measurement of CRP in clinical practice *(75)*. They have suggested that such testing should be limited to individuals assessed to be at intermediate risk by Framingham scoring, that is, those whose 10-year risk for coronary heart disease (CHD) is in the range of 10–20%. The purpose of CRP testing in an intermediate-risk patient is to find those with high CRP levels whose risk category subsequently could be raised to high. The practical consequences of elevating the risk category would be to intensify lifestyle therapies, make certain that low-dose aspirin is used, and set lower LDL goals. The magnitude of independent predictive power of elevated inflammatory cytokines and acute-phase proteins remains uncertain *(76, 77)*. In addition, whether interventions to lower CRP will lead to reduced CVD events remains unknown.

Other Conditions

The metabolic syndrome is associated with multiple additional clinical and laboratory changes. Several common conditions, which do not form part of the diagnostic criteria, have been associated with the metabolic syndrome and insulin resistance. Nonalcoholic steatohepatitis is increasingly recognized as the hepatic manifestation of the metabolic syndrome and is becoming a frequent cause of end-stage liver disease in western populations *(78, 79)*. In females, PCOS is also considered an insulin-resistant syndrome with increased risk of diabetes and CVD *(80, 81)*. Furthermore, interventions known to improve insulin resistance, such as weight loss and metformin, also improve ovarian function in this condition. Gout, although not part of modern diagnostic criteria, was one of the original metabolic disturbances described as part of the syndrome in the 1920s. We now know that the elevated uric acid levels are a result of insulin action on the renal tubular reabsorbtion of uric acid *(82)*. In nondiabetics of Asian and African ancestry, elevated serum uric acid was closely associated with components of the metabolic syndrome *(83)*. Whether uric acid levels provide additional information in predicting future CVD and diabetes need to be studied. Obstructive sleep apnea occurs commonly in individuals with the metabolic syndrome and has been independently associated with insulin resistance. This may be an effect mediated through the sympathetic nervous system or an effect of hypoxia to induce target organ insulin resistance *(84)*. Several cancers such as breast, colon, prostate, and endometrial cancer have also been associated with obesity and insulin resistance through an effect possibly mediated through reduced adiponectin levels or altered insulin and insulin-like growth factor levels *(85)*.

REFERENCES

1. Kahn R, Buse J, Ferrannini E, Stern M. The metabolic syndrome: time for a critical appraisal: joint statement from the American Diabetes Association and the European Association for the Study of Diabetes. *Diabetes Care* 2005; 28(9):2289–2304.
2. World Health Organisation. Defintion, diagnosis, and classification of diabetes mellitus and its complications: report of a WHO consultation, Part 1: diagnosis and classification of diabetes mellitus 1999.
3. Executive Summary of the Third Report of the National Cholesterol Education Program (NCEP). Expert Panel on Detection, Evaluation, and Treatment of High Blood Cholesterol in Adults (Adult Treatment Panel III). *JAMA* 2001; 285(19): 2486–2497.
4. Einhorn D, Reaven GM, Cobin RH et al. American College of Endocrinology position statement on the insulin resistance syndrome. *Endocr Pract* 2003; 9(3):237–252.
5. International Diabetes Federation consensus worldwide definition of the metabolic syndrome. 14 April, 2005.
6. Flegal KM, Carroll MD, Kuczmarski RJ, Johnson CL. Overweight and obesity in the United States: prevalence and trends, 1960–1994. *Int J Obes Relat Metab Disord* 1998; 22(1):39–47.
7. Gu D, Reynolds K, Wu X et al. Prevalence of the metabolic syndrome and overweight among adults in China. *Lancet* 2005; 365(9468):1398–1405.
8. Flegal KM. The obesity epidemic in children and adults: current evidence and research issues. *Med Sci Sports Exerc* 1999; 31(11 Suppl):S509–S514.
9. Ford ES. Prevalence of the metabolic syndrome defined by the International Diabetes Federation among adults in the U.S. *Diabetes Care* 2005; 28(11):2745–2749.
10. Cameron AJ, Shaw JE, Zimmet PZ. The metabolic syndrome: prevalence in worldwide populations. *Endocrinol Metab Clin North Am* 2004; 33(2):351–375.
11. Kanjilal S, Shanker J, Rao VS et al. Prevalence and component analysis of metabolic syndrome: an Indian atherosclerosis research study perspective. *Vasc Health Risk Manage* 2008; 4(1):189–197.
12. Morales DD, Punzalan FE, Paz-Pacheco E, Sy RG, Duante CA. Metabolic syndrome in the Philippine general population: prevalence and risk for atherosclerotic cardiovascular disease and diabetes mellitus. *Diab Vasc Dis Res* 2008; 5(1):36–43.
13. Boehm BO, Claudi-Boehm S, Yildirim S et al. Prevalence of the metabolic syndrome in southwest Germany. *Scand J Clin Lab Invest Suppl* 2005; 240:122–128.
14. Zimmet PZ. Kelly West Lecture 1991, Challenges in diabetes epidemiology from West to the rest. *Diabetes Care* 1992; 15(2):232–252.
15. Fujita T. The metabolic syndrome in Japan. *Nat Clin Pract Cardiovasc Med* 2008; 5 (Suppl 1):S15–S18.
16. Ford ES, Mokdad AH, Giles WH. Trends in waist circumference among U.S. adults. *Obes Res* 2003; 11(10):1223–1231.
17. Azizi F, Salehi P, Etemadi A, Zahedi-Asl S. Prevalence of metabolic syndrome in an urban population: Tehran Lipid and Glucose Study. *Diabetes Res Clin Pract* 2003; 61(1):29–37.
18. Harzallah F, Alberti H, Ben KF. The metabolic syndrome in an Arab population: a first look at the new International Diabetes Federation criteria. *Diabet Med* 2006; 23(4):441–444.

19. Kim HM, Kim DJ, Jung IH, Park C, Park J. Prevalence of the metabolic syndrome among Korean adults using the new International Diabetes Federation definition and the new abdominal obesity criteria for the Korean people. *Diabetes Res Clin Pract* 2007; 77(1):99106.
20. Dunaif A. Insulin resistance and the polycystic ovary syndrome: mechanism and implications for pathogenesis. *Endocr Rev* 1997; 18(6):774–800.
21. O'sullivan JB, Mahan CM. Criteria for the oral glucose tolerance test in pregnancy. *Diabetes* 1964; 13:278–285.
22. Lillioja S, Mott DM, Zawadzki JK et al. In vivo insulin action is familial characteristic in nondiabetic Pima Indians. *Diabetes* 1987; 36(11):1329–1335.
23. Troiano RP, Flegal KM. *Overweight prevalence among youth in the United States: why so many different numbers?* Int J Obes Relat Metab Disord 1999; 23(Suppl 2):S22–S27.
24. Weiss R, Dziura J, Burgert TS et al. Obesity and the metabolic syndrome in children and adolescents. *N Engl J Med* 2004; 350(23):2362–2374.
25. Cook S, Weitzman M, Auinger P, Nguyen M, Dietz WH. Prevalence of a metabolic syndrome phenotype in adolescents: findings from the third National Health and Nutrition Examination Survey, 1988–1994. *Arch Pediatr Adolesc Med* 2003; 157(8):821–827.
26. Rosenberg B, Moran A, Sinaiko AR. Insulin resistance (metabolic) syndrome in children. *Panminerva Med* 2005; 47(4):229–244.
27. Hanson RL, Narayan KM, McCance DR et al. Rate of weight gain, weight fluctuation, and incidence of NIDDM. *Diabetes* 1995; 44(3):261–266.
28. Colditz GA, Willett WC, Stampfer MJ et al. Weight as a risk factor for clinical diabetes in women. *Am J Epidemiol* 1990; 132(3):501–513.
29. bdul-Ghani MA, Tripathy D, DeFronzo RA. Contributions of beta-cell dysfunction and insulin resistance to the pathogenesis of impaired glucose tolerance and impaired fasting glucose. *Diabetes Care* 2006; 29(5):1130–1139.
30. Kim YB, Shulman GI, Kahn BB. Fatty acid infusion selectively impairs insulin action on Akt1 and protein kinase C lambda/zeta but not on glycogen synthase kinase-3. *J Biol Chem* 2002; 277(36):32915–32922.
31. Lee Y, Hirose H, Ohneda M, Johnson JH, McGarry JD, Unger RH. Beta-cell lipotoxicity in the pathogenesis of non-insulin-dependent diabetes mellitus of obese rats: impairment in adipocyte-beta-cell relationships. *Proc Natl Acad Sci USA* 1994; 91(23):10878–10882.
32. Stern MP, Williams K, Gonzalez-Villalpando C, Hunt KJ, Haffner SM. *Does the metabolic syndrome improve identification of individuals at risk of type 2 diabetes and/or cardiovascular disease?* Diabetes Care 2004; 27(11):2676–2681.
33. Protopsaltis I, Nikolopoulos G, Dimou E et al. Metabolic syndrome and its components as predictors of all-cause mortality and coronary heart disease in type 2 diabetic patients. *Atherosclerosis* 2006; 195(1), 189194.
34. Power D. Standards of medical care in diabetes. *Diabetes Care* 2006; 29(2):476–477.
35. Benjamin SM, Valdez R, Geiss LS, Rolka DB, Narayan KM. Estimated number of adults with prediabetes in the US in 2000: opportunities for prevention. *Diabetes Care* 2003; 26(3):645–649.
36. Cheng C, Kushner H, Falkner BE. The utility of fasting glucose for detection of prediabetes. *Metabolism* 2006; 55(4):434–438.
37. Wen CJ, Lee YS, Lin WY et al. The metabolic syndrome increases cardiovascular mortality in Taiwanese elderly. *Eur J Clin Invest* 2008; 38(7):469–475.
38. Morales DD, Punzalan FE, Paz-Pacheco E, Sy RG, Duante CA. Metabolic syndrome in the Philippine general population: prevalence and risk for atherosclerotic cardiovascular disease and diabetes mellitus. *Diab Vasc Dis Res* 2008; 5(1):36–43.
39. Shetty GK, Economides PA, Horton ES, Mantzoros CS, Veves A. Circulating adiponectin and resistin levels in relation to metabolic factors, inflammatory markers, and vascular reactivity in diabetic patients and subjects at risk for diabetes. *Diabetes Care* 2004; 27(10):2450–2457.
40. Stern MP, Williams K, Gonzalez-Villalpando C, Hunt KJ, Haffner SM. *Does the metabolic syndrome improve identification of individuals at risk of type 2 diabetes and/or cardiovascular disease?* Diabetes Care 2004; 27(11):2676–2681.
41. Sundstrom J, Riserus U, Byberg L, Zethelius B, Lithell H, Lind L. Clinical value of the metabolic syndrome for long term prediction of total and cardiovascular mortality: prospective, population based cohort study. *BMJ* 2006; 332(7546):878–882.
42. Eberly LE, Prineas R, Cohen JD et al. Metabolic syndrome: risk factor distribution and 18-year mortality in the multiple risk factor intervention trial. *Diabetes Care* 2006; 29(1):123–130.
43. Lakka HM, Laaksonen DE, Lakka TA et al. The metabolic syndrome and total and cardiovascular disease mortality in middle-aged men. *JAMA* 2002; 288(21):2709–2716.
44. Alexander CM, Landsman PB, Teutsch SM, Haffner SM. NCEP-defined metabolic syndrome, diabetes, and prevalence of coronary heart disease among NHANES III participants age 50 years and older. *Diabetes* 2003; 52(5):1210–1214.
45. Ninomiya JK, L'Italien G, Criqui MH, Whyte JL, Gamst A, Chen RS. Association of the metabolic syndrome with history of myocardial infarction and stroke in the Third National Health and Nutrition Examination Survey. *Circulation* 2004; 109(1):42–46.
46. Isomaa B, Almgren P, Tuomi T et al. Cardiovascular morbidity and mortality associated with the metabolic syndrome. *Diabetes Care* 2001; 24(4):683–689.
47. Hu G, Qiao Q, Tuomilehto J, Balkau B, Borch-Johnsen K, Pyorala K. Prevalence of the metabolic syndrome and its relation to all-cause and cardiovascular mortality in nondiabetic European men and women. *Arch Intern Med* 2004; 164(10):1066–1076.

48. Olefsky JM, Kolterman OG, Scarlett JA. Insulin action and resistance in obesity and noninsulin-dependent type II diabetes mellitus. *Am J Physiol* 1982; 243(1):E15–E30.

49. Muscelli E, Camastra S, Catalano C et al. Metabolic and cardiovascular assessment in moderate obesity: effect of weight loss. *J Clin Endocrinol Metab* 1997; 82(9):2937–2943.

50. Ruderman N, Chisholm D, Pi-Sunyer X, Schneider S. The metabolically obese, normal-weight individual revisited. *Diabetes* 1998; 47(5):699–713.

51. Vague J. The degree of masculine differentiation of obesities: a factor determining predisposition to diabetes, atherosclerosis, gout, and uric calculous disease. *Am J Clin Nutr* 1956; 4(1):20–34.

52. Kvist H, Chowdhury B, Grangard U, Tylen U, Sjostrom L. Total and visceral adipose-tissue volumes derived from measurements with computed tomography in adult men and women: predictive equations. *Am J Clin Nutr* 1988; 48(6):1351–1361.

53. Abate N, Burns D, Peshock RM, Garg A, Grundy SM. Estimation of adipose tissue mass by magnetic resonance imaging: validation against dissection in human cadavers. *J Lipid Res* 1994; 35(8):1490–1496.

54. Goodpaster BH, Kelley DE, Wing RR, Meier A, Thaete FL. Effects of weight loss on regional fat distribution and insulin sensitivity in obesity. *Diabetes* 1999; 48(4):839–847.

55. Cnop M, Landchild MJ, Vidal J et al. The concurrent accumulation of intra-abdominal and subcutaneous fat explains the association between insulin resistance and plasma leptin concentrations: distinct metabolic effects of two fat compartments. *Diabetes* 2002; 51(4):1005–1015.

56. Gale SM, Castracane VD. Mantzoros CS. Energy homeostasis, obesity and eating disorders: recent advances in endocrinology. *J Nutr* 2004; 134(2):295–298.

57. Gale SM, Castracane VD. Mantzoros CS. Energy homeostasis, obesity and eating disorders: recent advances in endocrinology. *J Nutr* 2004; 134(2):295–298.

58. Bluher M, Bullen JWJr. Lee JH et al. Circulating adiponectin and expression of adiponectin receptors in human skeletal muscle: associations with metabolic parameters and insulin resistance and regulation by physical training. *J Clin Endocrinol Metab* 2006; 91(6): 23102316.

59. Shetty GK, Economides PA, Horton ES, Mantzoros CS, Veves A. Circulating adiponectin and resistin levels in relation to metabolic factors, inflammatory markers, and vascular reactivity in diabetic patients and subjects at risk for diabetes. *Diabetes Care* 2004; 27(10):2450–2457.

60. Gazi IF, Filippatos TD, Tsimihodimos V et al. The hypertriglyceridemic waist phenotype is a predictor of elevated levels of small, dense LDL cholesterol. *Lipids* 2006; 41(7):647–654.

61. Nieves DJ, Cnop M, Retzlaff B et al. The atherogenic lipoprotein profile associated with obesity and insulin resistance is largely attributable to intra-abdominal fat. *Diabetes* 2003; 52(1):172–179.

62. Lewis GF, Steiner G. Acute effects of insulin in the control of VLDL production in humans. Implications for the insulin-resistant state. *Diabetes Care* 1996; 19(4):390–393.

63. Halle M, Berg A, Baumstark MW, Konig D, Huonker M, Keul J. Influence of mild to moderately elevated triglycerides on low density lipoprotein subfraction concentration and composition in healthy men with low high density lipoprotein cholesterol levels. *Atherosclerosis* 1999; 143(1):185–192.

64. Krauss RM. Dense low density lipoproteins and coronary artery disease. *Am J Cardiol* 1995; 75(6):53B–57B.

65. Deedwania P, Barter P, Carmena R et al. Reduction of low-density lipoprotein cholesterol in patients with coronary heart disease and metabolic syndrome: analysis of the Treating to New Targets Study. *Lancet* 2006; 368(9539):919–928.

66. Reaven GM. Insulin resistance/compensatory hyperinsulinemia, essential hypertension, and cardiovascular disease. *J Clin Endocrinol Metab* 2003; 88(6):2399–2403.

67. Hajjar I, Kotchen TA. Trends in prevalence, awareness, treatment, and control of hypertension in the United States, 1988–2000. *JAMA* 2003; 290(2):199–206.

68. Barbato A, Cappuccio FP, Folkerd EJ et al. Metabolic syndrome and renal sodium handling in three ethnic groups living in England. *Diabetologia* 2004; 47(1):40–46.

69. Anderson EA, Hoffman RP, Balon TW, Sinkey CA, Mark AL. Hyperinsulinemia produces both sympathetic neural activation and vasodilation in normal humans. *J Clin Invest* 1991; 87(6):2246–2252.

70. Tripathy D, Mohanty P, Dhindsa S et al. Elevation of free fatty acids induces inflammation and impairs vascular reactivity in healthy subjects. *Diabetes* 2003; 52(12):2882–2887.

71. Hanley AJ, Karter AJ, Festa A et al. Factor analysis of metabolic syndrome using directly measured insulin sensitivity: the Insulin Resistance Atherosclerosis Study. *Diabetes* 2002; 51(8):2642–2647.

72. Chobanian AV, Bakris GL, Black HR et al. The Seventh Report of the Joint National Committee on Prevention, Detection, Evaluation, and Treatment of High Blood Pressure: the JNC 7 report. *JAMA* 2003; 289(19):2560–2572.

73. Fernandez-Real JM, Ricart W. Insulin resistance and chronic cardiovascular inflammatory syndrome. *Endocr Rev* 2003; 24(3):278–301.

74. Grundy SM, Cleeman JI, Daniels SR et al. Diagnosis and management of the metabolic syndrome: an American Heart Association/National Heart, Lung, and Blood Institute Scientific Statement. *Circulation* 2005; 112(17):2735–2752.

75. Pearson TA, Mensah GA, Alexander RW et al. Markers of inflammation and cardiovascular disease: application to clinical and public health practice: a statement for healthcare professionals from the Centers for Disease Control and Prevention and the American Heart Association. *Circulation* 2003; 107(3):499–511.

76. Pepys MB, Hirschfield GM. C-reactive protein: a critical update. *J Clin Invest* 2003; 111(12):1805–1812.

77. Timpson NJ, Lawlor DA, Harbord RM et al. C-reactive protein and its role in metabolic syndrome: Mendelian randomisation study. *Lancet* 2005; 366(9501):1954–1959.
78. Musso G, Gambino R, Bo S, Cassader M. Should nonalcoholic fatty liver disease be included in the definition of metabolic syndrome? A cross-sectional comparison with adult treatment panel III criteria in nonobese nondiabetic subjects: response to Sookoian et al. *Diabetes Care* 2008; 31(5):e43.
79. Angulo P. Nonalcoholic fatty liver disease. *N Engl J Med* 2002; 346(16):1221–1231.
80. Cussons AJ, Watts GF, Burke V, Shaw JE, Zimmet PZ, Stuckey BG. Cardiometabolic risk in polycystic ovary syndrome: a comparison of different approaches to defining the metabolic syndrome. *Hum Reprod* 2008; 23(10):23522358.
81. Ehrmann DA, Liljenquist DR, Kasza K, Azziz R, Legro RS, Ghazzi MN. Prevalence and predictors of the metabolic syndrome in women with polycystic ovary syndrome. *J Clin Endocrinol Metab* 2006; 91(1):48–53.
82. Facchini F, Chen YD, Hollenbeck CB, Reaven GM. Relationship between resistance to insulin-mediated glucose uptake, urinary uric acid clearance, and plasma uric acid concentration. *JAMA* 1991; 266(21):3008–3011.
83. Nan H, Qiao Q, Soderberg S et al. Serum uric acid and components of the metabolic syndrome in non-diabetic populations in Mauritian Indians and Creoles and in Chinese in Qingdao, China. *Metab Syndr Relat Disord* 2008; 6(1):47–57.
84. Tassone F, Lanfranco F, Gianotti L et al. Obstructive sleep apnoea syndrome impairs insulin sensitivity independently of anthropometric variables. *Clin Endocrinol (Oxf)* 2003; 59(3):374–379.
85. Kelesidis I, Kelesidis T, Mantzoros CS. Adiponectin and cancer: a systematic review. *Br J Cancer* 2006; 94(9):1221–1225.

II PHYSIOLOGICAL EFFECTS OF EXERCISE IN TYPE 2 DIABETES

4

Exercise Performance and Effects of Exercise Training in Diabetes

Irene Schauer, Tim Bauer, Peter Watson, Judith G. Regensteiner, and Jane E.B. Reusch

CONTENTS

ABSTRACT

There is a well established relationship between physical activity, metabolism, diabetes, and cardiovascular risk. In fact, numerous prospective epidemiological studies demonstrate an inverse correlation between physical activity and mortality, both cardiovascular and all cause mortality. This association is plausible when considered in the context of the impact of physical activity upon metabolic parameters that modulate cardiovascular risk such as blood pressure, dyslipidemia, inflammatory markers, and carbohydrate tolerance. Exercise is also pivotal for weight maintenance and prevention of obesity, a leading cause of new onset diabetes, which in turn contributes significantly to cardiovascular disease burden and mortality, as well as to noncardiac and all cause mortality. Prospective studies demonstrate the ability of diet and exercise to prevent progression from impaired glucose tolerance to diabetes. Despite the salutary effects of exercise on diabetes and cardiovascular risk, recent literature indicates that people with diabetes do not exercise as much as those without. This failure to exercise is likely behavioral and functional. Our recent work demonstrates that there are defects in both maximal and submaximal exercise function in persons with type 2 diabetes mellitus. In this chapter, we will review the cardiovascular and metabolic impacts of exercise, the relationship of exercise to diabetes prevention, and work from our lab examining the impact of diabetes on exercise capacity with some insights into the general mechanisms likely to be involved. The later chapters in this section will outline the impact of exercise on body composition and on cardiac, skeletal muscle, and endothelial function in additional detail.

From: *Contemporary Diabetes: Diabetes and Exercise*
Edited by: J. G. Regensteiner et al. (eds.), DOI: 10.1007/978-1-59745-260-1_4
© Humana Press, a part of Springer Science+Business Media, LLC 2009

Key words: Diabetes; Exercise; Cardiovascular; Endothelial dysfunction; Insulin sensitivity; Myocardial dysfunction.

INTRODUCTION

Poor physical fitness is associated with increased morbidity and mortality. It has been observed consistently that low cardiorespiratory fitness and physical inactivity predict mortality in normal weight and obese men, in older men and women, and in men with Type 2 Diabetes Mellitus (T2DM) *(1–9)*. Sedentary behavior has been clearly implicated as a factor leading to the development of diabetes as well as the worsening of cardiovascular (CV) outcomes of diabetes. Physical inactivity has become so common that one group has coined the term "sedentary death syndrome" *(10)*. The sedentary death syndrome model proposes that evolution favored genes that support the physical activity required for long-term health in an agrarian society and that sedentary behavior is maladaptive.

Exercise has long been recognized as a cornerstone for the treatment of patients with T2DM. Over 80 years ago, Allen et al. reported that a single bout of exercise lowered the blood glucose concentration of persons with diabetes and improved glucose tolerance temporarily *(11)*. Since that observation, numerous studies have confirmed the beneficial effects of exercise for persons with T2DM *(12–17)*. Paradoxically, despite extensive data indicating the importance of physical activity and exercise, 60–80% of adults with T2DM do not exercise sufficiently, and adherence to exercise programs is low in these patients *(18, 19)*. One possible reason for this is that exercise performance is impaired in individuals with diabetes, even in early, uncomplicated T2DM *(20–23)*. This impairment will be discussed in detail in a later section.

BENEFITS OF ROUTINE PHYSICAL ACTIVITY

CV Disease and All-Cause Mortality

Meta-analyses covering over 2.6 million person-years of study provide indisputable support for the reduction in CV disease (CVD) risk associated with physical activity and with physical fitness. A 2001 meta-analysis of 23 studies representing more than 1.3 million person-years of follow up demonstrated a linear decrease in CVD risk with increased physical activity *(7)*. Relationship to fitness was more complex with a precipitous decline in CVD risk occurring before the 25th fitness percentile. In terms of mortality, one study found that low CV fitness predicted CV and all-cause mortality in a cohort of 25,714 healthy men (Fig. 1a) *(3)*. The same observation held true for a cohort of 1,263 diabetic men *(2)*, and the mortality benefit of CV fitness was observed even in obese subjects. The relationship between physical activity, obesity, and mortality has been addressed directly by Blair et al.. They examined subjects with body mass index (BMI) less than 25, 25–30, or greater than 30 and found that lower habitual physical activity was associated with increased mortality in all groups *(24)*. Similar benefits and a similar dose response have been demonstrated for people with diabetes (Fig. 1b) *(6, 8)*. A similar relationship between fitness and mortality was found among hypertensive men *(25)*, smokers and nonsmokers, and individuals with elevated and with normal cholesterol levels *(26)*. Furthermore, the increases in CVD and all-cause mortality associated with the metabolic syndrome and with obesity were eliminated or attenuated to less than statistical significance when mortality was adjusted for cardiorespiratory fitness, suggesting that the observed mortality effects of these conditions are largely explained by lower CV fitness in these groups *(4)*. In another epidemiological study, even occasional physical activity (one or less bouts per week) conferred a hazard ration of 0.70–0.59 compared with no physical activity *(5)*. This sort of evidence can be affected by selection bias and confounding variables. However, the consistency of the observations supports a cause and effect relationship between physical activity and decreased

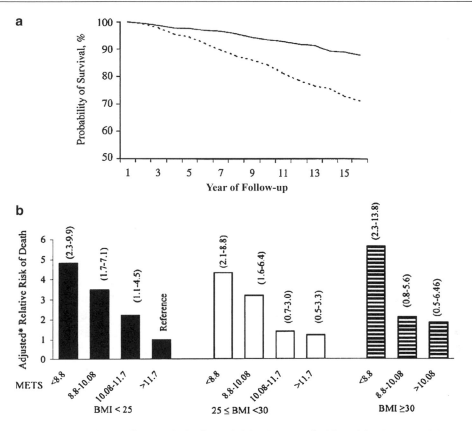

Fig. 1. (**a**) Improved survival in cardiovascularly fit (*solid line*) vs. unfit (*dotted line*) men with Type 2 Diabetes Mellitus (T2DM) over 12 years of follow-up in a cohort of 14,777 men *(2)*; (**b**) increased age-adjusted relative risk of all-cause mortality with decreased cardiovascular fitness in all weight categories in 2,196 diabetic men over 32,162 person-years of observation *(6)*. Reprinted with permission from *Diabetes Care and Ann Int Med.*

mortality, which is biologically plausible based on the impact of physical activity on lipids, blood pressure, endothelial function, carbohydrate tolerance, diabetes, and possibly inflammation and fibrinolysis.

Lipids

Results have been mixed in studies examining the effect of exercise interventions on lipid levels, as reviewed in *(27)*. In general, studies with longer interventions (greater than 6 months) of higher intensity have been most likely to show increases in HDL levels and reductions in cholesterol and triglyceride (TG) levels. For instance, in 111 sedentary, overweight men and women with mild to moderate dyslipidemia, Kraus et al. found significant reduction in LDL and TG levels and improvement in HDL level with their highest intensity intervention and increases in LDL particle size in all exercise groups after 6 months *(28)*. However, a recent study with a 9-month running intervention in young healthy adults showed only an insignificant trend toward LDL lowering and no effect on HDL or TG levels despite a 24% increase in peak VO$_2$ *(27)*. A significant reduction in apoB was reported, suggesting again that exercise may induce antiatherogenic changes in LDL particle size. A recent meta-analysis of studies of 2–12 months of exercise in subjects with T2DM found a significant decrease in TG levels, but no significant change in HDL or LDL *(29)*. Another study with a 31-week exercise intervention in subjects with T2DM did demonstrate a significant increase in HDL in addition to decreased TG, but stable LDL *(30)*. Unfortunately, the effects of diet have not been distinguished from those of exercise in most available studies.

Overall, HDL response to exercise training is variable and appears to depend upon multiple factors including dose, gender, and genetic background. As summarized by Ring-Dimitriou, studies support the need for longer duration, higher intensity exercise for significant HDL-raising effects *(27)*. They also suggest that gender differences may exist with greater benefit occurring in men than in women. This may reflect higher baseline HDL in female subjects. Recently it was reported that there may be genetic determinants of whether people will respond to exercise by increasing HDL cholesterol. A polymorphism in the PPAR delta receptor (more common in Causcasians) was associated with a significantly greater improvement in HDL with exercise training *(31)*. It is reasonable to conclude that exercise training may have a positive effect on lipids, but it should not be employed in lieu of lipid lowering phamacotherapy when indicated. At present it does represent one of the very few interventions, and arguably the safest intervention, with potential for raising HDL.

Fibrinolysis

In addition to the well-established risk factors, an elevated level of plasma fibrinogen has also been reported to be a CV risk factor. Acute exhaustive exercise stimulates both thrombosis and fibrinolysis with a net neutral effect on hemostasis in most populations *(32, 33)*. In the general population, the chronic and immediate postexercise responses in the thrombotic and fibrinolytic systems have been shown to be variable and reflect differing adaptations with ageing and responses to exercise protocols. In a recent study, investigators examined hemostatic variables including factor VII activity (FVIIa), tissue factor pathway inhibitor factor Xa complex (TFPI/Xa), and plasminogen activator inhibitor-1 (PAI-1) antigen activity after a high fat meal before and after exercise training *(34)*. They observed reduction in the potential for coagulation and improved fibrinolytic potential in trained subjects with the meal stimulation suggesting that under certain conditions (e.g., postprandially) exercise may have cardiovascularly beneficial effects on hemostasis.

In people with diabetes the results are similarly variable. Fibrinogen level is elevated in men and women with T2DM *(35)*. Results to date are not clear as to whether exercise training decreases fibrinogen level in the person with T2DM. Schneider et al. found that although VO_2max increased by 8% with 6 weeks of training, fibrinogen level did not change significantly in a group of sedentary persons with T2DM *(36)*. Conversely, Hornsby et al., found that a 12.5% increase in VO_2max after 12–14 weeks of training was associated with a significant decrease in fibrinogen level in sedentary persons with T2DM *(37)*. In the large Finnish Diabetes Prevention Study a combined diet and exercise intervention decreased PAI-1 level consistent with improved fibrinolysis *(38)*. Another recent study found improved fibrinolysis after 6 months of aerobic training in overweight to obese men and women *(39)*. Interestingly, improvements were significantly greater in men than in women and correlated closely with abdominal fat. Thus, the effect of exercise training on fibrinolysis appears to be generally salutary and may be mediated by changes in body composition, but this relationship requires further investigation.

Blood Pressure

High blood pressure is a leading contributor to CV mortality, and there is a consistent inverse relationship between physical activity and blood pressure in cross-sectional studies. The first study to examine the impact of training upon blood pressure was conducted by Jennings with a very rigorous exercise program in sedentary men *(40)*. Over the last few decades a dose–response effect of exercise on blood pressure has been observed in both men and women, including those with CV and metabolic comorbidities. A recent meta-analysis assessed 72 longitudinal intervention studies to determine the impact of exercise training on blood pressure *(41)*. Studies included both hypertensive and normotensive subjects. Overall the analysis demonstrated a small (3 mmHg), but clinically and statistically significant, decline in both systolic and diastolic average blood pressure, with a greater reduction in hypertensive subjects. They concluded that endurance training decreases blood pressure through a reduction in systemic vascular resistance secondary to decreased sympathetic nervous system and renin–angiotensin system activity. In a recent study of 30 obese T2DM subjects, a 3-month exercise intervention improved both systolic and diastolic blood pressure *(42)*. Overall, improvement of blood pressure with exercise training is the most consistently demonstrated benefit of physical activity on CV health.

Endothelial Function

Coronary and peripheral artery endothelial dysfunction (ED), most often measured as impaired vasodilator response to mechanical or pharmacologic stimuli, have been shown to correlate with CVD risk, cardiac events in known CVD, and poor prognosis in CVD *(43–48)*. Exercise training improves endothelial function in the context of metabolic disease and CVD. For instance, in a study of patients with congestive heart failure (CHF), 4 weeks of lower leg exercise training significantly improved upper extremity endothelium-dependent vasodilation, but not endothelium-independent responses *(49)*. Another study demonstrated improved flow-mediated dilatation (FMD) with a 12-week treadmill training program in hypertensive men *(50)*. Such responses to exercise training have also been demonstrated in insulin resistant and diabetic subjects. Kelly et al. showed that 8 weeks of stationary bike training significantly improved brachial artery FMD in a group of overweight children relative to a sedentary control group *(51)*. Similarly Meyer et al. found improved ED after 6 months of endurance training in obese sedentary children *(52)*. Two recent studies demonstrated improvement in endothelium dependent vascular reactivity after 8 weeks of exercise training in overweight and T2DM adult subjects *(53, 54)*. A third showed improvement in biomarkers of ED after 6 months of training in older patients with T2DM *(55)*. In contrast, in a study of T2DM subjects no improvement was seen in microvascular function as measured by maximum skin hyperemia after 6 months of aerobic exercise training *(56)*. Other studies have failed to find benefits of exercise on endothelial function in healthy individuals without baseline ED, for instance in healthy relatives of T2DM individuals *(57)* and in healthy middle aged men *(58)*. The weight of evidence suggests that exercise training does significantly improve impaired endothelial function, but has no significant impact in normal vessels.

Inflammation and Immunity

The relationship between exercise and immune function is reported to be a "J" shaped curve wherein increasing from sedentary to moderate activity improves immune function but exercise training in elite athletes may diminish immune function (especially in the first 24 h after a bout of exhaustive exercise) *(59)*. Regular performance of about 2 h of moderate exercise per day is associated with a reduction of risk for common viral infections of 29% compared to sedentary subjects *(60)*. In contrast, exhaustive exercise such as a marathon is associated with a 100–500% increase in the risk of viral infection *(61)*. It is worth noting that it is the rare individual who will exercise rigorously greater than 2 h per day, so the potential deleterious effects of exhaustive exercise are not likely to be observed in the general population.

Inflammation, the other face of the immune spectrum, is one of the universal mechanisms contributing to the initiation and progression of atherosclerosis *(62)* and the development of T2DM *(63, 64)*. In general short term moderate intensity exercise interventions have a modest positive impact on some subset of circulating cytokines such as IL-1, -6, and -18, CRP, and TNF-α; presumed anti-inflammatory markers such as adiponectin (and IL6?, see later); and inflammation-related cell adhesion molecules such as VCAM, ICAM, and the selectins *(55, 57, 65–68)*, but exact methods and results have been mixed. For instance, Zoppini et al. found stable CRP and decreased ICAM and P-selectin following 6 months of aerobic exercise in older, sedentary, overweight diabetics *(55)*. In contrast, Olson et al. found reduced CRP and increased adiponectin, but stable cell adhesion markers after 1 year of resistance training in overweight women *(65)*. In addition, there are studies that do not demonstrate any exercise-induced change in circulating inflammatory markers *(69)*. Thus, evidence regarding the effect of exercise on inflammation is mixed and apparently heavily dependent upon the baseline status of the population and on the nature, intensity, and regularity of the exercise intervention. It is likely that a muscle damaging level of exercise can cause inflammation while more modest or habitual exercise reduces systemic inflammation to some degree. The net result is therefore a balance of these two opposing forces. Further studies are clearly necessary for a better understanding of the effects of exercise on systemic inflammation.

A further complication to this question arises from the fact that one of the cytokines that is frequently measured in studies of inflammation in metabolic syndrome, obesity, and diabetes is IL-6. A large body of recent data suggests that IL-6 has pleiotropic effects that include significant metabolic and insulin sensitizing effects, as well as possible anti-inflammatory effects [reviewed in *(70, 71)*]. IL-6 is produced by skeletal muscle during sustained exercise and plasma levels of IL-6 are transiently dramatically elevated in response to exercise. Studies of IL-6-deficient mice have demonstrated that these animals have decreased exercise endurance, decreased O_2 consumption during exercise, and impaired fatty acid oxidation in response to exercise *(72)*. These effects appear to be mediated by a decrease in induction of AMP kinase activity and of fatty acid oxidation pathways in exercising muscle, by decreased lipolysis in adipocytes and glucose release from the liver, and by a decrease in sympathetic outflow during exercise *(70)*. Overall the literature is consistent with a crucial role for IL-6 in exercise performance and in the generation of a high turnover metabolic state during exercise and other forms of physical stress. Interestingly, by 9 months of age the IL-6-deficient mice are obese and have several features of metabolic syndrome including impaired glucose tolerance. Clearly, a full understanding of IL-6's complex role in exercise, metabolism, diabetes, and inflammation awaits further studies.

Obesity

Obesity is a common problem for persons with T2DM. Exercise conditioning may serve as an adjunct therapy especially when linked to diet. However, in the absence of diet exercise does not consistently lead to weight loss although body composition may be improved *(73)*. These changes in body composition include decreased visceral adiposity and thus may have significant beneficial effects on CV risk factors. However, exercise training without dietary change results in minimal absolute weight loss despite greater than 60–90-min a day of moderate activity *(74)*. In contrast to the limited impact of isolated exercise for weight loss, exercise is very effective for prevention of weight gain, acceleration of weight loss in combination with diet, and most importantly maintenance of weight loss. In a community-based study, introduction of walking and healthy snacks prevented weight gain *(75)*. Similarly, in the National Weight Control Registry, comparison of a group of subjects who have maintained a substantial weight loss for greater than 12 months with those who regained weight suggests that physical activity of greater than 2,000 calorie per week is a crucial element of long-term success *(76)*. When exercise mediation of weight loss has been examined prospectively, similar results are reported. For example, an intervention with diet with or without exercise for 12 weeks resulted in a weight loss of 10 kg with diet alone and 14 kg with diet plus exercise. After 12 weeks the dietary intervention was discontinued but the exercise intervention continued. At 36 weeks the diet group had regained all but

4 kg whereas the exercise group maintained 12 kg of weight loss *(77)*. It is critical to understand that exercise alone does not lead to weight loss and to convey this to patients so that they will have an appreciation of the role of exercise and not be discouraged by an apparent lack of weight loss results from their exercise regimen.

Glucose Regulation and Insulin Sensitivity

Glucose metabolism in response to exercise has been extensively studied as it poses an important clinical challenge. Exercise has two different impacts on carbohydrate metabolism, the bout effect and the training effect. The bout effect refers to the direct impact of an episode of exercise on glucose during the exercise and for an interval of 1–72 h after the exercise is complete. Exercise training is typically considered routine physical activity that increases functional exercise capacity for which the gold standard is maximal exercise capacity (VO_2max). Exercise training usually also effects body composition, especially lean body mass. The benefits of exercise for glycemia likely result from a combination of the bout and training effects.

It is well established that even a single bout of exercise has a pronounced effect on the metabolism of the person with T2DM. In fact, much of the benefit of training may be due to the most recent bout of exercise *(78, 79)*. In support of the concept that single bouts of exercise affect metabolic parameters, Devlin and others reported that a single bout of glycogen-depleting exercise in patients with T2DM significantly increased glucose disposal for up to 12–16 h postexercise due to an enhanced rate of nonoxidative glucose disposal *(78)*. This increase occurs at the level of both liver and muscle tissue *(80)*. Others have found that exercise conditioning for 1 week increases whole body insulin-mediated glucose disposal *(81)* and glucose tolerance *(12)* in patients with T2DM. It is not completely clear how much metabolic benefit is derived from a single bout of exercise versus the effect of cumulative bouts, but it is clear that the benefit of a bout of exercise is lost rather quickly so that repeated exercise, probably daily, is needed for long-term, bout effect benefits on glucose metabolism. In addition, a very brief period of exercise such as a single bout or even a week of exercise is clearly insufficient to cause increases in maximal oxygen consumption, changes in body composition, or improvement in other CV parameters, which are affected by longer periods of training and have clear independent mortality benefits, as well as potential independent effects on glucose metabolism.

The effects of exercise training or routine physical activity on insulin sensitivity are likely to be complex and multifactorial, and the relative roles of decreased visceral fat, CV fitness, and cumulative bout effects of exercise have yet to be defined [reviewed in *(82)*]. Recent studies clearly demonstrate that exercise training leading to increased fitness (generally defined as an increase in VO_2max) also results in improved insulin sensitivity as measured by the gold standard hyperinsulinemic euglycemic clamp *(83, 84)*. These studies also compared exercise regimens consisting of moderate versus high intensity activity but with equal exercise energy expenditure and found greater effects on insulin sensitivity with higher intensity physical activity despite similar effects on VO_2max. These results suggest that fitness per se may not correlate directly with insulin sensitivity. Others have asked whether the benefits of long-term exercise training (as opposed to the bout effect) on insulin sensitivity can be completely accounted for by changes in visceral adiposity and have had mixed results [reviewed in *(82)*].

The clinical implications were recently assessed in a meta-analysis that concluded that at least 12 weeks of exercise training, either aerobic, resistance, or combination training, results in a reduction in hemoglobin A1c of 0.8%, an effect that is comparable to the improvement typically achieved by dietary or single agent drug therapies *(85)*.

Prevention of Diabetes

The role of exercise in the prevention of diabetes is unequivocal but has been most often and best studied in the context of a combined diet and exercise intervention. Early epidemiological and sociological evidence demonstrated a strong inverse correlation between habitual physical activity and incidence of diabetes. This evidence included the change in incidence of diabetes with a move from a rural lifestyle, observed in American versus Mexican Pima Indians. This relationship has been observed across diverse populations including male college alumni, female college alumni, registered nurses, and British men [reviewed in *(86)*]. These observations were followed by a set of prospective studies, the Finnish Diabetes Prevention Study *(87)*, Da Qing Study *(88)*, and the Diabetes Prevention Program *(89)*. In all of these studies a diet and exercise intervention prevented transition from impaired glucose tolerance to diabetes in 50–60% of individuals. Only the Da Qing Study included an exercise alone arm. The preventative effect of exercise in this arm was similar to that observed with diet alone and was independent of weight loss, though body composition was not addressed. The success of exercise in diabetes prevention is likely to result from one or more of the effects described earlier, specifically improved insulin sensitivity, decreased visceral adiposity, and/or modulation of inflammation and oxidative stress.

EFFECTS OF T2DM ON EXERCISE PERFORMANCE

Introduction

Persons with T2DM are at higher risk than nondiabetics for coronary artery disease, stroke, and peripheral arterial disease due to accelerated atherosclerosis *(90)*. Exercise conditioning is thus likely to be especially beneficial in these individuals through the modification of CV risk factors discussed earlier *(79, 91)*. Furthermore, the observed beneficial effects of physical activity on insulin sensitivity and glucose metabolism make it clear that, in addition to reducing CV morbidity and mortality, exercise training, or even an increase in the level of habitual physical activity, has a key role in the management of diabetes. Yet the population studies described earlier indicate that people with T2DM are generally less active than nondiabetic people. While some aspects of this behavior may be accounted for by lifestyle choices that contribute to the initial development of diabetes, recent evidence suggests that pathophysiological factors may also contribute to this decrease in activity. This section will primarily address changes observed in subjects with T2DM in CV or cardiopulmonary exercise performance, defined by maximal oxygen consumption (VO_2max) and by kinetics of oxygen consumption during submaximal exercise. These data suggest that the cause and effect relationship of the correlation between low physical activity and diabetes may be bidirectional.

Maximal Exercise Capacity

Studies have clearly demonstrated that people with T2DM have a reduced CV exercise performance compared with nondiabetic persons matched for age, weight, and/or physical activity as evidenced by a lower VO_2max during incremental exercise (e.g., Table 1) *(15, 16, 22, 92–95)*. The overall difference in VO_2max between healthy persons and persons with T2DM is approximately 20%. The mechanisms for this impairment have not been completely elucidated. However, based upon available data, central cardiac and peripheral factors limiting systemic oxygen delivery, as well as defects in tissue oxygen extraction may all play a role (see later for potential mechanisms leading to exercise impairment). Interestingly, limited data suggest that although both men and women with T2DM demonstrate the exercise abnormality, women with T2DM may show worse CV exercise performance than male T2DM relative to their nondiabetic counterparts *(96)*. The gender relatedness of this preliminary observation in T2DM is currently under investigation.

Table 1
Maximal Exercise Capacity

	Lean control	Obese control	DM
Age (years)	36 ± 6	37 ± 6	42 ± 7
Fat free mass (kg)	42 ± 7	48 ± 5	47 ± 5
HgbA1c	6.0 ± 0.6	5.3 ± 0.5	9.0 ± 0.4*
Maximal exercise response			
VO_2max (pre)	25.1 ± 4.7	21.8 ± 2.9	17.7 ± 4.0*
(post)	26.0 ± 6.0	23.0 ± 1.8**	22.4 ± 5.5**
Maximal RER	1.13 ± 0.08	1.12 ± 0.06	1.16 ± 0.13

RER respiratory exchange ratio

*$P < 0.05$ for difference between T2DM and controls

**$P < 0.05$ for difference between pre and post training. Data are mean ± SD [Printed with permission from *J. Appl. Physiol. and Diab. Care (22, 92)*]

Submaximal Exercise Tolerance and Oxygen Uptake Kinetics (VO_2 Kinetics)

The exercise abnormality observed at maximal exercise in T2DM is also observed during less vigorous physical activity (i.e., submaximal exercise). During the early stages of an incremental exercise test, oxygen uptake (VO_2) increases with each increase in work rate. In nondiabetic individuals, there is a predictable increase in VO_2 to meet the metabolic demand for a given increase in workload (e.g., ~10.1 ml/min/W) *(97)*. The VO_2 to work load relationship thus describes an individual's overall ability to adjust to the exercise stress, and reductions in the slope of this relationship have been shown to effectively indicate abnormalities of cardiac output and gas exchange in cardiopulmonary and vascular diseases *(98)*.

Similar to persons who have overt CVD, the increase in VO_2 per unit of increase in workload is reduced in people with T2DM compared with healthy controls *(22)*. Potential mechanisms for this abnormal response include a decrease in oxygen delivery and decreased cardiac function, and/or an abnormality of muscle oxidative metabolism. To further evaluate this possibility, submaximal constant-load exercise has been employed. Unlike graded or incremental exercise, constant-load exercise is performed at a moderate workload below the individual's lactate threshold, where a steady-state VO_2 for a given work rate can be obtained.

Following the onset of exercise, VO_2 rises exponentially to steady state, the time course of which represents the VO_2 kinetic response. The VO_2 kinetics are determined by the systemic integration of muscle VO_2, CV adaptations of oxygen delivery, and pulmonary gas exchange. Three phases of the pulmonary VO_2 response to the change from rest to moderate constant-load exercise have been proposed *(99, 100)*. At the onset of exercise, pulmonary VO_2 in the lungs increases abruptly for the first 15–20 s as cardiac output and pulmonary blood flow initially increase (cardiodynamic phase or phase 1). Following a circulatory transit delay (usually about 20–40 s), VO_2 then increases exponentially (phase 2), reflecting the increase of muscle VO_2 as tissue oxygen extraction and blood flow increases to meet the exercise demand *(101, 102)*. This is the primary component of VO_2 kinetics and is described by a time constant (tau) reflecting the time to reach ~63% of the increase in VO_2. Phase 2 ends as muscle VO_2 and pulmonary gas exchange reach a steady state. Phase 3 is the steady-state VO_2 during moderate exercise.

In the healthy individual, VO_2 kinetics may be limited by either a maldistribution of blood flow to the working tissues limiting O_2 transfer or by the inertia of oxidative metabolism *(101, 103)*. In disease

Table 2
Submaximal Exercise Kinetics

	LC	OC	DM
VO$_2$ kinetics			
20 W Tau (s)	21.4 ± 8.9	18.4 ± 9.9	42.6 ± 23.8*
30 W Tau (s)	28.8 ± 5.3	27.8 ± 8.9	36.8 ± 6.2*
80 W Tau (s)	42.8 ± 7.5	41.2 ± 8.2	55.7 ± 20.6
Heart rate kinetics			
20 W Tau (s)	8.5 ± 4.6	10.6 ± 8.2	23.8 ± 16.2*
30 W Tau (s)	23.9 ± 13.8	14.2 ± 8.0	40.7 ± 11.9*
80 W Tau (s)	41.2 ± 14.8	43.3 ± 11.3	72.3 ± 21.5*

LC lean controls, *OC* overweight controls, *DM* T2 diabetes, *W* watts, *Tau* the monoexponential time constant of VO$_2$
*$P < 0.05$ difference between T2DM and both control groups. Data are mean ± SD
[Printed with permission from *J Appl. Physiol. (22)*]

states where oxygen delivery is compromised, as with CVDs, VO$_2$ kinetics are limited by the body's ability to deliver oxygen to working muscle, and therefore may directly reflect impaired oxygen delivery *(104, 105)*. Since impaired cardiac output and/or local distribution of blood flow to exercising muscles are components of the O$_2$ delivery process, VO$_2$ kinetics may thus provide a measure the effectiveness of the CV system in delivering sufficient oxygen to satisfy the requirements of muscle during exercise *(106)*. In this regard, the time constant of phase 2 VO$_2$ kinetics is prolonged in patient groups with abnormal CV responses to exercise, and in general is sensitive to alterations in oxygen exchange at the lungs, cardiac output, oxygen diffusion, and rates of tissue oxygen consumption.

We have observed that the VO$_2$ kinetic response is slowed in women with T2DM compared to nondiabetic women of similar BMI and physical activity levels in the absence of any clinical evidence of CVD (Table 2) *(22)*. To prospectively evaluate the effects of T2DM on maximal and submaximal exercise performance, we assessed exercise performance in 10 women with T2DM compared to groups of 10 lean and 10 obese nondiabetic women of similar age and physical activity levels *(22)*. We assessed VO$_2$max (see earlier Table 1), submax VO$_2$, VO$_2$ kinetic responses, and heart rate kinetic responses (measuring rate of rise of heart rate at the beginning of exercise). For constant load exercise, subjects performed transitions from rest to exercise for 6 min of constant work load cycle ergometer exercise at three workloads (two low work rates, 20 and 30 W, and one high work rate, 80 W). We found that women with T2DM had not only a lower VO$_2$max but also reduced VO$_2$ at all submaximal work loads (Fig. 2) and slower VO$_2$ kinetic and heart rate responses than either obese or lean nondiabetic controls (Table 2). These data suggested that diabetes, rather than obesity per se, is responsible for the observed exercise impairments. Additionally, our finding that heart rate kinetics are slowed in diabetes suggests a cardiac or "central" oxygen delivery component to the exercise impairment *(22)*.

More recently, we evaluated the T2DM VO$_2$ kinetic impairment in conjunction with measures of skeletal muscle oxygenation using near infrared spectroscopy in 11 T2DM and 11 healthy, sedentary subjects *(107)*. This combination of measurements allowed the investigation of changes in oxygen delivery relative to VO$_2$ at the level of the exercising muscle. We found slowed VO$_2$ kinetics and an altered profile of muscle deoxygenation following exercise onset in the T2DM subjects (Fig. 3). These data indicate a transient imbalance of muscle oxygen delivery relative to muscle VO$_2$ in T2DM consistent with subnormal microvascular blood flow increase in the skeletal muscle of T2DM subjects.

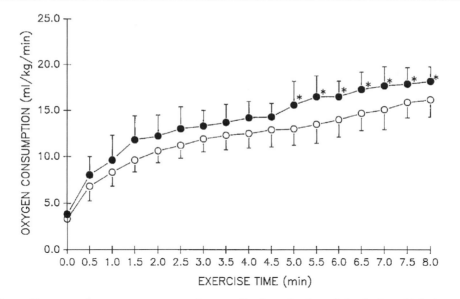

Fig. 2. This figure illustrates that oxygen consumption, at all submaximal work loads for which there are complete data, is reduced in persons with Type 2 Diabetes Mellitus (T2DM) (*open circles*) versus nondiabetic controls (*closed circles*) of similar age and activity levels during graded exercise testing *(23)*. Reprinted with permission from *Med Sci Sports Exerc.*

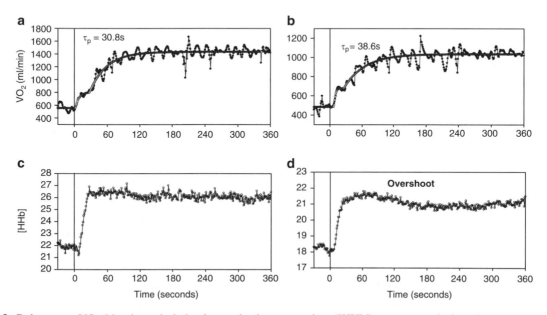

Fig. 3. Pulmonary VO$_2$ kinetic and skeletal muscle deoxygenation ([HHb]) responses during the transition from unloaded cycling to moderate constant work rate exercise in a healthy control (**a**, **c**) and T2DM subject (**b**, **d**). Loaded cycling begins at time = 0. τ_p, time constant of phase 2 pulmonary VO$_2$ kinetics. *Solid dark lines* represent curve fit of VO$_2$ kinetic response. Note slower VO$_2$ kinetics (**b**) and overshoot of [HHb] response (**d**) following onset of loaded exercise in the T2DM subject.

Interestingly, in this mixed set of men and women with T2DM, there were no differences in heart rate kinetics compared with sedentary control subjects, suggesting that the exercise abnormality during moderate exercise may be mediated by peripheral factors rather than central CV defects in oxygen delivery. Current studies are underway to investigate the roles of abnormal control of peripheral blood flow and muscle metabolism during exercise on the observed exercise impairment in T2DM.

POTENTIAL MECHANISMS LEADING TO EXERCISE IMPAIRMENT

There are several potential pathogenic mechanisms that may contribute to the decreased capacity for exercise in T2DM. These include metabolic and nonmetabolic sequelae of diabetes in the vasculature and in cardiac and skeletal muscle. These are discussed in the following sections.

Hyperglycemia

The relationship between markers of glucoregulation and exercise has been investigated to determine whether these factors are likely determinants of exercise performance. To date, associations have not been found between hemoglobin A1C or fasting serum glucose concentration and exercise performance (23, 94, 95, 108, 109). In other words, although a single bout of exercise improves glycemic control (albeit temporarily), changes in glycemic control, per se, do not appear to affect exercise performance.

Insulin Resistance

In contrast to hyperglycemia, various reports have suggested that insulin resistance (IR) is associated with reduced VO_2max in T2DM (110–121). IR has also been reported to be inversely correlated with VO_2max in several disease states in addition to diabetes, including heart failure and chronic renal failure (113, 114). That this decrease in exercise capacity is independent of other complications of diabetes or of the systemic illness associated with heart and renal failure is further supported by the recent finding of exercise defects in nondiabetic women with polycystic ovarian syndrome (PCOS) (115) and of exercise defects in the metabolic syndrome (116). The significant decline in VO_2max in subjects with PCOS compared to age- and weight-matched controls correlated with all measures of IR, but not with other reported measures including blood pressure, cholesterol, and androgen levels. In addition, there is an association between IR and low physical fitness level in normotensive men with a family history of hypertension (117).

The cause and effect relationship between IR and impaired exercise performance is not well understood and has been further addressed through the use of a pharmacological intervention to improve insulin sensitivity. In a study of 20 women with early, uncomplicated T2DM randomized to rosiglitazone or placebo, rosiglitazone treatment resulted in a significant improvement in VO_2max of 7%. This improvement correlated with both increased insulin sensitivity and improved endothelial function (110).

While the positive effects of exercise on insulin sensitivity are clear, the earlier results support the hypothesis that IR in turn negatively effects exercise capacity. Other literature lends support to multiple possible mechanisms for such a relationship including IR at the level of the vasculature leading to ED (in both peripheral and cardiac circulation), IR at the level of the muscle (cardiac and skeletal) leading to a decline in mitochondrial content and/or function, and IR at the level of the heart and/or skeletal muscle leading to inefficient substrate utilization. Recent attention has been focused on changes in substrate utilization and metabolic inflexibility in IR. Simply stated, insulin promotes carbohydrate utilization. In the absence of sufficient insulin signaling in IR, metabolism relies more heavily on fatty acids, a less oxygen efficient fuel source. These mechanisms and their potential relationship to exercise capacity are discussed further in the following sections.

ENDOTHELIAL DYSFUNCTION

One possible mechanism for the exercise abnormalities observed in persons with T2DM invokes ED as a contributing factor. The exercise abnormalities observed could reflect a deficient endothelial dilator response to metabolic demand in heart as well as peripheral skeletal muscle. In this scenario, exercise capacity would be limited by peripheral and/or coronary blood flow. It is well established that peripheral endothelial function and vascular reactivity in response to pharmacological vasodilators and to cuff ischemia at rest (118, 119) as well as in response to exercise are abnormal in adults with T2DM compared to nondiabetic controls (120, 121). Furthermore, insulin's physiologic ability to enhance endothelium-dependent vasodilation is markedly impaired in diabetic individuals compared with that of lean control subjects, and it has been proposed that IR at the level of the endothelial cell is invariably associated with ED (122). This is supported by the observation that obese subjects with and without T2DM have endothelium-dependent vasodilation that is reduced by 40–50% compared with lean control subjects (123). In addition, every insulin resistant state studied to date has been found to have associated ED (122). Thus, IR in T2DM results in ED and to impaired demand-mediated increases in muscle (and probably cardiac) blood flow, in addition to decreased glucose transport into muscle. Alternatively, the vascular dysfunction of T2DM and IR may be a direct result of IR at the level of the vascular smooth muscle cell causing altered substrate utilization with a greater reliance on less efficient fuels (fatty acids) and consequently impaired smooth muscle function. Finally, ED may result from the systemic inflammation and oxidative stress associated with IR and obesity. Prompted in part by findings in other disease states, such as heart failure, where an association between exercise performance and endothelial function has been reported (124), the relationship between endothelial function and the exercise abnormalities of T2DM is being investigated further.

Support for the ability of ED alone to cause exercise defects comes from the studies of Jones et al. using N-nitro-l-arginine methyl ester (l-NAME) to reduce nitric oxide (NO) levels prior to performing exercise. They found a decrease in maximal oxygen uptake (VO_2max), which correlated with the expected reduction in vasodilation and decreased perfusion of large muscle groups (125). However, in contrast to our studies with T2DM subjects, l-NAME induced an acceleration of the rate at which oxygen consumption increased with exercise (VO_2 kinetics) (125, 126). This could be explained by recent studies in animals and man demonstrating a role for NO in regulation of myocardial substrate utilization. Inhibition of NO synthase in dogs with l-NAME results in a marked increase in glucose oxidation and a decrease in fatty acid metabolism (127). It has been proposed that NO interferes with oxidative metabolism by competing for O_2 binding at cytochrome c oxidase in the mitochondrial electron transport chain (128–130). The result of such NO-mediated mitochondrial inhibition is to modulate muscle oxidative phosphorylation and muscle VO_2 kinetics. Thus, inhibition of NO synthesis alone appears to decrease VO_2max, but may speed VO_2 kinetics via the removal of NO-mediated effects on mitochondrial oxidative metabolism. The fact that both parameters are affected negatively in diabetes implies that changes in exercise parameters in diabetes cannot be fully explained by changes in NO synthesis or, presumably, ED alone.

MYOCARDIAL DYSFUNCTION

There are also likely to be cardiac factors contributing to the exercise abnormalities of T2DM. Evidence has accumulated for the existence of myocardial dysfunction that is unrelated to coronary artery disease in many individuals with diabetes, even early uncomplicated diabetes (e.g., 131–138).

This condition has been termed "diabetic cardiomyopathy" and generally refers to a finding of subclinically impaired left ventricular (LV) function at rest *(131, 134, 136, 137, 139, 177)* and/or during exercise *(133, 135)* in the absence of major coronary disease or hypertension. The earlier studies have demonstrated a predominant component of diastolic dysfunction in diabetic cardiomyopathy. Clinically it has been shown that cardiac diastolic dysfunction correlates closely with impairments in CV exercise capacity in heart failure *(124)*, in diabetes *(135, 139)*, and in normal subjects *(177)*. In our studies of exercise dysfunction in T2DM we have found a reduced cardiac output by right heart catheterization during exercise in persons with diabetes compared to nondiabetic, healthy, age- and weight-matched controls *(140)*. In addition, we have observed that pulmonary capillary wedge pressure rises more steeply and to a greater level with exercise in T2DM than in controls consistent with significant diastolic dysfunction during exercise *(140)* and that this presumed diastolic dysfunction correlates with the observed decrease in exercise capacity. Thus while the prevalence, etiology, and clinical significance remain unclear, it is possible that diabetic cardiomyopathy plays a significant role in the exercise defects seen in T2DM.

Finally, we have also observed that the cardiac diastolic dysfunction, which correlates with the decrease in exercise capacity in uncomplicated T2DM, also correlates with reduced myocardial perfusion (Regensteiner and Reusch, unpublished results). Based on these studies, impaired coronary artery endothelial function may be the mechanism for exercise impairment in T2DM via adverse effects on cardiac function. However, other data in the literature suggest the alternative or additional mechanisms discussed later.

Cardiac Substrate Utilization in Insulin Resistance

Cardiac energy production via preferential use of fat over glucose could contribute to exercise defects in diabetes. This model is supported by recent studies of cardiac substrate utilization in diabetes. Studies examining cardiac fuel utilization in IR DM rodents demonstrated a fixed, excess reliance on inefficient fat oxidation in the diabetic myocardium indicating metabolic inflexibility relative to nondiabetic controls *(141)*. Mazumder et al. characterized cardiac substrate utilization in mice and found that basal and palmitate-stimulated fatty acid utilization were 1.5–2-fold higher in IR ob/ob mice than in wild-type mice *(142)*. This fuel preference occurred at the expense of cardiac glucose oxidation and was accompanied by increased myocardial oxygen consumption with less ATP produced per unit of O_2 consumed, and impaired cardiac efficiency *(142)*. Similar results have been obtained in other IR animal models (db/db and ZDF) and in human subjects [reviewed in *(143)*]. For example, Peterson et al. demonstrated increased myocardial oxygen consumption, decreased cardiac efficiency, and increased cardiac fatty acid utilization in obese women compared to controls *(144)*. However, Knuuti et al. did not find changes in cardiac fatty acid utilization in a small study of men with impaired glucose tolerance *(145)*. Human studies demonstrate that a few days of high fat diet enhance fat oxidation and decrease mitochondrial efficiency (Ravussin E, Baton Rouge, LA, Personal communication). This is similar to the skeletal muscle mitochondrial dysfunction and inefficient glucose oxidation observed in subjects with T2DM and their relatives *(146, 147)*. Inefficient myocardial function usually leads to diastolic dysfunction, which is the defect our group has implicated in T2DM subjects with exercise intolerance.

Interestingly, increased fatty acid levels and utilization at the expense of glucose oxidation have also been demonstrated in ischemic myocardium in both animal models and humans [reviewed in *(148)*]. This fuel utilization preference has been shown to contribute to cellular acidosis and decreased cardiac efficiency in the ischemic heart and it is thought to play a role in ischemic and reperfusion injury. Pharmacological stimulation of glucose oxidation with dichloroacetate, an activator of the pyruvate dehydrogenase complex, rescues these defects in rat ischemic myocardium *(149)*. Similarly, agents that inhibit fatty acid oxidation (obliging reliance on glucose) decrease infarct size and troponin release in a rat ischemia/reperfusion model *(150)*, improve cardiac efficiency *(148)*, and are currently under investigation as antianginal agents *(151)*. Thus, the model of insulin resistance-induced myocardial substrate shifts may provide a mechanism not only for impaired exercise capacity but also for the worsened outcomes of acute coronary events in diabetes.

SKELETAL MUSCLE CHANGES IN DIABETES

The role of skeletal muscle in the impaired exercise responses of persons with T2DM has not been specifically elucidated. However, as skeletal muscle plays an integral role in IR, it is likely that changes in skeletal muscle structure and function may be associated with diminished exercise function. In our study of persons with T2DM in which VO_2max was lower, cardiac index was reduced by about 15% and yet arteriovenous oxygen extraction was the same in the T2DM subjects compared to obese controls *(140)*. Baldi et al. *(20)* also reported a reduced VO_2max, a trend toward lower cardiac output as measured by rebreathing techniques, and lower arteriovenous oxygen extraction in T2DM patients compared to controls. In their study VO_2max correlated with the arteriovenous oxygen difference, but not with cardiac output. The findings from both groups are interesting since even a modest reduction in cardiac output should increase reliance on arteriovenous oxygen extraction. The absence of an increase in this measure suggests that defects in oxygen transport to and/or oxidative capacity of the exercising skeletal muscle exist in T2DM and may contribute to the exercise defects seen in this population.

Related to these mechanisms, capillary density is reduced in T2DM skeletal muscle *(152)*, and basement membrane structures are altered *(153)*. These structural changes could directly contribute to alterations in microvascular hemodynamics that impair O_2 exchange from capillary to myocyte as suggested by the work in diabetic rodent models *(154–156)*. Indeed, the relationship between oxygen diffusion (potentially decreased in T2DM) and exercise performance in T2DM has not been extensively explored *(157, 158)*. However, microvascular complications of T2DM have been associated with abnormal vascular function and lowered exercise capacity *(159)* further suggesting this mechanism as a component to the exercise dysfunction in T2DM. There is currently debate regarding the potential for abnormalities of mitochondrial function *(21, 160–162)* and whether they relate to functional defects in exercise performance or simply reflect reduced content secondary to detraining *(163)*. To date, the available data are inconclusive, but rigorous studies are lacking. Nevertheless, adults with T2DM have been shown to demonstrate reduced skeletal muscle oxidative enzyme activity *(162)*, lower mitochondrial content *(161, 164)*, and an increased ratio of type IIb-to-type 1 muscle fiber ratio *(165)* compared with healthy subjects. Any of the factors may lead to reduced fractional oxygen extraction. Other, noncardiac components of oxygen delivery could also cause impairment in exercise performance in T2DM. Increased blood viscosity has been reported in persons with T2DM compared to nondiabetic individuals *(157, 158)*. However, we found that while average whole blood viscosity was higher in persons with T2DM than nondiabetic controls, there was not a statistical relationship between viscosity and exercise performance *(23)*. Overall it appears that the ability to deliver oxygen to the skeletal muscle as well as the ability of the muscle to utilize oxygen during exercise may be compromised in T2DM, and that this is another potential mechanism underlying the exercise defects seen in T2DM.

GENDER SPECIFICITY OF EFFECTS OF T2DM ON EXERCISE CAPACITY

Few previous studies have separately examined exercise performance in women with T2DM although it has been noted that they appear to have a reduced exercise performance compared to nondiabetic women *(121)*. In prior studies, we have observed that women with T2DM had a more impaired exercise performance relative to their nondiabetic female counterparts, than the men with T2DM compared to their nondiabetic male counterparts *(96)*. Maximal oxygen consumption was 26% lower in women with T2DM than nondiabetic women compared to 18% lower in men with T2DM compared to the nondiabetic men ($P < 0.05$). Although the small sample size makes these findings preliminary, the results are suggestive of possible sex-based differences in exercise performance between men and women with T2DM.

EFFECTS OF EXERCISE TRAINING ON EXERCISE PERFORMANCE IN T2DM

Exercise training can substantially improve exercise performance in individuals with T2DM *(15, 109, 166)*. Improvements in VO_2max in men and women with diabetes ranging from 8 to 30% have been documented *(92, 166, 167)*. In addition, a decreased heart rate per submaximal workload has been reported *(109)* suggesting an improved exercise efficiency, again similar to results in nondiabetic persons. Oxygen uptake kinetics and heart rate kinetics became faster after 4 months of exercise training in persons with T2DM although not in nondiabetic controls suggesting improvement in the rate of circulatory adjustment to the beginning of exercise *(92)*.

Exercise Training: Mechanisms of Improvement

Metabolic benefits in terms of how exercise improves insulin sensitivity are likely related to increased tissue sensitivity to insulin due to regular exercise conditioning *(168, 169)*. Studies have shown that insulin binding to monocytes *(170, 171)* and erythrocytes *(172)* is increased by exercise conditioning and decreased with inactivity. It is possible that exercise conditioning causes a diminished secretion of insulin in response to a particular glucose concentration *(173)*. Studies have suggested that exercise conditioning magnifies insulin-induced increases in the intrinsic activity of plasma membrane glucose transporters *(174)*.

As discussed earlier, T2DM may adversely affect exercise performance in part because of detrimental effects on diastolic function. Exercise training might be expected to improve diastolic dysfunction based on animal studies *(175)*, but randomized studies of exercise training are needed to confirm this benefit and provide the responsible mechanism.

Exercise and Endothelial Vasodilator Function

The beneficial effects of exercise on endothelial function have been suggested by both animal and human studies where exercise was associated with improved endothelial vasodilator function *(54, 176)*. In humans with T2DM, reactive hyperemic brachial artery vasodilation and forearm blood flow have been improved by exercise in contrast to the response in nondiabetic controls *(176)*. It is thought that the improvements represent a systemic rather than a local benefit of exercise since while the exercise was done using the lower body muscles, improvement in brachial artery reactivity in the arm was a primary outcome. Further research in this exciting area is underway.

SUMMARY

The relationship between CV exercise capacity and diabetes is complex and involves multiple physiological systems. Furthermore, the relationship is likely to represent bidirectional causality. The benefits of exercise (and, conversely, the ill effects of sedentary behavior) on CV risk factors, endothelial function, insulin sensitivity, diabetes prevention, and CV and all-cause mortality are clear. Other benefits including maintenance of mitochondrial health and number, and effects on hemostasis and systemic inflammation are likely, but less well defined. It also seems likely that further research will reveal other areas of benefit derived from regular exercise. On the other hand, individuals with T2DM who would be expected to benefit disproportionately from exercise have been shown to be relatively inactive and cardiovascularly unfit. While the increased risk of diabetes in sedentary individuals is undoubtedly one contributor to this relationship, recent evidence suggests that diabetes may itself cause defects in CV exercise capacity. These defects in turn may make exercise more difficult and uncomfortable and thus encourage sedentary behavior in the very population that would most benefit from exercise. The mechanism of decreased exercise capacity in T2DM is poorly understood, but appears to involve impaired oxygen delivery through cardiac and vascular mechanisms, as well as impaired oxygen utilization at the tissue level. A better understanding of these mechanisms and of the benefits of exercise in this population is essential and awaits further research.

REFERENCES

1. Blair SN, Wei M. Sedentary habits, health, and function in older women and men. *Am J Health Promot.* Sep–Oct 2000;15(1):1–8.
2. Wei M, Gibbons LW, Kampert JB, Nichaman MZ, Blair SN. Low cardiorespiratory fitness and physical inactivity as predictors of mortality in men with T2DM. *Ann Intern Med.* Apr 18 2000;132(8):605–611.
3. Wei M, Kampert JB, Barlow CE, et al. Relationship between low cardiorespiratory fitness and mortality in normal-weight, overweight, and obese men. *JAMA.* Oct 27 1999;282(16):1547–1553.
4. Katzmarzyk PT, Church TS, Janssen I, Ross R, Blair SN. Metabolic syndrome, obesity, and mortality: impact of cardiorespiratory fitness. *Diabetes Care.* Feb 2005;28(2):391–397.
5. Sundquist K, Qvist J, Sundquist J, Johansson SE. Frequent and occasional physical activity in the elderly: a 12-year follow-up study of mortality. *Am J Prev Med.* Jul 2004;27(1):22–27.
6. Church TS, Cheng YJ, Earnest CP, et al. Exercise capacity and body composition as predictors of mortality among men with diabetes. *Diabetes Care.* Jan 2004;27(1):83–88.
7. Williams PT. Physical fitness and activity as separate heart disease risk factors: a meta-analysis. *Med Sci Sports Exerc.* May 2001;33(5):754–761.
8. Gregg EW, Gerzoff RB, Caspersen CJ, Williamson DF, Narayan KM. Relationship of walking to mortality among US adults with diabetes. *Arch Intern Med.* Jun 23 2003;163(12):1440–1447.
9. Myers J, Kaykha A, George S, et al. Fitness versus physical activity patterns in predicting mortality in men. *Am J Med.* Dec 15 2004;117(12):912–918.
10. Lees SJ, Booth FW. Sedentary death syndrome. *Can J Appl Physiol.* Aug 2004;29(4):447–460; discussion 444–446.
11. Allen F, Stillman E, Fitz, R. Total dietary regulation in the treatment of diabetes. *Exercise*, Vol 11. NY: Rockefeller Institute of Medical Research; 1919:486–499.
12. Rogers MA, Yamamoto C, King DS, Hagberg JM, Ehsani AA, Holloszy JO. Improvement in glucose tolerance after 1 wk of exercise in patients with mild NIDDM. *Diabetes Care.* Sep 1988;11(8):613–618.
13. Wei M, Schwertner HA, Blair SN. The association between physical activity, physical fitness, and T2DM mellitus. *Compr Ther.* Fall 2000;26(3):176–182.
14. Ruderman N, Apelian AZ, Schneider SH. Exercise in therapy and prevention of type II diabetes. Implications for blacks. *Diabetes Care.* Nov 1990;13(11):1163–1168.
15. Schneider SH, Khachadurian AK, Amorosa LF, Clemow L, Ruderman NB. Ten-year experience with an exercise-based outpatient life-style modification program in the treatment of diabetes mellitus. *Diabetes Care.* Nov 1992;15(11):1800–1810.
16. Schneider SH, Elouzi EB. The role of exercise in type II diabetes mellitus. *Prev Cardiol.* Spring 2000;3(2):77–82.
17. Eves ND, Plotnikoff RC. Resistance training and T2DM: considerations for implementation at the population level. *Diabetes Care.* Aug 2006;29(8):1933–1941.
18. Morrato EH, Hill JO, Wyatt HR, Ghushchyan V, Sullivan PW. Physical activity in U.S. adults with diabetes and at risk for developing diabetes, 2003. *Diabetes Care.* Feb 2007;30(2):203–209.
19. Krug LM, Haire-Joshu D, Heady SA. Exercise habits and exercise relapse in persons with non-insulin-dependent diabetes mellitus. *Diabetes Educ.* May–Jun 1991;17(3):185–188.
20. Baldi JC, Aoina JL, Oxenham HC, Bagg W, Doughty RN. Reduced exercise arteriovenous O2 difference in T2DM. *J Appl Physiol.* Mar 2003;94(3):1033–1038.
21. Scheuermann-Freestone M, Madsen PL, Manners D, et al. Abnormal cardiac and skeletal muscle energy metabolism in patients with T2DM. *Circulation.* Jun 24 2003;107(24):3040–3046.

22. Regensteiner JG, Bauer TA, Reusch JE, et al. Abnormal oxygen uptake kinetic responses in women with type II diabetes mellitus. *J Appl Physiol.* Jul 1998;85(1):310–317.

23. Regensteiner JG, Sippel J, McFarling ET, Wolfel EE, Hiatt WR. Effects of non-insulin-dependent diabetes on oxygen consumption during treadmill exercise. *Med Sci Sports Exerc.* Jun 1995;27(6):875–881.

24. Blair SN, Kohl HW, III, Paffenbarger RS, Jr., Clark DG, Cooper KH, Gibbons LW. Physical fitness and all-cause mortality. A prospective study of healthy men and women. *JAMA.* Nov 3 1989;262(17):2395–2401.

25. Blair SN, Kohl HW, III, Barlow CE, Gibbons LW. Physical fitness and all-cause mortality in hypertensive men. *Ann Med.* Aug 1991;23(3):307–312.

26. Blair SN, Kampert JB, Kohl HW, III, et al. Influences of cardiorespiratory fitness and other precursors on cardiovascular disease and all-cause mortality in men and women. *JAMA.* Jul 17 1996;276(3):205–210.

27. Ring-Dimitriou S, von Duvillard SP, Paulweber B, et al. Nine months aerobic fitness induced changes on blood lipids and lipoproteins in untrained subjects versus controls. *Eur J Appl Physiol.* Feb 2007;99(3):291–299.

28. Kraus WE, Houmard JA, Duscha BD, et al. Effects of the amount and intensity of exercise on plasma lipoproteins. *N Engl J Med.* Nov 7 2002;347(19):1483–1492.

29. Thomas DE, Elliott EJ, Naughton GA. Exercise for T2DM mellitus. *Cochrane Database Syst Rev.* 2006;3:CD002968.

30. Krook A, Holm I, Pettersson S, Wallberg-Henriksson H. Reduction of risk factors following lifestyle modification programme in subjects with type 2 (non-insulin dependent) diabetes mellitus. *Clin Physiol Funct Imaging.* Jan 2003;23(1):21–30.

31. Hautala AJ, Leon A, Skinner JS, Rao DC, Bouchard C, Rankinen T. Peroxisome proliferator-activated receptor delta polymorphisms are associated with physical performance and plasma lipids: the HERITAGE family study. *Am J Physiol Heart Circ Physiol.* Jan 26 2007;292: H2498–H2505.

32. Bourey RE, Santoro SA. Interactions of exercise, coagulation, platelets, and fibrinolysis – a brief review. *Med Sci Sports Exerc.* Oct 1988;20(5):439–446.

33. Ribeiro J, Almeida-Dias A, Oliveira AR, Mota J, Appell HJ, Duarte JA. Exhaustive exercise with high eccentric components induces prothrombotic and hypofibrinolytic responses in boys. *Int J Sports Med.* Mar 2007;28(3):193–196.

34. Paton CM, Brandauer J, Weiss EP, et al. Hemostatic response to postprandial lipemia before and after exercise training. *J Appl Physiol.* Jul 2006;101(1):316–321.

35. Barazzoni R, Kiwanuka E, Zanetti M, Cristini M, Vettore M, Tessari P. Insulin acutely increases fibrinogen production in individuals with T2DM but not in individuals without diabetes. *Diabetes.* Jul 2003;52(7):1851–1856.

36. Schneider SH, Kim HC, Khachadurian AK, Ruderman NB. Impaired fibrinolytic response to exercise in type II diabetes: effects of exercise and physical training. *Metabolism.* Oct 1988;37(10):924–929.

37. Hornsby WG, Boggess KA, Lyons TJ, Barnwell WH, Lazarchick J, Colwell JA. Hemostatic alterations with exercise conditioning in NIDDM. *Diabetes Care.* Feb 1990;13(2):87–92.

38. Hamalainen H, Ronnemaa T, Virtanen A, et al. Improved fibrinolysis by an intensive lifestyle intervention in subjects with impaired glucose tolerance. The Finnish Diabetes Prevention Study. *Diabetologia.* Nov 2005;48(11):2248–2253.

39. Kulaputana O, Macko RF, Ghiu I, Phares DA, Goldberg AP, Hagberg JM. Human gender differences in fibrinolytic responses to exercise training and their determinants. *Exp Physiol.* Nov 2005;90(6):881–887.

40. Jennings G, Nelson L, Nestel P, et al. The effects of changes in physical activity on major cardiovascular risk factors, hemodynamics, sympathetic function, and glucose utilization in man: a controlled study of four levels of activity. *Circulation.* Jan 1986;73(1):30–40.

41. Fagard RH, Cornelissen VA. Effect of exercise on blood pressure control in hypertensive patients. *Eur J Cardiovasc Prev Rehabil.* Feb 2007;14(1):12–17.

42. Lazarevic G, Antic S, Cvetkovic T, Vlahovic P, Tasic I, Stefanovic V. A physical activity programme and its effects on insulin resistance and oxidative defense in obese male patients with T2DM mellitus. *Diabetes Metab.* Dec 2006;32(6):583–590.

43. Zeiher AM, Drexler H, Wollschlager H, Just H. Modulation of coronary vasomotor tone in humans. Progressive endothelial dysfunction with different early stages of coronary atherosclerosis. *Circulation.* Feb 1991;83(2):391–401.

44. Suwaidi JA, Hamasaki S, Higano ST, Nishimura RA, Holmes DR, Jr, Lerman A. Long-term follow-up of patients with mild coronary artery disease and endothelial dysfunction. *Circulation.* Mar 7 2000;101(9):948–954.

45. Chan NN, Colhoun HM, Vallance P. Cardiovascular risk factors as determinants of endothelium-dependent and endothelium-independent vascular reactivity in the general population. *J Am Coll Cardiol.* Dec 2001;38(7):1814–1820.

46. Thanyasiri P, Celermajer DS, Adams MR. Endothelial dysfunction occurs in peripheral circulation patients with acute and stable coronary artery disease. *Am J Physiol Heart Circ Physiol.* Aug 2005;289(2):H513–H517.

47. Neunteufl T, Heher S, Katzenschlager R, et al. Late prognostic value of flow-mediated dilation in the brachial artery of patients with chest pain. *Am J Cardiol.* Jul 15 2000;86(2):207–210.

48. Fichtlscherer S, Breuer S, Zeiher AM. Prognostic value of systemic endothelial dysfunction in patients with acute coronary syndromes: further evidence for the existence of the "vulnerable" patient. *Circulation.* Oct 5 2004;110(14):1926–1932.

49. Linke A, Schoene N, Gielen S, et al. Endothelial dysfunction in patients with chronic heart failure: systemic effects of lower-limb exercise training. *J Am Coll Cardiol.* Feb 2001;37(2):392–397.

50. Westhoff TH, Franke N, Schmidt S, et al. Beta-blockers do not impair the cardiovascular benefits of endurance training in hypertensives. *J Hum Hypertens.* Mar 1 2007;21(6):486–493.

51. Kelly AS, Wetzsteon RJ, Kaiser DR, Steinberger J, Bank AJ, Dengel DR. Inflammation, insulin, and endothelial function in overweight children and adolescents: the role of exercise. *J Pediatr.* Dec 2004;145(6):731–736.

52. Meyer AA, Kundt G, Lenschow U, Schuff-Werner P, Kienast W. Improvement of early vascular changes and cardiovascular risk factors in obese children after a six-month exercise program. *J Am Coll Cardiol.* Nov 7 2006;48(9):1865–1870.
53. De Filippis E, Cusi K, Ocampo G, et al. Exercise-induced improvement in vasodilatory function accompanies increased insulin sensitivity in obesity and T2DM mellitus. *J Clin Endocrinol Metab.* Dec 2006;91(12):4903–4910.
54. Maiorana A, O'Driscoll G, Cheetham C, et al. The effect of combined aerobic and resistance exercise training on vascular function in T2DM. *J Am Coll Cardiol.* Sep 2001;38(3):860–866.
55. Zoppini G, Targher G, Zamboni C, et al. Effects of moderate-intensity exercise training on plasma biomarkers of inflammation and endothelial dysfunction in older patients with T2DM. *Nutr Metab Cardiovasc Dis.* Dec 2006;16(8):543–549.
56. Middlebrooke AR, Elston LM, Macleod KM, et al. Six months of aerobic exercise does not improve microvascular function in T2DM mellitus. *Diabetologia.* Oct 2006;49(10):2263–2271.
57. Ostergard T, Nyholm B, Hansen TK, et al. Endothelial function and biochemical vascular markers in first-degree relatives of type 2 diabetic patients: the effect of exercise training. *Metabolism.* Nov 2006;55(11):1508–1515.
58. Maiorana A, O'Driscoll G, Dembo L, Goodman C, Taylor R, Green D. Exercise training, vascular function, and functional capacity in middle-aged subjects. *Med Sci Sports Exerc.* Dec 2001;33(12):2022–2028.
59. Gleeson M. Immune function in sport and exercise. *J Appl Physiol.* Feb 15 2007;103:693–699.
60. Matthews CE, Ockene IS, Freedson PS, Rosal MC, Merriam PA, Hebert JR. Moderate to vigorous physical activity and risk of upper-respiratory tract infection. *Med Sci Sports Exerc.* Aug 2002;34(8):1242–1248.
61. Nieman DC, Johanssen LM, Lee JW, Arabatzis K. Infectious episodes in runners before and after the Los Angeles Marathon. *J Sports Med Phys Fitness.* Sep 1990;30(3):316–328.
62. Libby P. Vascular biology of atherosclerosis: overview and state of the art. *Am J Cardiol.* Feb 6 2003;91(3A):3A–6A.
63. Festa A, D'Agostino R, Jr, Rich SS, Jenny NS, Tracy RP, Haffner SM. Promoter (4G/5G) plasminogen activator inhibitor-1 genotype and plasminogen activator inhibitor-1 levels in blacks, Hispanics, and non-Hispanic whites: the insulin resistance atherosclerosis study. *Circulation.* May 20 2003;107(19):2422–2427.
64. Festa A, Williams K, Tracy RP, Wagenknecht LE, Haffner SM. Progression of plasminogen activator inhibitor-1 and fibrinogen levels in relation to incident T2DM. *Circulation.* Apr 11 2006;113(14):1753–1759.
65. Olson TP, Dengel DR, Leon AS, Schmitz KH. Changes in inflammatory biomarkers following one-year of moderate resistance training in overweight women. *Int J Obes.* Feb 13 2007;31(6):996–1003.
66. Leick L, Lindegaard B, Stensvold D, Plomgaard P, Saltin B, Pilegaard H. Adipose tissue interleukin-18 mRNA and plasma interleukin-18: effect of obesity and exercise. *Obesity.* Feb 2007;15(2):356–363.
67. Mattusch F, Dufaux B, Heine O, Mertens I, Rost R. Reduction of the plasma concentration of C-reactive protein following nine months of endurance training. *Int J Sports Med.* Jan 2000;21(1):21–24.
68. Petersen AM, Pedersen BK. The role of IL-6 in mediating the anti-inflammatory effects of exercise. *J Physiol Pharmacol.* Nov 2006;57 Suppl 10:43–51.
69. Marcell TJ, McAuley KA, Traustadottir T, Reaven PD. Exercise training is not associated with improved levels of C-reactive protein or adiponectin. *Metabolism.* Apr 2005;54(4):533–541.
70. Ruderman NB, Keller C, Richard AM, et al. Interleukin-6 regulation of AMP-activated protein kinase: potential role in the systemic response to exercise and prevention of the metabolic syndrome. *Diabetes.* Dec 2006;55 Suppl 2:S48–S54.
71. Carey AL, Febbraio MA. Interleukin-6 and insulin sensitivity: friend or foe? *Diabetologia.* Jul 2004;47(7):1135–1142.
72. Faldt J, Wernstedt I, Fitzgerald SM, Wallenius K, Bergstrom G, Jansson JO. Reduced exercise endurance in interleukin-6-deficient mice. *Endocrinology.* Jun 2004;145(6):2680–2686.
73. Despres JP, Pouliot MC, Moorjani S, et al. Loss of abdominal fat and metabolic response to exercise training in obese women. *Am J Physiol.* Aug 1991;261(2 Part 1):E159–E167.
74. Zachwieja JJ. Exercise as treatment for obesity. *Endocrinol Metab Clin North Am.* Dec 1996;25(4):965–988.
75. Rodearmel SJ, Wyatt HR, Barry MJ, et al. A family-based approach to preventing excessive weight gain. *Obesity.* Aug 2006;14(8):1392–1401.
76. Phelan S, Wyatt HR, Hill JO, Wing RR. Are the eating and exercise habits of successful weight losers changing? *Obesity.* Apr 2006;14(4):710–716.
77. Pavlou KN, Krey S, Steffee WP. Exercise as an adjunct to weight loss and maintenance in moderately obese subjects. *Am J Clin Nutr.* May 1989;49(5 Suppl):1115–1123.
78. Devlin JT, Hirshman M, Horton ED, Horton ES. Enhanced peripheral and splanchnic insulin sensitivity in NIDDM men after single bout of exercise. *Diabetes.* Apr 1987;36(4):434–439.
79. Ruderman NB, Ganda OP, Johansen K. The effect of physical training on glucose tolerance and plasma lipids in maturity-onset diabetes. *Diabetes.* Jan 1979;28Suppl 1:89–92.
80. Galassetti P, Coker RH, Lacy DB, Cherrington AD, Wasserman DH. Prior exercise increases net hepatic glucose uptake during a glucose load. *Am J Physiol.* Jun 1999;276(6 Part 1):E1022–E1029.
81. O'Gorman DJ, Karlsson HK, McQuaid S, et al. Exercise training increases insulin-stimulated glucose disposal and GLUT4 (SLC2A4) protein content in patients with T2DM. *Diabetologia.* Dec 2006;49(12):2983–2992.
82. Gill JM. Physical activity, cardiorespiratory fitness and insulin resistance: a short update. *Curr Opin Lipidol.* Feb 2007;18(1):47–52.
83. Coker RH, Hays NP, Williams RH, et al. Exercise-induced changes in insulin action and glycogen metabolism in elderly adults. *Med Sci Sports Exerc.* Mar 2006;38(3):433–438.

84. DiPietro L, Dziura J, Yeckel CW, Neufer PD. Exercise and improved insulin sensitivity in older women: evidence of the enduring benefits of higher intensity training. *J Appl Physiol*. Jan 2006;100(1):142–149.

85. Snowling NJ, Hopkins WG. Effects of different modes of exercise training on glucose control and risk factors for complications in type 2 diabetic patients: a meta-analysis. *Diabetes Care*. Nov 2006;29(11):2518–2527.

86. Kelley DE, Goodpaster BH. Effects of exercise on glucose homeostasis in T2DM mellitus. *Med Sci Sports Exerc*. Jun 2001;33(6 Suppl):S495–S501; discussion S528–S599.

87. Tuomilehto J, Lindstrom J, Eriksson JG, et al. Prevention of T2DM mellitus by changes in lifestyle among subjects with impaired glucose tolerance. *N Engl J Med*. May 3 2001;344(18):1343–1350.

88. Pan XR, Li GW, Hu YH, et al. Effects of diet and exercise in preventing NIDDM in people with impaired glucose tolerance. The Da Qing IGT and Diabetes Study. *Diabetes Care*. Apr 1997;20(4):537–544.

89. Knowler WC, Barrett-Connor E, Fowler SE, et al. Reduction in the incidence of T2DM with lifestyle intervention or metformin. *N Engl J Med*. Feb 7 2002;346(6):393–403.

90. Ruderman NB, Haudenschild C. Diabetes as an atherogenic factor. *Prog Cardiovasc Dis*. Mar–Apr 1984;26(5):373–412.

91. Schneider SH, Vitug A, Ruderman N. Atherosclerosis and physical activity. *Diabetes Metab Rev*. 1986;1(4):513–553.

92. Brandenburg SL, Reusch JE, Bauer TA, Jeffers BW, Hiatt WR, Regensteiner JG. Effects of exercise training on oxygen uptake kinetic responses in women with T2DM. *Diabetes Care*. Oct 1999;22(10):1640–1646.

93. Kemmer FW, Tacken M, Berger M. Mechanism of exercise-induced hypoglycemia during sulfonylurea treatment. *Diabetes*. Oct 1987;36(10):1178–1182.

94. Kjaer M, Hollenbeck CB, Frey-Hewitt B, Galbo H, Haskell W, Reaven GM. Glucoregulation and hormonal responses to maximal exercise in non-insulin-dependent diabetes. *J Appl Physiol*. May 1990;68(5):2067–2074.

95. Schneider SH, Khachadurian AK, Amorosa LF, Gavras H, Fineberg SE, Ruderman NB. Abnormal glucoregulation during exercise in type II (non-insulin-dependent) diabetes. *Metabolism*. Dec 1987;36(12):1161–1166.

96. Saltin B, Lindgarde F, Houston M, Horlin R, Nygaard E, Gad P. Physical training and glucose tolerance in middle-aged men with chemical diabetes. *Diabetes*. Jan 1979;28Suppl 1:30–32.

97. Wasserman K, Hansen JE, Sue DY, Whipp BJ, Casaburi R. Principles of Exercise Testing and Interpretation, Second ed. London: Lea & Febiger, 1994.

98. Hansen JE, Sue DY, Oren A, Wasserman K. Relation of oxygen uptake to work rate in normal men and men with circulatory disorders. *Am J Cardiol*. Mar 1 1987;59(6):669–674.

99. Barstow TJ, Mole PA. Simulation of pulmonary O2 uptake during exercise transients in humans. *J Appl Physiol*. Dec 1987;63(6):2253–2261.

100. Whipp B, Mahler M. Dynamics of pulmonary gas exchange during exercise In: West J, ed. Pulmonary Gas Exchange, Vol 2. New York: Academic; 1980:33–96.

101. Grassi B, Poole DC, Richardson RS, Knight DR, Erickson BK, Wagner PD. Muscle O2 uptake kinetics in humans: implications for metabolic control. *J Appl Physiol*. Mar 1996;80(3):988–998.

102. Rossiter HB, Ward SA, Doyle VL, Howe FA, Griffiths JR, Whipp BJ. Inferences from pulmonary O2 uptake with respect to intramuscular [phosphocreatine] kinetics during moderate exercise in humans. *J Physiol*. Aug 1 1999;518 (Part 3):921–932.

103. Jones AM, Poole DC. Oxygen uptake dynamics: from muscle to mouth – an introduction to the symposium. *Med Sci Sports Exerc*. Sep 2005;37(9):1542–1550.

104. Sietsema KE. Oxygen uptake kinetics in response to exercise in patients with pulmonary vascular disease. *Am Rev Respir Dis*. May 1992;145(5):1052–1057.

105. Sietsema KE, Cooper DM, Perloff JK, et al. Dynamics of oxygen uptake during exercise in adults with cyanotic congenital heart disease. *Circulation*. Jun 1986;73(6):1137–1144.

106. Wasserman K. Overview and future directions. *Circulation*. Jan 1990;81(1 Suppl):II59–II64.

107. Bauer TA, Reusch JE, Levi M, Regensteiner JG. Skeletal muscle deoxygenation after the onset of moderate exercise suggests slowed microvascular blood flow kinetics in type 2 diabetes. *Diabetes Care*. Nov 2007; 30(11): 2880–2885.

108. Modan M, Meytes D, Rozeman P, et al. Significance of high HbA1 levels in normal glucose tolerance. *Diabetes Care*. May 1988;11(5):422–428.

109. Schneider SH, Amorosa LF, Khachadurian AK, Ruderman NB. Studies on the mechanism of improved glucose control during regular exercise in type 2 (non-insulin-dependent) diabetes. *Diabetologia*. May 1984;26(5):355–360.

110. Regensteiner JG, Bauer TA, Reusch JE. Rosiglitazone improves exercise capacity in individuals with T2DM. *Diabetes Care*. Dec 2005;28(12):2877–2883.

111. Reusch JE, Regensteiner JG, Watson PA. Novel actions of thiazolidinediones on vascular function and exercise capacity. *Am J Med*. Dec 8 2003;115 Suppl 8A:69S–74S.

112. Seibaek M, Vestergaard H, Burchardt H, et al. Insulin resistance and maximal oxygen uptake. *Clin Cardiol.* Nov 2003;26(11):515–520.

113. Eidemak I, Feldt-Rasmussen B, Kanstrup IL, Nielsen SL, Schmitz O, Strandgaard S. Insulin resistance and hyperinsulinaemia in mild to moderate progressive chronic renal failure and its association with aerobic work capacity. *Diabetologia.* May 1995;38(5):565–572.

114. Swan JW, Anker SD, Walton C, et al. Insulin resistance in chronic heart failure: relation to severity and etiology of heart failure. *J Am Coll Cardiol.* Aug 1997;30(2):527–532.

115. Orio F, Jr, Giallauria F, Palomba S, et al. Cardiopulmonary impairment in young women with polycystic ovary syndrome. *J Clin Endocrinol Metab.* Aug 2006;91(8):2967–2971.

116. Wong CY, O'Moore-Sullivan T, Fang ZY, Haluska B, Leano R, Marwick TH. Myocardial and vascular dysfunction and exercise capacity in the metabolic syndrome. *Am J Cardiol.* Dec 15 2005;96(12):1686–1691.

117. Endre T, Mattiasson I, Hulthen UL, Lindgarde F, Berglund G. Insulin resistance is coupled to low physical fitness in normotensive men with a family history of hypertension. *J Hypertens.* Jan 1994;12(1):81–88.

118. Williams SB, Cusco JA, Roddy MA, Johnstone MT, Creager MA. Impaired nitric oxide-mediated vasodilation in patients with non-insulin-dependent diabetes mellitus. *J Am Coll Cardiol.* Mar 1 1996;27(3):567–574.

119. McVeigh GE, Brennan GM, Johnston GD, et al. Impaired endothelium-dependent and independent vasodilation in patients with type 2 (non-insulin-dependent) diabetes mellitus. *Diabetologia.* Aug 1992;35(8):771–776.

120. Kingwell BA, Formosa M, Muhlmann M, Bradley SJ, McConell GK. Type 2 diabetic individuals have impaired leg blood flow responses to exercise: role of endothelium-dependent vasodilation. *Diabetes Care.* Mar 2003;26(3):899–904.

121. Regensteiner JG, Popylisen S, Bauer TA, et al. Oral l-arginine and vitamins E and C improve endothelial function in women with T2DM. *Vasc Med.* 2003;8(3):169–175.

122. Yki-Jarvinen H. Insulin resistance and endothelial dysfunction. *Best Pract Res Clin Endocrinol Metab.* Sep 2003;17(3):411–430.

123. Steinberg HO, Chaker H, Leaming R, Johnson A, Brechtel G, Baron AD. Obesity/insulin resistance is associated with endothelial dysfunction. Implications for the syndrome of insulin resistance. *J Clin Invest.* Jun 1 1996;97(11): 2601–2610.

124. Borlaug BA, Melenovsky V, Russell SD, et al. Impaired chronotropic and vasodilator reserves limit exercise capacity in patients with heart failure and a preserved ejection fraction. *Circulation.* Nov 14 2006;114(20):2138–2147.

125. Jones AM, Wilkerson DP, Campbell IT. Nitric oxide synthase inhibition with l-NAME reduces maximal oxygen uptake but not gas exchange threshold during incremental cycle exercise in man. *J Physiol.* Oct 1 2004;560 (Part 1):329–338.

126. Jones AM, Wilkerson DP, Koppo K, Wilmshurst S, Campbell IT. Inhibition of nitric oxide synthase by l-NAME speeds phase II pulmonary.VO2 kinetics in the transition to moderate-intensity exercise in man. *J Physiol.* Oct 1 2003;552 (Part 1):265–272.

127. Recchia FA, Osorio JC, Chandler MP, et al. Reduced synthesis of NO causes marked alterations in myocardial substrate metabolism in conscious dogs. *Am J Physiol Endocrinol Metab.* Jan 2002;282(1):E197–E206.

128. Xie YW, Shen W, Zhao G, Xu X, Wolin MS, Hintze TH. Role of endothelium-derived nitric oxide in the modulation of canine myocardial mitochondrial respiration in vitro. Implications for the development of heart failure. *Circ Res.* Sep 1996;79(3):381–387.

129. Shen W, Hintze TH, Wolin MS. Nitric oxide. An important signaling mechanism between vascular endothelium and parenchymal cells in the regulation of oxygen consumption. *Circulation.* Dec 15 1995;92(12):3505–3512.

130. Shen W, Zhang X, Zhao G, Wolin MS, Sessa W, Hintze TH. Nitric oxide production and NO synthase gene expression contribute to vascular regulation during exercise. *Med Sci Sports Exerc.* Aug 1995;27(8):1125–1134.

131. Baldi JC, Aoina JL, Whalley GA, et al. The effect of T2DM on diastolic function. *Med Sci Sports Exerc.* Aug 2006;38(8):1384–1388.

132. Bouchard A, Sanz N, Botvinick EH, et al. Noninvasive assessment of cardiomyopathy in normotensive diabetic patients between 20 and 50 years old. *Am J Med.* Aug 1989;87(2):160–166.

133. Mustonen JN, Uusitupa MI, Tahvanainen K, et al. Impaired left ventricular systolic function during exercise in middle-aged insulin-dependent and noninsulin-dependent diabetic subjects without clinically evident cardiovascular disease. *Am J Cardiol.* Dec 1 1988;62(17):1273–1279.

134. Poirier P, Bogaty P, Garneau C, Marois L, Dumesnil JG. Diastolic dysfunction in normotensive men with well-controlled T2DM: importance of maneuvers in echocardiographic screening for preclinical diabetic cardiomyopathy. *Diabetes Care.* Jan 2001;24(1):5–10.

135. Poirier P, Garneau C, Bogaty P, et al. Impact of left ventricular diastolic dysfunction on maximal treadmill performance in normotensive subjects with well-controlled T2DM mellitus. *Am J Cardiol.* Feb 15 2000;85(4):473–477.

136. Regan TJ, Lyons MM, Ahmed SS, et al. Evidence for cardiomyopathy in familial diabetes mellitus. *J Clin Invest.* Oct 1977;60(4):884–899.

137. Shimizu M, Sugihara N, Kita Y, Shimizu K, Shibayama S, Takeda R. Increase in left ventricular chamber stiffness in patients with non-insulin dependent diabetes mellitus. *Jpn Circ J.* Jul 1991;55(7):657–664.

138. Robillon JF, Sadoul JL, Jullien D, Morand P, Freychet P. Abnormalities suggestive of cardiomyopathy in patients with T2DM of relatively short duration. *Diabetes Metab.*Sep–Oct 1994;20(5):473–480.

139. Uusitupa M, Mustonen J, Laakso M, et al. Impairment of diastolic function in middle-aged type 1 (insulin-dependent) and type 2 (non-insulin-dependent) diabetic patients free of cardiovascular disease. *Diabetologia.* Nov 1988;31(11):783–791.

140. Regensteiner J, Groves, BM, Bauer, TA, Reusch JEB, Smith, SC, Wolfel, EE. Recently diagnosed T2DM mellitus adversely affects cardiac function during exercise. *Diabetes.* 2002;51 (Suppl):A59.

141. Oakes ND, Thalen P, Aasum E, et al. Cardiac metabolism in mice: tracer method developments and in vivo application revealing profound metabolic inflexibility in diabetes. *Am J Physiol Endocrinol Metab.* May 2006;290(5):E870–E881.

142. Mazumder PK, O'Neill BT, Roberts MW, et al. Impaired cardiac efficiency and increased fatty acid oxidation in insulin-resistant ob/ob mouse hearts. *Diabetes.* Sep 2004;53(9):2366–2374.

143. Carley AN, Severson DL. Fatty acid metabolism is enhanced in type 2 diabetic hearts. *Biochim Biophys Acta.* May 15 2005;1734(2):112–126.

144. Peterson LR, Herrero P, Schechtman KB, et al. Effect of obesity and insulin resistance on myocardial substrate metabolism and efficiency in young women. *Circulation.* May 11 2004;109(18):2191–2196.

145. Knuuti J, Takala TO, Nagren K, et al. Myocardial fatty acid oxidation in patients with impaired glucose tolerance. *Diabetologia.* Feb 2001;44(2):184–187.

146. Lowell BB, Shulman GI. Mitochondrial dysfunction and T2DM. *Science.* Jan 21 2005;307(5708):384–387.

147. Patti ME, Butte AJ, Crunkhorn S, et al. Coordinated reduction of genes of oxidative metabolism in humans with insulin resistance and diabetes: potential role of PGC1 and NRF1. *Proc Natl Acad Sci USA.* Jul 8 2003;100(14):8466–8471.

148. Folmes CD, Clanachan AS, Lopaschuk GD. Fatty acid oxidation inhibitors in the management of chronic complications of atherosclerosis. *Curr Atheroscler Rep.* Feb 2005;7(1):63–70.

149. Liu Q, Docherty JC, Rendell JC, Clanachan AS, Lopaschuk GD. High levels of fatty acids delay the recovery of intracellular pH and cardiac efficiency in post-ischemic hearts by inhibiting glucose oxidation. *J Am Coll Cardiol.* Feb 20 2002;39(4):718–725.

150. Zacharowski K, Blackburn B, Thiemermann C. Ranolazine, a partial fatty acid oxidation inhibitor, reduces myocardial infarct size and cardiac troponin T release in the rat. *Eur J Pharmacol.* Apr 20 2001;418(1–2):105–110.

151. Lopaschuk GD. Targets for modulation of fatty acid oxidation in the heart. *Curr Opin Investig Drugs.* Mar 2004;5(3):290–294.

152. He J, Watkins S, Kelley DE. Skeletal muscle lipid content and oxidative enzyme activity in relation to muscle fiber type in T2DM and obesity. *Diabetes.* Apr 2001;50(4):817–823.

153. Williamson JR, Kilo C. Capillary basement membranes in diabetes. *Diabetes.* May 1983;32 Suppl 2:96–100.

154. Behnke BJ, Kindig CA, McDonough P, Poole DC, Sexton WL. Dynamics of microvascular oxygen pressure during rest-contraction transition in skeletal muscle of diabetic rats. *Am J Physiol Heart Circ Physiol.* Sep 2002;283(3):H926–H932.

155. Kindig CA, Sexton WL, Fedde MR, Poole DC. Skeletal muscle microcirculatory structure and hemodynamics in diabetes. *Respir Physiol.* Feb 1998;111(2):163–175.

156. Padilla DJ, McDonough P, Behnke BJ, et al. Effects of Type II diabetes on capillary hemodynamics in skeletal muscle. *Am J Physiol Heart Circ Physiol.* Nov 2006;291(5):H2439–H2444.

157. MacRury SM, Small M, MacCuish AC, Lowe GD. Association of hypertension with blood viscosity in diabetes. *Diabetes Med.* Dec 1988;5(9):830–834.

158. McMillan DE. Exercise and diabetic microangiopathy. *Diabetes.* Jan 1979;28 Suppl 1:103–106.

159. Estacio RO, Regensteiner JG, Wolfel EE, Jeffers B, Dickenson M, Schrier RW. The association between diabetic complications and exercise capacity in NIDDM patients. *Diabetes Care.* Feb 1998;21(2):291–295.

160. Kelley DE, He J, Menshikova EV, Ritov VB. Dysfunction of mitochondria in human skeletal muscle in T2DM. *Diabetes.* Oct 2002;51(10):2944–2950.

161. Ritov VB, Menshikova EV, He J, Ferrell RE, Goodpaster BH, Kelley DE. Deficiency of subsarcolemmal mitochondria in obesity and T2DM. *Diabetes.* Jan 2005;54(1):8–14.

162. Simoneau JA, Kelley DE. Altered glycolytic and oxidative capacities of skeletal muscle contribute to insulin resistance in NIDDM. *J Appl Physiol.* Jul 1997;83(1):166–171.

163. Rabol R, Boushel R, Dela F. Mitochondrial oxidative function and T2DM. *Appl Physiol Nutr Metab.* Dec 2006;31(6):675–683.

164. Boushel R, Gnaiger E, Schjerling P, Skovbro M, Kraunsoe R, Dela F. Patients with T2DM have normal mitochondrial function in skeletal muscle. *Diabetologia*. Apr 2007;50(4):790–796.

165. Marin P, Andersson B, Krotkiewski M, Bjorntorp P. Muscle fiber composition and capillary density in women and men with NIDDM. *Diabetes Care*. May 1994;17(5):382–386.

166. Holloszy JO, Schultz J, Kusnierkiewicz J, Hagberg JM, Ehsani AA. Effects of exercise on glucose tolerance and insulin resistance. Brief review and some preliminary results. *Acta Med Scand Suppl.* 1986;711:55–65.

167. Verity LS, Ismail AH. Effects of exercise on cardiovascular disease risk in women with NIDDM. *Diabetes Res Clin Pract.* Jan 3 1989;6(1):27–35.

168. Berntorp K, Lindgarde F, Malmquist J. High and low insulin responders: relations to oral glucose tolerance, insulin secretion and physical fitness. *Acta Med Scand.* 1984;216(1):111–117.

169. King DS, Dalsky GP, Clutter WE, et al. Effects of exercise and lack of exercise on insulin sensitivity and responsiveness. *J Appl Physiol.* May 1988;64(5):1942–1946.

170. Heath GW, Gavin JR, III, Hinderliter JM, Hagberg JM, Bloomfield SA, Holloszy JO. Effects of exercise and lack of exercise on glucose tolerance and insulin sensitivity. *J Appl Physiol.* Aug 1983;55(2):512–517.

171. LeBlanc J, Nadeau A, Boulay M, Rousseau-Migneron S. Effects of physical training and adiposity on glucose metabolism and 125I-insulin binding. *J Appl Physiol.* Feb 1979;46(2):235–239.

172. Burstein R, Polychronakos C, Toews CJ, MacDougall JD, Guyda HJ, Posner BI. Acute reversal of the enhanced insulin action in trained athletes. Association with insulin receptor changes. *Diabetes.* Aug 1985;34(8):756–760.

173. Galbo H, Hedeskov CJ, Capito K, Vinten J. The effect of physical training on insulin secretion of rat pancreatic islets. *Acta Physiol Scand.* Jan 1981;111(1):75–79.

174. Douen AG, Ramlal T, Cartee GD, Klip A. Exercise modulates the insulin-induced translocation of glucose transporters in rat skeletal muscle. *FEBS Lett.* Feb 26 1990;261(2):256–260.

175. Brenner DA, Apstein CS, Saupe KW. Exercise training attenuates age-associated diastolic dysfunction in rats. *Circulation.* Jul 10 2001;104(2):221–226.

176. Sakamoto S, Minami K, Niwa Y, et al. Effect of exercise training and food restriction on endothelium-dependent relaxation in the Otsuka Long-Evans Tokushima Fatty rat, a model of spontaneous NIDDM. *Diabetes.* Jan 1998; 47(1):82–86.

177. Vanoverschelde JJ, Essamri B, Vanbutsele R, et al. Contribution of left ventricular diastolic function to exercise capacity in normal subjects. *J Appl Physiol.* May 1993;74(5):2225–2233.

5 The Cardiovascular Consequences of Type 2 Diabetes Mellitus

Sherita Hill Golden

CONTENTS

ABSTRACT

Atherosclerosis is the leading cause of death among individuals with type 2 diabetes, accounting for 80% of all mortality among affected individuals. The prediabetic state of insulin resistance, with its accompanying central adiposity, dyslipidemia, and hypertension, is thought to contribute to the development of cardiovascular disease in type 2 diabetes. This chapter summarizes (1) the pathophysiology of the prediabetic state, (2) use of the metabolic syndrome as a clinical proxy for the presence of insulin resistance, and (3) the prediabetic state (metabolic syndrome) as a predictor of cardiovascular disease, highlighting hypertension, dyslipidemia, and impaired glucose metabolism as the strongest predictors. Dyslipidemia, hypertension, and hyperglycemia are highlighted as important targets in cardiovascular disease prevention in type 2 diabetes. Current controversies regarding the glycemic target for cardiovascular disease prevention in diabetes are discussed in light of recently published clinical trials. Other direct cardiovascular effects of diabetes are highlighted, including left ventricular dysfunction, endothelial dysfunction, arterial stiffness, and systemic inflammation.

Key words: Cardiovascular disease; Metabolic syndrome; Dyslipidemia; Hypertension; Hyperglycemia.

From: *Contemporary Diabetes: Diabetes and Exercise*
Edited by: J. G. Regensteiner et al. (eds.), DOI: 10.1007/978-1-59745-260-1_5
© Humana Press, a part of Springer Science+Business Media, LLC 2009

BACKGROUND

Atherosclerosis is the leading cause of death among individuals with type 2 diabetes, accounting for 80% of all mortality among affected individuals. Approximately 75% of these deaths result from coronary atherosclerosis and 25% from cerebral or peripheral arterial disease. Greater than 75% of hospitalizations for diabetic complications are due to atherosclerosis (1). Mortality rates for ischemic heart disease are greater for individuals with diabetes than for unaffected individuals, and this difference is much greater for women. Although men with diabetes have a twofold greater risk of ischemic heart disease death compared with men without diabetes, women with diabetes have a fourfold greater risk of such deaths compared with women without diabetes (2). The decision to make diabetes a coronary heart disease risk equivalent is supported by a landmark study by Haffner et al. in 1998 (3), which showed that patients with diabetes who had never experienced a myocardial infarction had a comparable risk of cardiovascular disease mortality as individuals without diabetes who had experienced an infarction. This study formed the basis for the decision by the American Diabetes Association to intensify risk factor management, particularly cholesterol and hypertension control, in individuals with diabetes.

PATHOPHYSIOLOGY OF THE PREDIABETIC STATE

Insulin Resistance

It has traditionally been thought that type 2 diabetes is a direct risk factor for atherosclerosis and cardiovascular disease. However, there is growing evidence that both type 2 diabetes and cardiovascular disease spring from a "common soil" of metabolic antecedents, including impaired glucose tolerance, hypertension, dyslipidemia, and abdominal obesity (4–6) (see Fig. 1). The clustering of these cardiovascular risk factors results from an underlying insulin resistance syndrome, also known as metabolic syndrome or Syndrome X, that precedes the onset of type 2 diabetes (6–11). Reaven (7) first summarized the insulin resistance syndrome, or Syndrome X, as resistance to insulin-stimulated glucose uptake, hyperinsulinemia, impaired glucose tolerance, hyperglycemia, hypertension, elevated triglycerides, and decreased high-density lipoprotein (HDL) cholesterol. Since this initial description, multiple components of the insulin resistance syndrome, including hyperinsulinemia, impaired glucose tolerance, general and abdominal obesity, dyslipidemia (elevated triglycerides and low HDL), hypertension, elevated small dense LDL, elevated uric acid, and abnormal clotting factors, have been found to cluster in men and women in multiple ethnic groups (8–10, 12–31). Studies that assess insulin

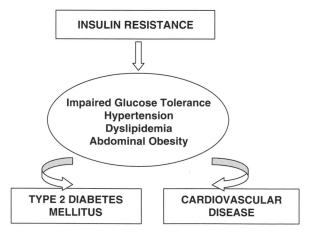

Fig. 1. The "common soil" from which type 2 diabetes and cardiovascular disease arise.

sensitivity by direct measures, such as the hyperinsulinemic euglycemic clamp and frequently sampled intravenous glucose tolerance test, show that reduced insulin sensitivity also clusters with the insulin resistance syndrome metabolic components *(32–38)*.

The presence of these cardiovascular risk factors related to insulin resistance prior to the onset of type 2 diabetes may explain why greater than 50% of patients with newly diagnosed type 2 diabetes already have evidence of coronary artery disease at the time of diagnosis *(1, 4)*. In the San Antonio Heart Study *(4)*, compared with individuals who remained nondiabetic, individuals who eventually developed diabetes had higher body mass index, triglycerides, blood pressure, fasting glucose, 2-h glucose, and fasting insulin as well as lower HDL-cholesterol several years prior to diagnosis. As noted earlier, the insulin resistance syndrome is also associated with other adverse cardiovascular risk factors in the prediabetic state, such as hypercoagulability, which can lead to atherosclerosis and clinical cardiovascular events.

The Metabolic Syndrome as a Proxy for Insulin Resistance

The best available measurements of insulin resistance used in the clinical setting, such as the glucose clamp, the insulin tolerance test, and the intravenous glucose tolerance test, are not practical for use in large epidemiological studies to detect patients at increased risk for cardiovascular disease *(39)*. Because the glucose clamp technique and other available techniques require dedicated equipment and trained personnel, most studies examining the relationship between insulin resistance and cardiovascular disease have used definitions of metabolic syndrome as a proxy for insulin resistance. There are currently at least five definitions of metabolic syndrome, as recently summarized by Grundy et al. *(40)* (see Table 1), and most population-based studies have examined these definitions in studies evaluating the risk of cardiovascular disease due to the insulin resistance/metabolic syndrome. Most commonly, these definitions include measures of insulin resistance and/or glucose, adiposity, dyslipidemia, and blood pressure. Although these definitions are readily available in population-based studies as well as clinical settings, a recent study found that the National Cholesterol Education Program (NCEP) definition of the metabolic syndrome had poor sensitivity in identifying insulin resistance assessed by the hyperinsulinemic-euglycemic clamp *(42, 43)*. This limitation should be kept in mind when using metabolic syndrome definitions as a proxy for insulin resistance as the presence of these definitions does not necessarily indicate the presence of directly measured insulin resistance.

Insulin Resistance and the Metabolic Syndrome as Predictors of Cardiovascular Disease

Epidemiological studies that have measured insulin resistance directly have shown that it is associated with coronary heart disease *(44–46)* and stroke *(47)* but not with femoral atherosclerosis *(48)*. We are unaware of studies showing that directly measured insulin resistance is a predictor of cardiovascular disease because too few large-scale studies have measured insulin resistance due to the cumbersome and invasive nature of assessing this parameter. Therefore, this is an area of active investigation. In the Framingham Offspring Cohort, increased insulin sensitivity, indirectly estimated from Gutt's insulin sensitivity index ($ISI_{0,120}$) derived from an oral glucose tolerance test, was found to be an independent predictor of incident cardiovascular disease *(49)*.

Clustering of dyslipidemia, abdominal obesity, hyperinsulinemia, impaired glucose tolerance, and hypertension have been associated with prevalent and incident atherosclerosis *(50)* and coronary heart disease *(51–57)*, coronary heart disease mortality *(58)*, femoral atherosclerosis *(48)*, claudication *(59)*, and stroke *(54, 60)*.

Table 1
Definitions of Metabolic Syndrome

Clinical measure	WHO (1998)	EGIR	ATP III (2001)	AACE (2003)	IDF (2005)
Insulin resistance	IGT, IFG, type 2 diabetes, or lowered insulin sensitivity[a] *Plus any 2 of the following*	Plasma insulin > 75th percentile *Plus any 2 of the following*	None *But any 3 of the following 5 features*	IGT or IFG *Plus any of the following based on clinical judgment*	None
Body weight	Men: WHR > 0.9 Women: WHR > 0.85 and/or BMI > 30 kg/m²	WC ≥ 94 cm in men WC ≥ 80 in women	WC ≥ 102 cm in men or ≥88 cm in women	BMI ≥ 25 kg/m²	↑ WC (population specific) *Plus any 2 of the following*
Lipid	TG ≥ 150 mg/dL and/or HDL-C < 35 mg/dL in men or <39 mg/dL in women	TG ≥ 150 mg/dL and or HDL-C < 39 mg/dL in men or women	TG ≥ 150 mg/dL HDL-C < 40 mg/dL in men or < 50 mg/dL in women	TG ≥ 150 mg/dL and HDL-C < 40 mg/dL in men or < 50 mg/dL in women	TG ≥ 50 mg/dL or on TG therapy HDL-C < 40 mg/dL in men or < 50 mg/dL in women or on HDL-C therapy
Blood pressure	≥140/90 mm Hg	≥140/90 mm Hg or on hypertension therapy	≥130/85 mm Hg	≥130/85 mm Hg	≥130 mm Hg systolic or ≥85 mm Hg diastolic or on hypertension therapy
Glucose	IGT, IFT, or type 2 diabetes	IFT or IFG (but not diabetes)	>110 mg/dL (included diabetes)[b]	IGT or IFG (but not diabetes)	≥100 mg/dL (includes diabetes)
Other	Microalbuminuria			Other features of insulin resistance[c]	

Reprinted with permission from Grundy et al.[40] © 2008, American Heart Association, Inc.

[a] Insulin sensitivity measured under hyperinsulinemic euglycemic conditions, glucose uptake lowest quartile for background population under investigation

[b] Modified in 2004 to be ≥100 mg/dL in accordance with the American Diabetes Association's updated IFG definitions (41)

[c] Family history of type 2 diabetes mellitus, polycystic ovary syndrome, sedentary lifestyle, advancing age, and ethnic groups susceptible to type 2 diabetes mellitus

Specific definitions of the metabolic syndrome, used as a proxy for insulin resistance in population-based studies, have also been shown to predict cardiovascular disease, although to varying degrees *(61)*. Ford et al. *(62)* recently reviewed prospective studies of the NCEP and World Health Organization (WHO) definitions of metabolic syndrome as predictors of cardiovascular disease from 1998 to 2004. They found that the aggregate relative risk estimate for cardiovascular disease from seven studies using the NCEP definition was 1.65 (95% CI: 1.38–1.99) and the aggregate risk from two studies using the WHO definition was 1.93 (95% CI: 1.39–2.67). In the remainder of this section, we will highlight a few of the studies included in Ford's review as well as some published more recently.

In a cross-sectional analysis, McNeill et al. found that individuals with metabolic syndrome, defined by the NCEP criteria, were two times as likely to have prevalent coronary heart disease and had thicker carotid intimal-medial thickness than those who did not have the syndrome in the Atherosclerosis Risk in Communities (ARIC) Study *(63)*. Compared to individuals without metabolic syndrome, those with metabolic syndrome only were 54% (OR = 1.54; 95% CI: 1.27–1.86) more likely and those with metabolic syndrome and diabetes were three times (OR = 3.28; 95% CI: 2.62–4.11) more likely to have prevalent coronary heart disease, respectively *(63)*.

Prospective analyses of the Kuopio Ischaemic Heart Disease Risk Factor Study demonstrated that the presence of metabolic syndrome predicted an increased risk of coronary heart disease, cardiovascular disease, and overall mortality over an average of 11.4 years of follow-up *(64)*. Among individuals who met the NCEP criteria of metabolic syndrome, there was a greater than fourfold increased risk of coronary heart disease death, following multivariate adjustment for other cardiovascular risk factors (HR = 4.26; 95% CI: 1.62–11.2) *(64)*. When metabolic syndrome was defined according to WHO criteria, there was a similarly increased risk of coronary heart disease mortality (HR = 3.32; 95% CI: 1.36–8.11) *(64)*.

Similarly, in the ARIC Study, individuals who met the NCEP criteria for metabolic syndrome had increased risk of CHD and stroke. Following adjustment for multiple cardiovascular risk factors, women with metabolic syndrome had a twofold increased risk of CHD (HR = 2.05; 95% CI: 1.59–2.64) and men with metabolic syndrome had a 50% increased risk of CHD (HR = 1.46; 95% CI: 1.23–1.74) compared to those without metabolic syndrome. Similar results were found for ischemic stroke, where women and men with metabolic syndrome had an increased risk of stroke compared to those without metabolic syndrome (HR = 1.96; 95% CI: 1.28–3.00 for women; HR = 1.42; 95% CI: 0.96–2.11 for men) *(65)*. Two other studies also found that metabolic syndrome, defined by NCEP criteria, predicted incident stroke *(66, 67)*. Koren-Morag et al. found that following multivariable adjustment, the presence of metabolic syndrome was associated with a 39% increased risk of ischemic stroke in men (OR = 1.39; 95% CI: 1.10–1.77) and a twofold increased risk in women (OR = 2.10; 95% CI: 1.26–3.51) *(67)*. In a case-control study of elderly patients with a first-ever acute ischemic nonembolic stroke, the adjusted odds ratio for metabolic syndrome in the stroke patients was 2.59 (95% CI: 1.24–5.42) *(66)*.

Which Metabolic Syndrome Risk Factor Clusters Are Most Associated with Atherosclerosis and Clinical Cardiovascular Events?

While specific definitions of metabolic syndrome appear to predict cardiovascular disease and may explain why individuals with diabetes are at such an increased risk of macrovascular disease, one important question is which components of the syndrome are most important in predicting cardiovascular disease risk. We have previously reviewed the literature in this area *(68)*. Among nearly 12,000 middle-aged adults in the ARIC Study without previously diagnosed diabetes, coronary artery disease, or dyslipidemia, we examined the association between various insulin resistance syndrome clusters and subclinical atherosclerosis, assessed by B-mode ultrasound measurements of carotid

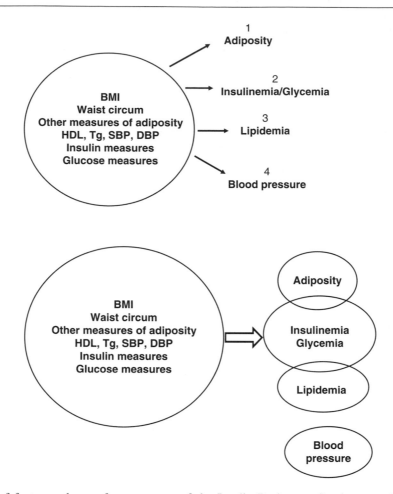

Fig. 2. Summary of factor analyses of components of the Insulin Resistance Syndrome and overlap among the physiological variables. *BMI* body mass index, *DBP* diastolic blood pressure, *HDL* HDL-cholesterol, *SBP* systolic blood pressure, *Tg* triglycerides. Reprinted with permission from Golden and Chong.[68] © 2004, Current Medicine Group, LLC, Philadelphia.

intimal-medial thickness *(50)*. We found that the insulin resistance syndrome clusters most strongly associated with excess carotid intimal-medial thickness all included hypertension and hypertrigly-ceridemia, indicating that the interaction between these two components are important in conferring cardiovascular risk. McNeill et al. also found that elevated blood pressure was significantly associated with incident coronary heart disease in ARIC, as was low HDL-cholesterol *(65)*. In the study by Koren-Morag et al., impaired fasting glucose and hypertension were the strongest predictors of ischemic stroke *(67)*.

Many epidemiological studies have used factor analysis to help reduce metabolic syndrome components into a better defined syndrome *(69)*. In factor analyses of metabolic syndrome in various populations, at least two factors have been identified as central to metabolic syndrome and most studies have identified three or four factors – adiposity, insulinemia/glycemia, lipidemia, and blood pressure *(69)* (see Fig. 2). Of note, there is overlap of these factors, with the insulin variables frequently included with measure of adiposity, glycemia, and lipidemia *(69)* (see Fig. 2). This suggests that insulin resistance and disordered glucose metabolism are central to the syndrome. In most studies, blood pressure appears

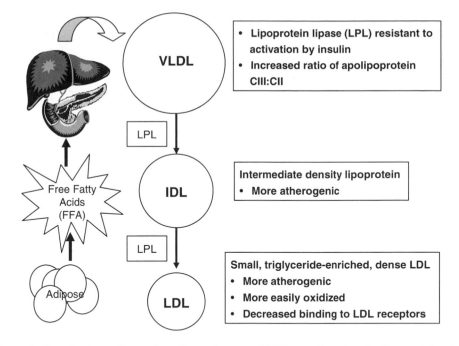

Fig. 3. Lipid metabolism in the setting of insulin resistance. *VLDL* very low-density lipoprotein cholesterol, *IDL* intermediate density lipoprotein cholesterol, *LDL* low density lipoprotein cholesterol.

to be a distinct factor that does not consistently overlap with the insulin resistance factors; hypertension, however, is still important in the pathogenesis of cardiovascular disease.

Four studies have employed factor analysis to determine which factors prospectively predict cardiovascular events *(54, 56, 58, 64)*, and each have identified insulinemia/glycemia, adiposity, and lipidemia as predictive factors. Two studies also found separate blood pressure factors *(56, 58)*. In general, the insulin resistance, blood pressure, and lipid factors predicted an increased risk of cardiovascular events in prospective analyses. Table 2 summarizes the risk of cardiovascular events according to the presence (vs. absence) of the various factors. Compared to individuals without the insulin resistance factor, those with the factor had a 28–43% increased risk of coronary heart disease death *(54, 56, 58, 64)*; however, in one study, the insulin resistance factor predicted a greater than threefold increased risk of coronary heart disease mortality *(64)*. The blood pressure and lipidemia factors predicted a similar 29–52% increased risk of coronary heart disease events, indicating that all of these factors are important in predicting cardiovascular disease risk *(68)*.

Does the Presence of Metabolic Syndrome Predict Cardiovascular Disease Beyond the Additive Effects of Its Individual Components?

If metabolic syndrome is related to an underlying pathophysiology of insulin resistance, one would expect the clustering of risk factors in the syndrome to predict cardiovascular disease beyond the additive effects of its individual components. In a cross-sectional analysis in the ARIC Study, clustering of metabolic syndrome components appeared to be synergistic and were associated with excess carotid atherosclerosis beyond the additive effects of its individual components *(50)*. However, in the same study population, McNeill et al. found that the CHD risk due to metabolic syndrome was not in excess of that predicted by its individual components *(65)*. These results were recently replicated in

Table 2
Insulin Resistance Syndrome Factors Predictive of Cardiovascular Disease Outcomes

Study	Components of factor	Risk of cardiovascular outcomes (risk estimate and 95% confidence interval)
Insulinemia factors		
Lempiainen et al.[56]	BMI, WHR, triglycerides, fasting plasma glucose, insulin	CHD death in men: RH = 1.33 (1.08–1.65)
Lehto et al.[58]	BMI, triglycerides, insulin, low HDL	CHD death in diabetics: RH = 1.43 (1.18–1.73)
Pyorala et al.[54]	BMI, subscapular skin fold, AUC insulin, AUC glucose, maximum O_2 uptake, mean BP, triglycerides	CHD: RH = 1.28 (1.10–1.50) Stroke: RH = 1.64 (1.29–2.08)
Lakka et al.[64]	BMI, WHR, fasting insulin, fasting glucose, triglycerides, HDL, systolic BP	CHD mortality: RR = 3.77 (1.74–8.17) CVD mortality: RR = 3.55 (1.96–6.43)
Blood pressure factors		
Lempiainen et al.[56]	Systolic BP, age, urinary micro-albumin/creatinine ratio, left ventricular hypertrophy	CHD death in men: RH = 1.52 (1.26–1.83) CHD death in women: RH = 1.44 (1.15–1.82)
Lehto et al.[58]	Hypertension, age, smoking	CHD death in diabetics: RH = 1.29 (1.07–1.56)
Lipidemia factors		
Pyorala et al.[54]	Cholesterol, triglycerides	CHD events: RH = 1.47 (1.26–1.71)
Lempiainen et al.[56]	Previous stroke, triglycerides, low HDL	CHD events in women only: RH = 1.34 (1.06–1.69)

Reprinted with permission from Golden and Chong.[68] © 2004, Current Medicine Group, LLC, Philadelphia

Abbreviations: *AUC* area under the curve, *BMI* body mass index, *BP* blood pressure, *CHD* coronary heart disease, *CVD* cardiovascular disease, *HDL* high-density lipoprotein, *RH* relative hazard, *RR* relative risk, *WHR* waist-to-hip ratio

a Swedish population that also showed that metabolic syndrome did not predict CVD mortality independently of its individual components *(70)*.

While there is controversy about whether metabolic syndrome is due to the underlying pathophysiology of insulin resistance, it is clear that the cardiovascular risk factors associated with the syndrome contribute to unfavorable cardiovascular outcomes in individuals with diabetes mellitus. We will now more closely examine three of those risk factors that need to be identified and treated aggressively in individuals with diabetes – dyslipidemia, hypertension, and hyperglycemia.

DYSLIPIDEMIA

Compared to individuals without diabetes, those with diabetes typically have elevated triglycerides and low HDL-cholesterol levels *(71)*. In studies of both diabetic and nondiabetic individuals, triglyceride levels are positively correlated with direct measures of insulin resistance *(35, 35–37)* as well as serum insulin levels *(22, 29)*. Individuals with type 2 diabetes have three characteristic abnormalities in their lipid profiles – (1) hypertriglyceridemia, (2) small, dense LDL-cholesterol, and (3) low HDL-cholesterol. In the Strong Heart Study, diabetic women had lower HDL-cholesterol levels compared to women without diabetes and both men and women with diabetes had lower LDL particle size than their nondiabetic counterparts *(37, 72)*. Type 2 diabetes is also associated with a higher prevalence of small, dense LDL-cholesterol *(73, 74)*.

Hypertriglyceridemia and Small, Dense LDL-Cholesterol

Insulin resistance is hypothesized to cause abnormalities in lipoprotein metabolism that lead to elevated triglyceride levels and atherogenesis, including impaired degradation of triglycerides in very low-density lipoprotein (VLDL) by lipoprotein lipase, increased hepatic VLDL synthesis, and increased free fatty acid (FFA) flux to the liver due to decreased FFA trapping by adipose tissue. Lipoprotein lipase, the enzyme responsible for triglyceride degradation, is activated by insulin; however, in the setting of diabetes and insulin resistance, lipoprotein lipase becomes resistant activation by insulin (see Fig. 3). In addition, the increased number of apoprotein CIII particles on triglyceride-rich VLDL particles also slows the degradation of triglycerides, as CIII is an inhibitor of lipoprotein lipase *(75)*. As a result, VLDLs are cleared more slowly leading to elevated levels of intermediate density lipoproteins, which are more atherogenic. Through the action of cholesterol ester transferase protein, these lipolytic products become triglyceride enriched, with hydrolysis of the triglycerides and phospholipids by hepatic lipase *(76, 77)*. The resultant LDL-cholesterol is smaller, triglyceride enriched, and denser. There are several mechanisms through which small, dense LDL particles promote atherosclerosis. They are more easily oxidized *(75, 76, 78)*, are cleared more slowly from the circulation due to decreased binding affinity for hepatic LDL receptors *(75, 76, 78)*, have greater propensity for transport into the subendothelial space *(76)*, enhance vascular permeability *(78)*, and are associated with increased binding to arterial wall proteoglycans *(76)*.

Other abnormalities in the setting of insulin resistance that lead to dyslipidemia include failure of insulin to suppress FFA release from adipose tissue and to stimulate FFA uptake in skeletal muscle, providing more substrate for hepatic triglyceride synthesis *(75, 76)* and increased hepatic triglyceride secretion through hyperinsulinemia-induced upregulation of fatty acid synthase and acetyl CoA carboxylase *(75)*. Hypertriglyceridemia is also associated with a proinflammatory state, including elevated levels of C-reactive protein, fibrinogen, plasminogen activator inhibitor-1, and interleukin-6, all of which are associated with atherosclerosis *(79)*.

Low HDL-Cholesterol

In the setting of insulin resistance, there is an increased transfer of cholesterol from HDL-cholesterol to triglyceride-enriched lipoproteins (i.e., VLDL-cholesterol) and a reciprocal transfer of triglycerides to HDL-cholesterol *(76)*. The triglycerides in these HDL-cholesterol particles are hydrolyzed by hepatic lipase, resulting in HDL-cholesterol that is more rapidly catabolized and cleared from the plasma. These HDL particles, which are subclasses 3b and 3c, are smaller and denser and likely do not have the same cardioprotective effect as the 2b subclass of HDL particles *(76)*.

Diabetic Dyslipidemia and Cardiovascular Events

The lipoprotein abnormalities outlined earlier have all been shown to be predictive of cardiovascular disease in epidemiological studies, although the majority of studies have not examined the role of dyslipidemia in predicting cardiovascular disease in individuals with diabetes specifically and this should be a focus of future epidemiological research. In a meta-analysis of 17 population-based studies *(80)*, each 1 mmol/L increase in plasma triglycerides was associated with a 32% increased risk of coronary heart disease in men and a 76% increased risk of coronary heart disease in women. Although these associations were attenuated following adjustment for HDL-cholesterol and other cardiovascular risk factors, they remained significant – 14% increased risk of coronary heart disease in men and a 37% increased risk of coronary heart disease in women for each 1 mmol/L increase in triglycerides. Although triglycerides were not predictive of coronary heart disease in patients with newly diagnosed type 2 diabetes in the United Kingdom Prospective Diabetes Study *(81)*, several other studies since the publication of the aforementioned meta-analysis have found hypertriglyceridemia to be a risk factor for coronary heart disease *(82–84)*.

In the United Kingdom Prospective Diabetes Study, in contrast to hypertriglyceridemia, low HDL cholesterol was a strong predictor of coronary heart disease in individuals with newly diagnosed type 2 diabetes *(81)*. Other studies have examined the ratio of total cholesterol to HDL-cholesterol (which may be relevant in individuals with type 2 diabetes) and the ratio of LDL- to HDL-cholesterol and have found that both are strong predictors of coronary heart disease *(81, 85–89)*. In addition, several epidemiological studies have shown that small, dense LDL-cholesterol is also predictive of coronary heart disease *(90–95)*.

HYPERTENSION

The prevalence of hypertension in diabetes mellitus is 1.5–3 times higher than it is in nondiabetic individuals *(96)*. Hypertension usually develops later in the course of type 1 diabetes in the setting of nephropathy; however, hypertension may be already present at the onset of type 2 diabetes as it is frequently present in the prediabetic state. While 30% of patients with type 1 diabetes will develop hypertension, approximately 20–60% of patients with type 2 diabetes will develop hypertension, depending on the patient population studied *(96)*.

As shown by Haffner et al., as well as others *(4, 97, 98)*, prediabetic individuals have higher blood pressure 3–16 years prior to the diagnosis of type 2 diabetes compared to individuals who remain nondiabetic, even within the normal range, which likely also contributes to diabetic cardiovascular disease. We studied a population of 1,152 white male medical students in the Johns Hopkins Precursors Study and found that compared to individuals who did not develop diabetes, those who developed type 2 diabetes had higher absolute systolic and diastolic blood pressure prior to their diagnosis and this difference was evident as early as 30 years of age (see Fig. 4a). In addition, the yearly rate of rise in systolic and diastolic blood pressure in those who developed diabetes compared to those who remained nondiabetic was significantly higher (see Fig. 4b) *(98)*. Thus, elevated blood pressure prior to the onset of type 2 diabetes contributes to the increased risk of cardiovascular disease.

Diabetic individuals with hypertension have a significantly increased risk of cardiovascular disease *(99)*. Factor analyses of the metabolic syndrome have also shown that blood pressure is important in predicting cardiovascular disease (see Table 2). Lempiainen et al. found that the blood pressure factor predicted a 52% increased risk of coronary heart disease death in men (RH = 1.52; 95% CI: 1.26–1.83) and a 44% increased risk in women (RH = 1.44; 95% CI: 1.15–1.82) *(56)*. Lehto et al. also found that their blood pressure factor predicted an increased risk of death in individuals with diabetes mellitus (RH = 1.29; 95% CI: 1.07–1.56) *(58)*. In the UKPDS, blood pressure was significantly associated with cardiovascular disease among individuals with type 2 diabetes. In that study, for every 10 mmHg reduction in systolic blood pressure, there was a 12% decrease in fatal and nonfatal MI, a 19% reduction in fatal and nonfatal stroke, and a 16% decrease in amputation or death from peripheral vascular disease *(100)*.

The pathophysiology of hypertension in the setting of diabetes and insulin resistance is somewhat complex. In the setting of nephropathy, hypertension likely results from increased extracellular fluid volume and total body sodium as well as decreased activity of the renin–angiotensin–aldosterone system (RAAS) *(96)*. The mechanisms linking hypertension to diabetes and insulin resistance in the

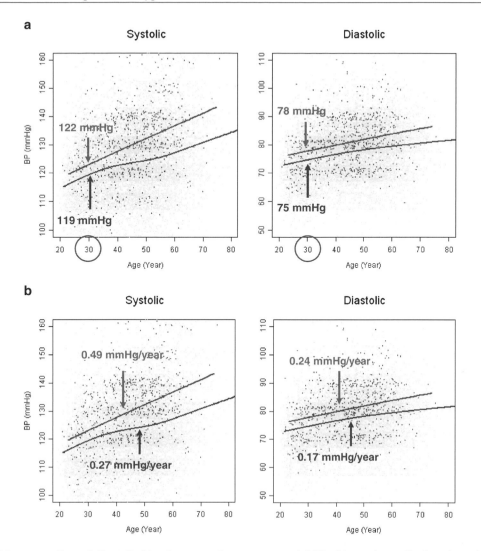

Fig. 4. (**a**) Mean systolic and diastolic blood pressure by age among 1,152 white male medical students in the Johns Hopkins Precursors Study (© 2003 American Diabetes Association). From *Diabetes Care*, Vol. 26; 1110–1115. Reprinted with permission from The American Diabetes Association. (**b**) Mean rate of change in systolic and diastolic blood pressure by age among 1,152 white male medical students in the Johns Hopkins Precursors Study.

nonnephropathy setting are thought to be different, with increased total body sodium in the setting of normal or low RAAS activity. Hyperinsulinemia and insulin resistance are postulated to contribute to hypertension in several ways, including increased renal sodium absorption *(96, 101)*, overactivity of the sympathetic nervous system *(102, 103)*, and decreased vasodilatory and increased vasopressor responses to skeletal muscle vasculature to insulin *(104)*. Epidemiological studies have shown that baseline plasma insulin levels predict incident hypertension in men and women as well as changes in blood pressure over time *(105)*. Although elevated blood pressure is not a consistent feature of the insulin resistance syndrome, the coexistence of insulin resistance in the setting of hypertension is likely a key risk factor in the etiology of cardiovascular disease in diabetes.

Table 3
Quantitative Summary of Meta-Analysis of Prospective Cohort
Studies Examining the Association Between Glycosylated
Hemoglobin and Cardiovascular Outcomes *(109)*

Type 1 Diabetes	Number of studies	Pooled relative risk (95% CI)
Coronary heart disease	3	1.15 (0.92–1.09)
Peripheral arterial disease	2	1.32 (1.19–1.45)
Type 2 Diabetes		
CHD and stroke combined (CVD)	10	1.18 (1.10–1.26)
CHD only	6	1.13 (1.06–1.20)
Stroke	3	1.17 (1.09–1.25)
Peripheral arterial disease	3	1.28 (1.18–1.39)

Abbreviations: *CI* Confidence interval, *CHD* coronary heart disease, *CVD* cardiovascular disease

HYPERGLYCEMIA

While the results from early clinical trials of glucose control which collected data on cardiovascular outcomes have been equivocal *(106)*, results of epidemiological studies suggest that hyperglycemia is associated with cardiovascular disease risk. Several meta-analyses have shown positive graded relations between fasting glucose and 2-h postprandial glucose levels and incident cardiovascular events extending below the threshold for a diagnosis of diabetes *(107, 108)*. A recent meta-analysis has also shown that hemoglobin A1c (Hb_{A1c}), a measure of chronic hyperglycemia, is also associated with an increased risk of cardiovascular disease (Table 3) *(109)*. Three studies in individuals with type 1 diabetes showed that there was a 15% increased risk of coronary heart disease for each 1% point increase in Hb_{A1c}, although the result was not statistically significant, likely due to the small sample size (RR = 1.15; 95% CI: 0.92–1.09). In contrast, two studies in individuals with type 1 diabetes showed that there was a significantly 32% increased risk of peripheral arterial disease for each 1% point increase in Hb_{A1c} (RR = 1.32; 95% CI: 1.19–1.45) *(109)*. There were ten studies identified in individuals with type 2 diabetes that evaluated Hb_{A1c} in relation to combined CHD or stroke and the pooled analysis showed an 18% increased risk of these events for each 1% point increase in Hb_{A1c} (RR = 1.18; 95% CI: 1.10–1.26) *(109)*. When examining individual cardiovascular disease endpoints in those with type 2 diabetes, there was a 13, 17, and 28% increased risk of coronary heart disease, stroke, and peripheral arterial disease, respectively, for each 1% point increase in Hb_{A1c} (Table 3) *(109)* This meta-analysis, while the most comprehensive to date, had several limitations. Several studies included glucose in models with Hb_{A1c}, leading to "overadjustment," which would underestimate the true effect of glycemic control on cardiovascular disease. In addition, many studies used automated selection strategies to select covariates to include in the final models. This relies on statistical cut points for model building instead of clinical and pathophysiological reasoning and as a result, only three studies included in the meta-analysis simultaneously adjusted for known risk factors for cardiovascular disease, such as age, sex, lipids, blood pressure, and smoking.

To address the concerns and limitations of the meta-analyses, an ancillary study in the ARIC Study measured Hb_{A1c} and examined it as a risk factor for coronary heart disease, stroke, and peripheral arterial disease during 8–10 years of follow-up (see Table 4). Following multivariable adjustment for multiple cardiovascular risk factors, including age, sex, race, smoking status, body mass index,

Table 4

Prospective Studies of Hemoglobin A1c as a Predictor of Cardiovascular Outcomes in Persons with Diabetes in the Atherosclerosis Risk in Communities Study

Study	Duration of follow-up	Number of subjects	Outcome	Adjusted relative risk (95% CI) for highest category compared with lowest
(110)	8–10 years	1,626	Coronary heart disease	≥8.2 vs. < 5.2% RR = 2.37 (1.50, 3.72) [RR = 1.14 (1.07, 1.21) per 1% point increase in HbA$_{1c}$]
(111)	8–10 years	1,635	Ischemic stroke	>6.8 vs. < 5.5% RR = 2.33 (1.29, 4.21)
(112)	8–10 years	1,894	Peripheral arterial disease	>7.5 vs. < 5.9% RR = 4.55 (1.52, 13.06) [intermittent claudication] RR = 4.56 (1.86, 11.18) [PAD hospitalization or amputation] RR = 1.64 (0.94, 2.87) [ankle brachial index < 0.9]

Reprinted with permission from Golden et al. Glycemic status and cardiovascular disease in type 2 diabetes mellitus: re-visiting glycated hemoglobin targets for cardiovascular disease prevention. *Diabetes, Obesity, and Metabolism* 2007; 9(6):792–798. © 2007 Wiley-Blackwell

Abbreviations: *MI* myocardial infarction, *CHD* coronary heart disease, *RR* relative risk, *CI* confidence interval

waist-to-hip ratio, blood pressure, and lipids, it was observed that individuals with diabetes in the highest quintile of Hb$_{A1c}$ had greater than twofold increased risk of coronary heart disease compared to those in the lowest quintile (RR = 2.42; 95% CI: 1.55–3.78; *p*-value for trend < 0.0001) *(110)*. In addition, among individuals with diabetes, the risk of coronary heart disease increased across the full range of Hb$_{A1c}$ values, such that there was a 14% increased risk of coronary heart disease for each 1% point increase in Hb$_{A1c}$ (RR = 1.14; 95% CI: 1.07–1.21) *(110)*. Similarly, there was an increased risk of stroke with increasing tertiles of Hb$_{A1c}$ among adults with diabetes (*p*-value for trend < 0.0001) with those in the upper two tertiles having a two- to fourfold increased risk of stroke compared to nondiabetic individuals in the lowest tertile of Hb$_{A1c}$ *(111)*. Finally, the risk of severe, symptomatic peripheral arterial disease was over fourfold greater in individuals with diabetes in the upper tertile of Hb$_{A1c}$ compared to the lowest tertile (RR = 4.56; 95% CI: 1.86–11.18) *(113)*. The results of these epidemiological studies, as well as epidemiological analyses of the United Kingdom Prospective Diabetes Study *(114, 115)*, suggest that HbA$_{1c}$ is linearly associated with an increased risk of cardiovascular disease, even below the current treatment threshold of 7% for prevention of microvascular diabetic complications. However, the results of two recent large clinical trials designed to examine intensive glucose control targeting an Hb$_{A1c}$ < 7% on risk of cardiovascular outcomes suggests that this may not be the case.

In the Action to Control Cardiovascular Risk in Diabetes (ACCORD) Trial *(116)*, 10,251 individuals with type 2 diabetes for an average of 10 years were randomized to receive intensive glucose lowering with a target Hb$_{A1c}$ of <6% versus a conventional Hb$_{A1c}$ target of 7.5%. The actual Hb$_{A1c}$ achieved in the intensive therapy group was 6.4%. Although there was not a significant reduction in the primary outcome (nonfatal MI, nonfatal stroke, and death from cardiovascular causes), there was a 24% reduction in nonfatal MI (HR = 0.76; 95% CI: 0.62–0.92). However, of concern was that there was a significantly increased risk of all-cause and cardiovascular mortality in the intensively treated group (HR = 1.22; 95% CI: 1.01–1.46 and HR = 1.35; 95% CI: 1.04–1.76, respectively). In the Action in Diabetes and Vascular Disease (ADVANCE) Study *(117)*, 11,140 individuals who had type 2 diabetes for an average duration of 8 years were randomized to intensive glucose control with a target HbA1c < 6.5% or to conventional glucose control with a target Hb_{A1c} of 7.0%. There was no significant reduction in major cardiovascular events (nonfatal MI, nonfatal stroke, or cardiovascular disease death), although there was not an increase in mortality in the intensively controlled group, in contrast to the ACCORD Study. These results indicate that targeting an Hb_{A1c} < 7% in individuals with type 2 diabetes of moderate duration does not reduce cardiovascular events and may increase risk for mortality. Further studies are needed to determine if there is a subgroup of patients who may still benefit from more intensive glucose control for cardiovascular disease prevention.

Acute Effects of Hyperglycemia

Acute effects of hyperglycemia can include several adverse vascular outcomes *(118)*. It can lead to endothelial dysfunction through inactivation of nitric oxide and by triggering production of reactive oxygen species. It also can have adverse cardiovascular effects, including impairment of ischemic preconditioning, increased cardiac myocycte death via apoptosis and exaggerated ischemia-reperfusion cellular injury, elevation of blood pressure, catecholamines, and natriuretic peptides, and promotion of platelet abnormalities and electrophysiological changes *(118)*. Hyperglycemia may act acutely to increase the propensity to thrombosis through increased synthesis of thromboxane and plasminogen activator inhibitor-1 and decreased synthesis of tissue plasminogen activator, all of which lead to decreased fibrinolytic activity *(118)*.

Levels of inflammatory cytokines, including interleukin-6, interleukin-8, and tumor necrosis factor-α, may be increased by acute hyperglycemia as well as induction of NF-kappa beta, a proinflammatory transcriptional factor. Interleukin-8 has been shown to destabilize plaques, which could lead to adverse cardiovascular consequences. In addition to causing inflammation, hyperglycemia leads to oxidative stress, with an increase in the generation of reactive oxygen species *(118)*.

Finally, acute hyperglycemia potentially has adverse effects on the brain. It may enhance neuronal damage following induced brain ischemia, especially in the ischemic penumbra, increase levels of glutamate in the neocortex, and lead to DNA fragmentation, disruption of the blood brain barrier, increase β-amyloid precursor protein, and increase superoxide levels. Hyperglycemia may also increase acidosis and lactate in the brain and levels of lactate-to-choline ratio, measured by proton magnetic resonance spectroscopy, predict clinical outcomes and infarct size in stroke *(118)*.

Chronic Effects of Hyperglycemia

Chronic hyperglycemia has known adverse effects on cardiovascular health in diabetes. Excess glucose is proposed to activate several pathways, as recently summarized by Sheetz et al. *(119)*, and outlined in Fig. 5. Activation of the aldolase reductase, advanced glycation endproduct, and reactive oxygen intermediate pathways leads to accumulation of glucotoxins. These glucotoxins, along with activation of the protein kinase C pathway, lead to activation of cell signaling molecules. These molecules alter gene expression and protein function, which ultimately leads to cellular dysfunction and damage, including abnormal angiogenesis, hyperpermeability, abnormal blood flow, contractility, cardiomyopathy, abnormal cell growth and survival, thrombosis, basement membrane thickening, and increased leukocyte adhesion *(119)*.

OTHER EFFECTS OF DIABETES ON THE CARDIOVASCULAR SYSTEM

As outlined in Fig. 6, there are several cardiovascular abnormalities that lead to cardiovascular disease in diabetes.

Left Ventricular Diastolic Dysfunction: Abnormalities in Early Diastolic Filling

Congestive heart failure is a frequent consequence of type 2 diabetes, independent of coronary heart disease *(120)*. Abnormalities in early left ventricular diastolic filling are seen in type 2 diabetes

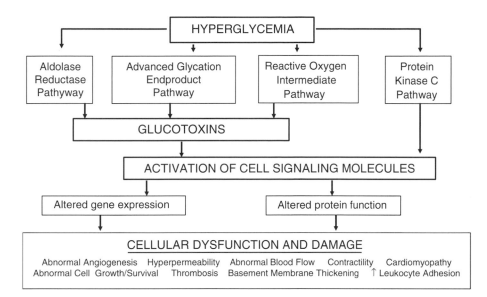

Fig. 5. Proposed mechanisms linking chronic hyperglycemia to adverse vascular outcomes. Adapted from Sheetz MJ and King GL, JAMA, 2003;289:1779–1788.

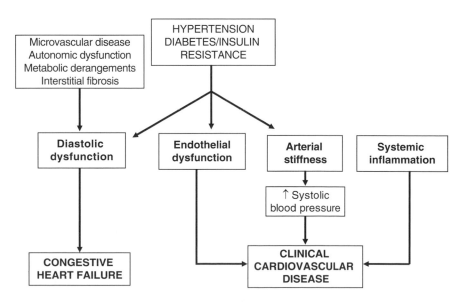

Fig. 6. Other adverse effects of diabetes on the cardiovascular system.

and may be due to reduced compliance or prolonged relaxation. There are several proposed mechanisms for this "diabetic cardiomyopathy," including myocardial microvascular disease, metabolic derangements associated with diabetes, interstitial fibrosis, hypertension, and autonomic dysfunction *(120)*. Cross sectionally, autonomic dysfunction is associated with hyperglycemia and diabetes *(121)* and it has also been shown on to be a predictor of incident type 2 diabetes in the ARIC Study *(122)*. Several studies have shown that diastolic dysfunction is present in diabetic individuals without clinical coronary heart disease *(123–126)* or hypertension *(127, 128)*. Left ventricular diastolic dysfunction, common in diabetes, is also associated with cardiac autonomic neuropathy, even in individuals free of coronary heart disease and independent of glycemic control *(129)*. Studies that have examined the efficacy of glycemic control in improving cardiac function have yielded mixed results *(120)*.

Endothelial Dysfunction

Type 2 diabetes is associated with impaired endothelium-dependent (nitric oxide-mediated) vasodilator function in the micro- and macrocirculation *(120)*. Endothelial dysfunction is also present in hypertension and in the metabolic syndrome, independent of hyperglycemia *(120)*. Kingwell et al. demonstrated that there was attenuation in leg blood flow due to impaired endothelium-dependent vasodilation and hypothesized that this may be important in determining leg ischemia in diabetic patients with peripheral arterial disease *(130)*.

Arterial Stiffness

There is a normal age-related increase in arterial stiffness that also occurs in the setting of hypertension; however, this process is accelerated in individuals with diabetes and insulin resistance *(120)*. Hyperglycemia, hyperinsulinemia, and hypertriglyceridemia are all thought to contribute to the increased arterial stiffness. In the setting of hyperglycemia, there is also glycation-induced cross-linking formation in the interstitial collagen of the vascular wall. These vascular changes may lead to elevated systolic blood pressure and an increased risk of atherosclerosis *(120)*.

Systemic Inflammation

Obesity, one of the most important risk factors for the development of type 2 diabetes, is associated with proinflammatory cytokines, including increased adipokines, tumor necrosis factor-alpha, interleukin-6, and plasminogen activator inhibitor-1 and decreased levels of adiponectin *(120)*. Both low-grade inflammation and specific inflammatory markers (interleukin-6 and C-reactive protein) have been shown to predict type 2 diabetes *(131, 132)* and higher adiponectin levels have been associated with a lower risk of developing type 2 diabetes *(133)*. Inflammatory cytokines have an adverse effect on insulin sensitivity as well as the vasculature and may be a mechanism by which known risk factors, such as hypertension, obesity, and smoking, promote cardiovascular disease in diabetes *(120)*.

SUMMARY

Cardiovascular disease remains the leading cause of death among individuals with diabetes mellitus. The prediabetic state, which includes impaired glucose metabolism, dyslipidemia, hypertension, and other cardiovascular risk factors and which proceeds the onset of type 2 diabetes by many years is a major contributor to elevated cardiovascular disease risk. Most of the research on cardiovascular disease risk reduction in diabetes has focused on treatment of hypertension and hyperlipidemia (primarily elevated LDL-cholesterol) and shown consistent beneficial effects. Thus, aggressive management of blood pressure and lipids remain the cornerstones of therapy for preventing cardiovascular disease in diabetes. There are several issues related to cardiovascular disease management in diabetes that require further investigation. First, the role of hyperglycemia in the development of the macrovascular complications of diabetes remains unresolved. The ACCORD and ADVANCE Trials did not show a benefit of intensive glucose control with an HbA$_{1c}$ of <7% in reducing cardiovascular outcomes in individuals with type 2 diabetes and in the ACCORD Trial, there was an increased risk of mortality, the etiology of which remains unclear. Other ongoing trials will provide additional information about whether specific glucose-lowering therapies may reduce cardiovascular risk in individuals with type 2 diabetes. Second, whether treatment of insulin resistance through pharmacologic or behavioral interventions will lower cardiovascular disease risk in diabetes remains unresolved as well. In the interim, cardiovascular risk factors should be treated aggressively with therapies aimed at lowering blood pressure, correcting dyslipidemia, and encouraging smoking cessation, physical activity, and aspirin use. These therapies are also known to improve systemic inflammation and endothelial dysfunction that contribute to cardiovascular disease in diabetes.

REFERENCES

1. National Diabetes Data Group: *Diabetes in America.* Bethesda, MD, National Institutes of Health, 1995.
2. Gu K, Cowie CC, Harris MI: Diabetes and decline in heart disease mortality in US adults. *JAMA* 281:1291–1297, 1999.
3. Haffner SM, Lehto S, Ronnemaa T, Pyorala K, Laakso M: Mortality from coronary heart disease in subjects with type 2 diabetes and in nondiabetic subjects with and without prior myocardial infarction. *N. Engl. J. Med.* 339:229–234, 1998.
4. Haffner SM, Stern MP, Hazuda HP, Mitchell BD, Patterson JK: Cardiovascular risk factors in confirmed prediabetic individuals. Does the clock for coronary heart disease start ticking before the onset of clinical diabetes? [see comments]. *JAMA* 263: 2893–2898, 1990.
5. Stern MP: Diabetes and cardiovascular disease. The "common soil" hypothesis. *Diabetes* 44:369–374, 1995.
6. Haffner SM, Mykkanen L, Festa A, Burke JP, Stern MP: Insulin-resistant prediabetic subjects have more atherogenic risk factors than insulin-sensitive prediabetic subjects: implications for preventing coronary heart disease during the prediabetic state [in process citation]. *Circulation* 101:975–980, 2000.
7. Reaven GM: Role of insulin resistance in human disease. *Diabetes* 37:1595–1607, 1988.
8. Liese AD, Mayer-Davis EJ, Chambless LE, Folsom AR, Sharrett AR, Brancati FL, Heiss G: Elevated fasting insulin predicts incident hypertension: the ARIC study. Atherosclerosis Risk in Communities Study Investigators. *J. Hypertens.* 17:1169–1177, 1999.
9. Meigs JB, D'Agostino RB, Sr., Wilson PW, Cupples LA, Nathan DM, Singer DE: Risk variable clustering in the insulin resistance syndrome. The Framingham Offspring Study. *Diabetes* 46:1594–1600, 1997.
10. Nabulsi AA, Folsom AR, Heiss G, Weir SS, Chambless LE, Watson RL, Eckfeldt JH: Fasting hyperinsulinemia and cardiovascular disease risk factors in nondiabetic adults: stronger associations in lean versus obese subjects. Atherosclerosis Risk in Communities Study Investigators. *Metabolism* 44:914–922, 1995.
11. Haffner SM, D'Agostino R, Jr., Mykkanen L, Tracy R, Howard B, Rewers M, Selby J, Savage PJ, Saad MF: Insulin sensitivity in subjects with type 2 diabetes. Relationship to cardiovascular risk factors: the Insulin Resistance Atherosclerosis Study. *Diabetes Care* 22:562–568, 1999.
12. Gaillard TR, Schuster DP, Bossetti BM, Green PA, Osei K: The impact of socioeconomic status on cardiovascular risk factors in African-Americans at high risk for type II diabetes. Implications for syndrome X. *Diabetes Care* 20:745–752, 1997.
13. Burchfiel CM, Hamman RF, Marshall JA, Baxter J, Kahn LB, Amirani JJ: Cardiovascular risk factors and impaired glucose tolerance: the San Luis Valley Diabetes Study. *Am. J. Epidemiol.* 131:57–70, 1990.
14. Edwards KL, Burchfiel CM, Sharp DS, Curb JD, Rodriguez BL, Fujimoto WY, LaCroix AZ, Vitiello MV, Austin MA: Factors of the insulin resistance syndrome in nondiabetic and diabetic elderly Japanese-American men. *Am. J. Epidemiol.* 147: 441–447, 1998.
15. Boyko EJ, Leonetti DL, Bergstrom RW, Newell-Morris L, Fujimoto WY: Low insulin secretion and high fasting insulin and C-peptide levels predict increased visceral adiposity. 5-Year follow-up among initially nondiabetic Japanese-American men. *Diabetes* 45:1010–1015, 1996.
16. Chien KL, Lee YT, Sung FC, Hsu HC, Su TC, Lin RS: Hyperinsulinemia and related atherosclerotic risk factors in the population at cardiovascular risk: a community-based study. *Clin. Chem.* 45:838–846, 1999.
17. Suehiro T, Ohguro T, Sumiyoshi R, Yasuoka N, Nakauchi Y, Kumon Y, Hashimoto K: Relationship of low-density lipoprotein particle size to plasma lipoproteins, obesity, and insulin resistance in Japanese men [see comments]. *Diabetes Care* 18:333–338, 1995.
18. Okosun IS, Cooper RS, Prewitt TE, Rotimi CN: The relation of central adiposity to components of the insulin resistance syndrome in a biracial US population sample. *Ethn. Dis.* 9:218–229, 1999.

19. Meigs JB, Nathan DM, Wilson PW, Cupples LA, Singer DE: Metabolic risk factors worsen continuously across the spectrum of nondiabetic glucose tolerance. The Framingham Offspring Study. *Ann. Intern. Med.* 128:524–533, 1998.

20. Lindahl B, Asplund K, Hallmans G: High serum insulin, insulin resistance and their associations with cardiovascular risk factors. The northern Sweden MONICA population study. *J. Intern. Med.* 234:263–270, 1993.

21. Laakso M, Pyorala K, Voutilainen E, Marniemi J: Plasma insulin and serum lipids and lipoproteins in middle-aged non-insulin-dependent diabetic and non-diabetic subjects. *Am. J. Epidemiol.* 125:611–621, 1987.

22. Laakso M, Barrett-Connor E: Asymptomatic hyperglycemia is associated with lipid and lipoprotein changes favoring atherosclerosis. *Arteriosclerosis* 9:665–672, 1989.

23. Kario K, Nago N, Kayaba K, Saegusa T, Matsuo H, Goto T, Tsutsumi A, Ishikawa S, Kuroda T, Miyamoto T, Matsuo T, Shimada K: Characteristics of the insulin resistance syndrome in a Japanese population. The Jichi Medical School Cohort Study. *Arterioscler. Thromb. Vasc. Biol.* 16:269–274, 1996.

24. Haffner SM, Valdez RA, Hazuda HP, Mitchell BD, Morales PA, Stern MP: Prospective analysis of the insulin-resistance syndrome (syndrome X). *Diabetes* 41:715–722, 1992.

25. Greenlund KJ, Valdez R, Casper ML, Rith-Najarian S, Croft JB: Prevalence and correlates of the insulin resistance syndrome among Native Americans. The Inter-Tribal Heart Project. *Diabetes Care* 22:441–447, 1999.

26. Gray RS, Robbins DC, Wang W, Yeh JL, Fabsitz RR, Cowan LD, Welty TK, Lee ET, Krauss RM, Howard BV: Relation of LDL size to the insulin resistance syndrome and coronary heart disease in American Indians. The Strong Heart Study. *Arterioscler. Thromb. Vasc. Biol.* 17:2713–2720, 1997.

27. Ferrannini E, Muscelli E, Stern MP, Haffner SM: Differential impact of insulin and obesity on cardiovascular risk factors in non-diabetic subjects [see comments]. *Int. J. Obes. Relat. Metab. Disord.* 20:7–14, 1996.

28. Chen W, Srinivasan SR, Elkasabany A, Berenson GS: Cardiovascular risk factors clustering features of insulin resistance syndrome (Syndrome X) in a biracial (Black-White) population of children, adolescents, and young adults: the Bogalusa Heart Study. *Am. J. Epidemiol.* 150:667–674, 1999.

29. Burchfiel CM, Abbott RD, Curb JD, Sharp DS, Rodriguez BL, Arakaki R, Yano K: Association of insulin levels with lipids and lipoproteins in elderly Japanese-American men. *Ann. Epidemiol.* 8:92–98, 1998.

30. Austin MA, Selby JV: LDL subclass phenotypes and the risk factors of the insulin resistance syndrome. *Int. J. Obes. Relat. Metab. Disord.* 19 Suppl 1:S22–S26, 1995.

31. Meigs JB, Mittleman MA, Nathan DM, Tofler GH, Singer DE, Murphy-Sheehy PM, Lipinska I, D'Agostino RB, Wilson PW: Hyperinsulinemia, hyperglycemia, and impaired hemostasis: the Framingham Offspring Study. *JAMA* 283:221–228, 2000.

32. Lind L, Lithell H, Pollare T: Is it hyperinsulinemia or insulin resistance that is related to hypertension and other metabolic cardiovascular risk factors? *J. Hypertens. Suppl.* 11:S11–S16, 1993.

33. Garg A, Helderman JH, Koffler M, Ayuso R, Rosenstock J, Raskin P: Relationship between lipoprotein levels and in vivo insulin action in normal young white men. *Metabolism* 37:982–987, 1988.

34. Lind L, Berne C, Lithell H: Prevalence of insulin resistance in essential hypertension. *J. Hypertens.* 13:1457–1462, 1995.

35. Laakso M, Sarlund H, Mykkanen L: Insulin resistance is associated with lipid and lipoprotein abnormalities in subjects with varying degrees of glucose tolerance. *Arteriosclerosis* 10:223–231, 1990.

36. Abbott WG, Lillioja S, Young AA, Zawadzki JK, Yki-Jarvinen H, Christin L, Howard BV: Relationships between plasma lipoprotein concentrations and insulin action in an obese hyperinsulinemic population. *Diabetes* 36:897–904, 1987.

37. Howard BV, Mayer-Davis EJ, Goff D, Zaccaro DJ, Laws A, Robbins DC, Saad MF, Selby J, Hamman RF, Krauss RM, Haffner SM: Relationships between insulin resistance and lipoproteins in nondiabetic African Americans, Hispanics, and non-Hispanic whites: the Insulin Resistance Atherosclerosis Study. *Metabolism* 47:1174–1179, 1998.

38. Karter AJ, Mayer-Davis EJ, Selby JV, D'Agostino RB, Jr., Haffner SM, Sholinsky P, Bergman R, Saad MF, Hamman RF: Insulin sensitivity and abdominal obesity in African-American, Hispanic, and non-Hispanic white men and women. The Insulin Resistance and Atherosclerosis Study. *Diabetes* 45:1547–1555, 1996.

39. Matsuda M, DeFronzo RA: In Vivo Measurement of Insulin Sensitivity in Humans. In Clinical Research in Diabetes and Obesity, Part I: Methods, Assessment, and Metabolic Regulation. Draznin B, Rizza R, Eds. Totowa, NJ, Humana, 1999, pp. 23–65.

40. Grundy SM, Cleeman JI, Daniels SR, Donato KA, Eckel RH, Franklin BA, Gordon DJ, Krauss RM, Savage PJ, Smith SC, Jr., Spertus JA, Costa F: Diagnosis and management of the metabolic syndrome: an American Heart Association/National Heart, Lung, and Blood Institute Scientific Statement. *Circulation* 112:2735–2752, 2005.

41. Grundy SM, Hansen B, Smith SC, Jr., Cleeman JI, Kahn RA: Clinical management of metabolic syndrome: report of the American Heart Association/National Heart, Lung, and Blood Institute/American Diabetes Association conference on scientific issues related to management. *Circulation* 109:551–556, 2004.

42. Liao Y, Kwon S, Shaughnessy S, Wallace P, Hutto A, Jenkins AJ, Klein RL, Garvey WT: Critical evaluation of adult treatment panel III criteria in identifying insulin resistance with dyslipidemia. *Diabetes Care* 27:978–983, 2004.

43. Cheal KL, Abbasi F, Lamendola C, McLaughlin T, Reaven GM, Ford ES: Relationship to insulin resistance of the adult treatment panel III diagnostic criteria for identification of the metabolic syndrome. *Diabetes* 53:1195–1200, 2004.

44. Shinozaki K, Suzuki M, Ikebuchi M, Hara Y, Harano Y: Demonstration of insulin resistance in coronary artery disease documented with angiography. *Diabetes Care* 19:1–7, 1996.

45. Bressler P, Bailey SR, Matsuda M, DeFronzo RA: Insulin resistance and coronary artery disease [published erratum appears in Diabetologia 1997 Mar;40(3):366]. *Diabetologia* 39:1345–1350, 1996.

46. Young MH, Jeng CY, Sheu WH, Shieh SM, Fuh MM, Chen YD, Reaven GM: Insulin resistance, glucose intolerance, hyperinsulinemia and dyslipidemia in patients with angiographically demonstrated coronary artery disease. *Am. J. Cardiol.* 72:458–460, 1993.

47. Matsumoto K, Miyake S, Yano M, Ueki Y, Miyazaki A, Hirao K, Tominaga Y: Insulin resistance and classic risk factors in type 2 diabetic patients with different subtypes of ischemic stroke. *Diabetes Care* 22:1191–1195, 1999.

48. Kekalainen P, Sarlund H, Farin P, Kaukanen E, Yang X, Laakso M: Femoral atherosclerosis in middle-aged subjects: association with cardiovascular risk factors and insulin resistance. *Am. J. Epidemiol.* 144:742–748, 1996.

49. Rutter MK, Meigs JB, Sullivan LM, D'Agostino RB, Sr., Wilson PW: Insulin resistance, the metabolic syndrome, and incident cardiovascular events in the Framingham Offspring Study. *Diabetes* 54:3252–3257, 2005.

50. Golden SH, Folsom AR, Coresh J, Sharrett AR, Szklo M, Brancati F: Risk factor groupings related to insulin resistance and their synergistic effects on subclinical atherosclerosis. The Atherosclerosis Risk in Communities Study. *Diabetes* 51:3069–3076, 2002.

51. Zavaroni I, Bonini L, Gasparini P, Barilli AL, Zuccarelli A, Dall'Aglio E, Delsignore R, Reaven GM: Hyperinsulinemia in a normal population as a predictor of non-insulin-dependent diabetes mellitus, hypertension, and coronary heart disease: the Barilla factory revisited. *Metabolism* 48:989–994, 1999.

52. Sheu WH, Jeng CY, Young MS, Le WJ, Chen YT: Coronary artery disease risk predicted by insulin resistance, plasma lipids, and hypertension in people without diabetes. *Am. J. Med. Sci.* 319:84–88, 2000.

53. Saku K, Zhang B, Shirai K, Jimi S, Yoshinaga K, Arakawa K: Hyperinsulinemic hypoalphalipoproteinemia as a new indicator for coronary heart disease. *J. Am. Coll. Cardiol.* 34:1443–1451, 1999.

54. Pyorala M, Miettinen H, Halonen P, Laakso M, Pyorala K: Insulin resistance syndrome predicts the risk of coronary heart disease and stroke in healthy middle-aged men: the 22-year follow-up results of the Helsinki Policemen Study. *Arterioscler. Thromb. Vasc. Biol.* 20:538–544, 2000.

55. Misra A, Reddy RB, Reddy KS, Mohan A, Bajaj JS: Clustering of impaired glucose tolerance, hyperinsulinemia and dyslipidemia in young north Indian patients with coronary heart disease: a preliminary case-control study. *Indian Heart J.* 51:275–280, 1999.

56. Lempiainen P, Mykkanen L, Pyorala K, Laakso M, Kuusisto J: Insulin resistance syndrome predicts coronary heart disease events in elderly nondiabetic men. *Circulation* 100:123–128, 1999.

57. Bergstrom RW, Leonetti DL, Newell-Morris LL, Shuman WP, Wahl PW, Fujimoto WY: Association of plasma triglyceride and C-peptide with coronary heart disease in Japanese-American men with a high prevalence of glucose intolerance. *Diabetologia* 33:489–496, 1990.

58. Lehto S, Ronnemaa T, Pyorala K, Laakso M: Cardiovascular risk factors clustering with endogenous hyperinsulinemia predict death from coronary heart disease in patients with Type II diabetes. *Diabetologia* 43:148–155, 2000.

59. Uusitupa MI, Niskanen LK, Siitonen O, Voutilainen E, Pyorala K: 5-Year incidence of atherosclerotic vascular disease in relation to general risk factors, insulin level, and abnormalities in lipoprotein composition in non-insulin-dependent diabetic and nondiabetic subjects. *Circulation* 82:27–36, 1990.

60. Folsom AR, Rasmussen ML, Chambless LE, Howard G, Cooper LS, Schmidt MI, Heiss G: Prospective associations of fasting insulin, body fat distribution, and diabetes with risk of ischemic stroke. The Atherosclerosis Risk in Communities (ARIC) Study Investigators. *Diabetes Care* 22:1077–1083, 1999.

61. Dekker JM, Girman C, Rhodes T, Nijpels G, Stehouwer CD, Bouter LM, Heine RJ: Metabolic syndrome and 10-year cardiovascular disease risk in the Hoorn Study. *Circulation* 112:666–673, 2005.

62. Ford ES: Risks for all-cause mortality, cardiovascular disease, and diabetes associated with the metabolic syndrome: a summary of the evidence. *Diabetes Care* 28:1769–1778, 2005.

63. McNeill AM, Rosamond WD, Girman CJ, Heiss G, Golden SH, Duncan BB, East HE, Ballantyne C: Prevalence of coronary heart disease and carotid arterial thickening in patients with the metabolic syndrome (the ARIC Study). *Am. J. Cardiol.* 94:1249–1254, 2004.

64. Lakka HM, Laaksonen DE, Lakka TA, Niskanen LK, Kumpusalo E, Tuomilehto J, Salonen JT: The metabolic syndrome and total and cardiovascular disease mortality in middle-aged men. *JAMA* 288:2709–2716, 2002.

65. McNeill AM, Rosamond WD, Girman CJ, Golden SH, Schmidt MI, East HE, Ballantyne CM, Heiss G: The metabolic syndrome and 11-year risk of incident cardiovascular disease in the atherosclerosis risk in communities study. *Diabetes Care* 28:385–390, 2005.

66. Milionis HJ, Rizos E, Goudevenos J, Seferiadis K, Mikhailidis DP, Elisaf MS: Components of the metabolic syndrome and risk for first-ever acute ischemic nonembolic stroke in elderly subjects. *Stroke* 36:1372–1376, 2005.

67. Koren-Morag N, Goldbourt U, Tanne D: Relation between the metabolic syndrome and ischemic stroke or transient ischemic attack: a prospective cohort study in patients with atherosclerotic cardiovascular disease. *Stroke* 36:1366–1371, 2005.

68. Golden SH, Chong R: Are there specific components of the insulin resistance syndrome that predict the increased atherosclerosis seen in type 2 diabetes mellitus? *Curr. Diab. Rep.* 4:26–30, 2004.

69. Meigs JB: Invited commentary: insulin resistance syndrome? Syndrome X? Multiple metabolic syndrome? A syndrome at all? Factor analysis reveals patterns in the fabric of correlated metabolic risk factors. *Am. J. Epidemiol.* 152:908–911, 2000.

70. Sundstrom J, Vallhagen E, Riserus U, Byberg L, Zethelius B, Berne C, Lind L, Ingelsson E: Risk associated with the metabolic syndrome versus the sum of its individual components. *Diabetes Care* 29:1673–1674, 2006.

71. Garg A, Grundy SM: Management of dyslipidemia in NIDDM. *Diabetes Care* 13:153–169, 1990.

72. Howard BV, Cowan LD, Go O, Welty TK, Robbins DC, Lee ET: Adverse effects of diabetes on multiple cardiovascular disease risk factors in women. The Strong Heart Study. Diabetes Care 21:1258–1265, 1998.

73. Feingold KR, Grunfeld C, Pang M, Doerrler W, Krauss RM: LDL subclass phenotypes and triglyceride metabolism in non-insulin-dependent diabetes. *Arterioscler. Thromb.* 12:1496–1502, 1992.

74. Selby JV, Austin MA, Newman B, Zhang D, Quesenberry CP, Jr., Mayer EJ, Krauss RM: LDL subclass phenotypes and the insulin resistance syndrome in women. *Circulation* 88:381–387, 1993.

75. Laws A: Insulin resistance and dyslipidemia. In Insulin Resistance. The Metabolic Syndrome X, 1st ed. Reaven GM, Laws A, Ed. Totowa, NJ, Humana, 1999, pp. 267–280.

76. Krauss RM: Lipids and lipoproteins in patients with type 2 diabetes. *Diabetes Care* 27:1496–1504, 2004.

77. Sniderman AD, Scantlebury T, Cianflone K: Hypertriglyceridemic hyperapob: the unappreciated atherogenic dyslipoproteinemia in type 2 diabetes mellitus. *Ann. Intern. Med.* 135:447–459, 2001.

78. Haffner SM: Lipoprotein disorders associated with type 2 diabetes mellitus and insulin resistance. *Am. J. Cardiol.* 90:55i–61i, 2002.

79. Temelkova-Kurktschiev T, Hanefeld M: The lipid triad in type 2 diabetes – prevalence and relevance of hypertriglyceridaemia/low high-density lipoprotein syndrome in type 2 diabetes. *Exp. Clin. Endocrinol. Diabetes* 112:75–79, 2004.

80. Hokanson JE, Austin MA: Plasma triglyceride level is a risk factor for cardiovascular disease independent of high-density lipoprotein cholesterol level: a meta-analysis of population-based prospective studies. *J. Cardiovasc. Risk* 3:213–219, 1996.

81. Turner RC, Millns H, Neil HA, Stratton IM, Manley SE, Matthews DR, Holman RR: Risk factors for coronary artery disease in non-insulin dependent diabetes mellitus: United Kingdom Prospective Diabetes Study (UKPDS: 23). *BMJ* 316:823–828, 1998.

82. Jeppesen J, Hein HO, Suadicani P, Gyntelberg F: Triglyceride concentration and ischemic heart disease: an eight-year follow-up in the Copenhagen Male Study. *Circulation* 97:1029–1036, 1998.

83. Iso H, Naito Y, Sato S, Kitamura A, Okamura T, Sankai T, Shimamoto T, Iida M, Komachi Y: Serum triglycerides and risk of coronary heart disease among Japanese men and women. *Am. J. Epidemiol.* 153:490–499, 2001.

84. Talmud PJ, Hawe E, Miller GJ, Humphries SE: Nonfasting apolipoprotein B and triglyceride levels as a useful predictor of coronary heart disease risk in middle-aged UK men. *Arterioscler. Thromb. Vasc. Biol.* 22:1918–1923, 2002.

85. Castelli WP, Garrison RJ, Wilson PW, Abbott RD, Kalousdian S, Kannel WB: Incidence of coronary heart disease and lipoprotein cholesterol levels. The Framingham Study. *JAMA* 256:2835–2838, 1986.

86. Goldbourt U, Yaari S: Cholesterol and coronary heart disease mortality. A 23-year follow-up study of 9902 men in Israel. *Arteriosclerosis* 10:512–519, 1990.

87. Assmann G, Schulte H, Funke H, von Eckardstein A: The emergence of triglycerides as a significant independent risk factor in coronary artery disease. *Eur. Heart J.* 19 Suppl M:M8–M14, 1998.

88. Assmann G, Schulte H: Relation of high-density lipoprotein cholesterol and triglycerides to incidence of atherosclerotic coronary artery disease (the PROCAM experience). Prospective Cardiovascular Munster study. *Am. J. Cardiol.* 70:733–737, 1992.

89. Huttunen JK, Manninen V, Manttari M, Koskinen P, Romo M, Tenkanen L, Heinonen OP, Frick MH: The Helsinki Heart Study: central findings and clinical implications. *Ann. Med.* 23:155–159, 1991.

90. Despres JP, Lamarche B, Mauriege P, Cantin B, Dagenais GR, Moorjani S, Lupien PJ: Hyperinsulinemia as an independent risk factor for ischemic heart disease. *N. Engl. J. Med.* 334:952–957, 1996.

91. Lamarche B, St Pierre AC, Ruel IL, Cantin B, Dagenais GR, Despres JP: A prospective, population-based study of low density lipoprotein particle size as a risk factor for ischemic heart disease in men. *Can. J. Cardiol.* 17:859–865, 2001.

92. Roheim PS, Asztalos BF: Clinical significance of lipoprotein size and risk for coronary atherosclerosis. *Clin. Chem.* 41:147–152, 1995.

93. Gardner CD, Fortmann SP, Krauss RM: Association of small low-density lipoprotein particles with the incidence of coronary artery disease in men and women. *JAMA* 276:875–881, 1996.

94. Stampfer MJ, Krauss RM, Ma J, Blanche PJ, Holl LG, Sacks FM, Hennekens CH: A prospective study of triglyceride level, low-density lipoprotein particle diameter, and risk of myocardial infarction. *JAMA* 276:882–888, 1996.

95. Blake GJ, Otvos JD, Rifai N, Ridker PM: Low-density lipoprotein particle concentration and size as determined by nuclear magnetic resonance spectroscopy as predictors of cardiovascular disease in women. *Circulation* 106:1930–1937, 2002.

96. Arauz-Pacheco C, Parrott MA, Raskin P: The treatment of hypertension in adult patients with diabetes. *Diabetes Care* 25:134–147, 2002.

97. McPhillips JB, Barrett-Connor E, Wingard DL: Cardiovascular disease risk factors prior to the diagnosis of impaired glucose tolerance and non-insulin-dependent diabetes mellitus in a community of older adults. *Am. J. Epidemiol.* 131:443–453, 1990.

98. Golden SH, Wang N, Klag MJ, Meoni LA, Brancati FL: Blood pressure in young adulthood and the risk of type 2 diabetes in middle age. *Diabetes Care* 26:1110–1115, 2003.

99. Knuiman MW, Welborn TA, McCann VJ, Stanton KG, Constable IJ: Prevalence of diabetic complications in relation to risk factors. *Diabetes* 35:1332–1339, 1986.

100. Adler AI, Stratton IM, Neil HA, Yudkin JS, Matthews DR, Cull CA, Wright AD, Turner RC, Holman RR: Association of systolic blood pressure with macrovascular and microvascular complications of type 2 diabetes (UKPDS 36): prospective observational study. *BMJ* 321:412–419, 2000.

101. Ferrannini E: Insulin resistance and blood pressure. In Insulin Resistance. The Metabolic Syndrome X, 1st ed. Reaven GM, Laws A, Ed. Totowa, NJ, Humana, 1999, pp. 281–308.

102. DeFronzo RA, Cooke CR, Andres R, Faloona GR, Davis PJ: The effect of insulin on renal handling of sodium, potassium, calcium, and phosphate in man. *J. Clin. Invest.* 55:845–855, 1975.

103. Rowe JW, Young JB, Minaker KL, Stevens AL, Pallotta J, Landsberg L: Effect of insulin and glucose infusions on sympathetic nervous system activity in normal man. *Diabetes* 30:219–225, 1981.

104. Laakso M, Edelman SV, Brechtel G, Baron AD: Decreased effect of insulin to stimulate skeletal muscle blood flow in obese man. A novel mechanism for insulin resistance. *J. Clin. Invest.* 85:1844–1852, 1990.

105. Reaven GM: Insulin resistance/compensatory hyperinsulinemia, essential hypertension, and cardiovascular disease. *J. Clin. Endocrinol. Metab.* 88:2399–2403, 2003.

106. Effect of intensive blood-glucose control with metformin on complications in overweight patients with type 2 diabetes (UKPDS 34). UK Prospective Diabetes Study (UKPDS) Group. *Lancet* 352:854–865, 1998.

107. Coutinho M, Gerstein HC, Wang Y, Yusuf S: The relationship between glucose and incident cardiovascular events. A metaregression analysis of published data from 20 studies of 95,783 individuals followed for 12.4 years. *Diabetes Care* 22:233–240, 1999.

108. Levitan EB, Song Y, Ford ES, Liu S: Is nondiabetic hyperglycemia a risk factor for cardiovascular disease? A meta-analysis of prospective studies. *Arch. Intern. Med.* 164:2147–2155, 2004.

109. Selvin E, Marinopoulos S, Berkenblit G, Rami T, Brancati FL, Powe NR, Golden SH: Meta-analysis: glycosylated hemoglobin and cardiovascular disease in diabetes mellitus. *Ann. Intern. Med.* 141:421–431, 2004.

110. Selvin E, Coresh J, Golden SH, Brancati FL, Folsom AR, Steffes MW: Glycemic control and coronary heart disease risk in persons with and without diabetes: the atherosclerosis risk in communities study. *Arch. Intern. Med.* 165:1910–1916, 2005.

111. Selvin E, Coresh J, Shahar E, Zhang L, Steffes M, Sharrett AR: Glycaemia (haemoglobin A(1c)) and incident ischaemic stroke: the Atherosclerosis Risk in Communities (ARIC) Study. *Lancet Neurol.* 4:821–826, 2005.

112. Selvin E, Wattanakit K, Steffes MW, Coresh J, Sharrett AR: HbA1c and peripheral arterial disease in diabetes: the atherosclerosis risk in communities study. *Diabetes Care* 29:877–882, 2006.

113. Selvin E, Wattanakit K, Steffes MW, Coresh J, Sharrett AR: HbA1c and peripheral arterial disease in diabetes: the atherosclerosis risk in communities study. *Diabetes Care* 29:877–882, 2006.

114. Stratton IM, Adler AI, Neil HA, Matthews DR, Manley SE, Cull CA, Hadden D, Turner RC, Holman RR: Association of glycaemia with macrovascular and microvascular complications of type 2 diabetes (UKPDS 35): prospective observational study. *BMJ* 321:405–412, 2000.

115. Adler AI, Stevens RJ, Neil A, Stratton IM, Boulton AJ, Holman RR: UKPDS 59: hyperglycemia and other potentially modifiable risk factors for peripheral vascular disease in type 2 diabetes. *Diabetes Care* 25:894–899, 2002.

116. Gerstein HC, Miller ME, Byington RP, Goff DC, Jr., Bigger JT, Buse JB, Cushman WC, Genuth S, Ismail-Beigi F, Grimm RH, Jr., Probstfield JL, Simons-Morton DG, Friedewald WT: Effects of intensive glucose lowering in type 2 diabetes. *N. Engl. J. Med.* 358:2545–2559, 2008.

117. Patel A, MacMahon S, Chalmers J, Neal B, Billot L, Woodward M, Marre M, Cooper M, Glasziou P, Grobbee D, Hamet P, Harrap S, Heller S, Liu L, Mancia G, Mogensen CE, Pan C, Poulter N, Rodgers A, Williams B, Bompoint S, de Galan BE, Joshi R, Travert F: Intensive blood glucose control and vascular outcomes in patients with type 2 diabetes. *N. Engl. J. Med.* 358:2560–2572, 2008.

118. Clement S, Braithwaite SS, Magee MF, Ahmann A, Smith EP, Schafer RG, Hirsch IB, Hirsh IB: Management of diabetes and hyperglycemia in hospitals. *Diabetes Care* 27:553–591, 2004.

119. Sheetz MJ, King GL: Molecular understanding of hyperglycemia's adverse effects for diabetic complications. *JAMA* 288:2579–2588, 2002.

120. Stewart KJ: Role of exercise training on cardiovascular disease in persons who have type 2 diabetes and hypertension. *Cardiol. Clin.* 22:569–586, 2004.

121. Liao D, Cai J, Brancati FL, Folsom A, Barnes RW, Tyroler HA, Heiss G: Association of vagal tone with serum insulin, glucose, and diabetes mellitus--The ARIC Study. *Diabetes Res. Clin. Pract.* 30:211–221, 1995.

122. Carnethon MR, Golden SH, Folsom AR, Haskell W, Liao D: Prospective investigation of autonomic nervous system function and the development of type 2 diabetes: the Atherosclerosis Risk In Communities study, 1987–1998. *Circulation* 107: 2190–2195, 2003.

123. Yasuda I, Kawakami K, Shimada T, Tanigawa K, Murakami R, Izumi S, Morioka S, Kato Y, Moriyama K: Systolic and diastolic left ventricular dysfunction in middle-aged asymptomatic non-insulin-dependent diabetics. *J. Cardiol.* 22:427–438, 1992.

124. Robillon JF, Sadoul JL, Jullien D, Morand P, Freychet P: Abnormalities suggestive of cardiomyopathy in patients with type 2 diabetes of relatively short duration. *Diabete Metab.* 20:473–480, 1994.

125. Takenaka K, Sakamoto T, Amano K, Oku J, Fujinami K, Murakami T, Toda I, Kawakubo K, Sugimoto T: Left ventricular filling determined by Doppler echocardiography in diabetes mellitus. *Am. J. Cardiol.* 61:1140–1143, 1988.

126. Tarumi N, Iwasaka T, Takahashi N, Sugiura T, Morita Y, Sumimoto T, Nishiue T, Inada M: Left ventricular diastolic filling properties in diabetic patients during isometric exercise. *Cardiology* 83:316–323, 1993.

127. Poirier P, Bogaty P, Garneau C, Marois L, Dumesnil JG: Diastolic dysfunction in normotensive men with well-controlled type 2 diabetes: importance of maneuvers in echocardiographic screening for preclinical diabetic cardiomyopathy. *Diabetes Care* 24:5–10, 2001.

128. Zabalgoitia M, Ismaeil MF, Anderson L, Maklady FA: Prevalence of diastolic dysfunction in normotensive, asymptomatic patients with well-controlled type 2 diabetes mellitus. *Am. J. Cardiol.* 87:320–323, 2001.

129. Poirier P, Bogaty P, Philippon F, Garneau C, Fortin C, Dumesnil JG: Preclinical diabetic cardiomyopathy: relation of left ventricular diastolic dysfunction to cardiac autonomic neuropathy in men with uncomplicated well-controlled type 2 diabetes. *Metabolism* 52:1056–1061, 2003.

130. Kingwell BA, Formosa M, Muhlmann M, Bradley SJ, McConell GK: Type 2 diabetic individuals have impaired leg blood flow responses to exercise: role of endothelium-dependent vasodilation. *Diabetes Care* 26:899–904, 2003.
131. Duncan BB, Schmidt MI, Pankow JS, Ballantyne CM, Couper D, Vigo A, Hoogeveen R, Folsom AR, Heiss G: Low-grade systemic inflammation and the development of type 2 diabetes: the atherosclerosis risk in communities study. *Diabetes* 52:1799–1805, 2003.
132. Pradhan AD, Manson JE, Rifai N, Buring JE, Ridker PM: C-reactive protein, interleukin 6, and risk of developing type 2 diabetes mellitus. *JAMA* 286:327–334, 2001.
133. Duncan BB, Schmidt MI, Pankow JS, Bang H, Couper D, Ballantyne CM, Hoogeveen RC, Heiss G: Adiponectin and the development of type 2 diabetes: the atherosclerosis risk in communities study. *Diabetes* 53:2473–2478, 2004.

6   Endothelial Dysfunction, Inflammation, and Exercise

John Doupis, Jordan C. Schramm, and Aristidis Veves

CONTENTS

ABSTRACT

Vascular endothelial function is essential for the maintenance of health of the vessel wall and for the vasomotor control in both conduit and resistance vessels. These functions are due to the production of numerous vasomodulators, of which nitric oxide (NO) has been the most significant and the most widely studied. Endothelial function deteriorates with age and in the presence of several other risk factors for atherosclerosis, including diabetes, obesity, hypercholesterolemia, hypertension, hyperhomocysteinemia, and smoking. In addition, endothelial dysfunction is highly related with chronic vascular inflammation and is considered to be an independent risk factor for atherosclerosis. Physical training has beneficial effects on multiple cardiovascular risk factors, such as dyslipidemia, hypertension, diabetes, and cardiovascular events, by augmenting endothelial, NO-dependent vasodilation in both large and small arteries. In addition, physical activity shows beneficial effect on the chronic vascular inflammation, reducing most of the biochemical inflammation markers.

Key words: Diabetes; Exersice; Endothelial Dysfunction.

INTRODUCTION

The main reason for increased morbidity and mortality in patients with type 1 or 2 diabetes is cardiovascular disease. The relationship between diabetes and cardiovascular disease is so intimate that diabetes itself may be considered a cardiovascular disease *(1)*. A considerable body of evidence in humans indicates that endothelial dysfunction is closely associated with the development of micro

From: *Contemporary Diabetes: Diabetes and Exercise*
Edited by: J. G. Regensteiner et al. (eds.), DOI: 10.1007/978-1-59745-260-1_6
© Humana Press, a part of Springer Science+Business Media, LLC 2009

and macrovascular diseases in both type 1 and type 2 diabetes *(2)*. In addition, recent compelling evidence has shown the significant and independent role of inflammation, insulin resistance, and subsequent endothelial dysfunction in the initiation and progression of atherosclerosis, superimposed on traditional risk factors *(3–6)*.

Exercise is currently considered as the cornerstone of the prevention and management of type 2 diabetes. Although there is no evidence that exercise can prevent type 1 diabetes, there is evidence from cohort studies that regular physical activity is associated with reduced mortality in both type 1 and type 2 diabetes *(7)*. Given the abundant data linking diabetes, endothelial dysfunction, inflammation, and atherosclerosis, the present chapter will focus on the effects of exercise on endothelial reactivity and systemic inflammation in diabetic patients.

ENDOTHELIUM

The vascular endothelium is a large paracrine organ that secretes numerous factors regulating vascular tone, cell growth, platelet and leukocyte interactions, and thrombogenicity. The endothelium senses and responds to a myriad of internal and external stimuli through complex cell membrane receptors and signal transduction mechanisms, leading to the synthesis and release of various vasoactive, thromboregulatory, and growth factor substances *(8–16)*. The normal, healthy endothelium regulates vascular tone and structure while exerts anticoagulant, antiplatelet, and fibrinolytic properties. Under normal conditions, shear stress created by laminar blood flow through the vessel lumen stimulates a G protein-mediated signaling pathway in endothelial cells. The maintenance of vascular tone is accomplished by the release of numerous dilator and constrictor substances. Arginine is used as a substrate by endothelial nitric oxide synthase (eNOS) to produce nitric oxide (NO), the most potent vasodilatory molecule, originally identified as endothelium-derived relaxing factor (EDRF) (Fig. 1. Other endothelium-derived

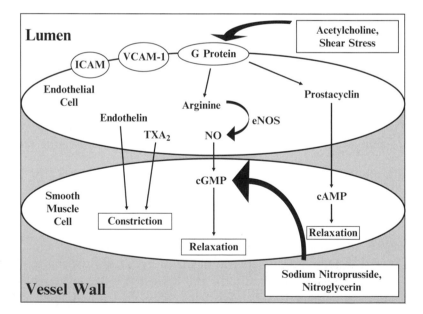

Fig. 1. Physiology of endothelium and vascular smooth muscle in maintaining vascular tone. The endothelium acts as a paracrine organ, secreting vasodilator substances [nitric oxide *(NO)* and prostacyclin] and vasoconstrictor substances (endothelin and TXA2), which diffuse and act on the adjacent smooth muscle. Shear stress and acetylcholine are capable of producing endothelium-dependent vasodilation, while sodium nitroprusside *(SNP)* and nitroglycerin *(NTG)* -elicit endothelium-independent vasodilation.

vasodilators are prostacyclin and bradykinin *(17)*. ProstaIcyclin acts synergistically with NO to inhibit platelet aggregation *(18)*. Bradykinin stimulates release of NO, prostacyclin, and endothelium-derived hyperpolarizing factor, another vasodilator, which contributes to inhibition of platelet aggregation *(17)*. Bradykinin also stimulates production of tissue plasminogen activator (t-PA), thus, may play an important role in fibrinolysis. The endothelium also produces vasoconstrictor substances, such as endothelin (the most potent endogenous vasoconstrictor identified to date) and angiotensin II. Angiotensin II not only acts as a vasoconstrictor but also as a prooxidant stimulating the production of endothelin *(1)*. Endothelin and angiotensin II promote the proliferation of smooth muscle cells and, thereby, contribute to the formation of plaque *(17)*. Activated macrophages and vascular smooth muscle cells, which are characteristic cellular components of atherosclerotic plaque, produce large amounts of endothelin-1 *(19)*.

Endothelium-Dependent vs. Independent Vasodilation

Endothelial-derived vasoactive substances produce their effects on smooth muscle cells through various intracellular signaling pathways. The details of these pathways will not be discussed here in full, except to note that the NO pathway uses the second messenger cyclic guanosine monophosphate (cGMP) while the prostacyclin pathway involves the second messenger cyclic adenosine monophosphate (cAMP) (Fig. 1). Additionally, vascular smooth muscle is influenced by many other factors (e.g., neural, endocrine) other than the paracrine influences from the endothelium *(12, 13)*. Vasodilation can hence be categorized as either endothelium dependent or endothelium independent. Physiologically, all of these mechanisms of vascular control work in concert, but experimentally they can be isolated and studied.

Endothelium-dependent vasodilation can be isolated for study in two convenient ways. In one method, which will be discussed in detail later, flow-mediated vasodilation (FMD) is measured after a 5-min inclusion of the branchial artery. This technique is very attractive, because it is noninvasive and allows repeated measurements. An alternative invasive method relies on the intra-arterial administration of agents that are capable of activating the same G-protein pathway as shear stress, mainly acetylcholine chloride or metacholine, and causes endothelium-dependent vasodilation *(20–22)*.

Endothelium-independent vasodilation is elicited with the administration of two similarly acting compounds, nitroglycerin (NTG) sublingually or sodium nitroprusside (SNP) topically. These drugs are NO donors and increase the production of cGMP in the vascular smooth muscle cells directly and independently from any endothelial action. In this way, the endothelium is bypassed, resulting in vasodilation that is completely independent of the endothelium *(20, 22)*.

Initial studies reported impaired endothelium-dependent vasodilation in diabetes while the endothelium independent was normal. However, subsequent studies, especially in the microcirculation, have shown that both the endothelium-dependent and independent vasodilation are impaired, indicating that diabetes affects both the endothelial and vascular smooth muscle cell *(20–25)*.

Micro vs. Macrocirculation

Diabetes affects the macrocirculation in a similar way that other proatherogenic conditions do. As a result, there are no major differences in the development of macrovascular disease between diabetic and nondiabetic patients. In the lower extremity, a minor difference is that diabetes tends to affect more often the arteries below the knee while in nondiabetic patients the femoral artery is more commonly affected *(26–30)*.

The microcirculation is almost exclusively affected by diabetes and leads to the development of the long-term diabetic complications (nephropathy, retinopathy, and neuropathy). Usually, there are no clinical manifestations of microcirculation complications in nondiabetic patients with atherosclerosis *(31–34)*.

In 1959, an occlusive "small vessel disease" was described in a retrospective histological study and was suggested as the main mechanism for the development of diabetic microvascular disease *(26)*. However, it was subsequently shown that the microcirculation does not suffer from an occlusive disorder analogous to the atherosclerotic disease that affects the capillaries or arterioles *(27–30)*. Instead, convincing evidence has shown that the main changes in the microcirculation are functional rather than structural, such as increased vascular permeability and impaired autoregulation of blood flow and vascular tone, with hyperglycemia and insulin resistance likely working synergistically to bring about these changes. It should be noted though that while the disease process differs between micro and macrocirculation, in both cases, the regulation of vascular tone that depends on the normal function of the endothelial cell – vascular smooth muscle cell axis is impaired, and that this impairment is the first step for the development of vascular disease *(25, 31, 34)*.

Evaluation of the Macrocirculation Vascular Reactivity

The most common method for evaluating the vascular reactivity in the macrocirculation is by ultrasonographic imaging, which is a noninvasive technique. The brachial artery is one of the most convenient to work with because FMD can be easily induced at this location *(35)*. Subject preparation is critical because there are many factors (e.g., temperature, food, drugs, sympathetic stimuli, and menstrual cycle) that can affect flow-mediated vascular reactivity. Therefore, subjects should fast for at least 8–12 h before the study, which must be taken place in a quiet, temperature-controlled room. A continuous two-dimensional grayscale ultrasound image is taken in the longitudinal plane of the brachial artery in the area above the antecubital fossa with the patient in the supine position, using a high-resolution ultrasound machine. Electrocardiogram (EKG) should be used in conjunction with ultrasound so that analysis can be done at a consistent time in the cardiac cycle.

A baseline image is first taken, followed by occlusion of the brachial artery by inflation of a sphygmomanometric cuff placed either above or below the antecubital fossa (Fig. 2). The cuff is typically inflated to 50 mmHg above systolic pressure for 5 min, during which the resultant ischemia causes dilation of downstream blood vessels. When the cuff is deflated there is an increased flow in the brachial artery because of hypoxia-induced reactive hyperemia. This results in increased shear stress, leading to vasodilation. Ultrasound image acquisition begins a few seconds before release of the cuff and continues for at least 1 min after. Several studies have suggested that the maximal increase in diameter occurs ~60 s after the release of the occlusive cuff (Fig. 3). FMD is calculated as the percent change between poststimulus and baseline diameter *(35)*.

Assessment of the endothelium-independent vasodilation is performed by sublingual administration of NTG. This is performed after a resting period of at least 15 min after the FMD evaluation that allows the vessel diameter to return to baseline. Images of the brachial artery are recorded at baseline, prior to administration of NTG, and during peak vasodilation that typically occurs 3–4 min after the administration of NTG (Fig. 3). The endothelium-independent vasodilation is calculated as the percent change between poststimulus and baseline diameter *(35)*.

Evaluation of the Microcirculation Vascular Reactivity

The most widely accepted technique for evaluating blood flow in the skin microcirculation is the use of laser Doppler flowmetry in conjunction with iontophoresis. Laser Doppler flowmetry uses a red laser that is transmitted to the skin. Red blood cells moving in the skin back-scatter light from the laser, causing a frequency shift in the light that is sensed by the probe and used as a measure of

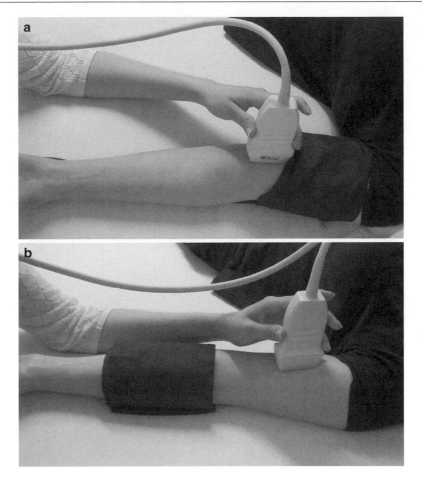

Fig. 2. Technique for obtaining ultrasonographic images of the left brachial artery. The patient lies in the supine position while the technician obtains an image in the longitudinal plane of the brachial artery in the area above the antecubital fossa. The sphygmomanometric cuff, which is used in the assessment of endothelium-dependent flow-mediated vasodilation (*FMD*), can be placed either above (**a**) or below (**b**) the antecubital fossa.

superficial microvascular perfusion *(23, 36)*. There are two types of laser probes available for use: single-point laser probes and real-time laser scanners.

One of the major limitations of using single-point laser probes is that skin exhibits a heterogeneous hyperemic response across its surface. The method of real-time laser scanning can overcome this limitation by evaluating the entire area of skin rather than single points. In this procedure, a laser Doppler perfusion imager is used to sequentially scan an area of skin with a 1-mW helium–neon laser beam of 633-nm wavelength (Fig. 4). The blood flow in the skin is recorded by the scanner and expressed in volts.

The iontophoresis technique is used to apply vasoactive substances to a localized area of the skin. In this technique, a delivery vehicle device is attached firmly to the skin with double-sided adhesive tape. The device contains two chambers that accommodate two single-point laser probes. A small quantity of 1% Ach solution or 1% of SNP solution is placed in the iontophoresis chamber and a constant current of 200 mA is applied for 60 s, achieving a dose of 6 mC/cm^2 between the iontophoresis

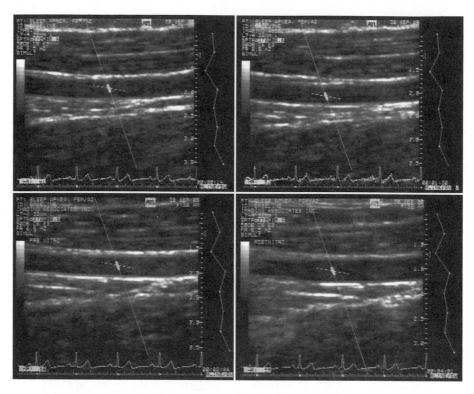

Fig. 3. Ultrasonographic images of endothelium-dependent vasodilation, before and 5 min after the cuff release (*up*), and images of endothelium-independent vasodilation before and 3 min after the nitroglycerin (*NTG*) administration (*down*).

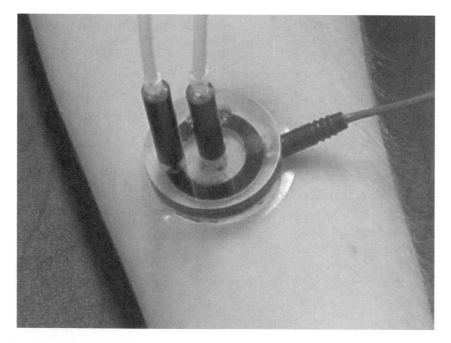

Fig. 4. An iontophoresis chamber with two single-point laser probes in position on the forearm. Probe 1 (in the periphery of the circular chamber) measures the direct effect of vasoactive substance on the microvasculature, while probe 2 (in the center of the chamber) measures the indirect effect of vasoactive substance on the microvasculature (the nerve-axon related hyperemic response). In this method of laser Doppler flowmetry, it is possible to evaluate endothelium-dependent vasodilation with the use of acetylcholine chloride solution as the vasoactive substance, and endothelium-independent vasodilation with the use of sodium nitroprusside (*SNP*) solution as the vasoactive substance.

chamber and a second nonactive electrode placed 10–15 cm proximal to the chamber. This current causes a movement of solution to be iontophoresed toward the skin, resulting in vasodilatation *(36)*.

A baseline scan is taken and iontophoresis is performed as described above. Following the completion of the iontophoresis, a second scan is taken. The difference in blood flow between the two scans represents the increase in the blood flow (Figs. 5 and 6) *(36)*.

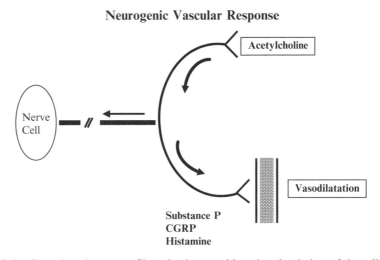

Fig. 5. Stimulation of the C-nociceptive nerve fibers leads to antidromic stimulation of the adjacent C fibers, which secrete substance P, calcitonin gene-related peptide (*CGRP*), and histamine that cause vasodilatation and increased blood flow.

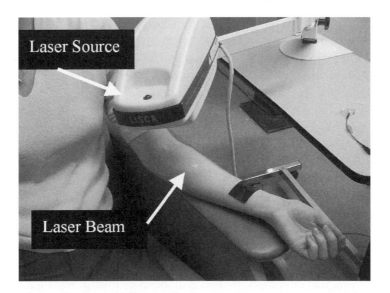

Fig. 6. A laser Doppler perfusion imager, which sequentially scans selected areas of skin in real time. This method allows for the evaluation of the hyperemic response to vasoactive substance over the entire area of skin rather than at a single point.

Biochemical and Cellular Markers of Endothelial Dysfunction

Endothelial cells produce a wide array of vasoactive factors. Under normal conditions, these factors are present in small concentrations in the systemic circulation but during endothelial injury their levels increase considerably. These molecules can therefore serve as biochemical markers for endothelial dysfunction, some of which will be discussed below.

Cellular adhesion molecules (CAMs) are produced by endothelial cells and inserted into their apical membrane in response to inflammatory stimuli. As their name implies, CAMs are involved in the adhesion of circulating leukocytes to endothelial cells and play a role in transmigration. Pathologically, CAMs play a significant role in the development of atherosclerosis as they facilitate the migration of monocytes to the vascular intima where they phagocytize oxidized low-density lipoprotein (ox-LDL) and become foam cells *(4, 5)*.

In addition to the membrane-bound form, CAMs are also produced in the soluble form, and as such, they can be measured in the plasma. Soluble intercellular adhesion molecules (sICAMs) at increased concentrations have been shown to correlate with a higher risk of future cardiovascular disease *(37)*. Endothelial cells express CAMs when incubated in high glucose conditions in vitro *(38)*, and elevated levels of CAMs have been observed in patients both with impaired glucose tolerance (IGT) and with diabetes *(39, 40)*. Furthermore, in the vitreous, levels of vascular cell adhesion molecule-1 (VCAM-1) and vascular endothelial growth factor (VEGF) directly correlate in patients with proliferative diabetic retinopathy (PDR) *(41)*.

Von Willebrand factor (vWF), a multimeric glycoprotein synthesized principally by endothelial cells, is involved in platelet adhesion and aggregation. It also acts as the carrier of coagulation factor VIII in the plasma. Damage to endothelial cells induces the release of increased amounts of vWF into the bloodstream, and this has been found in association with atherosclerosis *(42)* and diabetes *(42–44)*. Notably, plasma vWF concentration increases later in disease progression than does the plasma concentration of sCAMs *(45)*. As a result, vWF is increasingly being used as a late marker of endothelial dysfunction *(45)*.

ENDOTHELIAL DYSFUNCTION DIABETES AND CARDIOVASCULAR DISEASE

Endothelial dysfunction is a term that implies diminished production or availability of NO and/or an imbalance in the endothelium-derived relaxing and contractive factors. In nondiabetic subjects, endothelial dysfunction is present long before atherosclerosis appears and can serve as an independent predictor of future cardiovascular disease *(46–48)*. Diabetes – both type1 and type 2 – along with obesity and hyperlipidemia are the most significant factors for endothelial dysfunction. Other factors that induce endothelial dysfunction are hyperhomocysteinemia, smoking, and high caffeine consumption *(49, 50)*.

In type 1 diabetes, endothelial dysfunction is present in the early stages, usually within 5 years after the diagnosis of the disease, and is progressively deteriorating. When the first stages of microvascular complications present themselves, especially microalbuminuria, endothelial impairment is fully established and manifests itself by impaired endothelium-dependent vasodilation and increased serum levels of markers of endothelial dysfunction, such as vWF and CAMs *(51–53)*.

The role of endothelial impairment in type 2 diabetes is more complicated. In type 2 diabetic patients, markers of endothelial dysfunction are often elevated years before any evidence of macroangiopathy becomes evident *(54–62)*. The effects of aging hyperlipidemia, hypertension, and other factors add to the complexity of the problem.

A major pathophysiological alteration of type 2 diabetes is insulin resistance. There is a growing body of evidence that demonstrates the coexistence of insulin resistance and endothelial dysfunction. Insulin-induced vasodilation, which is partially regulated by NO release, is impaired in obese nondiabetic individuals who display insulin resistance *(63)*. Data from a large number of clinical studies suggest that endothelial dysfunction occurs in a concomitant manner with insulin resistance and antedates overt hyperglycemia in patients with type 2 diabetes. Furthermore, additional studies have shown that, endothelial dysfunction is present early in individuals at risk of developing type 2 diabetes, even at a stage when normal glucose tolerance and insulin sensitivity exists *(64, 65)*.

ROLE OF INFLAMMATION IN CARDIOVASCULAR DISEASE

Over the last decade, an abundance of evidence has emerged demonstrating a central role for inflammation in all phases of the atherosclerotic disease process, from lesion initiation to progression and, finally, to plaque rupture and the consecutive complications of cardiovascular disease. Thus, a large number of population-based epidemiological and clinical studies have shown strong and consistent relationships between markers of inflammation and impaired carbohydrate and lipids metabolism, endothelial dysfunction, and atherosclerosis. The results of these studies have increased interest in the potential use of inflammatory biomarkers to predict the risk for cardiovascular events, while they also raise the possibility that inflammatory factors may serve as targets of therapy *(66–88)*.

The Role of Inflammation in the Pathogenesis of Atherosclerosis

Inflammation is a major factor that causes endothelial dysfunction and leads to the expression of CAMs, cytokines, and chemokines which facilitate adherence and endothelial transmigration of leukocytes (monocytes and T-helper lymphocytes). Monocytes residing in the arterial wall become activated by proinflammatory cytokines and differentiate into macrophages. Activated macrophages and lymphocytes increase the expression of CAMs, cytokines, growth factors, and metalloproteinases which result in recruitment of more leukocytes into the arterial wall, activate the complement pathways of the immune system and the acute phase response, stimulate proliferation and migration of smooth muscle cells (SMCs), and promote fibrous tissue deposition *(4, 88)*.

The next step involves the development of the early atherosclerotic lesion. During this phase, ox-LDL are taken up by macrophages via the scavenger receptor lectin-like oxidized low-density lipoprotein receptor-1 (LOX-1) leading to foam cells formation which characterize early atheroma *(89)*. Within the developing atheroma, the foam cells secrete proinflammatory cytokines [such as tumor necrosis factor alpha (TNF-α) and interleukin (IL)-1]. Apart from macrophages, T-lymphocytes are also present in the arterial intima and their activation also results in the secretion of cytokines, chemokines, and growth factors and triggers the CD40/CD40L signaling pathway *(90, 91)*. Thus, inflammation plays an important role in both the early and late stages of the development of the atherosclerotic plaque.

Serum Markers of Inflammation

A number of biomarkers that appear to be linked to inflammation and atherogenesis have being identified, while others are still under evaluation. The most significant of them are briefly analyzed below.

C-Reactive Protein

C-reactive protein (CRP) was originally discovered by Tillett and Francis in 1930 and is an early acute-phase reactant that is produced in response to acute injury, infection, or other acute inflammatory stimuli. Although the main source for CRP production is the liver, recent studies have shown that arterial tissue can also produce CRP *(92)*. IL-1, IL-6, and TNF-α are the main cytokines that stimulate CRP synthesis by inducing hepatic gene expression *(93)*.

Current clinical evidence supports that CRP is a strong and independent predictor of atherosclerotic risk and it may be used as a tool for determining the risk for acute coronary syndromes as it strongly predicts future cardiovascular events *(66–75)*. In addition, several studies have demonstrated relationships between CRP and the metabolic syndrome *(94, 95)*, while other studies suggest that CRP is not only a serum biomarker for atherosclerosis but is also involved in the process of atherosclerosis through the promotion of endothelial dysfunction. There is also evidence that early CRP deposition on arterial wall induces ICAM-1, VCAM-1, and monocyte chemoattractant protein (MCP-1) production by endothelial cells. More recently, CRP has been demonstrated to inhibit the survival and differentiation of bone marrow-derived endothelial progenitor cells, which play a key role in postnatal neovascularization *(96–100)*. Conditions, activities, and medications that affect levels of CRP are summarized in Table 1.

Cytokines and Chemokines

Cytokines are small, nonstructural proteins with molecular weights ranging from 8 to 40,000 Da. Originally called lymphokines and monokines to indicate their cellular sources, it became clear that the term "cytokine" is the best description, since nearly all nucleated cells are capable of synthesizing these proteins and, in turn, of responding to them.

There are presently 18 cytokines with the name IL. Other cytokines have retained their original biological description, such as TNF. Some cytokines clearly promote inflammation and are characterized as proinflammatory cytokines, whereas other cytokines suppress the activity of proinflammatory cytokines and are characterized as antiinflammatory cytokines. For example, IL-4, IL-10, and IL-13 are potent activators of B lymphocytes but at the same time they are also potent antiinflammatory agents as they suppress the expression of proinflammatory cytokines.

The main proinflammatory cytokines are IL-1, IL-6, and TNF-α. IL-1 and IL-6 are pleiotropic cytokines with a broad range of humoral and cellular immune effects relating to inflammation, host defense, and tissue injury. Serum levels of the proinflammatory cytokines IL-1, IL-6, TNF-α are elevated in hypercholesterolemic patients *(101)*. In addition, several clinical studies have shown an association between the plasma levels of these cytokines and cardiovascular risk *(102–105)*.

Table 1
Conditions, Activities, and Medications that Affect Levels of C-Reactive Protein

Increase levels	*Decrease levels*
Inflammation – bacterial infection	Inhibitory cytokinesis
Coronary artery disease	Exercise
Obesity	
Sepsis	
Smoking	
Vasculitis	
Inhibitory cytokinesis	
Malignancy	
Connective tissue disease	
Allograft vasculopathy and graft occlusion	

Chemokines are small proteins involved in the chemotaxis of monocytes and lymphocytes in the early stages of atherosclerosis. In particular, MCP-1 has been postulated as a major signal for the accumulation of mononuclear leukocytes. MCP-1 is produced by a variety of cells – including leukocytes, endothelial cells, and fibroblasts – in response to ox-LDL and proinflammatory cytokines. Enhanced levels of MCP-1 have been found in patients with cardiovascular risk factors, such as hyperlipidemia. In these patients, serum concentrations of MCP-1 were significantly correlated with LDL cholesterol. Furthermore, this chemokine is upregulated in human atherosclerotic plaque and in the arteries of primates fed a high-cholesterol diet. Increased MCP-1 expression has been found in patients with coronary artery disease *(89, 104, 105)*.

In conclusion, it seems that proinflammatory cytokines and chemokines are taking a great part in the process of atherogenesis and they could possibly be promising markers of atherosclerosis.

Adiponectin

Adiponectin is an adipocyte-derived 244 amino acid adipokine that is synthesized and secreted by adipocytes and presents well-established antiatherogenic and insulin-sensitizing properties. Low levels of adiponectin have been associated with obesity, the metabolic syndrome, and type 2 diabetes *(106)*. Other studies suggest that low levels of adiponectin have also been associated with CVD in different patient populations, independently of traditional risk factors *(107–109)*.

Cell biology and animal studies suggest that adiponectin plays an important role in both glucose/insulin/fatty acid metabolism and inflammation. Whereas initial studies demonstrated that adiponectin suppresses the production of the potent proinflammatory cytokine TNF-α, recent studies have showed that this adipokine also induces various antiinflammatory cytokines, such as IL-10 or IL-1 receptor antagonists. Considering that adiponectin appears to be a modulator of lipid metabolism and systemic inflammation, it has been proposed as a novel predictor of individuals at risk for the metabolic syndrome and possibly type 2 diabetes.

Others

Other serum markers of inflammation are CD40 and CD40, lipoprotein-associated phospholipase A2, myeloperoxidase, neopterin, defensins, and cathelicidins. All the above, have been shown to contribute to the progression of atherosclerosis and cardiovascular disease *(89, 105)*.

EXERCISE AND ENDOTHELIAL FUNCTION

Exercise is known to reduce cardiovascular disease as it increases blood flow, and, therefore, it shears stress, through the large and small vessels; it has been suggested that it affects its beneficial effects through endothelial stimulation and improvement of the endothelial function *(110)*. However, most of the studies that included healthy subjects showed that training of small or large groups of muscles had no effect on endothelial function while a few studies suggested a beneficial effect *(111–116)*. Given the fact that healthy subjects already have normal endothelial function, the lack of any exercise benefit on the endothelial function is not surprising, as a further increase of it to supraphysiological levels seems not feasible. More realistically, it would be expected that in healthy subjects, exercise averts the decline of endothelial function and, therefore, prevents the development of cardiovascular disease. Support to this hypothesis is provided by numerous epidemiologic studies that have clearly demonstrated that daily physical aerobic exercise prevents the cardiovascular mortality and morbidity and that physical inactivity (sedentary state) per se is a risk factor for cardiovascular diseases *(117–119)*.

In contrast to studies that involved healthy subjects, studies in subjects with cardiovascular disease, congestive heart failure *(120, 121)*, and type 2 diabetes *(122)* showed that regular exercise had a significant increase in flow-mediated endothelium-dependent and -independent vasodilation. The beneficial effects were seen both during exercise of localized muscle groups, mainly in lower limbs, *(123–125)* or whole body exercise *(120–122, 126–129)*.

Although the mechanism of improvement in endothelial function during exercise has not been fully clarified, it is thought that regular aerobic exercise increases NO production through the upregulation of eNOS gene expression and VEGF-induced angiogenesis. In addition, exercise decreases NO inactivation through the augmentation of superoxide dismutase (SOD) and glutathione peroxidase (GPx) and attenuation of nicotinamide adenine dinucleotide/nicotinamide adenine dinucleotide phosphate (NADH/NADPH) oxidase activity, leading to an increase in NO bioavailability *(130)*.

EXERCISE AND INFLAMMATION

Large epidemiological studies have shown that regular exercise is associated with reduced inflammation *(131–133)*. Thus, increased physical activity is associated with reduced CRP levels, fibrinogen, coagulation factors VIII and IX, vWF, fibrin d-dimer, and t-PA antigen. Furthermore, an interventional study showed that regular daily exercise leads to the reduction of the CRP serum levels In the same study, the monocyte production of proinflammatory TNF-α and IL-6 cytokines levels was also reduced while the production of antiatherogenic and antiinflammatory cytokines such as IL-4, IL-10, and transforming growth factor-β (TGF-β) was increased *(134–136)*.

The exact mechanisms that are related to the reduced inflammation in subjects who exercise regularly are not clear. However, acute exercise has been shown to increase the levels of IL-10 and IL-1ra *(134–136)*. Furthermore, it inhibits the production of TNF-α, at least partly through the suppressive action of IL-10 and the muscle-derived IL-6 *(137)*. Other possible mechanisms include alterations in the balance between the sympathetic and parasympathetic nervous systems, reduced expression of toll-like receptor 4 (TLR4) and changes in the innate immunity *(138)*.

REFERENCES

1. Grundy SM, Benjamin IJ, Burke GL, Chait A, Eckel RH, Howard BV, Mitch W, Smith SC Jr, Sowers JR. Diabetes and cardiovascular disease: a statement for healthcare professionals from the American Heart Association. *Circulation* 1999;100:1134–46.
2. Tuomilehto J, Lindstrom J, Eriksson JG, Valle TT, Hamalainen H, Ilanne-Parikka P, Keinanen-Kiukaanniemi S, Laakso M, Louheranta A, Rastas M, Salminen V, Uusitupa M. Finnish Diabetes Prevention Study Group. Prevention of type 2 diabetes mellitus by changes in lifestyle among subjects with impaired glucose tolerance. *N Engl J Med.* 2001;344:1343–50.
3. Quinones MJ, Nicholas SB, Lyon CJ. Insulin resistance and the endothelium. *Curr Diab Rep.* 2005;5(4):246–53.
4. Libby P, Aikawa M, Jain MK. Vascular endothelium and atherosclerosis. *Handb Exp Pharmacol.* 2006;176 (Pt. 2):285–306.
5. Glasser SP, Selwyn AP, Ganz P. Atherosclerosis: risk factors and the vascular endothelium. *Am Heart J.* 1996; 131:379–84.
6. Libby P. Inflammation and cardiovascular disease mechanisms. *Am J Clin Nutr.* 2006;83(2):456S–60S.
7. Haffner SM. The metabolic syndrome: inflammation, diabetes mellitus, and cardiovascular disease. *Am J Cardiol.* 2006;97(2A):3A–11A.
8. Key NS. Scratching the surface: endothelium as a regulator of thrombosis, fibrinolysis, and inflammation. *J Lab Clin Med.* 1992;120(2):184–6.
9. Anggard EE. J Endocrinol. *The endothelium – the body's largest endocrine gland? J Endocrinol.* 1990;127(3):371–5.
10. Inagami T, Naruse M, Hoover R. Endothelium as an endocrine organ. *Annu Rev Physiol.* 1995;57:171–89.
11. Baumgartner-Parzer SM, Waldhausl WK. The endothelium as a metabolic and endocrine organ: it's relation with insulin resistance. *Exp Clin Endocrinol Diabetes* 2001;109(Suppl. 2):S166–79.

12. Fleming I, Bauersachs J, Busse R. Paracrine functions of the coronary vascular endothelium. *Mol Cell Biochem.* 1996;157(1–2):137–45.

13. Triggle CR, Ding H, Anderson TJ, Pannirselvam M. The endothelium in health and disease: a discussion of the contribution of non-nitric oxide endothelium-derived vasoactive mediators to vascular homeostasis in normal vessels and in type II diabetes. *Mol Cell Biochem.* 2004;263:21–7.

14. Henrich WL. The endothelium – a key regulator of vascular tone. *Am J Med Sci.* 1991;302(5):319–28.

15. Davignon J, Ganz P. Role of endothelial dysfunction in atherosclerosis. *Circulation.* 2004;109(23 Suppl. 1):III27–32.

16. Kitamoto S, Egashira K. Endothelial dysfunction and coronary atherosclerosis. *Curr Drug Targets Cardiovasc Haematol Disord.* 2004;4(1):13–22.

17. Harris MI, Flegal KM, Cowie CC, Eberhardt MS, Goldstein DE, Little RR, Wiedmeyer HM, Byrd-Holt DD. Prevalence of diabetes, impaired fasting glucose, and impaired glucose tolerance in U.S. adults. The Third National Health and Nutrition Examination Survey, 1988–1994. *Diabetes Care* 1998;21:518–24.

18. Mokdad AH, Bowman BA, Ford ES, Vinicor F, Marks JS, Koplan JP. The continuing epidemics of obesity and diabetes in the United States. *JAMA* 2001;286:1195–200.

19. Knowler WC, Barrett-Connor E, Fowler SE, Hamman RF, Lachin JM, Walker EA, Nathan DM. Diabetes Prevention Program Research Group. Reduction in the incidence of type 2 diabetes with lifestyle intervention or metformin. *N Engl J Med.* 2002;346:393–403.

20. Dogra G, Rich L, Stanton K, Watts GF. Endothelium-dependent and independent vasodilation studies at normoglycaemia in type I diabetes mellitus with and without microalbuminuria. *Diabetologia* 2001;44:593–601.

21. Meeking DR, Cummings MH, Thorne S, Donald A, Clarkson P, Crook JR, Watts GF, Shaw KM. Endothelial dysfunction in type 2 diabetic subjects with and without microalbuminuria. *Diabet Med.* 1999;16:841–7.

22. McVeigh GE, Brennan GM, Johnston GD, McDermott BJ, McGrath LT, Henry WR, Andrews JW, Hayes JR. Impaired endothelium-dependent and independent vasodilation in patients with type 2 (non-insulin-dependent) diabetes mellitus. *Diabetologia* 1992;35:771–6.

23. Veves A, Akbari CM, Primavera J, Donaghue VM, Zacharoulis D, Chrzan JS, DeGirolami U, LoGerfo FW, Freeman R. Endothelial dysfunction and the expression of endothelial nitric oxide synthetase in diabetic neuropathy, vascular disease and foot ulceration. *Diabetes* 1998;47:457–63.

24. Koitka A, Abraham P, Bouhanick B, Sigaudo-Roussel D, Demiot C, Saumet JL. Impaired pressure-induced vasodilation at the foot in young adults with type 1 diabetes. *Diabetes* 2004;53:721–5.

25. Schalkwijk CG, Stehouwer CD. Vascular complications in diabetes mellitus: the role of endothelial dysfunction. *Clin Sci (Lond).* 2005;109(2):143–59.

26. Goldenberg S, Alex M, Joshi RA, Blumenthal HT. Nonatheromatous peripheral vascular disease of the lower extremity in diabetes mellitus. *Diabetes* 1959;8:261–73.

27. Strandness DE Jr, Priest RE, Gibbons GE. Combined clinical and pathological study of diabetic and nondiabetic peripheral arterial disease. *Diabetes* 1964;13:366–72.

28. Conrad MC. Large and small artery occlusion in diabetics and nondiabetics with severe vascular disease. *Circulation* 1967;36:83–91.

29. Barner HB, Kaiser GC, Willman VL. Blood flow in the diabetic leg. *Circulation* 1971;43:391–4.

30. LoGerfo FW, Coffman JP. Current concepts. Vascular and microvascular disease of the foot in diabetes. Implications for foot care. *N Engl J Med.* 1984;311:1615–9.

31. Cypress M, Tomky D. Microvascular complications of diabetes. *Nurs Clin North Am.* 2006;41(4):719–36.

32. He Z, King GL. Microvascular complications of diabetes. *Endocrinol Metab Clin North Am.* 2004;33(1):215–38.

33. Veldman BA, Vervoort G. Pathogenesis of renal microvascular complications in diabetes mellitus. *Neth J Med.* 2002;60(10):390–6.

34. Theuma P, Fonseca VA. Novel cardiovascular risk factors and macrovascular and microvascular complications of diabetes. *Curr Drug Targets.* 2003;4(6):477–86.

35. Corretti MC, Anderson TJ, Benjamin EJ, Celermajer D, Charbonneau F, Creager MA, Deanfield J, Drexler H, Gerhard-Herman M, Herrington D, Vallance P, Vita J, Vogel R. Guidelines for the ultrasound assessment of endothelial-dependent flow-mediated vasodilation of the brachial artery: a report of the International Brachial Artery Reactivity Task Force. *J Am Coll Cardiol.* 2002;39:257–65.

36. Akbari CM, Saouaf R, Barnhill DF, Newman PA, LoGerfo FW, Veves A. Endothelium-dependent vasodilatation is impaired in both micro- and macrocirculation during acute hyperglycemia. *J Vasc Surg* 1998;28:687–94.

37. Ridker PM, Hennekens CH, Roitman-Johnson B, Stampfer MJ, Allen J. Plasma concentration of soluble intercellular adhesion molecule 1 and risks of future myocardial infarction in apparently healthy men. *Lancet* 1998;351:88–92.

38. Altannavch TS, Roubalova K, Kucera P, Andel M. Effect of high glucose concentrations on expression of ELAM-1, VCAM-1 and ICAM-1 in HUVEC with and without cytokine activation. *Physiol Res.* 2004;53:77–82.

39. Ferri C, Desideri G, Baldoncini R, Bellini C, De Angelis C, Mazzocchi C, Santucci A. Early activation of vascular endothelium in nonobese, nondiabetic essential hypertensive patients with multiple metabolic abnormalities. *Diabetes* 1998;47:660–7.

40. Otosuki M, Hashimoto K, Morimoto Y, Kishimoto T, Kasayama S. Circulating vascular cell adhesion molecule-1 (V CAM-1) in atherosclerotic NIDDM patients. *Diabetes* 1997;46:2096–101.

41. Hernandez C, Burgos R, Canton A, Garcia-Arumi J, Segura RM, Simo R. Vitreous levels of vascular cell adhesion molecule and vascular endothelial growth factor in patients with proliferative diabetic retinopathy: a case-control study. *Diabetes Care* 2001;24:516–21.

42. Tull SP, Anderson SI, Hughan SC, Watson SP, Nash GB, Rainger GE. Cellular pathology of atherosclerosis: smooth muscle cells promote adhesion of platelets to cocultured endothelial cells. *Circ Res.* 2006;98:98–104.

43. Verrotti A, Greco R, Basciani F, Morgese G, Chiarelli F. von Willebrand factor and its propeptide in children with diabetes. Relation between endothelial dysfunction and microalbuminuria. *Pediatr Res.* 2003;53:382–6.

44. Economides PA, Caselli A, Zuo CS, Khaodhiar L, Sparks C, Katsilambros N, Horton ES, Veves A. Kidney oxygenation during water diuresis and endothelial function in patients with type 2 diabetes and subjects at risk to develop diabetes. *Metabolism* 2004;53:222–7.

45. Lim SC, Caballero AE, Smakowski P, LoGerfo FW, Horton ES, Veves A. Soluble intercellular adhesion molecule, vascular cell adhesion molecule, and impaired microvascular reactivity are early markers of vasculopathy in type 2 diabetic individuals without microalbuminuria. *Diabetes Care.* 1999;22(11):1865–70.

46. Elliott HL. *Endothelial dysfunction in cardiovascular disease: risk factor, risk marker, or surrogate end point? J Cardiovasc Pharmacol.* 1998;32(Suppl. 3):S74–7.

47. Feener EP, King GL. Endothelial dysfunction in diabetes mellitus: role in cardiovascular disease. *Heart Fail Monit.* 2001;1(3):74–82.

48. Sherman DL, Loscalzo J. Endothelial dysfunction and cardiovascular disease. *Cardiologia* 1997;42(2):177–87.

49. Pittilo MR. Cigarette smoking, endothelial injury and cardiovascular disease. *Int J Exp Pathol.* 2000;81(4):219–30.

50. Doupis J, Tentolouris N, Perrea D, Zacharopoulou O, Kyriaki D, Katsilambros N. Acute methionine-induced hyperhomocysteinaemia causes endothelial dysfunction in patients with type 2 diabetes. *Diabetes* 2003;52(Suppl. 1):A153–4.

51. Van Ittersum FJ, Spek JJ, Praet IJ et al.. Ambulatory blood pressures and autonomic nervous function in normoalbuminuric type I diabetic patients. *Nephrol Dial Transplant.* 1998;13:326–32.

52. Schalkwijk CG, Poland, DC, van Dijk W et al.. Plasma concentration of C-reactive protein is increased in type I diabetic patients without clinical macroangiopathy and correlates with markers of endothelial dysfunction: evidence for chronic inflammation. *Diabetologia* 1999;42: 351–7.

53. Wetzels, JF. Transcapillary escape rate of albumin is increased and related to haemodynamic changes in normoalbuminuric type 1 diabetic patients. *J. Hypertens.* 1999;17:1911–6.

54. Cosentino F, Luscher TF. Endothelial dysfunction in diabetes mellitus. *J Cardiovasc Pharmacol* 1998;32(Suppl. 3):S54–61.

55. De Mattia G, Bravi MC, Laurenti O, Cassone-Faldetta M, Proietti A, De Luca O, Armiento A, Ferri C. Reduction of oxidative stress by oral *N*-acetyl-l-cysteine treatment decreases plasma soluble vascular cell adhesion molecule-1 concentrations in nonobese, non-dyslipidaemic, normotensive patients with non-insulin-dependent diabetes. *Diabetologia* 1998;41:1392–6.

56. Gazis A, White DJ, Page SR, Cockcroft JR. Effect of oral vitamin E (a-tocopherol) supplementation on vascular endothelial function in type 2 diabetes mellitus. *Diabet Med.* 1999;16:304–11.

57. Bloomgarden ZT. Endothelial dysfunction, neuropathy and the diabetic foot, diabetic mastopathy, and erectile dysfunction. *Diabetes Care* 1998;21:183–9.

58. Hsueh WA, Anderson PW. Hypertension, the endothelial cell, and the vascular complications of diabetes mellitus [clinical conference]. *Hypertension* 1992;20:253–63.

59. Janka HU. Platelet and endothelial function tests during metformin treatment in diabetes mellitus. Horm Metab Res. 1985;(Suppl. 15):120–122.

60. Neri S, Bruno CM, Leotta C, D'Amico RA, Pennisi G, Ierna D. Early endothelial alterations in non-insulin-dependent diabetes mellitus. *Int J Clin Lab Res.* 1998;28:100–3.

61. Watts GF, Playford DA. Dyslipoproteinaemia and hyperoxidative stress in the pathogenesis of endothelial dysfunction in non-insulin dependent diabetes mellitus: a hypothesis. *Atherosclerosis* 1998;141:17–30.

62. Escandon JC, Cipolla M. Diabetes and endothelial dysfunction: a clinical perspective. *Endocr Rev.* 2001; 22(1):36–52.

63. Ridker PM, Cushman M, Stampfer MJ, Tracy R, Hennekens CH. Inflammation, aspirin, and the risk of cardiovascular disease in apparently healthy men. *N Engl J Med.* 1997;336:973–9.

64. Caballero AE, Arora S, Saouaf R, Lim SC, Smakowski P, Park JY, King GL, LoGerfo FW, Horton ES, Veves A. Microvascular and macrovascular reactivity is reduced in subjects at risk for type 2 diabetes. *Diabetes* 1999; 48(9):1856–62.

65. Goldfine AB, Beckman JA, Betensky RA, Devlin H, Hurley S, Varo N, Schonbeck U, Patti ME, Creager MA. Family history of diabetes is a major determinant of endothelial function. *J Am Coll Cardiol.* 2006;47(12):2456–61.

66. Ridker PM, Glynn RJ, Hennekens CH. C-reactive protein adds to the predictive value of total and HDL cholesterol in determining risk of first myocardial infarction. *Circulation* 1998;97:2007–11.

67. Ridker PM, Cushman M, Stampfer MJ, Tracy RP, Hennekens CH. Plasma concentration of C-reactive protein and risk of developing peripheral vascular disease. *Circulation* 1998;97:425–8.

68. Ridker PM, Buring JE, Shih J, Matia M, Hennekens CH. Prospective study of C-reactive protein and the risk of future cardiovascular events among apparently healthy women. *Circulation* 1998;98:731–3.

69. MRFIT Research Group. Relationship of C-reactive protein and coronary heart disease in the MRFIT nested case-control study. *Am J Epidemiol.* 1996;144:537–47.

70. Tracy RP, Lemaitre RN, Psaty BM, et al. Relationship of C-reactive protein to risk of cardiovascular disease in the elderly: results from the Cardiovascular Health Study and the Rural Health Promotion Project. *Arterioscler Thromb Vasc Biol.* 1997;17:1121–7.

71. Liuzzo G, Biasucci LM, Gallimore JR, et al. The prognostic value of C-reactive protein and serum amyloid A protein in severe unstable angina. *N Engl J Med.* 1994;331:417–24.

72. Thompson SG, et al.. European Concerted Action on Thrombosis and Disabilities Angina Pectoris Study Group. Hemostatic factors and the risk of myocardial infarction or sudden death in patients with angina pectoris. *N Engl J Med.* 1995;332:635–41.

73. European Concerted Action on Thrombosis, and Disabilities Angina Pectoris Study Group. Production of C-reactive protein and risk of coronary events in stable and unstable angina. *Lancet* 1997;349:462–6.

74. Ridker PM, Rifai N, Pfeffer MA, et al. Inflammation, pravastatin, and the risk of coronary events after myocardial infarction in patients with average cholesterol levels. *Circulation* 1998;98:839–44.

75. Ridker PM, Rifai N, Rose MA, Buring JE, Cook NR. Comparison of C-reactive protein and low-density lipoprotein cholesterol levels in the prediction of first cardiovascular events. *N Engl J Med.* 2002;347:1557–65.

76. Pischon T, Girman CJ, Hotamisligil GS, et al. Plasma adiponectin levels and risk of myocardial infarction in men. *JAMA* 2004;291:1730–7.

77. Hotta K, Funahashi T, Arita Y, et al. Plasma concentrations of a novel, adipose-specific protein, adiponectin, in type 2 diabetic patients. *Arterioscler Thromb Vasc Biol* 2000;20:1595–9.

78. Kumada M, Kihara S, Sumitsuji S, et al. Association of hypoadiponectinemia with coronary artery disease in men. *Arterioscler Thromb Vasc Biol.* 2003;23:85–9.

79. Kojima S, Funahashi T, Sakamoto T, et al. The variation of plasma concentrations of a novel, adipocyte derived protein, adiponectin, in patients with acute myocardial infarction. *Heart* 2003;89:667.

80. Kowalski J, Okopien B, Madej A, et al. Levels of sICAM-1, sVCAM-1 and MCP-1 in patients with hyperlipoproteinemia IIa and -IIb. *Int J Clin Pharmacol Ther.* 2001;39:48–52.

81. Matsumori A, Furukawa Y, Hashimoto T, et al. Plasma levels of the monocyte chemotactic and activating factor/monocyte chemoattractant protein-1 are elevated in patients with acute myocardial infarction. *J Mol Cell Cardiol.* 1997;29:419–23.

82. Schonbeck U, Varo N, Libby P, Buring J, Ridker PM. Soluble CD40L and cardiovascular risk in women. *Circulation* 2001;104:2266–8.

83. Kinlay S, Schwartz GG, Olsson AG, et al. Effect of atorvastatin on risk of recurrent cardiovascular events after an acute coronary syndrome associated with high soluble CD40 ligand in the Myocardial Ischemia Reduction with Aggressive Cholesterol Lowering (MIRACL) Study. *Circulation* 2004;110:386–91.

84. Caslake MJ, Packard CJ, Suckling KE, et al. Lipoprotein-associated phospholipase A2, platelet-activating factor acetylhydrolase: a potential new risk factor for coronary artery disease. *Atherosclerosis* 2000;150:413–9.

85. Packard CJ, et al. West of Scotland Coronary Prevention Study Group. Lipoprotein-associated phospholipase A2 as an independent predictor of coronary heart disease. *N Engl J Med.* 2000;343:1148–55.

86. Blake GJ, Dada N, Fox JC, Manson JE, Ridker PM. A prospective evaluation of lipoproteinassociated phospholipase A2 levels and the risk of future cardiovascular events in women. *J Am Coll Cardiol.* 2001;38:1302–6.

87. Ballantyne CM, Hoogeveen RC, Bang H, et al. Lipoprotein associated phospholipase A2, high-sensitivity C-reactive protein, and risk for incident coronary heart disease in middle-aged men and women in the Atherosclerosis Risk in Communities (ARIC) Study. *Circulation* 2004;109:837–42.

88. Ballantyne CM, Nambi V. Markers of inflammation and their clinical significance. *Atherosclerosis* 2005;6:21–9.

89. Francisco G, Hernandez C, Simo R. Serum markers of vascular inflammation in dyslipemia. *Clin Chim Acta.* 2006;369(1):1–16.

90. Stemme S, Faber B, Holm J, Wiklund O, Witztum JL, Hansson GK. T lymphocytes from human atherosclerotic plaques recognize oxidized low density lipoprotein. *Proc Natl Acad Sci USA* 1995;92:3893–7.

91. Li D, Liu L, Chen H, Sawamura T, Mehta JL. LOX-1, an oxidized LDL endothelial receptor, induces CD40/CD40L signaling in human coronary artery endothelial cells. *Arterioscler Thromb Vasc Biol.* 2003;23:816–21.

92. Yasojima K, Shwab C, McGeer EG, McGeer PL. Generation of C-reactive protein and complement components in atheroscleroticplaques. *Am J Pathol.* 2001;158:1039–51.

93. Albert MA. The role of C-reactive protein in cardiovascular disease risk. *Curr Cardiol Rep.* 2000;2(4):274–9.

94. Ridker PM, Buring JE, Cook NR, Rifai N. C-reactive protein, the metabolic syndrome, and risk of incident cardiovascular events: an 8-year follow-up of 14719 initially healthy American women. *Circulation* 2003;107:391–7.

95. Rutter MK, Meigs JB, Sullivan LM, D'Agostino Sr RB, Wilson PW. C-reactive protein, the metabolic syndrome, and prediction of cardiovascular events in the Framingham Offspring Study. *Circulation* 2004;110:380–5.

96. Verma S, Wang CH, Li SH, Dumont AS, Fedak PW, Badiwala MV, Dhillon B, Weisel RD, Li RK, Mickle DA, Stewart DJ. A self-fulfilling prophecy: C-reactive protein attenuates nitric oxide production and inhibits angiogenesis. *Circulation* 2002;106(8):913–9.

97. Verma S, Kuliszewski MA, Li SH, Szmitko PE, Zucco L, Wang CH, Badiwala MV, Mickle DA, Weisel RD, Fedak PW, Stewart DJ, Kutryk MJ. C-reactive protein attenuates endothelial progenitor cell survival, differentiation, and function: further evidence of a mechanistic link between C-reactive protein and cardiovascular disease. *Circulation* 2004; 109(17):2058–67.

98. Verma S. C-reactive protein incites atherosclerosis. *Can J Cardiol.* 2004;20(Suppl. B):29B–31B.

99. Manolov DE, Koenig W, Hombach V, Torzewski J. C-reactive protein and atherosclerosis. *Is there a causal link? Histol Histopathol.* 2003;18(4):1189–93.

100. Torzewski M, Rist C, Mortensen RF, Zwaka TP, Bienek M, Waltenberger J, Koenig W, Schmitz G, Hombach V, Torzewski J. C-reactive protein in the arterial intima: role of C-reactive protein receptor-dependent monocyte recruitment in atherogenesis. *Arterioscler Thromb Vasc Biol.* 2000;20(9):2094–9.

101. Ferroni P, Basili S, Vieri M, et al. Soluble P-selectin and proinflammatory cytokines in patients with polygenic type IIa hypercholesterolemia. *Haemostasis* 1999;29:277–85.

102. Ridker PM, Hennekens CH, Buring JE, Rifai N. C-reactive protein and other markers of inflammation in the prediction of cardiovascular disease in women. *N Engl J Med.* 2000;342:836–43.

103. Harris TB, Ferrucci L, Tracy RP, et al. Associations of elevated interleukin-6 and C-reactive protein levels with mortality in the elderly. *Am J Med.* 1999;106:506–12.

104. Verma S, Szmitko PE, Wang CH, Li SH, Weisel RD, De Almeida JR, Todd J. New markers of inflammation and endothelial cell activation: part I. *Circulation* 2003;108;1917–23.

105. De Martinis M, Franceschi C, Monti D, Ginaldi L. Inflammation markers predicting frailty and mortality in the elderly. *Exp Mol Pathol.* 2006;80:219–27.

106. Arita Y, Kihara S, Ouchi N, et al. Paradoxical decrease of an adiposespecific protein, adiponectin, in obesity. *Biochem Biophys Res Commun.* 1999;257:79–83.

107. Hotta K, Funahashi T, Arita Y, et al. Plasma concentrations of a novel, adipose-specific protein, adiponectin, in type 2 diabetic patients. *Arterioscler Thromb Vasc Biol.* 2000;20:1595–9.

108. Buras J, Reenstra WR, Orlow D, Horton ES, Veves A. Changes in adiponectin levels related to treatment with troglitazone do not affect endothelial function in type 2 diabetes. *Obes Res.* 2005;13:1167–74.

109. Shetty GK, Economides PA, Horton ES, Mantzoros CS, Veves A. Circulating adiponectin and resistin levels in relation to metabolic factors, inflammatory markers, and vascular reactivity in diabetic patients and subjects at risk for diabetes. *Diabetes Care* 2004;27:2450–7.

110. Green DJ, Maiorana A, O'Driscoll G, Taylor R. *Effect or exercise training on endothelium-derived nitric oxide function in humans J Physiol.* 2004;561(Pt. 1):1–25.

111. Green DJ, Fowler DT, O' Driscoll JG, Blanksby BA, Taylor RR. Endothelium derived notric oxide activity in forearm vessels of tennis players. *J Appl Physiol.* 1996;81:943–8.

112. Green DJ, O' Driscoll, Blanksby BA, Taylor RR. Effects of casting on forearm resistance vessels in young men. *Med Sci Sports Exerc.* 1997;29:1325–31.

113. Green DJ, Cable NT, Fox C, Rankin JM, Taylor RR. Modification of forearm resistance vessels by exercise. *J Appl Physiol.* 2004;77:1929–33.

114. Kingwell BA, Sherrard B, Jennings GL, Dart AM. Four weeks of cycle training increases basal production of nitric oxide from the forearm. *Am J Physiol.* 1997;272:H1070–7.

115. Clarkson P, Montgomery HE, Mullen MJ, Donald AE, Powe AJ, Bull T, Jubb M, World M, Deanfield JE. Exercise training enhances endothelial function in young men. *J Am Coll Cardiol*. 1999;33:1379–85.

116. Maiorana A, O'Driscoll G, Dembo L, Cheetham C, Goodman C, Taylor R, Green D. Exercise training, vascular function and functional capacity in middle aged subjects. *Med Sci Sports Exerc*. 2001;33:2022–8.

117. Castelli WP. Epidemiology of coronary heart disease: the Framingham study. *Am J Med* 1984;76:4–12.

118. Paffenbarger RS, Hyde RT, Wing AL, et al. The association of changes in physical-activity level and other lifestyle characteristics with mortality among men. *N Engl J Med*. 1993;328:538–45.

119. Blair SN, Goodyear NN, Gibbons LW, Cooper, KH. Physical fitness and incidence of hypertension in healthy normotensive men and women. *JAMA* 1984;252:487–90.

120. Maiorana A, O'Driscoll G, Dembo L, Cheetham C, Goodman C, Taylor R, Green D. Effect of aerobic and resistance exercise training on vascular function in heart failure. *Am J Physiol*. 2000;279:H1999–2005.

121. Linke A, Schoene N, Gielen S, Hofer J, Erbs S, Schuler G, Hambrecht R. Endothelial dysfunction in patients with chronic heart failure: systemic effect of lower limb exercise training. *J Am Coll Cardiol*. 2001;37:392–7.

122. Cohen ND, Dunstan DW, Robinson C, Vulikh E, Zimmet PZ, Shaw JE. Improved endothelial function following a 14-month resistance exercise training program in adults with type 2 diabetes. *Diabetes Res Clin Pract*. 2008;79(3):405–11.

123. Horning B, Maier V, Dreler H. Physical training improves endothelial function in patients with chronic heart failure. *Circulation* 1996;93:210–4.

124. Katz SD, Yuen J, Bijou R, Lejemtel TH. Training improves endothelium dependent vasodilation in resistance vessels of patients with heart failure. *J Appl Physiol*. 1997;82:1488–92.

125. Hambrecht R, Hilbrich L Erbs S, Gielen S, Fiehn E, Schoene N, Schuler G. Corrections of endothelial dysfunction in chronic heart failure: additional effects of exercise training and oral l-arginine supplementation. *J Am Coll Cardiol*. 2000;35:706–13.

126. Hambrecht R, Fiehn E, Weigl C, Gielen S, Hamman C, Kaiser R, Yu J, Adams V, Niebauer J, Schuler G. Regular physical exercise corrects endothelial dysfunction and improves exercise capacity in patients with chronic heart failure. *Circulation* 1998;98:2709–15.

127. Hambrecht R, Wolf A, Gielen S, Linke A, Hofer J, Erbs S, Schoene N, Schuler G. Effect of exercise on coronary endothelial function in patients with coronary heart disease. *N Eng J Med*. 2000;342:454–60.

128. Hambrecht R, Adams V, Erbs S, Linke a Krankel N, Shu Y, Baither Y, Gielen S, Thiele H, Gummert JF, Mohr FW, Schuler G. Regular physical activity improves endothelial function in patients with coronary artery disease by increasing phosphorylation of endothelial nitric oxide synthase. *Circulation* 2003;107:3152–8.

129. Higashi Y, Sasaki S, Kurisu S, Yoshimizu A, Sasaki N, Matsuura H, Kajiyama G, Oshima T. Regular aerobic exercise augments endothelium dependent vascular relaxation in normotensive as well as hypertensive subjects. *Circulation* 1999;30:252–8.

130. Higashi Y, Yoshizumi M. Exersise and endothelial function: role of endothelium-derived nitric oxide and oxidative stress in healthy subjects and hypertensive patients. *Pharm Ther*. 2004;102:87–96.

131. Geffken DF, Cushman M, Burke GL, Polak JF, Sakkinen PA, Tracy RP. Association between physical activity and markers of inflammation in a healthy elderly population. *Am J Epidemiol*. 2001;153:242–50.

132. Abramson JL, Vaccarino V. Relationship between physical activity and inflammation among apparently healthy middle-aged and older US adults. *Arch Intern Med*. 2002;162:1286–92.

133. Wannamethee SG, Lowe GD, Whincup PH, Rumley A, Walker M, Lennon L. Physical activity and hemostatic and inflammatory variables in elderly men. *Circulation* 2002;105:1785–90.

134. Smith JK, Dykes R, Douglas JE, Krishnaswamy G, Berk S. Long-term exercise and atherogenic activity of blood mononuclear cells in persons at risk of ischemic heart disease. *JAMA* 1999;281:1722.

135. Das UN. Free radicals, cytokines, and nitric oxide in cardiac failure and myocardial infarction. *Mol Cell Biochem*. 2000;215:145.

136. Das UN. Is obesity an inflammatory condition? *Nutrition*. 2001;17:953.

137. Febbraio MA, Pedersen BK. Muscle-derived interleukin-6: mechanisms for activation and possible biological roles. *FASEB J*. 2002;16:1335–47.

138. Woods JA, Vieira VJ, Keylock KT. Exercise, inflammation, and innate immunity. *Neurol Clin*. 2006;24:585–99.

7

Exercise, Adiposity, and Regional Fat Distribution

Kerry J. Stewart

ABSTRACT

Being overweight or obese and physical inactivity markedly increases the risk of developing cardiovascular and other complications in persons with type 2 diabetes. Growing evidence highlights the adverse effect of having abdominal obesity on cardiometabolic health. There is also an increasing prevalence of non-alcoholic fatty liver disease, which also contributes to increased cardiometabolic risk among diabetics. Increasing levels of physical activity contribute to weight reduction, along with dietary interventions. However, independent of total body weight loss, exercise reduces abdominal obesity, and along with the concomitant benefits on multiple cardiometabolic risk factors such as hypertension, insulin resistance, hyperlipidemia, among others, plays a central role in reducing the complications of diabetes. There is some but not entirely conclusive evidence, mainly because of the lack of randomized, controlled trials, that exercise also reduces hepatic fat. Though exercise has been widely recognized as an cornerstone treatment in the medical management for type 2 diabetes, its benefits go beyond the established benefits on fitness levels. The discussion in this chapter focuses on the benefits of exercise on favorable altering body composition, which can occur largely independent of weight change. The resulting reduction in regional fat depots is an important benefit of regular physical activity. For most individuals with diabetes, participation in both aerobic and resistance exercise is recommended to maximize benefits on body composition. These benefits consist of reduction in fat and increased in lean mass.

Key words: Exercise; Physical activity; Obesity; Abdominal obesity; Overweight; Type 2 diabetes; Metabolic syndrome.

From: *Contemporary Diabetes: Diabetes and Exercise*
Edited by: J. G. Regensteiner et al. (eds.), DOI: 10.1007/978-1-59745-260-1_7
© Humana Press, a part of Springer Science+Business Media, LLC 2009

The type 2 diabetes epidemic is largely attributable to being overweight or obese and being physically inactivie *(1, 2)*. The consequences of obesity are severe, affecting the health, quality of life, and economics of the nation *(3)*. On the basis of the body mass index (BMI), the 2001 National Health Interview Survey *(4)* reported that 36% of adults were overweight (BMI > 25) and 23% were obese (BMI > 30). The mean yearly change in these rates increased from 0.61% during the period from 1986 to 1995 to 0.95% from 1997 to 2002 *(5)*. The June 2007 Consumer Reports health survey indicated that 41% of the adult US population is trying to lose weight. Sixty-three percent of people polled responded that they have dieted at some point in their lives. Besides being a risk factor for type 2 diabetes *(6)*, obesity, one of the ten leading US health indicators, is also associated with increased risk for hypertension, dyslipidemia, coronary heart disease, stroke, and certain cancers *(7)*. The Chicago Heart Association Detection Project in Industry study *(8)*, after a mean follow-up of 32 years, showed that individuals with no cardiovascular risk factors as well as for those with one or more risk factors at baseline, and those who were obese in middle age had a higher risk of hospitalization and mortality from cardiovascular disease and diabetes in older age than those who were of normal weight. Some studies have shown that abdominal obesity may be a better predictor than overall obesity for disease risks and all-cause mortality *(9)*. Data from the National Health and Nutrition Examination Survey between the periods of 1988–1994 and 2003–2004 have shown that the age-adjusted waist circumference increased from 96.0 to 100.4 cm among men ($p < 0.001$) and from 89.0 to 94.0 cm among women ($p < 0.001$) and that the age-adjusted prevalence of abdominal obesity increased from 29.5% to 42.4% among men ($p < 0.001$) and from 47.0% to 61.3% among women ($p < 0.001$). Thus, the mean waist circumference and the prevalence of abdominal obesity among US adults have increased markedly during the past 15 years, and over one-half of US adults had abdominal obesity in the period of 2003–2004.

Unfortunately, the problem of increasing levels of obesity is also a growing concern in children. In the National Heart, Lung and Blood Institute Growth and Health Study *(10)*, 1,166 Caucasian and 1,213 African-American girls, were followed longitudinally between age 9 or 10 and 18 years, and self-reported measures were obtained at age 21–23 years. The rates of overweight increased through adolescence from 7 to 10% in the Caucasian girls and from 17 to 24% in the African-American girls. Girls who were overweight during childhood were 11–30 times more likely to be obese in young adulthood. Being overweight was significantly associated with an increased prevalence of cardiovascular disease risk factors including systolic and diastolic blood pressure, high-density lipoprotein cholesterol, and triglyceride levels. Similar to adults, the mean waist circumference and waist-height ratio and the prevalence of abdominal obesity among US children and adolescents greatly increased between 1988–1994 and 1999–2004 *(11)*. Using the 90th percentile values of waist circumference for gender and age, the prevalence of abdominal obesity increased by 65.4% (from 10.5% to 17.4%) and 69.4% (from 10.5% to 17.8%) for boys and girls, respectively. Another study *(12)* of 9- to 11.5-year-old obese and lean children found that higher levels of total body fat and waist circumference were associated with increased levels of fasting insulin, C-reactive protein, and triglycerides and lower HDL cholesterol. Increased waist circumference and reduced cardiorespiratory fitness were strongly associated with increased insulin resistance. Clearly, interventions are needed to reduce fatness and increase fitness in children as these modifiable risk factors markedly increase their future risk of developing type 2 diabetes.

Nevertheless, whether obesity or fitness and activity level are more important to developing diabetes and diabetes-related cardiovascular complications is not entirely clear. In the Medical Expenditure Panel Survey, *(1)* type 2 diabetes and cardiovascular disease risk increased with a higher BMI regardless of activity level and increased with inactivity regardless of BMI. Thus, both physical inactivity and obesity seem to be strongly and independently associated with these conditions. In the Nurses' Health Study *(13)*, sedentary behaviors, especially TV watching, were associated with significantly

Table 1
Classification of Weight Status by Body Mass Index

BMI	Classification
Below 18.5	Underweight
18.5–24.9	Healthy weight
25.0–29.9	Overweight
30 or higher	Obese

On the basis of body mass index, this table categorizes individuals into different weight classifications

elevated risk of obesity and type 2 diabetes, whereas even light to moderate activity was associated with substantially lower risk. In a 2007 report from the Nurses' Health Study *(14)*, among 68,907 female nurses who had no history of diabetes, cardiovascular disease, or cancer at baseline, during 16 years of follow-up, the risk of developing type 2 diabetes increased progressively with increasing BMI and waist circumference and with decreasing physical activity levels. In combined analyses, obesity and physical activity independently contributed to the development of diabetes; however, the magnitude of the risk contributed by obesity appeared to be greater than that imparted by physical activity.

OVERWEIGHT AND OBESITY DEFINED

The most prevalent method for determining overweight and obesity classification is the BMI. BMI is calculated as weight in kilograms divided by the square of height in meters and is expressed as kg/m^2. According to the National Institutes of Health's Clinical Guidelines on the Identification, Evaluation, and Treatment of Overweight and Obesity in Adults *(15)* and as shown in Table 1, an individual with a BMI greater than 25 kg/m^2 is considered overweight whereas the threshold for obesity begins above 30 kg/m^2. Although the BMI is readily obtainable and widely used in clinical settings and in population studies, it does not specify body fat distribution.

Fat distribution, particularly the accumulation of abdominal visceral fat, may be a more powerful determinant of metabolic disease and cardiovascular disease risk than being merely overweight or obese. A recent study of 164 adult patients with established diabetes who have a history of poor glycemic control found that waist circumference by itself, independent of other risk factors comprising the metabolic syndrome, was a strong predictor of future glycemic control *(16)*. Fat distributed in the arms and legs, however, appears to impose little or no risk *(17, 18)*. Nevertheless, a recent study in men found that 6 months of exercise combined with weight loss was efficacious for reducing intramuscular lipids, which correlated with improvements in glucose tolerance *(19)*. After accounting for intramuscular lipid, the changes in other regional fat depots did not independently add to the prediction of changes in glucose tolerance. Further research is needed to fully clarify these mechanisms.

For abdominal obesity, waist circumference correlates strongly with abdominal fat content as determined by imaging methods *(20)* and provides a good quality clinical measurement for determining abdominal obesity. Among most adults with a BMI of 25–34.9 kg/m^2, sex-specific cut points for waist circumference have been identified for an increased relative risk for the development of obesity-associated risk factors *(15)*. A waist circumference greater than 102 cm (40 in.) among men and greater than 88 cm (35 in.) among women indicates an increased risk. Of note, waist circumference cut points tend to lose their incremental predictive power in individuals with a BMI >35 kg^2 because they will typically exceed the waist circumference cut points noted.

Despite the detrimental effects of abdominal obesity on cardiometabolic health, the Shape of the Nations survey *(21)*, which was performed to assess knowledge and understanding of the increased risk associated with abdominal obesity, showed the need to improve efforts for education and action to increase awareness of this health risk. On average, 39% of all people visiting a primary care physician worldwide were overweight or obese. In North America, this proportion was 49%. Abdominal obesity was recognized by 58% of primary care physicians worldwide as a significant risk factor for heart disease; an equal proportion considered high BMI to be a risk factor. Worldwide, 45% of all physicians reported never measuring waist circumference and 52% overestimated the waist circumference that puts their patients at risk. In the general population, 42% were aware of the association between abdominal obesity and risk, but only 60% considered high BMI an important risk factor. Only a small proportion of the general population knew their waist circumference or knew the waist circumference that is considered to confer significantly increased risk. More than half (59%) of at-risk patients had not been informed by their physicians about the association of abdominal obesity with heart disease.

A BRIEF REVIEW OF MECHANISMS LINKING OBESITY WITH TYPE 2 DIABETES

A summary of several of the mechanisms leading to the development of diabetes and the risk of developing cardiovascular disease complications from diabetes related to adiposity and inactivity is shown in Fig. 1. A key physiological mechanism in this pathway is that increased general and abdominal obesity is strongly associated with insulin resistance, which represents the principal underlying

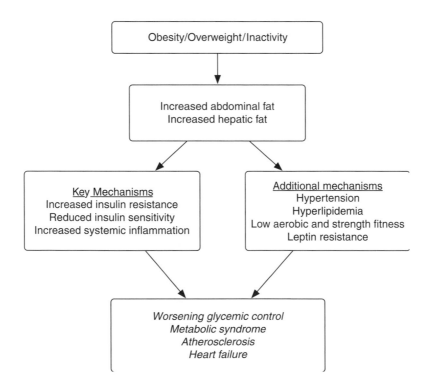

Fig. 1. A summary of several mechanisms leading to the development of diabetes and the risk of developing cardiovascular disease complications from diabetes related to adiposity and inactivity.

defect leading to type 2 diabetes. Consequently, there is a gradual rise in insulin production, which eventually cannot compensate for increasing levels of insulin resistance, which can lead to a complete halt in the ability to produce insulin in patients who do not take action such as exercise or weight loss to reduce their insulin resistance. According to Lazar *(22)*, the epidemic of obesity-associated diabetes is a major crisis in modern societies, in which food is plentiful and exercise is optional. The relationship between obesity and diabetes is of such interdependence that the term 'diabesity' has been coined *(23)*. Insulin resistance is a central pathogenic factor for the metabolic syndrome and is associated with both generalized obesity and the accumulation of fat in the omental and intramyocellular compartments *(24)*. The accumulation of intramyocellular lipids may be due to reduced lipid oxidation capacity *(23)*. In the context of the current obesity epidemic, it is imperative to consider interventions that promote weight loss and ameliorate insulin resistance *(24)*.

Adipose tissue is a dynamic endocrine organ that secretes a number of factors that are increasingly recognized to contribute to systemic and vascular inflammation *(25–27)*. Many of these factors, collectively referred to as adipokines, appear to regulate, directly or indirectly, a number of the processes that contribute to the development of atherosclerosis, including hypertension, endothelial dysfunction, insulin resistance, and vascular remodeling. Several adipokines are preferentially expressed in visceral adipose tissue, and the secretion of proinflammatory adipokines is elevated with increasing adiposity. Biomarkers of inflammation including leukocyte count, tumor necrosis factor-alpha (TNF-alpha), interleukin 6 (IL-6), and C-reactive protein, among others, are associated with insulin resistance and predict the development of type 2 diabetes and cardiovascular disease *(28)*. Among 44 men and women, AT IL-18 mRNA content and plasma IL-18 concentration were higher in the obese group than in the nonobese group, and these were positively correlated with insulin resistance *(29)*. Visceral fat accumulation appears to accelerate the adverse effects of these processes leading to the development of diabetes and atherosclerosis. Adiponectin, which is a protein that has both anti-inflammatory and insulin-sensitizing effects, is downregulated in obesity *(28)*. Some consider adiponectin to be the "common soil" linking type 2 diabetes and coronary heart disease *(30)*. Among 3,640 nondiabetic men aged 60–79 years, lower levels of adiponectin were associated with increased waist circumference and decreased levels of alcohol intake and physical activity. Lower adiponectin level was also associated with increased levels of insulin resistance, triglyceride, C-reactive protein, tissue plasminogen activator, and alanine aminotransferase and with lower levels of HDL-cholesterol and Factor VIII, factors associated with diabetes. The risk of having metabolic syndrome status decreased significantly with increasing adiponectin. Among 148 women, aged 18–81 years with a BMI range of 17.2–44.3 kg/m^2, plasma adiponectin did not change with age but lower levels were associated with increased general and abdominal obesity, insulin levels, and glucose utilization during hyperinsulinemic-euglycemic clamp studies *(31)*. Taken together, all of these data suggest that adiponectin may be a strong marker of risk for diabetes.

Leptin, a protein hormone that plays a central role in regulating energy intake and energy expenditure, is secreted from adipose tissue. Although leptin is a signaling protein that reduces appetite, obese persons appear to be resistant to the effects of leptin. As circulating leptin levels increase, cells that respond to leptin become desensitized to its effects. Thus, a cycle is created, which leads to worsening insulin resistance and obesity, and eventually diabetes. Obesity is also associated with an increase in adipose tissue macrophages, which also participate in the inflammatory process through the elaboration of cytokines *(28)*. In a 10-year prospective longitudinal study of 748 adults, baseline leptin levels predicted the development of obesity, and after adjustment for obesity, the development of glucose intolerance, insulin resistance, and metabolic syndrome *(32)*. Inflammation is closely associated with endothelial dysfunction and is recognized as one of the cardiovascular risk factors clustering in metabolic syndrome *(27)*. Obesity is also associated with oxidative stress, and the oxidation of LDL contributes to the development of atherosclerotic lesions. Among 586 men and women enrolled in a population-based study conducted in Spain *(33)*, increased BMI and waist circumference were each associated with increased levels of oxidized-LDL and C-reactive protein, independent of traditional cardiovascular disease risk factors. Of note, the risk of high oxidized-LDL was more strongly and independently associated with increased waist circumference independently of BMI in the population. These data further emphasize the high risk conferred by high levels of abdominal fat deposition.

HEPATIC FAT

Nonalcoholic fatty liver disease (NAFLD) is a chronic liver disease that can progress to cirrhosis and hepatocellular carcinoma *(34)*. The incidence of NAFLD is increasing due to its prevalence in obesity, diabetes, and insulin-resistance syndrome *(35, 36)*, though some patients have normal glucose tolerance or body weight *(36)*. According to the third National Health and Nutrition Examination Survey, more than 6.4 million adults in the USA have NAFLD *(37)*. Its prevalence increases steadily to 70–90% in obesity or type 2 diabetes *(38)*. Cross-sectional data show that NAFLD is associated with systemic inflammation and insulin resistance *(39)*. A study of 30 healthy normal and moderately overweight nondiabetic men found that fat accumulation in the liver is, independent of BMI and intra-abdominal and overall obesity, characterized by several features of insulin resistance *(40)*. In a 2007 review, Targher *(38)* notes the association of NAFLD with multiple classical and unclassical cardiometabolic risk factors, including an association of increased NAFLD with greater carotid artery intima-media thickness and plaque, and impaired endothelial function, independent of obesity and other metabolic syndrome components. These findings suggest that NAFLD might be an early mediator of cardiovascular disease. Overall, there is limited randomized trial data on lifestyle interventions for reducing hepatic fat *(34)*. In a 12-week study, adolescents with NAFLD at baseline showed significant differences in body mass, BMI, and visceral and subcutaneous fat versus controls *(35)*. A diet, exercise, and counseling program reduced glucose, abdominal fat, and NAFLD. In a small nonrandomized study, ten volunteers had significant reductions of hepatic fat in 10 days *(41)*. In another nonrandomized study of eight obese diabetics, dietary weight loss of 8 kg was associated with reduced hepatic fat, hepatic insulin resistance, and normalization of basal glucose production *(42)*. A 6-month study of caloric restriction with or without exercise found that either intervention lead to reduced lipid deposition in visceral and hepatic tissue and reduced insulin resistance *(43)*. Clearly, additional research is needed to delineate the role of exercise and weight loss for reducing hepatic fat.

PHYSICAL ACTIVITY FOR MANAGING OBESITY AND ALTERING BODY COMPOSITION

Although many individuals with type 2 diabetes clearly need to reduce their overall body weight, not all individuals who are overweight or obese will develop the full range of obesity-related metabolic complications *(44)*. Variations in body fat distribution, and particularly those with increased abdominal fat accumulation, seem to be at a high risk for developing type 2 diabetes and its complications. It is well established that physical activity improves fitness, reduces cardiovascular and metabolic disease risk factors, and is effective for increasing insulin sensitivity and reducing A1C. Exercise training does not typically result in substantial weight loss in relatively short periods of time. Successful programs for weight loss and maintenance most often rely on a combination of diet, exercise, and behavior modification. Exercise alone, without concomitant dietary caloric restriction and behavior modification tends to produce only modest weight loss in the range of 2 kg *(45)*. Weight loss may be modest because overweight and obese persons may not be able to carry out enough exercise to burn a sufficient number of calories to markedly effect energy balance. Furthermore, the caloric expenditure with exercise can be easily counterbalanced by eating more or becoming less active outside of structured exercise sessions *(45)*. Attaining greater amounts of weight loss requires a high volume of exercise. In a randomized study of diet and exercise, exercise of 700 kcal/day, which requires about an hour of moderate to intense aerobic exercise, produced as much fat loss as what might be expected from a 700 kcal/day dietary deficit *(46)*. A recent randomized study tested the effect of a 25% energy deficit by diet alone or diet plus exercise on body composition and fat distribution *(47)*. After 6 months the calculated energy deficit across the intervention was not different between caloric restriction and caloric restriction plus exercise. Overall, participants lost 10% of their body weight, about 24% of their fat mass, and 27% of their abdominal visceral fat. Thus, exercise can play an equivalent role to caloric restriction in terms of energy balance but it also has the advantage of increasing aerobic fitness, which has other beneficial effects on cardiometabolic health.

Less appreciated is the fact that maintaining a high level of physical activity will result in favorable alterations in body composition, independent of total weight loss. More specifically, exercise training has been consistently shown to reduce abdominal obesity, and resistance training will preserve or increase lean mass. This benefit of exercise is of clinical importance since abdominal obesity is at the core of the diabetes epidemic. Among men who participated in 13 weeks of supervised exercise, regular exercise without weight loss was associated with a substantial reduction in total and visceral fat and in skeletal muscle lipid in both obesity and type 2 diabetes *(48)*. Combined with the observation that abdominal obesity conveys a significant health risk, and that increased fitness is associated with reduced morbidity and mortality independent of BMI, these findings have important clinical and public health implications. The important role of exercise was also demonstrated in a study *(49)* in which modest weight loss by diet or diet plus exercise for 14 weeks resulted in similar improvements in total abdominal subcutaneous fat, and glycemic status in older women with type 2 diabetes; however, exercise was necessary for abdominal visceral fat loss. In healthy persons, exercise reduced abdominal fat *(50–53)*, with some data suggesting a preferential loss of visceral fat *(46, 51, 53)*. In a randomized controlled trial involving obese, sedentary, postmenopausal women aged 50–75 years, exercisers showed significant differences from controls in baseline to 12-month changes in body weight, total body fat, intra-abdominal, and subcutaneous abdominal fat *(53)*. Of note, a dose response for greater body fat loss was observed with increasing duration of exercise. Conversely, a review of exercise and changes in body composition reported that although well-controlled short-term studies suggest a dose-response relationship between exercise and abdominal fat loss, there is insufficient evidence of such a relationship for long term *(54)*. In a 3-month study involving obese men, weight loss induced by increased daily physical activity without caloric restriction substantially reduced obesity (particularly abdominal obesity) and insulin resistance *(46)*. Among older persons with hypertension, many of whom had metabolic syndrome, a 6-month exercise training program was associated with reductions in total abdominal fat of 12%, abdominal visceral fat of 18%, and abdominal subcutaneous fat of 9%, despite a modest 2.2 kg weight loss. Changes in abdominal fatness were the strongest determinants of improvements in metabolic syndrome *(55)*. Among diabetics *(56)*, aerobic fitness increased by 41% and insulin sensitivity by 46% after 2 months of exercise. There was a 48% loss of visceral fat and an 18% loss of subcutaneous fat despite no total body weight loss. Among lean and obese men with and without diabetes, 13 weeks of supervised exercise, five times per week at a moderate intensity, did not result in a body weight change *(48)*. However, significant reductions in total, abdominal subcutaneous, and visceral fat were observed in all groups. The reduction in total and abdominal subcutaneous fat was not different between groups; however, the reduction in visceral fat was greater in the obese and type 2 diabetic groups by comparison to the lean group. A significant increase in total skeletal muscle, high-density muscle area, and mean muscle attenuation was observed independent of group. Among men with and without diabetes, a 12-week program of aerobic exercise produced a reduction in waist circumference and fasting IL-6 concentrations, suggesting clinically relevant improvements in cardiometabolic risk factors despite no change in body weight *(57)*.

TYPE OF EXERCISE

Aerobic exercises entail rhythmic repetitive movements of large muscle groups against small resistance. Such activities can be performed for a relatively long time at a low or moderate intensity. They include walking, jogging, swimming, cycling, rowing, jumping rope, skating, running, and cross-country skiing. These activities increase the demand for oxygen, and the muscles adapt by enhanced extraction of oxygen, which is the reason they are called *aerobic activities*. Sustained slow-movement activity, often involving small muscle groups against high resistance, is known as *static activity* or *resistive exercise*. Examples are weight lifting, pushups, sit-ups, carrying heavy packages, and handgrips. Most activities requiring lifting and straining, such as shoveling, have a large static component.

Although most studies on the treatment and prevention of obesity have focused mainly on aerobic activities, resistance training is a behaviorally feasible alternative for weight control *(58)*. As stated earlier, aerobic exercise by itself does not typically result in marked reductions in weight loss although abdominal fat loss can be substantial. The American Diabetes Association consensus statement on physical activity/exercise and type 2 diabetes says that a program of weight control is recommended and this should include aerobic exercise and, in the absence of contraindications, should also include resistance exercise *(45)*. Resting energy expenditure decreases with aging and this decrease is closely correlated to losses in skeletal muscle mass *(59)*. Exercise training that includes a resistance component should also preserve or increase lean body mass. This benefit of resistance training is particularly important in older persons since the mechanical stimuli provided by the task of daily living are not sufficient to offset the loss of skeletal mass and function with aging *(58)*.

Resistance exercise increases muscle mass by a minimum of 1–2 kg after a few months duration *(60)*. Theoretically, a gain of 1 kg in muscle mass should result in an resting energy expenditure increase of about 21 kcal/kg of new muscle *(61)*. Resistance training studies report resting energy expenditure increases in the range of 28–218 kcal/kg of muscle *(62–65)*. Thus, when sustained over years or decades, this mode of exercise can make clinically important differences in daily energy expenditure.

Resistance training can reduce total body fat mass in men *(66, 67)* and women *(66, 68–70)*, independent of dietary caloric restriction. Several studies have demonstrated decreases in visceral adipose tissue after resistance exercise programs *(66, 67, 70–72)*.

Treuth and coworkers assessed body composition in older men using dual energy X-ray absorptiometry *(67)* and in older women using computed tomography *(70)* and observed significant decreases in visceral fat following 16 weeks of resistance training. Ross et al. *(71, 72)* used magnetic resonance imaging to measure regional fat losses after exercise combined with diet interventions. In their first study *(71)*, both diet plus aerobic exercise *and* diet plus resistance training elicited similar losses of visceral fat that were greater than losses of whole body subcutaneous fat. In a follow-up study *(72)* they isolated the effects of endurance exercise training and resistance exercise by comparing the responses to diet alone and diet combined with each training modality in middle-aged obese men. All three groups lost significant amounts of total body fat, and all three groups experienced a significantly greater visceral fat loss compared with whole body subcutaneous fat loss. The changes amounted to a 40% reduction in visceral fat in the resistance training and diet group, 39% in the endurance training and diet group, and a 32% reduction in the diet-only group.

As reviewed by Braith and Stewart *(58)*, resistance training plays an important role in glycemic control. Muscle contraction increases glucose uptake in skeletal muscle. While aerobic exercise uses large muscle groups for long periods of time, resistance training that uses the major muscle groups may provide comparable or even greater recruitment of muscle mass during an exercise workout session. Although there are little data that resistance training prevents type 2 diabetes, this mode of exercise reduces acute insulin responses during oral glucose tolerance testing in healthy persons, diabetic men and women, and improves insulin sensitivity in persons with diabetes and insulin resistance. Among older men who were overweight or obese *(73)*, participation in aerobic versus resistance exercise for 6 months resulted in comparable improvements in glucose metabolism in older men, whereas an increase in insulin activation of glycogen synthase occurred only with aerobic exercise.

The American College of Sports Medicine has recommended the use of progressive resistance training as part of a well-rounded exercise program for individuals with type 2 diabetes *(74)*. Similarly, in the absence of contraindications, the American Diabetes Association *(45)* also recommends resistance training for those with type 2 diabetes. These recommendations are supported by evidence that resistance is an integral component in the therapeutic management of glycemic control in type 2 diabetics *(75, 76)*, particularly if the resistance training is performed in a supervised versus home-based program *(77)*. Among older men with type 2 diabetes who participated in a 16-week progressive resistance training supervised program *(76)*, though there was no weight loss, there were reductions in visceral and subcutaneous fat, which were accompanied by increased insulin sensitivity and decreased fasting blood glucose.

Although performing resistance training by itself rather than in combination with aerobic exercise appears to contribute to some aspects of improving body composition such as reducing abdominal fatness and increasing lean tissue, the available evidence does not support its exclusive use without aerobic exercise. Thus, for the overweight or obese individual with type 2 diabetes whose goals include weight and fat reduction as well as improved glycemic control, a combined exercise routine consisting of both aerobic and resistance remains the primary recommendation for most patients. Specific guidelines for patients with type 2 diabetes can be found in Chap. 9, and guidelines for medical screening for participation in exercise training can be found in Chap. 12.

SUMMARY

Being overweight or obese and physical inactivity markedly increases the risk of developing cardiovascular and other complications in persons with type 2 diabetes. Growing evidence highlights the particularly adverse effect of having abdominal obesity on cardiometabolic health. There is also an increasing prevalence of NAFLD, which also contributes to increased cardiometabolic risk among diabetics. Many studies show that increasing levels of physical activity and participation in exercise training programs contribute to weight reduction, along with dietary interventions. However, independent of total body weight loss, exercise reduces abdominal obesity, and along with the concomitant benefits on multiple cardiometabolic risk factors such as hypertension, insulin resistance, hyperlipidemia, among others, plays a central role in reducing the complications of diabetes. There is some but not entirely conclusive evidence, mainly because of the lack of randomized, controlled trials showing that exercise also reduces hepatic fat. Although exercise has been widely recognized as an important component of the overall medical management for type 2 diabetes, its benefits go beyond the established benefits on fitness levels. The evidence as discussed in this chapter clearly notes the benefits of exercise on favorable alterations in body composition, which can occur independent of weight change. The resulting reduction in regional fat depots is an especially important result of regular physical activity. For most individuals with diabetes, participation in both aerobic and resistance exercise is recommended to maximize benefits on body composition. These benefits consist of reduction in fat and increase in lean mass.

REFERENCES

1. Sullivan PW, Morrato EH, Ghushchyan V, Wyatt HR, Hill JO. Obesity, inactivity, and the prevalence of diabetes and diabetes-related cardiovascular comorbidities in the U.S., 2000–2002. *Diabetes Care*. 2005;28(7):1599–603. Cited in PubMed; 15983307.
2. Fox CS, Pencina MJ, Meigs JB, Vasan RS, Levitzky YS, D'Agostino RB Sr. Trends in the incidence of type 2 diabetes mellitus from the 1970s to the 1990s. The Framingham Heart Study. *Circulation*. 2006;113:2914–18. Cited in PubMed; 16785337.
3. Hill JO, Catenacci V, Wyatt HR. Obesity: overview of an epidemic. *The Psychiatric clinics of North America*. 2005;28(1):1–23, vii. Cited in PubMed; 15733608.
4. Lucas JW, Schiller JS, Benson V. Summary health statistics for U.S. adults: National Health Interview Survey, 2001. *Vital Health Stat* 10. 2004(218):1–134. Cited in PubMed; 15791758.
5. Caban AJ, Lee DJ, Fleming LE, Gomez-Marin O, LeBlanc W, Pitman T. Obesity in US workers: The National Health Interview Survey, 1986 to 2002. *Am J Public Health*. 2005;95(9):1614–22. Cited in PubMed; 16051934.
6. Mokdad AH, Ford ES, Bowman BA, Dietz WH, Vinicor F, Bales VS, et al. Prevalence of obesity, diabetes, and obesity-related health risk factors, 2001. *JAMA*. 2003;289(1):76–9. Cited in PubMed; 12503980.
7. State-specific prevalence of obesity among adults – United States, 2005. MMWR Morb Mortal Wkly Rep. 2006;55 (36):985–8. Cited in PubMed; 16971886.
8. Yan LL, Daviglus ML, Liu K, Stamler J, Wang R, Pirzada A, et al. Midlife body mass index and hospitalization and mortality in older age. *JAMA*. 2006;295(2):190–8.
9. Li C, Ford ES, McGuire LC, Mokdad AH. Increasing trends in waist circumference and abdominal obesity among US adults. *Obesity*. 2007;15(1):216–24. Cited in PubMed; 17228050.
10. Thompson DR, Obarzanek E, Franko DL, Barton BA, Morrison J, Biro FM, et al. Childhood overweight and cardiovascular disease risk factors: the National Heart, Lung, and Blood Institute Growth and Health Study. *J Pediatr*. 2007;150(1):18–25. Cited in PubMed; 17188606.
11. Li C, Ford ES, Mokdad AH, Cook S. Recent trends in waist circumference and waist-height ratio among US children and adolescents. *Pediatrics*. 2006;118(5):e1390–e1398. Cited in PubMed; 17079540.
12. Krekoukia M, Nassis GP, Psarra G, Skenderi K, Chrousos GP, Sidossis LS. Elevated total and central adiposity and low physical activity are associated with insulin resistance in children. *Metabolism*. 2007;56(2):206–13. Cited in PubMed; 17224334.
13. Hu FB, Li TY, Colditz GA, Willett WC, Manson JE. Television watching and other sedentary behaviors in relation to risk of obesity and type 2 diabetes mellitus in women. *JAMA*. 2003;289(14):1785–91. Cited in PubMed; 12684356.
14. Rana JS, Li TY, Manson JE, Hu FB. Adiposity compared with physical inactivity and risk of type 2 diabetes in women. *Diabetes Care*. 2007;30(1):53–8. Cited in PubMed; 17192333.
15. Stewart KJ, McFarland LD, Weinhofer JJ, Cottrell E, Brown CS, Shapiro EP. Safety and efficacy of weight training soon after acute myocardial infarction. *J Cardiopulm Rehabil*. 1998;18(1):37–44. Cited in PubMed; 9494881.
16. Blaha MJ, Gebretsadik T, Shintani A, Elasy TA. Waist circumference, not the metabolic syndrome, predicts glucose deterioration in type 2 diabetes. *Obesity*. 2008;16(4):869–74. Cited in PubMed; 18277389.
17. Williams MJ, Hunter GR, Kekes-Szabo T, Snyder S, Treuth MS. Regional fat distribution in women and risk of cardiovascular disease. *Am J Clin Nutr*. 1997;65(3):855–60. Cited in PubMed; 9062540.
18. Hunter GR, Kekes-Szabo T, Snyder SW, Nicholson C, Nyikos I, Berland L. Fat distribution, physical activity, and cardiovascular risk factors. *Med Sci Sports Exerc*. 1997;29(3):362–9. Cited in PubMed; 9139175.
19. Prior SJ, Joseph LJ, Brandauer J, Katzel LI, Hagberg JM, Ryan AS. Reduction in midthigh low-density muscle with aerobic exercise training and weight loss impacts glucose tolerance in older men. *J Clin Endocrinol Metab*. 2007;92(3):880–6. Cited in PubMed; 17200170.
20. Stewart KJ, DeRegis JR, Turner KL, Bacher AC, Sung J, Hees PS, et al. Usefulness of anthropometrics and dual-energy X-ray absorptiometry for estimating abdominal obesity measured by magnetic resonance imaging in older men and women. *J Cardiopulm Rehabil*. 2003;23(2):109–14. Cited in PubMed; 12668933.
21. Smith SC Jr, Haslam D. Abdominal obesity, waist circumference and cardio-metabolic risk: awareness among primary care physicians, the general population and patients at risk – the Shape of the Nations survey. *Curr Med Res Opin*. 2007;23(1):29–47. Cited in PubMed; 17261236.

22. Lazar MA. How obesity causes diabetes: not a tall tale. *Science*. 2005;307(5708):373–5. Cited in PubMed; 15662001.
23. Golay A, Ybarra J. Link between obesity and type 2 diabetes. *Best Pract Res Clin Endocrinol Metab*. 2005;19(4):649–63. Cited in PubMed; 16311223.
24. Lara-Castro C, Garvey WT. Diet, insulin resistance, and obesity: zoning in on data for Atkins dieters living in South Beach. *J Clin Endocrinol Metab*. 2004;89(9):4197–205. Cited in PubMed; 15356006.
25. Lyon CJ, Law RE, Hsueh WA. Minireview: adiposity, inflammation, and atherogenesis. *Endocrinology*. 2003;144(6):2195–200. Cited in PubMed; 12746274.
26. Van Gaal LF, Mertens IL, De Block CE. Mechanisms linking obesity with cardiovascular disease. *Nature*. 2006;444(7121):875–80. Cited in PubMed; 17167476.
27. Schernthaner GH, Schernthaner G. Insulin resistance and inflammation in the early phase of type 2 diabetes: potential for therapeutic intervention. *Scand J Clin Lab Invest Suppl*. 2005;240:30–40. Cited in PubMed; 16112958.
28. Lee YH, Pratley RE. The evolving role of inflammation in obesity and the metabolic syndrome. *Curr Diab Rep*. 2005;5(1):70–5. Cited in PubMed; 15663921.
29. Leick L, Lindegaard B, Stensvold D, Plomgaard P, Saltin B, Pilegaard H. Adipose tissue interleukin-18 mRNA and plasma interleukin-18: effect of obesity and exercise. *Obesity*. 2007;15(2):356–63. Cited in PubMed; 17299108.
30. Wannamethee SG, Tchernova J, Whincup P, Lowe GD, Rumley A, Brown K, et al. Associations of adiponectin with metabolic and vascular risk parameters in the British Regional Heart Study reveal stronger links to insulin resistance-related than to coronary heart disease risk-related parameters. Int J Obes. 2007;1089–1098. Cited in PubMed; 17264850.
31. Ryan AS, Berman DM, Nicklas BJ, Sinha M, Gingerich RL, Meneilly GS, et al. Plasma adiponectin and leptin levels, body composition, and glucose utilization in adult women with wide ranges of age and obesity. *Diabetes care*. 2003; 26(8):2383–8. Cited in PubMed; 12882866.
32. Franks PW, Brage S, Luan J, Ekelund U, Rahman M, Farooqi IS, et al. Leptin predicts a worsening of the features of the metabolic syndrome independently of obesity. *Obes Res*. 2005;13(8):1476–84. Cited in PubMed; 16129731.
33. Weinbrenner T, Schroder H, Escurriol V, Fito M, Elosua R, Vila J, et al. Circulating oxidized LDL is associated with increased waist circumference independent of body mass index in men and women. *Am J Clin Nutr*. 2006;83(1):30–5; quiz 181–2. Cited in PubMed; 16400046.
34. Clark JM. Weight loss as a treatment for nonalcoholic fatty liver disease. *J Clin Gastroenterol*. 2006;40(3 Suppl 1): S39–S43. Cited in PubMed; 16540766.
35. de Piano A, Prado WL, Caranti DA, Siqueira KO, Stella SG, Lofrano M, et al. Metabolic and nutritional profile of obese adolescents with nonalcoholic fatty liver disease. *J Pediatr Gastroenterol Nutr*. 2007;44(4):446–52. Cited in PubMed; 17414142.
36. Marchesini G, Brizi M, Morselli-Labate AM, Bianchi G, Bugianesi E, McCullough AJ, et al. Association of nonalcoholic fatty liver disease with insulin resistance. *Am J Med*. 1999;107(5):450–5. Cited in PubMed; 10569299.
37. Clark JM, Brancati FL, Diehl AM. The prevalence and etiology of elevated aminotransferase levels in the United States. *Am J Gastroenterol*. 2003;98(5):960–7. Cited in PubMed; 12809815.
38. Targher G. Non-alcoholic fatty liver disease, the metabolic syndrome and the risk of cardiovascular disease: the plot thickens. *Diabet Med*. 2007;24(1):1–6. Cited in PubMed; 17227317.
39. Park SH, Kim BI, Yun JW, Kim JW, Park DI, Cho YK, et al. Insulin resistance and C-reactive protein as independent risk factors for non-alcoholic fatty liver disease in non-obese Asian men. *J Gastroenterol Hepatol*. 2004;19(6):694–8. Cited in PubMed; 15151626.
40. Seppala-Lindroos A, Vehkavaara S, Hakkinen AM, Goto T, Westerbacka J, Sovijarvi A, et al. Fat accumulation in the liver is associated with defects in insulin suppression of glucose production and serum free fatty acids independent of obesity in normal men. *J Clin Endocrinol Metab*. 2002;87(7):3023–8. Cited in PubMed; 12107194.
41. Hollingsworth KG, Abubacker MZ, Joubert I, Allison ME, Lomas DJ. Low-carbohydrate diet induced reduction of hepatic lipid content observed with a rapid non-invasive MRI technique. *Br J Radiol*. 2006;79(945):712–15. Cited in PubMed; 16940371.
42. Petersen KF, Dufour S, Befroy D, Lehrke M, Hendler RE, Shulman GI. Reversal of nonalcoholic hepatic steatosis, hepatic insulin resistance, and hyperglycemia by moderate weight reduction in patients with type 2 diabetes. *Diabetes*. 2005;54(3):603–8. Cited in PubMed; 15734833.
43. Larson-Meyer DE, Heilbronn LK, Redman LM, Newcomer BR, Frisard MI, Anton S, et al. Effect of calorie restriction with or without exercise on insulin sensitivity, beta-cell function, fat cell size, and ectopic lipid in overweight subjects. *Diabetes care*. 2006;29(6):1337–44. Cited in PubMed; 16732018.
44. Sims EA. Are there persons who are obese, but metabolically healthy? *Metabolism*. 2001;50(12):1499–504. Cited in PubMed; 11735101.

45. Sigal RJ, Kenny GP, Wasserman DH, Castaneda-Sceppa C, White RD. Physical activity/exercise and type 2 diabetes: a consensus statement from the American Diabetes Association. *Diabetes Care*. 2006;29(6):1433–8. Cited in PubMed; 16732040.

46. Ross R, Dagnone D, Jones PJ, Smith H, Paddags A, Hudson R, et al. Reduction in obesity and related comorbid conditions after diet-induced weight loss or exercise-induced weight loss in men. A randomized, controlled trial. *Ann Intern Med*. 2000;133(2):92–103. Cited in PubMed; 10896648.

47. Redman LM, Heilbronn LK, Martin CK, Alfonso A, Smith SR, Ravussin E. Effect of calorie restriction with or without exercise on body composition and fat distribution. *J Clin Endocrinol Metab*. 2007;92(3):865–72. Cited in PubMed; 17200169.

48. Lee S, Kuk JL, Davidson LE, Hudson R, Kilpatrick K, Graham TE, et al. Exercise without weight loss is an effective strategy for obesity reduction in obese individuals with and without type 2 diabetes. *J Appl Physiol*. 2005;99(3):1220–5. Cited in PubMed; 15860689.

49. Giannopoulou I, Ploutz-Snyder LL, Carhart R, Weinstock RS, Fernhall B, Goulopoulou S, et al. Exercise is required for visceral fat loss in postmenopausal women with type 2 diabetes. *J Clin Endocrinol Metab*. 2005;90(3):1511–18. Cited in PubMed; 15598677.

50. Schwartz RS, Cain KC, Shuman WP, Larson V, Stratton JR, Beard JC, et al. Effect of intensive endurance training on lipoprotein profiles in young and older men. *Metabolism*. 1992;41(6):649–54.

51. Schwartz RS, Shuman WP, Larson V, Cain KC, Fellingham GW, Beard JC, et al. The effect of intensive endurance exercise training on body fat distribution in young and older men. *Metabolism*. 1991;40(5):545–51.

52. Despres JP. Abdominal obesity as important component of insulin-resistance syndrome. *Nutrition*. 1993;9(5):452–9.

53. Irwin ML, Yasui Y, Ulrich CM, Bowen D, Rudolph RE, Schwartz RS, et al. Effect of exercise on total and intra-abdominal body fat in postmenopausal women: a randomized controlled trial. *JAMA*. 2003;289(3):323–30. Cited in PubMed; 12525233.

54. Ross R, Janssen I. Physical activity, total and regional obesity: dose-response considerations. *Med Sci Sports Exerc*. 2001;33(6 Suppl):S521–7; discussion S8–S9. Cited in PubMed; 11427779.

55. Stewart KJ, Bacher AC, Turner K, Lim JG, Hees PS, Shapiro EP, et al. Exercise and risk factors associated with metabolic syndrome in older adults. *Am J Prev Med*. 2005;28(1):9–18. Cited in PubMed; 15626550.

56. Mourier A, Gautier JF, De Kerviler E, Bigard AX, Villette JM, Garnier JP, et al. Mobilization of visceral adipose tissue related to the improvement in insulin sensitivity in response to physical training in NIDDM. Effects of branched-chain amino acid supplements. *Diabetes Care*. 1997;20(3):385–91. Cited in PubMed; 9051392.

57. Dekker MJ, Lee S, Hudson R, Kilpatrick K, Graham TE, Ross R, et al. An exercise intervention without weight loss decreases circulating interleukin-6 in lean and obese men with and without type 2 diabetes mellitus. *Metabolism*. 2007;56(3):332–8. Cited in PubMed; 17292721.

58. Braith RW, Stewart KJ. Resistance exercise training: its role in the prevention of cardiovascular disease. *Circulation*. 2006;113(22):2642–50. Cited in PubMed; 16754812.

59. Vaughan L, Zurlo F, Ravussin E. Aging and energy expenditure. *Am J Clin Nutr*. 1991;53(4):821–5. Cited in PubMed; 2008859.

60. Fleck SJ, Kraemer WJ. Designing Resistance Taining Programs, 2nd ed. Champaign, IL: Human Kinetics Books; 1997.

61. Weinsier RL, Schutz Y, Bracco D. Reexamination of the relationship of resting metabolic rate to fat-free mass and to the metabolically active components of fat-free mass in humans. *Am J Clin Nutr*. 1992;55(4):790–4. Cited in PubMed; 1550060.

62. Broeder CE, Burrhus KA, Svanevik LS, Wilmore JH. The effects of either high-intensity resistance or endurance training on resting metabolic rate. *Am J Clin Nutr*. 1992;55(4):802–10. Cited in PubMed; 1550062.

63. Campbell WW, Crim MC, Young VR, Evans WJ. Increased energy requirements and changes in body composition with resistance training in older adults. *Am J Clin Nutr*. 1994;60(2):167–75. Cited in PubMed; 8030593.

64. Ryan AS, Pratley RE, Elahi D, Goldberg AP. Resistive training increases fat-free mass and maintains RMR despite weight loss in postmenopausal women. *J Appl Physiol*. 1995;79(3):818–23. Cited in PubMed; 8567523.

65. Taaffe DR, Pruitt L, Reim J, Butterfield G, Marcus R. Effect of sustained resistance training on basal metabolic rate in older women. *J Am Geriatr Soc*. 1995;43(5):465–71. Cited in PubMed; 7730525.

66. Hunter GR, Bryan DR, Wetzstein CJ, Zuckerman PA, Bamman MM. Resistance training and intra-abdominal adipose tissue in older men and women. *Med Sci Sports Exerc*. 2002;34(6):1023–8. Cited in PubMed; 12048332.

67. Treuth MS, Ryan AS, Pratley RE, Rubin MA, Miller JP, Nicklas BJ, et al. Effects of strength training on total and regional body composition in older men. *J Appl Physiol*. 1994;77(2):614–20. Cited in PubMed; 8002507.

68. Schmitz KH, Jensen MD, Kugler KC, Jeffery RW, Leon AS. Strength training for obesity prevention in midlife women. *Int J Obes Relat Metab Disord*. 2003;27(3):326–33. Cited in PubMed; 12629559.

69. Prabhakaran B, Dowling EA, Branch JD, Swain DP, Leutholtz BC. Effect of 14 weeks of resistance training on lipid profile and body fat percentage in premenopausal women. *Br J Sports Med*. 1999;33(3):190–5. Cited in PubMed; 10378072.

70. Treuth MS, Hunter GR, Kekes-Szabo T, Weinsier RL, Goran MI, Berland L. Reduction in intra-abdominal adipose tissue after strength training in older women. *J Appl Physiol*. 1995;78(4):1425–31. Cited in PubMed; 7615451.

71. Ross R, Rissanen J. Mobilization of visceral and subcutaneous adipose tissue in response to energy restriction and exercise. *Am J Clin Nutr*. 1994;60(5):695–703. Cited in PubMed; 7942575.

72. Ross R, Rissanen J, Pedwell H, Clifford J, Shragge P. Influence of diet and exercise on skeletal muscle and visceral adipose tissue in men. *J Appl Physiol*. 1996;81(6):2445–55. Cited in PubMed; 9018491.

73. Ferrara CM, Goldberg AP, Ortmeyer HK, Ryan AS. Effects of aerobic and resistive exercise training on glucose disposal and skeletal muscle metabolism in older men. *J Gerontol A Biol Sci Med Sci*. 2006;61(5):480–7. Cited in PubMed; 16720745.

74. Albright A, Franz M, Hornsby G, Kriska A, Marrero D, Ullrich I, et al. American College of Sports Medicine position stand. Exercise and type 2 diabetes. *Med Sci Sports Exerc*. 2000;32(7):1345–60. Cited in PubMed; 10912903.

75. Cornelissen VA, Fagard RH. Effect of resistance training on resting blood pressure: a meta-analysis of randomized controlled trials. *J Hypertens*. 2005;23(2):251–9. Cited in PubMed; 15662209.

76. depIbanez J, Izquierdo M, Arguelles I, Forga L, Larrion JL, Garcia-Unciti M, et al. Twice-weekly progressive resistance training decreases abdominal fat and improves insulin sensitivity in older men with type 2 diabetes. *Diabetes Care*. 2005;28(3):662–7. Cited in PubMed; 15735205.

77. Dunstan DW, Zimmet PZ, Welborn TA, De Courten MP, Cameron AJ, Sicree RA, et al. The rising prevalence of diabetes and impaired glucose tolerance: the Australian Diabetes, Obesity and Lifestyle Study. *Diabetes Care*. 2002;25(5):829–34. Cited in PubMed; 11978676.

8 Diabetes Mellitus and Exercise Physiology in the Presence of Diabetic Comorbidities

Amy G. Huebschmann and Judith G. Regensteiner

CONTENTS

ABSTRACT

While uncomplicated type 2 diabetes mellitus (T2DM) is already associated with an impaired exercise capacity, the presence of other comorbidities appears to further worsen exercise capacity in T2DM. Common diabetic comorbidities such as hypertension, arterial stiffness, cardiovascular disease, systolic dysfunction, diastolic dysfunction, and diabetic nephropathy are all associated with worse exercise capacity in T2DM. Benefits of exercise training programs for those with T2DM and certain comorbidities (e.g., hypertension, increased arterial stiffness, or post-myocardial infarction) have been shown to include improved exercise capacity. Further study is warranted to determine the specific benefits and risks of exercise training in subpopulations of T2DM such as those with T2DM and either congestive heart failure or microvascular complications of diabetes.

Key words: Diabetes mellitus; Exercise capacity; Hypertension; Arterial stiffness; Cardiovascular disease; Diabetic microvascular complications.

INTRODUCTION

People with type 2 diabetes mellitus (T2DM), even when uncomplicated, have been shown to have decreased exercise capacity when compared with age and weight-matched nondiabetic subjects *(1–4)* as detailed in Chap. 1 of this book. In the presence of diabetic comorbidities, such as nephropathy or retinopathy, maximal exercise capacity is further reduced *(5)*. Since the prevalence of comorbidities

From: *Contemporary Diabetes: Diabetes and Exercise*
Edited by: J. G. Regensteiner et al. (eds.), DOI: 10.1007/978-1-59745-260-1_8
© Humana Press, a part of Springer Science+Business Media, LLC 2009

Table 1
Prevalence of Selected Comorbidities in People with T2DM

Comorbidity	HTN (%)	CHF (%)	CAD (%)	PAD (%)	Nephropathy (%)	Retinopathy (%)
T2DM	39–71[a–c]	11.8[d]	27–55[e,f]	1.2–12.5[g]	7–30[h]	3–27[i]

T2DM type 2 diabetes mellitus, *HTN* hypertension, *CHF* congestive heart failure, *CAD* coronary artery disease, *PAD* peripheral arterial disease
[a] Albright et al. 1995 *(6)*
[b] Geiss et al. 2002 *(7)*
[c] HDS I 1993 *(8)*
[d] Nichols et al. 2001 *(9)*
[e] Anand et al. *(10)*
[f] Fein S. *(11)*
[g] Adler et al. 2002 *(12)*
[h] Adler et al. 2003 *(13)*
[i] Brown et al. 2003 *(14)*

is relatively high in the diabetic population (Table 1)), the impact of comorbidities on exercise performance is of major concern. Since exercise has a central therapeutic role in diabetes, it is important to recognize how differences in exercise physiology in the presence of diabetic comorbidities may impact upon exercise recommendations to this population. This chapter will describe the exercise abnormalities correlated with the common diabetic comorbidities of hypertension, arterial stiffness, congestive heart failure (CHF, including systolic and diastolic dysfunction), as well as macrovascular and microvascular disease. Certainly, many diabetics with complications will have more than one of these entities simultaneously, but the changes in exercise physiology attendant to these comorbidities will be addressed individually. This chapter will also discuss the available data on the particular benefits of exercise training with each comorbidity when those data are available. The focus will be on exercise pathophysiology in subjects with T2DM, with type 1 diabetes mellitus (T1DM) included as well, although the data in T1DM are more limited.

As context for this chapter's discussion of diabetic comorbidities impact upon exercise impairment, it is useful to quickly review the exercise abnormalities in uncomplicated diabetes. Subjects with T1DM have been shown in two small studies to have no exercise impairment (as assessed by maximal exercise capacity) in comparison with similarly active nondiabetic controls matched for age, sex, and body weight *(15, 16)*. However, exercise impairment has been shown in subjects with uncomplicated T2DM and will be briefly discussed.

Despite a lack of microvascular or macrovascular complications, subjects with T2DM have ~20% worse maximal exercise capacity when compared with control subjects *(1–4)*. This impairment appears to be caused by slowed oxygen delivery to working muscles of both "central" (cardiac) and "peripheral" (exercising muscle) origins. The peripheral causes of decreased exercise capacity may include endothelial dysfunction (precluding appropriate vasodilation to increase perfusion of exercising muscle), decreased oxygen diffusion, or decreased oxygen extraction *(17)*. The central causes may include endothelial dysfunction [precluding appropriate vasodilation of coronary arteries in response to increased myocardial workload *(17)*], decreased cardiac output during exercise *(18)*, and exercise-associated impaired left ventricular function *(19)*. Exercise-associated impaired left ventricular function (also termed "diabetic cardiomyopathy") is not present in all subjects with T2DM, but is relatively common, and will be discussed separately in the "Congestive Heart Failure" section of this chapter.

HYPERTENSION AND ARTERIAL STIFFNESS

Hypertension and arterial stiffness both reflect similar vascular pathophysiology relating to increased peripheral vascular resistance and/or cardiac output. Both may play important roles in altering usual exercise physiology. It is important to consider how these pathophysiologic factors may impact on exercise, since the prevalence of hypertension in subjects with T2DM ranges from 39% to 71% *(6–8)* and arterial stiffness has been shown to be 13% higher in subjects with T2DM than nondiabetics *(20)*. This section will review how hypertension and arterial stiffness impair exercise performance in diabetes, the methods by which routine exercise training can remediate these deficits, and the attendant benefits to exercise in diabetics beyond improving exercise performance.

Effects of Hypertension on Exercise Performance in DM

The addition of hypertension to diabetes has been shown to decrease exercise capacity. One small Austrian study showed a significantly decreased maximal oxygen consumption (VO_2max) in eight subjects with T2DM and hypertension when compared with six normotensive T2DM subjects, eight nondiabetic hypertensive subjects, and eight age, sex, and body mass index (BMI)-matched controls ($p < 0.01$ vs. normotensive T2DM, nondiabetic hypertensives, and controls) *(21)*. Babalola et al. showed a tendency toward a lower exercise time in diabetic hypertensives (289 ± 110 s) compared with diabetics without hypertension (321 ± 119 s), hypertensives who did not have diabetes (309 ± 73 s), and healthy controls (490 ± 156 s) using a modified Bruce protocol treadmill test *(22)*. This study lacked sample size to differentiate between the diabetic and diabetic-hypertensive groups. However, there was a statistically significant difference in exercise duration between the four groups ($p < 0.05$), and a rank-order trend suggested the worst exercise capacity (as measured by maximal exercise time) was in the diabetic-hypertensive group.

Effects of Hypertension on Exaggerated Sympathetic Nervous System Response to Exercise in T2DM

The greater response of the sympathetic nervous system to exercise in people with diabetes and comorbid hypertension is of interest for three reasons. First, it is known that the sympathetic nervous system is already more active in resting subjects with diabetes or hypertension than in nondiabetic or nonhypertensive subjects *(23–26)*. This raises the question how that elevated baseline activity will impact sympathetic activity with exercise. Second, it is known that exercise induces an increase in sympathetic nervous system activity and catecholamine release in all subjects, but that during exercise there are feedback mechanisms, which further mediate sympathoadrenal activity levels *(27)*. Since catecholamines induce lipolysis, the insulin resistance-induced impairment of lipolysis in adipocytes is one such diabetic maladaptation, which may result in positive feedback to the sympathoadrenal axis during exercise *(28)*. The existence of greater sympathetic activation with exercise in subjects with both diabetes and hypertension encourages the investigation of other possible contributors to this positive feedback. Third, it is of clinical interest to know that catecholamine levels become higher with exercise in diabetic hypertensives than in diabetic nonhypertensive individuals due to a more robust sympathoadrenal response. Future research may explore to what degree the exaggerated sympathoadrenal response to exercise in diabetes is a beneficial compensatory adaptation or a maladaptive response due to abnormal metabolic and circulatory factors.

Sympathoadrenal overactivity has been demonstrated in subjects with T2DM and comorbid hypertension as expressed by the increased release of catecholamines with exercise. One study looked at differences in exercise-induced catecholamine response between four groups: T2DM with hypertension,

T2DM without hypertension, hypertension without T2DM, and control subjects *(21)*. Each subject performed a stationary bicycling exercise for 15 min with 5-min incremental workload steps of 25%, 50%, and 75% of individually measured VO_2max. Blood pressure and plasma catecholamine measurements were obtained 10 min prior to exercise, then at each 5-min workload, and at timed intervals during recovery. This study showed greater exercise-induced unconjugated normetanephrine levels in the hypertensive T2DM subjects as compared with their age, sex, and BMI-matched controls (2,156 ± 373 pg/ml/min vs. 1,133 ± 180 pg/ml/min, $p = 0.04$) with no change in the normotensive T2DM or nondiabetic hypertensive subjects as compared with controls *(21)*. At baseline, unconjugated metanephrines were lower in hypertensive T2DM and normotensive T2DM subjects ($p = 0.03$ and 0.04, respectively) than in their respective controls. Although there was a lower VO_2max in the T2DM hypertensives than in the other groups ($p < 0.01$ vs. normotensive T2DM, nondiabetic hypertensives, and controls), no tests of correlation were performed between the unconjugated metanephrine levels and exercise capacity. The authors of this study concluded that the excessive response of plasma unconjugated normetanephrines may serve as a marker of exaggerated sympathoadrenal function in hypertensive T2DM *(21)*. Previous studies have found that subjects with excessive sympathoadrenal activity had elevated noradrenaline levels during exercise testing but not at baseline *(29, 30)*. It is not yet certain if the elevated catecholamine response to exercise is due to sympathoadrenal overactivity or to a greater catecholamine response requirement *(31)* to maintain cardiac output and glucose homeostasis with exercise. Again, this suggests further research is warranted into the mechanisms of exaggerated exercise-induced sympathetic outflow as well as whether this greater sympathetic activity is beneficial or only maladaptive.

Arterial Stiffness in the Presence of Hypertension and T2DM

Increased arterial stiffness (also termed "decreased elasticity" or "decreased vascular compliance") is an ubiquitous endpoint of many disease processes. Not only diabetes but also arterial hypertension, hyperlipidemia, CHF, and chronic uremia have all been shown to lead to decreased elasticity in large arteries *(32)*. However, arterial stiffness may be particularly pronounced in T2DM. Given that arterial stiffness is a newer physiologic measure as yet without well-defined reference normal levels, the prevalence of arterial stiffness in T2DM is uncertain. However, one epidemiologic study showed a 13% increase in arterial stiffness (as measured by pulse pressure/stroke volume) in T2DM subjects as compared with controls *(20)*.

Increased arterial stiffness results from three general types of changes to arterial structure and function *(32)*. Structural arterial changes include smooth muscle cell hypertrophy, increased collagen matrix deposits, and abnormal proteoglycan metabolism *(32)*. Functional abnormalities such as endothelial dysfunction and abnormal vasa vasorum microcirculation also increase arterial wall stiffness *(32)*. Finally, increased permeability of vessel walls leads to disruption of the interstitial matrix *(32)*. Thus, arterial stiffness results from a combination of structural and functional processes.

The degree of arterial stiffness observed is determined by the timing and magnitude of reflected waves from the peripheral vasculature as well as the cardiac output and central arterial vascular resistance *(33, 34)*. Noninvasive measurements of arterial stiffness include: pulse pressure, pulse pressure/stroke volume, augmentation index, pulse wave velocity, and ultrasound stiffness index β. For each of these metrics, higher measurements indicate greater stiffness. Like hypertension, increased arterial stiffness is related to increased vascular resistance, but is felt to reflect central aortic blood pressure as opposed to the peripheral blood pressure measured with a sphygmomanometer *(35)*. Though a paucity of data exist to compare the utility of lowering arterial stiffness versus treating blood pressure with regard to morbidity, a large randomized controlled trial illustrated that improved arterial stiffness between groups correlated with better cardiovascular outcomes (decreased cardiovascular events/ procedures and/or decreased renal impairment) despite equivalent blood pressures between the amlodipine and atenolol-based regimens *(36)*. This illustrates that although arterial stiffness is related to hypertension, vascular compliance may have additional physiologic relevance beyond hypertension. The next section will review the implications of arterial stiffness upon exercise performance in subjects with T2DM.

Effects of Arterial Stiffness on Exercise Performance in DM

Increased arterial stiffness in diabetes causes abnormalities in the vascular circulation with exercise in subjects with T1DM and T2DM. Arterial stiffness (as measured by ultrasound with stiffness "β") independently predicted decreased peripheral circulation to the foot during exercise (as measured by the well-validated transcutaneous oxygen tension index *(37–39)* in Japanese subjects with T2DM and normal peripheral circulation [ankle-brachial index (ABI) > 0.9] *(40)*. This study is the only one to date to examine arterial stiffness and circulation in T2DM subjects, but other studies have examined this in the T1DM population. Subjects with T1DM maintained a higher peripheral vascular resistance during bicycle ergometry as compared with control subjects ($p < 0.01$) with an associated greater rise in diastolic blood pressure ($p < 0.01$, T1DM vs. controls) *(41)*. Other studies have also confirmed an exaggerated diastolic blood pressure rise with exercise in T1DM subjects versus controls *(42, 43)*. In T1DM adolescents with increased arterial stiffness, elevated diastolic blood pressure with exercise and endothelial dysfunction (as measured by impaired forearm vasodilator response to brachial ischemia) were present and correlated with diabetes duration and glycemic control *(43)*.

Benefits of Exercise Training in Persons with Diabetes Mellitus and Hypertension or Arterial Stiffness

Aerobic exercise has been repeatedly shown to lower blood pressure in nondiabetic hypertensive individuals by an average of 5–6 (systolic) and/or 4–5 (diastolic) mmHg *(44, 45)*. Even lower-intensity exercise such as regular walking has been shown to lower blood pressure by 3 (systolic) and/or 2 (diastolic) mmHg *(46)*. Less information is present on benefits in subjects with diabetes and comorbid hypertension, but the available data will be reviewed.

In older nondiabetic individuals with mild to moderate hypertension, exercise training for 7 months reduced systolic blood pressure as well as decreased left ventricular mass *(47)*, both of which have been shown to reduce mortality and cardiovascular morbidity *(48–53)*. To our knowledge, there has only been one randomized-controlled trial of exercise training in human subjects with both diabetes mellitus (DM) and hypertension *(54)*. This trial aimed to provide consensus guidelines to enable improved control of glucose levels, blood pressure, and lipid levels in an "intensively treated" group with uncontrolled T2DM (HbA1c > 8%) vs. a comparable T2DM control group receiving "usual care" *(54)*. Over 85% of both study groups had comorbid hypertension with a similar degree of hypertensive control at baseline *(54)*. The exercise intervention consisted of a recommended aerobic exercise bicycling regimen as well as resistance exercises with elastic exercise bands. The exercise training frequency (three to five times per week), duration (45–55 min), and intensity (50–80% of maximal heart rate) were adjusted for each subject based on their baseline exercise test performance and were increased over the course of the study. The control group did not receive the exercise intervention. Over 12 months in subjects with T2DM, weekly exercise levels increased 2.5-fold in the intervention group (from 7.5 to 19.7 METs) with no significant change in the control group *(54)*. There was no increase in the use of antihypertensive agents from baseline in either the intervention or the control groups, but yet there was a significant 12-month improvement in the intervention group's mean blood pressure from 144/85 to 130/76 ($p < 0.005$) *(54)*. It is implied that, in the absence of prescription antihypertensive medication changes, the exercise regimen led to this blood pressure improvement *(54)*. More convincingly, over the 6 months following this intervention the exercise level worsened significantly in the intervention group (from 19.7 to 9.1 METs) and the accompanying increased systolic blood pressure and weight in that group correlated negatively to amount of time spent on exercise ($r = 0.43$ for systolic blood pressure, $r = 0.363$ for weight, both $p < 0.05$) *(54)*. The benefits of consistent exercise during the trial (mean blood pressure decrease of 14/9 mmHg) are confirmed by the worsened blood pressure when exercise compliance declined.

The impact of exercise training on arterial stiffness has also been examined in both rats and humans *(55, 56)*. Diabetic rats that performed 16 weeks of regular exercise on running wheels had better measures of left ventricular stiffness as compared with sedentary diabetic control rats ($p < 0.01$) *(55)* The authors hypothesized that the improved myocardial compliance was due to a change in functional wall properties because markers of increased structural rigidity (e.g., myocardial hydroxyproline concentration, advanced glycation end product fluorescence) were not different between groups *(55)*. In a cohort of 23 human subjects with T2DM, 3 weeks of moderate exercise training for all subjects resulted in lessened arterial stiffness (as measured by ultrasound stiffness index β) at the carotid ($p = 0.020$) and femoral ($p < 0.001$) arteries *(56)*. In this study, improved insulin resistance resulting from exercise training correlated with decreased arterial stiffness at the carotid ($p = 0.040$) and femoral artery ($p = 0.016$) *(56)*. In contrast, despite increasing VO_2max, another small crossover human study did not show an improvement in arterial stiffness or blood pressure after 8 weeks of bicycle exercise training (thrice weekly at 60% maximum heart rate) in five men and women with T2DM and isolated systolic hypertension *(57)*.

In summary, hypertension and arterial stiffness are related abnormal pathophysiological processes which are prevalent in diabetes. Arterial stiffness is a much newer physiologic measurement than hypertension, and so the clinical consequences of its presence and treatment are generally less well-known than that of hypertension. Comorbid hypertension has been shown to impair exercise capacity and increase catecholamine release with exercise in subjects with T2DM. Arterial stiffness has been correlated with decreased peripheral muscle perfusion during exercise in T2DM persons with normal peripheral circulation as well as increased peripheral vascular resistance with exercise in T1DM. In the majority of studies done to date, both hypertension and arterial stiffness are at least partially remediable with exercise training. The benefits of lowering blood pressure and arterial stiffness in diabetic-hypertensive subjects and lack of harmful side effects with appropriate prescreening of subjects is encouraging enough to recommend exercise routinely to patients with DM and comorbid hypertension.

CONGESTIVE HEART FAILURE

This section is divided into two parts. The first describes the prevalence and relevance of diastolic dysfunction in T2DM and how CHF due to diabetic diastolic dysfunction affects exercise capacity. The second section focuses on how CHF due to systolic dysfunction impairs exercise capacity.

Effects of Impaired Diastolic Dysfunction on Exercise Performance in T2DM

In 1972, Rubler et al. described four diabetic subjects with CHF despite normal coronary arteries and no convincing etiology for their cardiomyopathy *(58)*. Further recognition of "diabetic cardiomyopathy" followed, with prevalence rate estimates of diastolic dysfunction in diabetic subjects ranging from 30% in studies using conventional echocardiography *(59–61)* to 52–60% with more detailed

Doppler echocardiograms using Valsalva maneuvers and pulmonary venous recordings *(62, 63)*. Some studies have shown that diastolic dysfunction is already present with 30% prevalence even early after the time of T2DM diagnosis *(59, 60)*. Since its discovery three decades ago, greater understanding has developed as to the characteristics and causes of diabetic cardiomyopathy, though it is still incompletely understood. Current theory holds that diabetic cardiomyopathy is caused by hyperglycemia-induced myocardial fibrosis due to a variety of factors at the myocardial level which may include increased oxidative stress, endothelial dysfunction, advanced glycation end products, activated protein kinase C-β, and elevated free fatty acids *(64)*. Physiologically, diastolic dysfunction is a cardinal feature of the diabetic cardiomyopathy *(64–66)*.

Diastolic dysfunction is usually asymptomatic unless accompanied by other comorbidities *(64)*. In the presence of comorbid hypertension or myocardial ischemia, clinical features of CHF may develop from diastolic dysfunction despite the maintenance of a normal ejection fraction *(65, 66)*. Several studies have shown that asymptomatic subjects with T2DM and diastolic dysfunction still remain at higher risk to develop CHF *(64, 66)* and also appear to have lower exercise capacity than diabetic subjects without diastolic dysfunction *(67–69)*.

Four studies to date have correlated diastolic dysfunction with exercise impairment. Poirier et al., showed worse maximal exercise treadmill performance in men with well-controlled uncomplicated T2DM and diastolic dysfunction ($n = 10$) as compared with age, weight, and clinically matched T2DM controls without diastolic dysfunction ($n = 9$) *(19)*. In this study, the diabetics with resting diastolic dysfunction had a decreased duration of exercise time on a modified Bruce protocol (662 s vs. 803 s, $p < 0.02$) and decreased metabolic equivalents ("METs") of 11.4 vs. 9.5 METs ($p < 0.02$) *(19)*. A correlation was also seen between the E_m/A_m ratio (echocardiographic marker of diastolic dysfunction as defined by the ratio of early and late mitral valve wave-filling velocities) and exercise duration ($r = 0.64$, $p = 0.004$) and METs ($r = 0.66$, $p = 0.003$) *(19)*. A group of both T1DM and T2DM subjects (69.6% T2DM) performed symptom-limited Bruce protocol exercise tests. In this study, exercise performance in METs was lower in the diabetics with diastolic dysfunction versus diabetics without diastolic dysfunction (8.56 vs 10.32 METs, $p < 0.05$) *(68)*. Irace et al. performed ergometer exercise stress tests in 38 subjects with T2DM and compared the presence of diastolic dysfunction in the subjects with a symptom-limited stress test (prior to reaching maximal predicted heart rate) versus the subjects who completed ergometer tests to maximal predicted heart rate *(69)*. The 24 T2DM subjects with symptom-limited ergometer exercise stress tests had a correlation between decreased diastolic function and exercise duration *(69)*. However, no significant correlation between diastolic dysfunction and exercise duration was found in the 14 subjects with T2DM who were able to complete ergometer exercise stress tests to maximal predicted heart rate *(69)*. In comparing 170 subjects with T2DM and normal exercise capacity ($n = 52$) or abnormal exercise capacity ($n = 118$), Fang et al. showed that preserved diastolic function (as defined by maximal early mitral valve wave filling velocity $= E_m$) was correlated with better maximal exercise treadmill capacity ($r = 0.43$, $p < 0.001$) and remained an independent predictor of exercise capacity after multivariate analysis ($p < 0.05$) *(70)*. In summary, diastolic dysfunction has been repeatedly correlated to decreased exercise capacity in T2DM.

Though diastolic dysfunction is certainly a cardinal feature of "diabetic cardiomyopathy," some evidence is mounting that a subclinical depression of systolic function may also be present in some diabetics. Despite maintaining categorically "normal" systolic function, subjects with T2DM have been shown to have significantly lower cardiac ejection fractions as compared to nondiabetic subjects. Sasso et al. found that subjects with well-controlled, recent onset T2DM (3.9-year mean duration of diabetes) have lower ejection fractions both at rest (57% vs 67%, $p < 0.001$) and during exercise (64% vs. 72%, $p < 0.001$) than age, gender, and BMI-matched control subjects *(71)*. Amongst the T2DM subjects, greater insulin sensitivity was correlated with higher rest and exercise ejection fractions ($r = 0.59$, $p < 0.004$ for rest, $r = 0.58$, $p < 0.005$ for exercise) *(71)*.

No studies to date have examined the impact of exercise training in diabetes upon diastolic dysfunction. However, two studies have shown improvement in diastolic filling after exercise training in nondiabetic subjects with diastolic dysfunction *(72, 73)*, providing plausibility that training may work in diabetics, as well.

Impairment of Exercise Performance in Diabetes Mellitus with Comorbid CHF Due to Systolic Cardiomyopathy

CHF due to systolic cardiomyopathy has an estimated prevalence of 11.8% in T2DM *(9)*. Several studies have shown that diabetes in conjunction with systolic cardiomyopathy (T2DM–CHF) leads to worse exercise performance even when compared to subjects with CHF due to systolic cardiomyopathy alone. In 20 subjects with tightly controlled T2DM (HbA1c < 7%) and moderate CHF symptoms, peak exercise performance yielded a VO_2max nearly 20% less than nondiabetic age and gender-matched subjects with moderate CHF (left ventricular ejection fraction, LVEF < 40%) *(74)*. Multivariate linear regression further determined that the strongest predictor of VO_2max in the DM-CHF subjects was alveolar-capillary membrane conductance [which determines the diffusing capacity of the lung (DL_{CO}) along with pulmonary capillary blood volume]. The authors suggested that the T2DM–CHF subjects may have a pulmonary angiopathy which allows leakage across the alveolar-capillary membrane as exercise raises the capillary pulmonary pressure *(74)*. Tibb et al. found a 30% reduction in VO_2max in 78 subjects with systolic cardiomyopathy (defined by LVEF < 40%) and comorbid T2DM as compared with 78 similarly sedentary age and gender-matched controls (Fig. 1) *(75)*. Ingle et al. showed that 6-min walk distances are impaired in subjects with T2DM–CHF

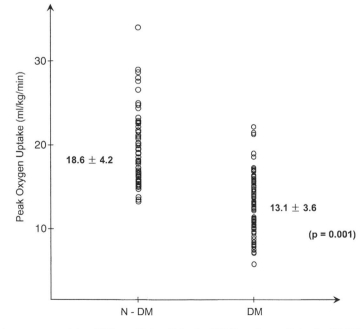

Fig. 1. Individual peak oxygen uptake (*VO₂peak*) in diabetic (*DM*) and nondiabetic (*N-DM*) patients with chronic heart failure due to left ventricular systolic dysfunction. Mean VO₂peak is significantly lower in DM than in N-DM patients. Reprinted from Tibb et al. *(75)*, with permission from American College of Cardiology Foundation.

as compared with age and gender-matched nondiabetic CHF patients (238 m vs. 296 m, $p = 0.005$) *(76)*. In both the Tibb and Ingle studies *(75, 76)*, there was a higher prevalence of coronary artery disease (CAD) in the T2DM subjects, but the Ingle study performed a subanalysis matching only subjects with CAD and the walking distance remained statistically impaired (231 m vs. 283 m, $p = 0.001$) *(76)*. Prevalence of angiotension-converting enzyme inhibitor, angiotensin-II receptor blocker, and beta-blocker usage between groups was analyzed in all three studies and no differences were observed. In summary, subjects with T2DM and CHF from systolic cardiomyopathy have a greater exercise impairment than nondiabetic subjects with systolic cardiomyopathy alone; however, the reasons for this difference are not fully understood.

Theoretically, insulin may improve exercise tolerance in DM–CHF subjects by increasing the ejection fraction. Insulin has been shown to have a direct inotropic effect on the myocardium in animals *(77, 78)*, and to increase resting left ventricular ejection fraction in normal human subjects (54% vs. 47%, $p < 0.01$) *(79)*. When an insulin-dextrose infusion was administered to T2DM and nondiabetic subjects (both groups with preserved systolic function), the left ventricular ejection fraction rose both at baseline and with exercise in T2DM *(71)*. In the nondiabetic subjects given insulin-dextrose, the LVEF rose with exercise but not at baseline *(71)*. The exact physiologic mechanisms whereby insulin is able to increase LVEF without provoking hypoglycemia are still uncertain.

One study has shown that insulin administration may improve maximal exercise capacity in T2DM–CHF subjects by other mechanisms than increased LVEF. Guazzi postulated that insulin administration may improve exercise capacity in T2DM–CHF subjects in part by ameliorating pulmonary angiopathy, and, therefore, looked at the impact of insulin therapy on VO_2max and alveolar-capillary membrane diffusing capacity (DL_{CO}) in T2DM–CHF subjects *(80)*. Using a parallel crossover design with subjects acting as their own controls, they found administration of insulin improved VO_2max by 13.5% ($p < 0.01$) and improved ventilatory efficiency (slope of ventilation/carbon dioxide production decreased by 18%, $p < 0.01$) *(80)*. Changes in both VO_2max and ventilatory efficiency after insulin administration correlated strongly with a better alveolar-capillary membrane diffusing capacity ($r = 0.67$, $p = 0.002$ for VO_2max and DL_{CO}, $r = -0.73$, $p < 0.001$ for ventilatory efficiency and DL_{CO}) *(80)*. These changes were present both 1 h and 6 h after a 60-min insulin infusion, but had resolved within 24 h after the insulin *(80)*. The changes from insulin were not due to glycemic changes (dextrose counter-infusions maintained glucose homeostasis) or from a change in ejection fraction in these subjects *(80)*. In summary, insulin therapy has been shown to improve exercise capacity in subjects with T2DM and CHF from systolic cardiomyopathy, at least in part by improving pulmonary angiopathy and seemingly without any changes in glycemic control or ejection fraction. However, it is unlikely that insulin would be utilized clinically to increase exercise capacity alone, as its side effect profile creates an unfavorable risk-benefit ratio.

Rigorous studies have not been performed to look at the physiologic impact of exercise training in subjects with T2DM and systolic cardiomyopathy *(81)*.

MACROVASCULAR DISEASE

Impairment of Exercise Performance in Diabetes Mellitus with Comorbid Coronary Artery Disease

The incidence of CAD in subjects with DM (both type 1 and type 2) is – two to three times increased over that of the general population *(82–84)* and diabetics' mortality following acute myocardial infarction (MI) is double that of nondiabetic controls similar in age *(84, 85)*. Importantly, it has been shown that post-MI subjects with greater peak VO_2max levels achieved through cardiac rehabilitation have lower cardiovascular mortality and morbidity *(86, 87)*. Given the above data, this section will review the impact of DM (which generally lowers maximal exercise capacity) on VO_2max in post-MI subjects with and without cardiac rehabilitation.

The limited studies available have differed on whether T2DM impairs maximal exercise capacity in post-MI subjects (without cardiac rehabilitation) as compared with nondiabetic post-MI subjects without cardiac rehabilitation. Izawa et al. found that the maximal exercise capacity was impaired in 30 post-MI T2DM subjects as opposed to 41 nondiabetic controls (22.6 ml/min/kg vs. 26.1 ml/min/kg, $p < 0.01$) despite similar resting ejection fractions between groups *(88)*. However, another study found no difference in exercise capacity (without cardiac rehabilitation) between 59 post-MI subjects with T2DM and 36 post-MI nondiabetic controls (20.2 ml/min/kg vs. 22.4 ml/min/kg, p = NS) *(89)*. Izawa et al. found an impaired chronotropic response to exercise which correlated with impaired VO_2max in post-MI subjects with diabetes as compared with the nondiabetic post-MI controls *(88)*. The chronotropic response to exercise was measured by the change in heart rate from baseline to peak exercise (delta heart rate (HR)) divided by the change in serum norepinephrine concentration (delta norepinephrine (NE)) from baseline to peak exercise (delta HR/delta NE). This ratio of delta HR/delta NE has been shown by Colucci et al. to inversely correspond to impaired VO_2max in nondiabetic subjects with systolic cardiomyopathy *(90)*. The data from Colucci et al. in nondiabetics with CHF also suggested their chronotropic inhibition results from postsynaptic beta-adrenergic desensitization. Apart from lowering VO_2max, an inhibited chronotropic response has been shown elsewhere to predict cardiovascular events within a T2DM cohort *(91)*. In the study by Izawa et al., other possible predictors of an impaired VO_2max besides impaired sympathetic responsiveness were not analyzed, but the groups had no significant differences in age, BMI, ejection fraction, extent and location of infarction, or medication usage (beta blockers were exclusion criteria and subjects were matched for angiotension-converting enzyme, nitrate, and calcium-channel blocker use). The subjects with T2DM were well controlled with an average HbA1c of 6.9%, and only one subject required insulin therapy. Given the small sample sizes of the two studies looking at this issue and their discordant results, more studies are needed to determine if there are differences in exercise capacity caused by diabetes added to post-MI status.

Exercise rehabilitation has been shown to improve mortality in post-MI patients by 20% *(92, 93)*, but benefits may be attenuated in T2DM subjects whose exercise training response appears inhibited. A cohort of 59 T2DM subjects and 36 well-matched nondiabetic subjects were followed after a cardiac rehabilitation program performed for indications of acute MI or unstable angina in the month prior to enrollment *(89)*. At study entry, the two groups showed no difference in their VO_2max or duration of exercise on a maximal exercise test (graded bicycle ergometer) *(89)*. Both groups then compliantly participated in a 2-month cardiac rehabilitation program consisting of three 1-h moderate exercise training sessions per week. The maximal stress test was repeated at completion of the rehabilitation program. The T2DM group did show improvement with the cardiac rehabilitation program, including an increased VO_2max of 13% from study entry, but their improvement was drastically attenuated as compared with the nondiabetic subjects *(89)*. Despite no difference between groups VO_2max at study entry, at completion of the study the nondiabetic subjects had a higher VO_2max (28.8 vs. 22.6, $p < 0.001$), peak workload (139 W vs. 120 W, $p = 0.009$), and longer duration of exercise (13.7 min vs. 11.8 min, $p = 0.017$) than the subjects with T2DM *(89)*. Linear regression was performed to determine predictors of change in VO_2max in the T2DM group. This analysis showed that the change in VO_2max was independently associated with fasting blood glucose ($p = 0.001$) and a trend toward association with BMI ($p = 0.056$), but was not associated with age, insulin resistance (determined by HOMA), duration of DM, microalbuminuria, left ventricular ejection fraction, or insulin therapy *(89)*. To our knowledge, no other studies have been performed looking specifically at differences in exercise response to cardiac rehabilitation between post-MI subjects with and without DM. No studies to date have compared mortality after cardiac rehabilitation in post-MI nondiabetic subjects versus those with T2DM.

In summary, data are insufficient to clearly determine if diabetic subjects post-MI have an impaired maximal exercise capacity prior to cardiac rehabilitation as compared to similar nondiabetic post-MI individuals. Any true differences may be mediated by an impaired chronotropic response normalized for the degree of sympathetic activity (delta HR/delta NE). After standard cardiac rehabilitation, the limited data in T2DM post-MI subjects show less improvement in exercise capacity as compared to nondiabetic post-MI subjects. Fasting glucose levels were the best predictor of improved exercise capacity after cardiac rehabilitation in T2DM post-MI subjects. More study is warranted to determine the impact of exercise training on outcomes such as mortality and cardiovascular morbidity in subjects with T2DM and comorbid CAD.

Impairment of Exercise Performance in Diabetes Mellitus with Comorbid Peripheral Arterial Disease

DM is a strong risk factor for the development of peripheral arterial disease (PAD). The cumulative incidence of PAD was 11% over 18 years following T2DM diagnosis in the United Kingdom Prospective Diabetes Study (UKPDS) cohort (Fig. 2)) *(12)*. In the UKPDS study, a multivariate model examined the relative contributions of different risks for PAD in this diabetic cohort, and the strongest predictors were cardiovascular disease and current smoking which both ascribed threefold odds of PAD. Lesser, but distinct risk, was ascribed to worse glycemic control, higher systolic blood pressure, and lower high-density lipoprotein (HDL) levels.

There are conflicting results in the small studies to date comparing exercise capacity in subjects with PAD and comorbid DM to nondiabetic PAD subjects *(94–97)*. Oka et al. found a decreased maximal walking distance (279 m vs. 461 m, $p = 0.01$), and decreased distance to onset of claudication (127 m vs. 187 m, $p = 0.01$) in patients with DM and PAD as compared with PAD alone *(95)*. Both groups were well-matched for ABI, cholesterol, and systolic blood pressure levels and had similar prevalence of known CAD *(95)*. Similarly, Dolan et al. showed DM subjects with PAD had a shorter 6-min walk distance (1,040 ft vs. 1,168 ft, $p < 0.001$) and slower walking velocity (0.83 m/s vs. 0.90 m/s, $p < 0.001$) despite age adjustment between groups and similar baseline ABI and physical activity levels *(94)*. A multivariate linear regression model in this study found diabetes-associated neuropathy, greater exertional leg symptomatology, and greater comorbid cardiovascular disease to be predictive of the worsened exercise capacity in the diabetic group *(94)*. In Dolan et al.'s

Fig. 2. Prevalence of peripheral arterial disease at diagnosis and at 3-year intervals over 18 years. Prevalence reported as mean with 95% confidence intervals as error bars. Peripheral arterial disease defined as any two of the following: ankle brachial index <0.8, absence of both dorsalis pedis and posterior tibial pulses to palpation in at least one leg, intermittent claudication. Reproduced with permission from Adler et al. *(12)*.

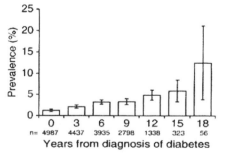

study, there was a greater BMI in the diabetic subjects as compared to the nondiabetic subjects (94). However, in subjects with a comparable BMI, ABI, and blood pressure levels, Katzel et al. found no difference in either age-adjusted VO$_2$max or onset of claudication time between 47 diabetic and 72 nondiabetic subjects with PAD (1.16 L/min in diabetics vs. 1.12 L/min in nondiabetics) (96). Green et al. furthered the concept of BMI as an explanatory variable of exercise performance (97). In their study, there was a significant difference in maximal exercise time between 12 T2DM PAD subjects and 12 age- and gender-matched leaner nondiabetic PAD subjects, but no difference between maximal walking time between the 12 T2DM PAD subjects and 7 nondiabetic subjects matched for BMI (median 845 s T2DM, 915 s "heavy" nondiabetics, 1,448 s "leaner" nondiabetics) (97). No difference was found between the three groups for pain-free exercise time, maximum cycling time, or VO$_2$max, although trends toward significance were seen in the latter two parameters for "leaner" nondiabetics versus both T2DM and "heavy" nondiabetics. Maximal walking time was significantly negatively correlated with BMI ($r = -0.38$, $p < 0.05$) as well as with the VO$_2$ time constant, tau ($r = -0.49$, $p > 0.05$). The time constant, tau, reflects the rapidity with which VO$_2$ responds to exercise and was significantly worse in T2DM subjects as compared to both the "heavy" and "lean" nondiabetic groups [$p < 0.05$, 71 s (T2DM) vs. 38 s ("heavy") vs. 37 s ("lean"), respectively] (97). The longer tau in T2DM and its inverse correlation with maximal walking time suggests the greater time for working muscles to receive steady-state oxygen distribution may decrease walking time in T2DM separately from BMI. A significant limitation of this study is the greater female distribution in the "heavy" control group as compared to both the T2DM and "lean" control groups, which may have lowered the exercise capacity in the "heavy" control group (97). Thus, current limited evidence suggests a greater BMI and longer VO$_2$ time constant, tau, may play a role in the impaired maximal exercise times for T2DM subjects with PAD found in some studies.

The optimal form of exercise for subjects with T2DM and symptomatic PAD is a supervised exercise rehabilitation program with therapeutic modality of walking to near-maximal claudication pain over 6 months (98). It has been recommended that subjects with PAD and comorbid conditions that limit weight-bearing exercise consider low-impact activities, such as stationary bicycling or aquatic exercise, although improvements in walking may be less (6, 99).

Data are lacking on the impact of exercise training on exercise capacity in subjects with DM and comorbid PAD; only limited subgroup analyses have been made to date. Sanderson et al. studied 42 subjects with PAD, 33% of whom had diabetes, and randomized the subjects (stratified for age, gender, and DM2) to 6 weeks of treadmill exercise training at 80% of subject's VO$_2$max ($n = 13$), 6 weeks of bicycle exercise training at 80% of subject's VO$_2$max ($n = 15$), or no exercise therapy. Both the treadmill exercise training and cycling training regimens improved VO$_2$max in this study (99). The treadmill training regimen increased the mean duration of walking exercise time (mean increase 240 s, $p < 0.05$), and this change in walking time was significantly correlated with the training-induced improvement in peak VO$_2$ ($r = 0.77$, $p < 0.05$) and change in peak heart rate ($r = 0.54$, $p < 0.05$) (99). The bicycling regimen of exercise training increased mean cycling time by 93 s, but this change was not correlated with other measured parameters (99). A subgroup analysis showed more severe pain in the symptomatic limb was the only baseline characteristic to differentiate "exercise responders" who increased their mean cycling or walking times from the entire sample; therefore, diabetes did not appear to play a role in the likelihood of a subject to respond. Ekroth et al. showed a mean 234% improved walking distance after 4–6 months of training in PAD subjects that was independent of the presence of DM (100). Beyond these subgroup analyses, we are not aware of any studies designed to differentiate the response to exercise training in subjects with PAD and comorbid DM as compared to nondiabetic PAD controls.

MICROVASCULAR DISEASE

Impaired Exercise Capacity from Microvascular Complications in Diabetes Mellitus

Microvascular complications of T2DM include nephropathy, neuropathy, and retinopathy, and all of these have an increasing incidence with greater duration of T2DM. The prevalence of nephropathy and retinopathy in T2DM have been reported to range from 7% to 30% (13) and from 3% to 27% (14), respectively. Given their occurrence later in the course of diabetes, microvascular complications are present at a more advanced stage of diabetic pathophysiology. As such, it is reasonable to consider that they may be explicitly associated with increased exercise impairment, and also present simultaneously with other abnormalities that impair exercise capacity [e.g., nephropathy in the form of microalbuminuria has been linked with the presence of diastolic dysfunction (101)]. This section will review the evidence in the literature that microvascular complications are correlated with exercise impairment.

Diabetic Nephropathy Decreases Exercise Capacity

Diabetic nephropathy has been shown to adversely affect exercise capacity in both T1DM and T2DM subjects. Jensen et al. found a 25–30% reduction in maximal exercise capacity when comparing normoalbuminuric T1DM subjects and T1DM subjects with either microalbuminuria (30–300 mg/day) or macroalbuminuria (>300 mg/day) (102). In an earlier nonexercise-related study by this group, resting left ventricular function was also found to be impaired in T1DM subjects with microalbuminuria and macroalbuminuria as evidenced by greater left-ventricular end-diastolic volume ($p < 0.05$), lower stroke volumes ($p < 0.05$), and a trend toward decreased cardiac output ($p = 0.10$ for macroalbuminuric subjects and $p < 0.05$ for microalbuminuric subjects) (103) The Strong Heart study also showed a correlation between the severity of microalbuminuria and the degree of diastolic dysfunction (101). Lau et al. also showed a decrement in maximal exercise capacity in T2DM subjects with microalbuminuria (30–300 mg/day of microalbumin) as compared with normoalbuminuric T2DM subjects ($p = 0.015$) and nondiabetic control subjects ($p < 0.001$). The authors hypothesized that pulmonary microangiopathy and diastolic dysfunction may partially explain this exercise decrement, as their subjects had worsened gas exchange with exercise ($p = 0.019$ for group trend between control, T2DM, and T2DM with nephropathy for minute ventilation/carbon dioxide production) and a greater frequency of diastolic dysfunction that normoalbuminuric T2DM subjects ($p = 0.013$) (104). Thus, diabetic nephropathy was clearly correlated with exercise impairment (102), and comorbid diastolic dysfunction (101, 103, 104) as well as pulmonary angiopathy (104) may partially explain this impairment.

Effects of End-Stage Renal Disease on Exercise Performance in T2DM

End-stage renal disease (ESRD) from T2DM has been shown to occur in only 0.8% of a cohort of T2DM patients followed for 10 years; however, incidence does continue to increase with time. Accordingly, diabetic nephropathy was the single most common cause of new-onset ESRD in the United States in 2002 (45% of incident dialysis patients). Given the multiple comorbidities associated with ESRD (105), it is understandable that it would correspond to even greater decreased exercise capacity than non-ESRD nephropathy. In both diabetic and nondiabetic subjects with ESRD on dialysis, maximal exercise capacity has been shown to be about 60% that of age-matched control subjects (106–108). Moderate anemia (hematocrit < 30%) has been shown to lower VO_2max, and is improved with erythropoietin administration (109). However, other factors which depress exercise capacity are felt to be numerous and have not yet been specified (110). More intensive hemodialysis sessions (five to six nocturnal sessions per week lasting 6–8 h per session) led to significant improvements in

VO_2max 3–6 months after the transition from thrice-weekly conventional hemodialysis *(111)*. Also, 1 month after renal transplant, VO_2max showed improvement to nearly that expected for sedentary age-matched subjects *(107, 112)*. These improvements in VO_2max either from more intensive hemo-dialysis or after renal transplant occurred despite the absence of any exercise training or significant improvements in anemia in these studies *(107, 111, 112)*. Such findings further specify that as yet undefined factors related to ESRD significantly depress exercise capacity in both diabetic and nondiabetic subjects with ESRD.

Exercise training studies have not been done in the population with diabetes and comorbid renal failure. More studies in this population would be of benefit given the debilitating effects of renal disease on functional capacity.

Limited Data on Exercise Capacity Association with Retinopathy or Neuropathy

Diabetic retinopathy has also been associated with reductions in exercise capacity in T2DM subjects. Despite adjusting for known predictors of exercise capacity such as age and duration of diabetes in a regression analysis, the VO_2max in the Appropriate Blood Pressure Control in Diabetes (ABCD) trial subjects with T2DM was independently reduced by the presence of diabetic nephropathy ($p = 0.04$) and retinopathy ($p = 0.026$) *(5)*. Other studies have not explicitly looked at the relationship between diabetic retinopathy and exercise capacity or the causes of this abnormality. To our knowledge, no studies have explored any potential associations between diabetic neuropathy and exercise capacity.

Hazards of Exercise Training with Diabetic Microvascular Complications

Although exercise training is highly beneficial to most participants, the presence of microvascular complications raises some safety considerations. Diabetic retinopathy may lead to adverse outcomes with vigorous exercise. Diabetic subjects with active proliferative diabetic retinopathy (PDR) are at higher risk for vitreous hemorrhage or retinal detachment *(113)*. Subjects with PDR or moderate to severe nonproliferative retinopathy are recommended to avoid strenuous exercise, Valsalva maneuvers, and jarring activities per the most recent American Diabetes Association (ADA) position statements (Table 2)) *(31, 114)*. In addition to retinopathy potentially leading to adverse outcomes, diabetic neuropathy and nephropathy also may be hazards.

The most recent ADA position statement on DM and exercise suggests that "significant peripheral neuropathy is an indication to limit weight-bearing exercise" such as jogging or pro-longed walking *(114)*. This contraindication is motivated by risk to patients of foot ulceration and fractures due to their impaired sensation and proprioception. The ADA suggests nonweight-bearing exercises such as swimming, bicycling, or rowing for affected patients with significant neuropathy *(114)*.

Some experts have discouraged strenuous physical activity in subjects with diabetic nephropathy given the propensity for exaggerated blood pressure elevations with high-intensity exercise *(115)* and proteinuria *(116–120)* associated with acute exercise-induced blood pressure excursions *(114)*. Results have been mixed on whether microalbuminuria increases to a significant degree in subjects without baseline nephropathy *(118, 121, 122)*.

However, the most recent ADA guidelines emphasizes that aerobic exercise training has been shown to decrease urinary protein excretion *(123, 124)*, and, therefore, recommended no specific exercise restrictions for people with diabetic kidney disease. The guidelines do recommend strong consideration of exercise stress testing prior to an aerobic exercise program in previously sedentary individuals with diabetic kidney disease given their significant prevalence of CAD *(114)*.

Table 2
Considerations for Activity Limitation in DR

Level of DR	Acceptable activities	Discouraged activities
No DR	Dictated by medical status	Dictated by medical status
Mild NPDR	Dictated by medical status	Dictated by medical status
Moderate NPDR	Dictated by medical status	Activities that dramatically elevate blood pressure Power lifting Heavy Valsalva
Severe NPDR	Dictated by medical status	Activities that substantially increase systolic blood pressure, Valsalva maneuvers, and active jarring Boxing Heavy competitive sports
PDR	Low-impact, cardiovascular conditioning Swimming Walking Low-impact aerobics Stationary cycling Endurance exercises	Strenuous activities, Valsalva maneuvers, pounding, or jarring Weight lifting Jogging High-impact aerobics Racquet sports Strenuous trumpet playing

Reproduced with permission from Zinman et al. *(31)*
DR diabetic retinopathy, *NPDR* nonproliferative diabetic retinopathy, *PDR* proliferative diabetic retinopathy

Separate from safety considerations, high-intensity exercise may be precluded by pain or early fatigue from comorbid diabetic neuropathy *(125–127)*, musculoskeletal pain/osteoarthritis *(125, 128–130)*, renal osteodystrophy *(131)*, or myopathy *(131)*, especially in subjects with ESRD *(131)*.

No studies have looked at the impact of exercise training on the remediation of microvascular complications in humans.

SPECIAL CASES

Exercise Impairment with Diabetes Mellitus and Atrial Fibrillation

Subjects with T2DM have been shown to develop atrial fibrillation more often than nondiabetics *(132, 133)*. The prevalence of comorbid diabetes was recently found to be 23% in a trial of elderly subjects with atrial fibrillation *(134)*. Physiologically, these two diseases may be linked as cardiovascular abnormalities that predict the development of atrial fibrillation *(132)*, and diabetes confers a significant risk of cardiovascular morbidity *(82, 135, 136)*.

One small trial compared the VO_2max before and after direct current cardioversion to establish sinus rhythm in subjects with atrial fibrillation without comorbidity ("lone atrial fibrillation"), atrial fibrillation and hypertension, or atrial fibrillation and diabetes *(137)*. This study found no improvement in VO_2max or subject-measured effort of exercise (Borg scale) in subjects with diabetes and atrial fibrillation after cardioversion, despite an improvement in VO_2max and subject-measured effort of exercise in lone atrial fibrillation and, to a lesser degree, in subjects with hypertension and atrial fibrillation. The authors theorized the lack of improvement in diabetes and atrial fibrillation corresponded to the lack of improved endothelial function, as this had improved in both the hypertensive and lone atrial fibrillation groups.

SUMMARY

There is a high prevalence of hypertension, arterial stiffness, vascular disease, and diastolic and systolic dysfunction which deleteriously impact exercise capacity in diabetes. Hypertension and arterial stiffness may both be improved in diabetes by exercise training programs *(54–56)*, and should be recommended. Subjects who have suffered an MI and have T2DM have been shown to rehabilitate to a lesser degree than nondiabetic post-MI subjects *(89)*. Data on the impact of exercise training for diabetics with diastolic dysfunction, systolic cardiomyopathy, and peripheral arterial disease are only available from subgroup analyses or nondiabetic populations. Since it is recognized that mortality is generally lower in the diabetic population with better exercise capacity *(138)*, exercise training to raise the exercise capacity is worthwhile, at least in theory, in diabetics with all comorbid conditions. However, more studies are needed to explicitly clarify the benefits of exercise training in the diabetic with diastolic or systolic dysfunction, CAD (without recent MI), or PAD.

The presence of diabetic nephropathy has been consistently associated with decreased exercise capacity, while possible associations between exercise capacity and either diabetic retinopathy or diabetic neuropathy are understudied. Existing diabetic retinopathy, nephropathy, or neuropathy may pose safety concerns to the diabetic planning to institute a new exercise regimen more intense than brisk walking. Given the lack of randomized trial data, the recommendations given in the ADA position statement *(114)* should be followed with regards to exercise precautions in the diabetic person with microvascular disease. More study in the area of safety and efficacy of exercise training in the diabetic with microvascular disease is also warranted.

In summary, exercise training is quite important to treat the metabolic and cardiovascular abnormalities associated with T2DM. Clinicians should work to insure that their diabetic patients may exercise safely to achieve these goals.

REFERENCE

1. Schneider, SH, Khachadurian, AK, Amorosa, LF, Clemow, L, Ruderman, NB: Ten-year experience with an exercise-based outpatient life-style modification program in the treatment of diabetes mellitus. *Diabetes Care* 15:1800–1810, 1992

2. Kjaer, M, Hollenbeck, CB, Frey-Hewitt, B, Galbo, H, Haskell, W, Reaven, GM: Glucoregulation and hormonal responses to maximal exercise in non-insulin-dependent diabetes. *J Appl Physiol* 68:2067–2074, 1990

3. Regensteiner, JG, Sippel, J, McFarling, ET, Wolfel, EE, Hiatt, WR: Effects of non-insulin-dependent diabetes on oxygen consumption during treadmill exercise. *Med Sci Sports Exerc* 27:875–881, 1995

4. Regensteiner, JG, Bauer, TA, Reusch, JE, Brandenburg, SL, Sippel, JM, Vogelsong, AM, Smith, S, Wolfel, EE, Eckel, RH, Hiatt, WR: Abnormal oxygen uptake kinetic responses in women with type II diabetes mellitus. *J Appl Physiol* 85:310–317, 1998

5. Estacio, RO, Regensteiner, JG, Wolfel, EE, Jeffers, B, Dickenson, M, Schrier, RW: The association between diabetic complications and exercise capacity in NIDDM patients. *Diabetes Care* 21:291–295, 1998

6. Albright, A, Franz, M, Hornsby, G, Kriska, A, Marrero, D, Ullrich, I, Verity, LS: American College of Sports Medicine position stand. Exercise and type 2 diabetes. *Med Sci Sports Exerc* 32:1345–1360, 2000

7. Geiss, LS, Rolka, DB, Engelgau, MM: Elevated blood pressure among U.S. adults with diabetes, 1988–1994. *Am J Prev Med* 22:42–48, 2002

8. Hypertension in Diabetes Study (HDS): I. Prevalence of hypertension in newly presenting type 2 diabetic patients and the association with risk factors for cardiovascular and diabetic complications. *J Hypertens* 11:309–317, 1993

9. Nichols, GA, Hillier, TA, Erbey, JR, Brown, JB: Congestive heart failure in type 2 diabetes: prevalence, incidence, and risk factors. *Diabetes Care* 24:1614–1619, 2001

10. Anand, DV, Lim, E, Hopkins, D, Corder, R, Shaw, LJ, Sharp, P, Lipkin, D, Lahiri, A: Risk stratification in uncomplicated type 2 diabetes: prospective evaluation of the combined use of coronary artery calcium imaging and selective myocardial perfusion scintigraphy. *Eur Heart J* 27:713–721, 2006

11. Fein, F, Scheur, J: Heart disease in diabetes mellitus: theory and practice. Rifkin H, Porte D Jr., Eds. New York, Elsevier, 1990, pp. 812–823

12. Adler, AI, Stevens, RJ, Neil, A, Stratton, IM, Boulton, AJ, Holman, RR: UKPDS 59: hyperglycemia and other potentially modifiable risk factors for peripheral vascular disease in type 2 diabetes. *Diabetes Care* 25:894–899, 2002

13. Adler, AI, Stevens, RJ, Manley, SE, Bilous, RW, Cull, CA, Holman, RR: Development and progression of nephropathy in type 2 diabetes: the United Kingdom Prospective Diabetes Study (UKPDS 64). *Kidney Int* 63:225–232, 2003

14. Brown, JB, Pedula, KL, Summers, KH: Diabetic retinopathy: contemporary prevalence in a well-controlled population. *Diabetes Care* 26:2637–2642, 2003

15. Veves, A, Saouaf, R, Donaghue, VM, Mullooly, CA, Kistler, JA, Giurini, JM, Horton, ES, Fielding, RA: Aerobic exercise capacity remains normal despite impaired endothelial function in the micro- and macrocirculation of physically active IDDM patients. *Diabetes* 46:1846–1852, 1997

16. Rowland, TW, Martha, PM, Jr., Reiter, EO, Cunningham, LN: The influence of diabetes mellitus on cardiovascular function in children and adolescents. *Int J Sports Med* 13:431–435, 1992

17. Regensteiner, JG: Type 2 diabetes mellitus and cardiovascular exercise performance. *Rev Endocr Metab Disord* 5:269–276, 2004

18. Regensteiner, JG, Groves, BM, Bauer, TA, Reusch, JEB, Smith, SC, Wolfel, EE: Recently diagnosed type 2 diabetes mellitus adversely affects cardiac function during exercise (abstract). *Diabetes* 51(Suppl. 2):A59, 2002

19. Poirier, P, Garneau, C, Bogaty, P, Nadeau, A, Marois, L, Brochu, C, Gingras, C, Fortin, C, Jobin, J, Dumesnil, JG: Impact of left ventricular diastolic dysfunction on maximal treadmill performance in normotensive subjects with well-controlled type 2 diabetes mellitus. *Am J Cardiol* 85:473–477, 2000

20. Devereux, RB, Roman, MJ, Paranicas, M, O'Grady, MJ, Lee, ET, Welty, TK, Fabsitz, RR, Robbins, D, Rhoades, ER, Howard, BV: Impact of diabetes on cardiac structure and function: the strong heart study. *Circulation* 101:2271–2276, 2000

21. Raber, W, Raffesberg, W, Waldhausl, W, Gasic, S, Roden, M: Exercise induces excessive normetanephrine responses in hypertensive diabetic patients. *Eur J Clin Invest* 33:480–487, 2003

22. Babalola, RO, Ajayi, AA: A cross-sectional study of echocardiographic indices, treadmill exercise capacity and microvascular complications in Nigerian patients with hypertension associated with diabetes mellitus. *Diabet Med* 9:899–903, 1992

23. Esler, M: The sympathetic system and hypertension. *Am J Hypertens* 13:99S–105S, 2000

24. Esler, M, Rumantir, M, Kaye, D, Lambert, G: The sympathetic neurobiology of essential hypertension: disparate influences of obesity, stress, and noradrenaline transporter dysfunction? *Am J Hypertens* 14:139S–146S, 2001

25. Esler, M, Rumantir, M, Wiesner, G, Kaye, D, Hastings, J, Lambert, G: Sympathetic nervous system and insulin resistance: from obesity to diabetes. *Am J Hypertens* 14:304S–309S, 2001

26. Johnson, RJ, Rodriguez-Iturbe, B, Kang, DH, Feig, DI, Herrera-Acosta, J: A unifying pathway for essential hypertension. *Am J Hypertens* 18:431–440, 2005

27. Christensen, NJ, Galbo, H: Sympathetic nervous activity during exercise. *Annu Rev Physiol* 45:139–153, 1983

28. Sullivan, L: Obesity, diabetes mellitus and physical activity – metabolic responses to physical training in adipose and muscle tissues. *Ann Clin Res* 14(Suppl. 34):51–62, 1982

29. Goldstein, DS: Plasma catecholamines and essential hypertension. An analytical review. *Hypertension* 5:86–99, 1983

30. Goldstein, DS: Plasma norepinephrine during stress in essential hypertension. *Hypertension* 3:551–556, 1981

31. Zinman, B, Ruderman, N, Campaigne, BN, Devlin, JT, Schneider, SH: Physical activity/exercise and diabetes. *Diabetes Care* 27(Suppl. 1):S58–S62, 2004

32. Et-Taouil, K, Safar, M, Plante, GE: Mechanisms and consequences of large artery rigidity. *Can J Physiol Pharmacol* 81:205–211, 2003

33. Nichols, WW, O'Rourke, M: McDonald's blood flow in arteries: theoretical, experimental and clinical principles. 2005. London, UK

34. Mitchell, GF, Lacourciere, Y, Ouellet, JP, Izzo, JL, Jr., Neutel, J, Kerwin, LJ, Block, AJ, Pfeffer, MA: Determinants of elevated pulse pressure in middle-aged and older subjects with uncomplicated systolic hypertension: the role of proximal aortic diameter and the aortic pressure-flow relationship. *Circulation* 108:1592–1598, 2003

35. Chobanian, AV, Bakris, GL, Black, HR, Cushman, WC, Green, LA, Izzo, JL, Jr., Jones, DW, Materson, BJ, Oparil, S, Wright, JT, Jr., Roccella, EJ: The Seventh Report of the Joint National Committee on Prevention, Detection, Evaluation, and Treatment of High Blood Pressure: the JNC 7 report. *JAMA* 289:2560–2572, 2003

36. Williams, B, Lacy, PS, Thom, SM, Cruickshank, K, Stanton, A, Collier, D, Hughes, AD, Thurston, H, O'Rourke, M: Differential impact of blood pressure-lowering drugs on central aortic pressure and clinical outcomes: principal results of the Conduit Artery Function Evaluation (CAFE) study. *Circulation* 113:1213–1225, 2006

37. Franzeck, UK, Talke, P, Bernstein, EF, Golbranson, FL, Fronek, A: Transcutaneous PO2 measurements in health and peripheral arterial occlusive disease. *Surgery* 91:156–163, 1982

38. Wyss, CR, Matsen, FA, III, Simmons, CW, Burgess, EM: Transcutaneous oxygen tension measurements on limbs of diabetic and nondiabetic patients with peripheral vascular disease. *Surgery* 95:339–346, 1984

39. Rooke, TW, Osmundson, PJ: The influence of age, sex, smoking, and diabetes on lower limb transcutaneous oxygen tension in patients with arterial occlusive disease. *Arch Intern Med* 150:129–132, 1990

40. Kizu, A, Koyama, H, Tanaka, S, Maeno, T, Komatsu, M, Fukumoto, S, Emoto, M, Shoji, T, Inaba, M, Shioi, A, Miki, T, Nishizawa, Y: Arterial wall stiffness is associated with peripheral circulation in patients with type 2 diabetes. *Atherosclerosis* 170:87–91, 2003

41. Matthys, D, Craen, M, De Wolf, D, Vande, WJ, Verhaaren, H: Reduced decrease of peripheral vascular resistance during exercise in young type I diabetic patients. *Diabetes Care* 19:1286–1288, 1996

42. Rubler, S, Arvan, SB: Exercise testing in young asymptomatic diabetic patients. *Angiology* 27:539–548, 1976

43. Newkumet, KM, Goble, MM, Young, RB, Kaplowitz, PB, Schieken, RM: Altered blood pressure reactivity in adolescent diabetics. *Pediatrics* 93:616–621, 1994

44. Whelton, SP, Chin, A, Xin, X, He, J: Effect of aerobic exercise on blood pressure: a meta-analysis of randomized, controlled trials. *Ann Intern Med* 136:493–503, 2002

45. Kelley, GA, Kelley, KA, Tran, ZV: Aerobic exercise and resting blood pressure: a meta-analytic review of randomized, controlled trials. *Prev Cardiol* 4:73–80, 2001

46. Kelley, GA, Kelley, KS, Tran, ZV: Walking and resting blood pressure in adults: a meta-analysis. *Prev Med* 33:120–127, 2001

47. Turner, MJ, Spina, RJ, Kohrt, WM, Ehsani, AA: Effect of endurance exercise training on left ventricular size and remodeling in older adults with hypertension. *J Gerontol A Biol Sci Med Sci* 55:M245–M251, 2000

48. Domanski, M, Mitchell, G, Pfeffer, M, Neaton, JD, Norman, J, Svendsen, K, Grimm, R, Cohen, J, Stamler, J: Pulse pressure and cardiovascular disease-related mortality: follow-up study of the Multiple Risk Factor Intervention Trial (MRFIT). *JAMA* 287:2677–2683, 2002

49. Benetos, A, Thomas, F, Bean, K, Gautier, S, Smulyan, H, Guize, L: Prognostic value of systolic and diastolic blood pressure in treated hypertensive men. *Arch Intern Med* 162:577–581, 2002

50. Turnbull, F: Effects of different blood-pressure-lowering regimens on major cardiovascular events: results of prospectively-designed overviews of randomised trials. *Lancet* 362:1527–1535, 2003

51. Levy, D, Salomon, M, D'Agostino, RB, Belanger, AJ, Kannel, WB: Prognostic implications of baseline electrocardiographic features and their serial changes in subjects with left ventricular hypertrophy. *Circulation* 90:1786–1793, 1994

52. Mathew, J, Sleight, P, Lonn, E, Johnstone, D, Pogue, J, Yi, Q, Bosch, J, Sussex, B, Probstfield, J, Yusuf, S: Reduction of cardiovascular risk by regression of electrocardiographic markers of left ventricular hypertrophy by the angiotensin-converting enzyme inhibitor ramipril. *Circulation* 104:1615–1621, 2001

53. Devereux, RB, Wachtell, K, Gerdts, E, Boman, K, Nieminen, MS, Papademetriou, V, Rokkedal, J, Harris, K, Aurup, P, Dahlof, B: Prognostic significance of left ventricular mass change during treatment of hypertension. *JAMA* 292:2350–2356, 2004

54. Menard, J, Payette, H, Baillargeon, JP, Maheux, P, Lepage, S, Tessier, D, Ardilouze, JL: Efficacy of intensive multitherapy for patients with type 2 diabetes mellitus: a randomized controlled trial. *CMAJ* 173:1457–1466, 2005

55. Woodiwiss, AJ, Kalk, WJ, Norton, GR: Habitual exercise attenuates myocardial stiffness in diabetes mellitus in rats. *Am J Physiol* 271:H2126–H2133, 1996

56. Yokoyama, H, Emoto, M, Fujiwara, S, Motoyama, K, Morioka, T, Koyama, H, Shoji, T, Inaba, M, Nishizawa, Y: Short-term aerobic exercise improves arterial stiffness in type 2 diabetes. *Diabetes Res Clin Pract* 65:85–93, 2004

57. Ferrier, KE, Waddell, TK, Gatzka, CD, Cameron, JD, Dart, AM, Kingwell, BA: Aerobic exercise training does not modify large-artery compliance in isolated systolic hypertension. *Hypertension* 38:222–226, 2001

58. Rubler, S, Dlugash, J, Yuceoglu, YZ, Kumral, T, Branwood, AW, Grishman, A: New type of cardiomyopathy associated with diabetic glomerulosclerosis. *Am J Cardiol* 30:595–602, 1972

59. Di Bonito, P, Cuomo, S, Moio, N, Sibilio, G, Sabatini, D, Quattrin, S, Capaldo, B: Diastolic dysfunction in patients with non-insulin-dependent diabetes mellitus of short duration. *Diabet Med* 13:321–324, 1996

60. Beljic, T, Miric, M: Improved metabolic control does not reverse left ventricular filling abnormalities in newly diagnosed non-insulin-dependent diabetes patients. *Acta Diabetol* 31:147–150, 1994

61. Nicolino, A, Longobardi, G, Furgi, G, Rossi, M, Zoccolillo, N, Ferrara, N, Rengo, F: Left ventricular diastolic filling in diabetes mellitus with and without hypertension. *Am J Hypertens* 8:382–389, 1995

62. Redfield, MM, Jacobsen, SJ, Burnett, JC, Jr., Mahoney, DW, Bailey, KR, Rodeheffer, RJ: Burden of systolic and diastolic ventricular dysfunction in the community: appreciating the scope of the heart failure epidemic. *JAMA* 289:194–202, 2003

63. Poirier, P, Bogaty, P, Garneau, C, Marois, L, Dumesnil, JG: Diastolic dysfunction in normotensive men with well-controlled type 2 diabetes: importance of maneuvers in echocardiographic screening for preclinical diabetic cardiomyopathy. *Diabetes Care* 24:5–10, 2001

64. Bell, DS: Diabetic cardiomyopathy. *Diabetes Care* 26:2949–2951, 2003

65. Bell, DS: Diabetic cardiomyopathy. A unique entity or a complication of coronary artery disease? *Diabetes Care* 18:708–714, 1995
66. Trost, S, LeWinter, M: Diabetic cardiomyopathy. *Curr Treat Options Cardiovasc Med* 3:481–492, 2001
67. Salmasi, AM, Rawlins, S, Dancy, M: Left ventricular hypertrophy and preclinical impaired glucose tolerance and diabetes mellitus contribute to abnormal left ventricular diastolic function in hypertensive patients. *Blood Press Monit* 10:231–238, 2005
68. Saraiva, RM, Duarte, DM, Duarte, MP, Martins, AF, Poltronieri, AV, Ferreira, ME, Silva, MC, Hohleuwerger, R, Ellis, A, Rachid, MB, Monteiro, CF, Kaiser, SE: Tissue Doppler imaging identifies asymptomatic normotensive diabetics with diastolic dysfunction and reduced exercise tolerance. *Echocardiography* 22:561–570, 2005
69. Irace, L, Iarussi, D, Guadagno, I, De Rimini, ML, Lucca, P, Spadaro, P, Romano, A, Mansi, L, Iacono, A: Left ventricular function and exercise tolerance in patients with type II diabetes mellitus. *Clin Cardiol* 21:567–571, 1998
70. Fang, ZY, Sharman, J, Prins, JB, Marwick, TH: Determinants of exercise capacity in patients with type 2 diabetes. *Diabetes Care* 28:1643–1648, 2005
71. Sasso, FC, Carbonara, O, Cozzolino, D, Rambaldi, P, Mansi, L, Torella, D, Gentile, S, Turco, S, Torella, R, Salvatore, T: Effects of insulin-glucose infusion on left ventricular function at rest and during dynamic exercise in healthy subjects and noninsulin dependent diabetic patients: a radionuclide ventriculographic study. *J Am Coll Cardiol* 36:219–226, 2000
72. Levy, WC, Cerqueira, MD, Abrass, IB, Schwartz, RS, Stratton, JR: Endurance exercise training augments diastolic filling at rest and during exercise in healthy young and older men. *Circulation* 88:116–126, 1993
73. Belardinelli, R, Georgiou, D, Cianci, G, Berman, N, Ginzton, L, Purcaro, A: Exercise training improves left ventricular diastolic filling in patients with dilated cardiomyopathy. Clinical and prognostic implications. *Circulation* 91:2775–2784, 1995
74. Guazzi, M, Brambilla, R, Pontone, G, Agostoni, P, Guazzi, MD: Effect of non-insulin-dependent diabetes mellitus on pulmonary function and exercise tolerance in chronic congestive heart failure. *Am J Cardiol* 89:191–197, 2002
75. Tibb, AS, Ennezat, PV, Chen, JA, Haider, A, Gundewar, S, Cotarlan, V, Aggarwal, VS, Talreja, A, Le Jemtel, TH: Diabetes lowers aerobic capacity in heart failure. *J Am Coll Cardiol* 46:930–931, 2005
76. Ingle, L, Reddy, P, Clark, AL, Cleland, JG: Diabetes lowers six-minute walk test performance in heart failure. *J Am Coll Cardiol* 47:1909–1910, 2006
77. Lee, JC, Downing, SE: Effects of insulin on cardiac muscle contraction and responsiveness to norepinephrine. *Am J Physiol* 230:1360–1365, 1976
78. Downing, SE, Lee, JC: Myocardial and coronary vascular responses to insulin in the diabetic lamb. *Am J Physiol* 237:H514–H519, 1979
79. Fisher, BM, Gillen, G, Dargie, HJ, Inglis, GC, Frier, BM: The effects of insulin-induced hypoglycaemia on cardiovascular function in normal man: studies using radionuclide ventriculography. *Diabetologia* 30:841–845, 1987
80. Guazzi, M, Tumminello, G, Matturri, M, Guazzi, MD: Insulin ameliorates exercise ventilatory efficiency and oxygen uptake in patients with heart failure-type 2 diabetes comorbidity. *J Am Coll Cardiol* 42:1044–1050, 2003
81. McGavock, JM, Eves, ND, Mandic, S, Glenn, NM, Quinney, HA, Haykowsky, MJ: The role of exercise in the treatment of cardiovascular disease associated with type 2 diabetes mellitus. *Sports Med* 34:27–48, 2004
82. Stamler, J, Vaccaro, O, Neaton, JD, Wentworth, D: Diabetes, other risk factors, and 12-yr cardiovascular mortality for men screened in the Multiple Risk Factor Intervention Trial. *Diabetes Care* 16:434–444, 1993
83. Garcia, MJ, McNamara, PM, Gordon, T, Kannel, WB: Morbidity and mortality in diabetics in the Framingham population. Sixteen year follow-up study. *Diabetes* 23:105–111, 1974
84. Rytter, L, Troelsen, S, Beck-Nielsen, H: Prevalence and mortality of acute myocardial infarction in patients with diabetes. *Diabetes Care* 8:230–234, 1985
85. Granger, CB, Califf, RM, Young, S, Candela, R, Samaha, J, Worley, S, Kereiakes, DJ, Topol, EJ: Outcome of patients with diabetes mellitus and acute myocardial infarction treated with thrombolytic agents. The Thrombolysis and Angioplasty in Myocardial Infarction (TAMI) Study Group. *J Am Coll Cardiol* 21:920–925, 1993
86. Kavanagh, T, Mertens, DJ, Hamm, LF, Beyene, J, Kennedy, J, Corey, P, Shephard, RJ: Prediction of long-term prognosis in 12 169 men referred for cardiac rehabilitation. *Circulation* 106:666–671, 2002
87. Vanhees, L, Fagard, R, Thijs, L, Amery, A: Prognostic value of training-induced change in peak exercise capacity in patients with myocardial infarcts and patients with coronary bypass surgery. *Am J Cardiol* 76:1014–1019, 1995
88. Izawa, K, Tanabe, K, Omiya, K, Yamada, S, Yokoyama, Y, Ishiguro, T, Yagi, M, Hirano, Y, Kasahara, Y, Osada, N, Miyake, F, Murayama, M: Impaired chronotropic response to exercise in acute myocardial infarction patients with type 2 diabetes mellitus. *Jpn Heart J* 44:187–199, 2003
89. Verges, B, Patois-Verges, B, Cohen, M, Lucas, B, Galland-Jos, C, Casillas, JM: Effects of cardiac rehabilitation on exercise capacity in type 2 diabetic patients with coronary artery disease. *Diabet Med* 21:889–895, 2004

90. Colucci, WS, Ribeiro, JP, Rocco, MB, Quigg, RJ, Creager, MA, Marsh, JD, Gauthier, DF, Hartley, LH: Impaired chronotropic response to exercise in patients with congestive heart failure. Role of postsynaptic beta-adrenergic desensitization. *Circulation* 80:314–323, 1989

91. Endo, A, Kinugawa, T, Ogino, K, Kato, M, Hamada, T, Osaki, S, Igawa, O, Hisatome, I: Cardiac and plasma catecholamine responses to exercise in patients with type 2 diabetes: prognostic implications for cardiac-cerebrovascular events. *Am J Med Sci* 320:24–30, 2000

92. Oldridge, NB, Guyatt, GH, Fischer, ME, Rimm, AA: Cardiac rehabilitation after myocardial infarction. Combined experience of randomized clinical trials. *JAMA* 260:945–950, 1988

93. O'Connor, GT, Buring, JE, Yusuf, S, Goldhaber, SZ, Olmstead, EM, Paffenbarger, RS, Jr., Hennekens, CH: An overview of randomized trials of rehabilitation with exercise after myocardial infarction. *Circulation* 80:234–244, 1989

94. Dolan, NC, Liu, K, Criqui, MH, Greenland, P, Guralnik, JM, Chan, C, Schneider, JR, Mandapat, AL, Martin, G, McDermott, MM: Peripheral artery disease, diabetes, and reduced lower extremity functioning. *Diabetes Care* 25:113–120, 2002

95. Oka, RK, Sanders, MG: The impact of type 2 diabetes and peripheral arterial disease on quality of life. *J Vasc Nurs* 23:61–66, 2005

96. Katzel, LI, Sorkin, JD, Powell, CC, Gardner, AW: Comorbidities and exercise capacity in older patients with intermittent claudication. *Vasc Med* 6:157–162, 2001

97. Green, S, Askew, CD, Walker, PJ: Effect of type 2 diabetes mellitus on exercise intolerance and the physiological responses to exercise in peripheral arterial disease. *Diabetologia* 50:859–866, 2007

98. Gardner, AW, Poehlman, ET: Exercise rehabilitation programs for the treatment of claudication pain. A meta-analysis. *JAMA* 274:975–980, 1995

99. Sanderson, B, Askew, C, Stewart, I, Walker, P, Gibbs, H, Green, S: Short-term effects of cycle and treadmill training on exercise tolerance in peripheral arterial disease. *J Vasc Surg* 44:119–127, 2006

100. Ekroth, R, Dahllof, AG, Gundevall, B, Holm, J, Schersten, T: Physical training of patients with intermittent claudication: indications, methods, and results. *Surgery* 84:640–643, 1978

101. Liu, JE, Robbins, DC, Palmieri, V, Bella, JN, Roman, MJ, Fabsitz, R, Howard, BV, Welty, TK, Lee, ET, Devereux, RB: Association of albuminuria with systolic and diastolic left ventricular dysfunction in type 2 diabetes: the Strong Heart Study. *J Am Coll Cardiol* 41:2022–2028, 2003

102. Jensen, T, Richter, EA, Feldt-Rasmussen, B, Kelbaek, H, Deckert, T: Impaired aerobic work capacity in insulin dependent diabetics with increased urinary albumin excretion. *Br Med J (Clin Res Ed)* 296:1352–1354, 1988

103. Kelbaek, H, Jensen, T, Feldt-Rasmussen, B, Christensen, NJ, Richter, EA, Deckert, T, Nielsen, SL: Impaired left-ventricular function in insulin-dependent diabetic patients with increased urinary albumin excretion. *Scand J Clin Lab Invest* 51:467–473, 1991

104. Lau, AC, Lo, MK, Leung, GT, Choi, FP, Yam, LY, Wasserman, K: Altered exercise gas exchange as related to microalbuminuria in type 2 diabetic patients. *Chest* 125:1292–1298, 2004

105. Zoccali, C, Mallamaci, F, Tripepi, G: Traditional and emerging cardiovascular risk factors in end-stage renal disease. *Kidney Int Suppl* 63:S105–S110, 2003

106. Johansen, KL: Physical functioning and exercise capacity in patients on dialysis. *Adv Ren Replace Ther* 6:141–148, 1999

107. Painter, P, Messer-Rehak, D, Hanson, P, Zimmerman, SW, Glass, NR: Exercise capacity in hemodialysis, CAPD, and renal transplant patients. *Nephron* 42:47–51, 1986

108. Moore, GE, Brinker, KR, Stray-Gundersen, J, Mitchell, JH: Determinants of VO2peak in patients with end-stage renal disease: on and off dialysis. *Med Sci Sports Exerc* 25:18–23, 1993

109. Mayer, G, Thum, J, Cada, EM, Stummvoll, HK, Graf, H: Working capacity is increased following recombinant human erythropoietin treatment. *Kidney Int* 34:525–528, 1988

110. Painter, P, Moore, G, Carlson, L, Paul, S, Myll, J, Phillips, W, Haskell, W: Effects of exercise training plus normalization of hematocrit on exercise capacity and health-related quality of life. *Am J Kidney Dis* 39:257–265, 2002

111. Chan, CT, Notarius, CF, Merlocco, AC, Floras, JS: Improvement in exercise duration and capacity after conversion to nocturnal home haemodialysis. *Nephrol Dial Transplant* 22:3285–3291, 2007

112. Painter, P, Hanson, P, Messer-Rehak, D, Zimmerman, SW, Glass, NR: Exercise tolerance changes following renal transplantation. *Am J Kidney Dis* 10:452–456, 1987

113. Sigal, RJ, Kenny, GP, Wasserman, DH, Castaneda-Sceppa, C: Physical activity/exercise and type 2 diabetes. *Diabetes Care* 27:2518–2539, 2004

114. Sigal, RJ, Kenny, GP, Wasserman, DH, Castaneda-Sceppa, C, White, RD: Physical activity/exercise and type 2 diabetes: a consensus statement from the American Diabetes Association. *Diabetes Care* 29:1433–1438, 2006

115. Mogensen, CE: Nephropathy: early. In *Handbook of Exercise in Diabetes*. 2nd ed. Ruderman N, Devlin JT, Schneider SH, Kriska A, Eds. Alexandria, VA, American Diabetes Association, 2002, pp. 433–449

116. Romanelli, G, Giustina, A, Cravarezza, P, Caldonazzo, A, Agabiti-Rosei, E, Giustina, G: Albuminuria induced by exercise in hypertensive type I and type II diabetic patients: a randomised, double-blind study on the effects of acute administration of captopril and nifedipine. *J Hum Hypertens* 5:167–173, 1991

117. Hoogenberg, K, Dullaart, RP: Abnormal plasma noradrenaline response and exercise induced albuminuria in type 1 (insulin-dependent) diabetes mellitus. *Scand J Clin Lab Invest* 52:803–811, 1992

118. Viberti, GC, Jarrett, RJ, McCartney, M, Keen, H: Increased glomerular permeability to albumin induced by exercise in diabetic subjects. *Diabetologia* 14:293–300, 1978

119. Tuominen, JA, Ebeling, P, Koivisto, VA: Long-term lisinopril therapy reduces exercise-induced albuminuria in normoalbuminuric normotensive IDDM patients. *Diabetes Care* 21:1345–1348, 1998

120. Poulsen, PL, Ebbehoj, E, Mogensen, CE: Lisinopril reduces albuminuria during exercise in low grade microalbuminuric type 1 diabetic patients: a double blind randomized study. *J Intern Med* 249:433–440, 2001

121. Lane, JT, Ford, TC, Larson, LR, Chambers, WA, Lane, PH: Acute effects of different intensities of exercise in normoalbuminuric/normotensive patients with type 1 diabetes. *Diabetes Care* 27:28–32, 2004

122. Huttunen, NP, Kaar, M, Puukka, R, Akerblom, HK: Exercise-induced proteinuria in children and adolescents with type 1 (insulin dependent) diabetes. *Diabetologia* 21:495–497, 1981

123. Ward, KM, Mahan, JD, Sherman, WM: Aerobic training and diabetic nephropathy in the obese Zucker rat. *Ann Clin Lab Sci* 24:266–277, 1994

124. Albright, AL, Mahan, JD, Ward, KM, Sherman, WM, Roehrig, KL, Kirby, TE: Diabetic nephropathy in an aerobically trained rat model of diabetes. *Med Sci Sports Exerc* 27:1270–1277, 1995

125. Davison, SN: Pain in hemodialysis patients: prevalence, cause, severity, and management. *Am J Kidney Dis* 42:1239–1247, 2003

126. Parving, HH, Hommel, E, Mathiesen, E, Skott, P, Edsberg, B, Bahnsen, M, Lauritzen, M, Hougaard, P, Lauritzen, E: Prevalence of microalbuminuria, arterial hypertension, retinopathy and neuropathy in patients with insulin dependent diabetes. *Br Med J (Clin Res Ed)* 296:156–160, 1988

127. Cohen, JA, Jeffers, BW, Faldut, D, Marcoux, M, Schrier, RW: Risks for sensorimotor peripheral neuropathy and autonomic neuropathy in non-insulin-dependent diabetes mellitus (NIDDM). *Muscle Nerve* 21:72–80, 1998

128. Kay, J, Bardin, T: Osteoarticular disorders of renal origin: disease-related and iatrogenic. *Baillieres Best Pract Res Clin Rheumatol* 14:285–305, 2000

129. Kart-Koseoglu, H, Yucel, AE, Niron, EA, Koseoglu, H, Isiklar, I, Ozdemir, FN: Osteoarthritis in hemodialysis patients: relationships with bone mineral density and other clinical and laboratory parameters. *Rheumatol Int* 25:270–275, 2005

130. Naidich, JB, Mossey, RT, McHeffey-Atkinson, B, Karmel, MI, Bluestone, PA, Mailloux, LU, Stein, HL: Spondyloarthropathy from long-term hemodialysis. *Radiology* 167:761–764, 1988

131. Evans, N, Forsyth, E: End-stage renal disease in people with type 2 diabetes: systemic manifestations and exercise implications. *Phys Ther* 84:454–463, 2004

132. Kannel, WB, Abbott, RD, Savage, DD, McNamara, PM: Epidemiologic features of chronic atrial fibrillation: the Framingham study. *N Engl J Med* 306:1018–1022, 1982

133. Strongin, LG, Korneva, KG, Panova, EI: Disturbances of cardiac rhythm and metabolic control in patients with type-2 diabetes. *Kardiologiia* 45:46–49, 2005

134. Douketis, JD, Arneklev, K, Goldhaber, SZ, Spandorfer, J, Halperin, F, Horrow, J: Comparison of bleeding in patients with nonvalvular atrial fibrillation treated with ximelagatran or warfarin: assessment of incidence, case-fatality rate, time course and sites of bleeding, and risk factors for bleeding. *Arch Intern Med* 166:853–859, 2006

135. Haffner, SM, Lehto, S, Ronnemaa, T, Pyorala, K, Laakso, M: Mortality from coronary heart disease in subjects with type 2 diabetes and in nondiabetic subjects with and without prior myocardial infarction. *N Engl J Med* 339:229–234, 1998

136. Kannel, WB, McGee, DL: Diabetes and cardiovascular risk factors: the Framingham study. *Circulation* 59:8–13, 1979

137. Guazzi, M, Belletti, S, Bianco, E, Lenatti, L, Guazzi, MD: Endothelial dysfunction and exercise performance in lone atrial fibrillation or associated with hypertension or diabetes: different results with cardioversion. *Am J Physiol Heart Circ Physiol* 291:H921–H928, 2006

138. Wei, M, Gibbons, LW, Kampert, JB, Nichaman, MZ, Blair, SN: Low cardiorespiratory fitness and physical inactivity as predictors of mortality in men with type 2 diabetes. *Ann Intern Med* 132:605–611, 2000

III   Management and Treatment

9 Prescribing Exercise for Patients with Diabetes

Dalynn T. Badenhop

ABSTRACT

Exercise prescription for patients with diabetes follows guidelines regarding frequency, intensity, duration, and mode of exercise established for patients participating in a medically supervised exercise program. Physicians and health care professionals should devise an exercise care plan that maximizes the benefits and minimizes the risks for each patient. The distinction between prescribing exercise for patients with T1DM and patients with T2DM with and without DRCs is reviewed. The question whether to exercise or not based on hyperglycemia /hypoglycemia is presented. It is highly recommended that health care professionals incorporate progressive resistance training and lifestyle-based physical activity into the exercise prescription for patients with diabetes. Health care professionals should be knowledgeable about diabetic medications to avoid the potential for hypoglycemia associated with exercise.

Key words: Exercise prescription; Progressive resistance training; Lifestyle-based physical activity; Self blood glucose monitoring.

From: *Contemporary Diabetes: Diabetes and Exercise*
Edited by: J. G. Regensteiner et al. (eds.), DOI: 10.1007/978-1-59745-260-1_9
© Humana Press, a part of Springer Science+Business Media, LLC 2009

INTRODUCTION

Prescribing exercise for most patients with diabetes is closely aligned with guidelines for apparently healthy persons *(1)*. However, exercise recommendations for patients who have diabetes-related complications (DRCs) parallel those of patients participating in a medically supervised exercise program *(2, 3)*. One of the challenges patients with diabetes face is how to comply with complex treatment regimens. Health care professionals are in a key position to help monitor and motivate patient compliance with medications, diet, and exercise routines. Working closely with the patient's primary care physician or endocrinologist, health care professionals need to consider all aspects of this complicated medical condition and devise an exercise recommendation that maximizes the benefits and minimizes the risks of exercise in a given patient. In addition to discussing the basic principles of exercise prescription for patients with diabetes, this chapter will also cover the following topics:

- Distinguishing between the exercise prescription for patients with Type 1 diabetes mellitus (T1DM) and Type 2 diabetes mellitus (T2DM) with and without DRCs
- Hypoglycemia, hyperglycemia, ketosis, and the importance of self-blood glucose monitoring
- Incorporation of progressive resistance training into the exercise prescription for patients with diabetes
- Lifestyle-based physical activity interventions for patients with diabetes
- Guidelines regarding frequency, intensity, duration, and mode of exercise
- Special considerations to avoid hypoglycemia when using certain medications that are prescribed for managing diabetes

Although food intake and the timing of meals is an important consideration when prescribing exercise for patients with diabetes, this topic will be discussed only briefly in this chapter. For further information please refer to Chapter 11.

BENEFITS OF REGULAR EXERCISE IN PATIENTS WITH T2DM

The benefits of exercise, one of the cornerstones of diabetes therapy, for the patient with T2DM are substantial and recent studies strengthen the importance of long-term exercise programs for the treatment and prevention of this common metabolic abnormality and its complications *(4–7)*. The low-cost, nonpharmacological nature of physical activity further enhances its therapeutic appeal. Regular exercise by patients with T2DM improves glycemic control, reduces the risk for cardiovascular disease (CVD) and its complications, improves overall health and wellness, and prevents or delays the onset of T2DM in patients prone to the disease *(8–12)* (Table 1).

Until recently, T2DM almost entirely had its onset in adulthood but now is increasing in prevalence in youth. T2DM is often attributable to obesity and physical inactivity, and is commonly accompanied by hypertension, abnormal lipids, and clotting abnormalities. The risk of myocardial infarction is 50%

Table 1
**Key Mechanisms by Which Exercise Contributes
To Effective Diabetes Management**

Improved sensitivity to insulin in the peripheral tissues
Reduced levels of blood glucose
Reduced dosages or need for insulin or oral hypoglycemics
Decreased plasma insulin levels
Enhanced glucose tolerance
Reduced hemoglobin A_{1C} levels

Table 2
The Role of Exercise in Reducing the Risk for Cardiovascular Disease and its Complications

Improved functional capacity
Improved lipid profile (decrease in triglycerides, VLDL,
    and small dense subclass of LDL-cholesterol; increase in HDL-cholesterol)
Increased weight loss, particularly intra-abdominal fat
Lowered systolic and diastolic blood pressure
Increased fibrinolytic activity
Decreased susceptibility to serious ventricular arrhythmias

Table 3
The Role of Exercise in Improving Overall Health and Wellness

Reduced incidence of depression and anxiety
Improved quality of life
Better management of life, family, societal, and work stressors

higher in men with diabetes and 150% higher in women with diabetes compared with nondiabetics *(13–15)*. The risk of death from cardiovascular causes is doubled in men with diabetes and is four times higher in women with diabetes compared with patients without diabetes *(13–15)*. Among patients with diabetes, coronary heart disease and stroke are the major causes of morbidity and mortality *(16)*. Hypertension and peripheral arterial disease are among the major vascular comorbidities of T2DM *(15, 16)*. The improvement in many of the risk factors for CVD has been linked to a decrease in plasma insulin levels and the improved insulin sensitivity associated with exercise *(17)*, thereby improving glycemic control. Exercise is effective in glucose control because of its insulin-like effect that enhances the uptake of glucose even in the presence of insulin deficiency. The role of physical activity is of great importance for the management of T2DM because it is the only intervention that directly affects cardiorespiratory fitness. This is important because of the strong association between higher levels of cardiorespiratory fitness and reduced cardiovascular mortality in people without diabetes, even after adjustment for other known risk factors *(18)* (Tables 2 and 3).

BENEFITS OF LIFESTYLE-BASED PHYSICAL ACTIVITY INTERVENTIONS

Few patients with diabetes participate in regular physical activity, and in those who do the level of intensity is low *(19, 20)*. Findings from the third National Health and Nutrition Examination Survey reported that of individuals with T2DM, 31% reported no regular physical activity and another 38% reported less than recommended levels of physical activity *(21)*.

Because long-term adherence to structured endurance exercise programs is problematic for individuals with T2DM, the focus of those seeking to introduce physical activity interventions has recently broadened to include not only structured and supervised fitness classes but also toward lifestyle-based physical activity interventions. This approach gives patients confidence that they will obtain significant health benefits from less strenuous and less-structured physical activity *(22)*. The goal is for patients to more easily incorporate this type of physical activity into their daily lives. These interventions place no specific emphasis on the intensity component of their exercise but focus on attaining a desired level of total energy expenditure on either a daily or weekly basis. An example of a lifestyle activity is taking frequent short walks during the day to accumulate 30 min of activity rather than a structured program in which the individual would spend 30 min on a treadmill in the gym.

Two studies evaluated the effects of a lifestyle-based physical activity intervention in individuals with T2DM. Yamanouchi et al. *(22)* evaluated the effects of walking combined with diet therapy on insulin sensitivity in obese noninsulin-dependent diabetes mellitus patients (average age = 41.5 years). The diet and exercise group was instructed to walk at least 10,000 steps/day. On average, this group of subjects walked 19,200 steps/day. The diet only group was told to maintain a normal daily routine. This group walked an average of 4,500 steps/day for 8 weeks. Body weight reduction was greater in the diet and exercise group than the diet only group. After training, glucose infusion rate and metabolic clearance rate increased in the diet and exercise group but not in the diet only group. Analysis also showed a significant correlation between the change in metabolic clearance rate and the average steps per day. These results provide evidence that walking can be recommended as an adjunct therapy for body weight reduction and improvement in insulin sensitivity in obese patients with diabetes who are not using insulin. The fact that the average number of steps performed on a daily basis far exceeded the prescribed number of steps suggests that this population was agreeable and able to perform this amount of daily physical activity.

Walker et al. *(23)* examined the impact of a 12-week walking program on body composition and risk factors for CVD in overweight and obese women who either had T2DM or were nondiabetic but had first-degree relatives with diabetes (average age = 57 years of age). Subjects in both groups were asked to walk 1 hour per day on 5 days each week for 12 weeks. Both groups increased their maximal aerobic capacity. In the diabetic women, abdominal body fat decreased along with fasting blood glucose, total cholesterol, and low-density lipoprotein-cholesterol. The nondiabetic women with normal resting glucose levels failed to lose body fat. However, their HbA_{1c}, total cholesterol, and LDL-cholesterol decreased. Thus, 12 weeks of walking increased the fitness of the women. Their improved fitness was not related to their improvement in abdominal body fat but their improvement in fasting blood glucose was related to the loss of abdominal body fat.

These studies also showed that walking is a form of moderate exercise that can be safely performed by middle-aged and older persons and can readily be incorporated into a daily routine. Clinically, these two studies support the notion that walking is an effective means of treatment in obese or overweight patients with diabetes.

BENEFITS OF PROGRESSIVE RESISTANCE TRAINING IN PATIENTS WITH DIABETES

The regular participation in aerobic exercise is often hindered in many patients with T2DM because of advancing age, obesity, and other comorbid conditions. Obese, diabetic patients are often unable to perform weight-bearing exercise because of the stress and strain on their musculoskeletal system. In addition, they are unable to use their large muscle groups for an extended period of time. Weight lifting or progressive resistance training offers an effective complement to aerobic exercise for these patients because it can use smaller isolated muscle groups for a shorter period. Resistance training reduces acute insulin responses during glucose tolerance testing in diabetics and improves insulin sensitivity. Resistance training decreases glycosylated hemoglobin levels in diabetic men and women regardless of age *(24)*. Two clinical trials support the value of resistance training in older patients with T2DM. Dunstan et al. *(25)* examined the effect of high-intensity progressive resistance training combined with moderate weight loss on glycemic control and body composition in older Type 2 diabetics. Thirty-six overweight men and women with T2DM were randomized to resistance training and moderate weight loss (resistance training plus weight loss) or a moderate weight loss control group (weight loss). HbA_{1c} fell significantly more in the resistance training plus weight loss group than in the weight loss group at 3 and 6 months. Lean body mass increased in the combined group and decreased in the weight loss group. There were no differences between the groups for fasting glucose or insulin levels. Thus, resistance training in combination with moderate weight loss was effective in improving glycemic control in older patients with T2DM. Increased lean body mass in the resistance training plus weight loss group was an additional benefit from resistance training in managing older patients with T2DM.

Castaneda et al. *(26)* investigated the effect of high-intensity resistance training on glycemic control in 62 Latino older adults with T2DM randomly assigned to a 16-week supervised resistance training or a control group. The resistance training group exhibited a reduction in plasma glycosylated hemoglobin levels, increased muscle glycogen stores, and a reduction in their dose of prescribed diabetes medication. Control subjects showed no change in HbA_{1c}, a reduction in muscle glycogen, and a 42% increase in diabetes medications. Compared to control subjects, the resistance-trained group increased lean mass, reduced systolic blood pressure, and decreased trunk fat mass. Thus, resistance training appears to be feasible and effective in improving glycemic control and reducing the risk factors associated with the metabolic syndrome/diabetes in older diabetic patients.

These studies add to the rationale that resistance training performed on a regular basis has clinically important therapeutic value and should be incorporated into the plan of care for managing glycemic control in older patients with T2DM. However, resistance training has not been routinely used in the clinical management of diabetes, despite recommendations for this in recent position statements from the American Diabetes Association (ADA) *(2, 3)* and the American College of Sports Medicine *(9)*. Unfortunately, this form of exercise has not been routinely recommended by many clinicians to older adults and those with diseases such as diabetes, hypertension, and CVD *(27)*. Their main concern is that acute rises in blood pressure associated with resistance training might be harmful, possibly provoking stroke, myocardial ischemia, or retinal hemorrhage *(2, 3)*. In research studies of resistance training in patients with T2DM, there is no evidence that moderate-intensity resistance training increases these risks *(25, 26, 28–31)*. Although it is well known that blood pressure rises while lifting a heavy weight, blood pressure can also rise considerably while performing aerobic exercise *(2, 3)*. Similarly, there is no evidence that these acute rises in blood pressure during moderate-intensity aerobic exercise are associated with adverse outcomes. More important, participation in regular aerobic and resistance exercise does lead to reductions in resting blood pressure. Benn et al. *(32)* demonstrated that in healthy older men, the myocardial demands of high-intensity resistance exercise were comparable to those occasionally needed for activities of daily living, such as climbing stairs, walking up a hill, or carrying 20–30 lbs of groceries. These studies support the safety of resistance training in older adults, including those with ischemic heart disease, suggesting that resistance training should be a component of an overall fitness program, along with aerobic training in many clinical populations *(27)*.

EXERCISE AND T1DM

T1DM is usually manifest at a much younger age, is generally not associated with obesity, and is less responsive to exercise training. Those with T1DM are prone to hypoglycemia during and immediately after exercise. Exercise can lead to excessive swings in plasma glucose levels that are unacceptable for the management of the disease. However, people with uncomplicated T1DM do not have to restrict physical activity, provided blood sugar levels are monitored regularly and controlled appropriately. Many athletes who have T1DM have trained and competed successfully. Monitoring blood sugars levels in an exercising person with T1DM is important so that diet and insulin dosages can be adjusted accordingly. Exercise will nonetheless increase glucose disposal and diminish insulin requirements on exercise days *(33)*.

Exercise is not considered a primary component of treatment in T1DM to improve glycemic control. Several studies have failed to show an independent effect of exercise training on improving glycemic control as measured by HbA_{1c} in patients with T1DM, although more studies of this subject would be beneficial *(34–36)*. Patients with T1DM are nonetheless encouraged to exercise to gain the wide-ranging benefits of exercise in improving known risk factors for coronary artery disease. The same logic can be applied for reducing the risk for cerebrovascular and peripheral arterial disease, although this has not been studied. Health care professionals need to advise patients with T1DM about safe and enjoyable physical activities that are consistent with their lifestyle and culture *(37)*. Patients with T1DM who exercise on a regular basis will also feel an improvement in their quality of life and an enhancement of their self-esteem and sense of well-being *(37)*.

RISKS OF EXERCISE IN PATIENTS WITH DIABETES

The risk-to-benefit ratio of exercise is highly favorable for most patients with diabetes. However, exercise is not entirely without risk and health care professionals should be aware of the risks to maximize patient safety *(38)*. Before prescribing a physical activity regimen, patients should be assessed for metabolic control, complication status, and any other medical indications not to exercise. Refer to Tables 4 and 5.

Table 4
Risks Associated with Exercise in Patients with Diabetes

Cardiovascular risks
   Cardiac dysfunction and arrhythmias due to ischemic heart disease (often silent ischemia)
   Excessive rises or falls in blood pressure or heart rate due to autonomic neuropathy
   Postexercise orthostatic hypotension and postural hypotension due to autonomic neuropathy
   Cardiomyopathy due to long-standing diabetes
   Screening for ischemic heart disease is recommended for patients with diabetic autonomic neuropathy *(39)*

Metabolic risks
   Worsening of hyperglycemia and development of ketosis (primarily in Type 1)
   Hypoglycemia in patients on insulin or oral hypoglycemic agents (Type 1 and Type 2 diabetes)

Musculoskeletal and traumatic risks
   Foot ulcers, skin breakdown, and infection (especially in the presence of neuropathy) *(40)*
   Orthopedic injuries related to peripheral neuropathy
   Accelerated degenerative joint disease (Charcot joint destruction)

Microvascular risks
   Retinopathy – Patients who have proliferative or severe nonproliferative diabetic retinopathy should avoid
      anaerobic exercise and exercise that involves excessive straining, jarring, or valsalva-like maneuvers
      because of the potential risk of triggering vitreous hemorrhage or retinal detachment *(41)*
   Nephropathy – There is no need for any specific exercise restrictions for people with diabetic kidney
      disease *(42)*
   Neuropathy – Peripheral neuropathy is an indication to limit weight-bearing exercise (*see* Table 5)

Table 5
Exercise for Diabetic Patients with Loss
of Protective Sensation

Contraindicated	Recommended
Treadmill	Swimming
Prolonged walking	Bicycling
Jogging	Rowing
Step exercises	Chair exercises
	Arm exercises
	Other nonweight-bearing exercises

SCREENING PATIENTS WITH DIABETES FOR EXERCISE PROGRAMS

The recommendation that people with diabetes participate in an exercise program is based on considerable evidence that the benefits outweigh the risks *(37, 38)*. In order to maximize the risk to benefit ratio, it is necessary to provide appropriate screening of patients, program design, monitoring, and patient education. The chronic hyperglycemia of diabetes is associated with long-term damage, dysfunction, and failure of various organs, especially the eyes, kidneys, nerves, heart, and blood vessels *(43)*. In screening patients for an exercise program, Schneider found the prevalence of previously undiagnosed disease as follows: 6% ischemic heart disease, 14% peripheral vascular disease, 42% hypertension, 8% proteinuria, and 16% with background retinopathy *(44)*. Effective screening of patients with diabetes prior to initiating an exercise program should include the following:

Evaluate for vascular and neurological complications

- Peripheral vascular disease
- Retinopathy
- Nephropathy
- Peripheral neuropathy
- Autonomic neuropathy

Screen patients for knowledge level and current control of diabetes

- Insulin and oral hypoglycemics
- Self-monitoring of blood sugar levels
- Dietary habits
- Current level of regular physical activity

Refer to Table 6 on precautions and special instructions for patients with diabetes.

EXERCISE TESTING IN PATIENTS WITH DIABETES

The prevalence of premature coronary artery disease is high in patients with diabetes but a majority of cases occur in the absence of typical signs and symptoms *(45, 46)*. Thus, formal exercise testing is often advisable if previously sedentary diabetics are to undertake a moderate- or high-intensity exercise program *(2, 3)*. A more detailed discussion of guidelines for exercise testing in patients with diabetes can be found in Chapter 12.

Table 6
Precautions and Special Instructions for Patients with Diabetes (37)

Exercising late in the evening increases the risk of nocturnal hypoglycemia

Avoid strenuous exercise until diabetes is under control

Know the signs, symptoms, and management of hypoglycemia such as confusion, weakness, fatigue, loss of consciousness, and convulsions

Episodes of hypoglycemia may occur as late as 24–48 hours postexercise

Certain medications tend to mask or exacerbate the effect of hypoglycemia with exercise
  – β-Blockers
  – Coumadin
  – Calcium channel blockers
  – Diuretics
  – Nicotinic acid

Carry a carbohydrate source during exercise

Avoid exercise at time of peak insulin effect or do one of the following:
  – Use a carbohydrate snack 30 min prior to exercise
  – Decrease insulin or oral hypoglycemic dosage prior to exercise

Test blood glucose frequently. Glycemic responses to different circumstances are individual

Schedule exercise 1–2 h after meals, not at peak insulin time

Drink plenty of water before, during, and after exercise

Take caution when exercising in hot weather. Heat loss is less efficient in many patients with diabetes due to poor peripheral circulation and failure of the sweating mechanism

Monitor patients with diabetes for hypertension during exercise and hypotension after exercise

Carry an identification card that indicates that the patient has diabetes

Carry change for a phone call or carry a cell phone

Exercising extremities should not be used as insulin injection sites
  – Inject insulin into the abdomen if exercise will begin 30 min after injection
  – When insulin is injected into the active muscle, muscle glucose is used more rapidly and the elevated insulin levels will inhibit glucose production resulting in hypoglycemia

Patients with peripheral neuropathy will require an alternative method to pulse taking (e.g., RPE)

Abnormal pulse rates and blood pressure responses will be exhibited by those patients with autonomic neuropathy. These patients should also avoid rapid changes in position

Patients with peripheral neuropathy must wear proper shoes and inspect their feet daily for blisters, sores, and ulcers

EXERCISE PRESCRIPTION FOR PATIENTS WITH DIABETES

Prescribing exercise and increasing daily physical activity for people with diabetes must be individualized according to medication schedule, presence and severity of diabetic complications, presence or severity of comorbidities such as CVD or peripheral arterial disease, and goals and expected benefits of the program. As part of instructions offered to the patient regarding an exercise program, the timing and quantity of food intake must also be considered. The goals of patients participating in an exercise program should include:

• Normalization of blood sugar levels
• Minimizing diabetic complications
• Management of body weight
• Incorporating daily physical activity into their lifestyle
• Improving cardiovascular fitness, strength, flexibility, and CVD risk factors

The formulation and components of an exercise prescription for a patient with diabetes are similar to the standard exercise prescription for healthy people but health care professionals need to consider all aspects of this complicated medical condition and analyze and apply the risks and benefits of exercise in a given patient *(38, 47)*.

Mode of Exercise

For those with T2DM, it is important to identify a mode of exercise that can safely and effectively allow for reaching desired levels of exercise intensity that can be maintained. For example, walking is a convenient, low-cost, and low-impact mode of physical activity for those with diabetes. Slow jogging or a combination of walking and jogging may be appropriate for low-risk patients who are not overweight. The speed of walking can be adjusted to the prescribed intensity, based on what is appropriate for the individual patient. Although walking is appropriate for many patients, it may not be feasible for obese patients and those who have DRCs such as peripheral neuropathy or lower-extremity microvascular disease. These patients may require alternative modes that are nonweight-bearing such as stationary cycling, swimming, rowing ergometers, or an exercise modality that offers a seated combination of arm and leg ergometry (e.g., Nu-Step®, Ann Arbor, MI; AirDyne®, Schwinn Fitness, Vancouver, WA; BioStep®, Biodex Medical Systems, Shirley, NY).

Frequency, intensity, and duration of exercise are dependent on one another to produce the desired therapeutic impact on patients with diabetes. Most research would support the notion that the total volume (i.e., number of minutes per week at a minimal intensity) of structured aerobic or resistance exercise training and/or physical activity may be the most important factor to produce the desired results. A consensus statement from the ADA makes the following recommendations regarding volume of exercise *(2, 3)*:

- To improve glycemic control, assist with weight management and reduce risk of CVD, perform 150 min/week of moderate-intensity aerobic physical activity and/or at least 90 min/week of vigorous aerobic exercise.
- Perform >4 hours/week of moderate to vigorous physical activity to achieve greater CVD risk reduction.
- To achieve long-term maintenance of weight loss, 7 hours/week of moderate to vigorous aerobic physical activity may be necessary.

Frequency of Exercise

Exercising ≤2 days/week has minimal effect or benefit and there is little additional cardiovascular benefit from exercising >5 days/week. The duration of glycemic improvement after the last bout of exercise in patients with diabetes is >12 but <72 hours. As a result, it is recommended that for most patients with diabetes, their physical activity should be distributed over 3–5 days/week with no more than two consecutive days without physical activity. Patients on insulin may need to exercise daily in order to lessen the difficulty of balancing caloric needs with insulin dosage. Obese patients may need to participate in daily physical activity to achieve long-term weight loss *(2, 3)*.

Intensity of Exercise

Persons with diabetes who have been inactive should initially engage in physical activity of a low-to-moderate intensity. Higher intensity exercise is associated with greater cardiovascular risk, greater chance for injury, and lower compliance than lower intensity exercise. Monitoring the intensity of physical activity in persons with diabetes may require the use of heart rate and/or ratings of perceived

160 BPM – Peak HR on exercise test

<u>60 BPM</u> – Standing resting HR

100 BPM – Heart rate range

$$100 \times .40 = 40 \text{ BPM};\qquad 100 \times .60 = 60 \text{ BPM}$$
$$\underline{+\quad 60 \text{ BPM}}\qquad\qquad\underline{+\quad 60 \text{ BPM}}$$
$$\text{THRR} = 100 \text{ BPM}\qquad \text{to}\qquad 120 \text{ BPM}$$

Fig. 1. Calculation of a target heart rate range.

Rating	Perceived Exertion
6	
7	Very, very light
8	
9	Very light
10	
11	Fairly light
12	
13	Somewhat hard
14	
15	Hard
16	
17	Very hard
18	
19	Very, very hard
20	

Fig. 2. Borg Scale for rating of perceived exertion.

exertion (RPE). It is imperative that those using the RPE scale become familiar with its use for accurate documentation of a patient's intensity of exercise (9). If a patient with diabetes has a low functional capacity and/or suffers from DRCs (e.g., peripheral neuropathy, autonomic neuropathy, and morbid obesity), it is recommended that exercise generally be prescribed at an intensity corresponding to 40–60% of heart rate reserve (HRR) (*see* Fig. 1) or an RPE of 12–13 (*see* Fig. 2). Patients whose history does not include any complications and whose function is not limited may exercise at intensities corresponding to 50–75% of HRR or an RPE of 13–15. Young patients with T1DM and patients with T2DM who have high functional capacities should be able to exercise at intensities equal to 60–85% of HRR or an RPE of 14–16. Table 7 summarizes these recommendations.

Patients with diabetes should perform an adequate warm-up and cooldown associated with their exercise regimen. Warm-up should be with low-intensity aerobic exercise that raises their heart rate to within 10–20 beats/min of the lower limit of their target heart rate range. At the end of the aerobic conditioning phase of their workout, patients should reduce their intensity for at least 5–10 min before stopping completely. This cooldown helps ensure the gradual return of the heart rate and blood pressure to near-resting levels and reduces the potential for postexercise hypotension and arrhythmias (1).

Table 7
Classification of Intensity of Exercise Based on History of Diabetes-Related Complications (Drcs) and Functional Capacity

History and functional capacity	Heart rate reserve (%)	Ratings of perceived exertion	Intensity
DRCs and/or low function	40–60	12–13	Moderate
No DRCs with preserved function	50–75	13–15	Moderate–hard
High functioning without DRCs	60–85	14–16	Hard

Duration of Exercise

The duration of physical activity for persons with diabetes is directly related to the caloric expenditure requirements and inversely related to the intensity. Initially, those with DRCs and/or who have lower functional capacities should engage in shorter sessions of activity (e.g., 10–15 min) *(38)*. The long-term goal for most patients would be to exercise for 30–45 min for 3–5 days/week *(38)*. Physical activity can be divided into two or three 10–15 min sessions per day to achieve the desired energy expenditure results. For patients who have a goal of weight loss, the intensity should be low to moderate (40–75% HRR) and the duration needs to be incrementally increased to approximately 60 min/day to achieve the goals of 7 h/week of physical activity and of long-term maintenance of major weight loss. But health care professionals should be aware that longer exercise sessions may result in a higher incidence of musculoskeletal injury and lower compliance long term *(1–3)*.

Rate of Progression

Exercise programs for patients with diabetes should gradually increase frequency or duration of exercise initially instead of intensity. It is recommended to avoid having beginning exercisers perform too much exercise too soon. Given that older age and obesity are common elements of T2DM, it may take months rather than weeks for these patients to adapt to a recommended physical activity program. After the desired duration of the activity is achieved, any increase in intensity should be small and approached with caution *(1)*. It is also important to closely monitor the patient's signs, symptoms, and response to exercise as they progress.

PRESCRIBING PROGRESSIVE RESISTANCE TRAINING FOR PATIENTS WITH DIABETES

Progressive resistance training should be included in the treatment regimen of patients with diabetes because it improves physiological and psychological function, increases or preserves lean body mass, and improves glucose homeostasis. In the absence of contraindications *(27)* (*see* Table 8), people with diabetes should be encouraged to perform resistance training as a part of their therapeutic plan. Specific recommendations for safe and effective resistance training are outlined in Table 9 *(27)*.

Caution should be used in cases of advanced retinal and cardiovascular complications. Modifications such as lowering the intensity of lifting, preventing exercise to the point of exhaustion, and eliminating the amount of sustained gripping or isometric contractions should be advised *(9)*. To ensure resistance, exercises are performed correctly, maximize the health benefits and minimize the risk of injury, it is recommended that initial supervision and periodic reassessments are conducted by an experienced clinical exercise physiologist.

Table 8
Medical Contraindications to Resistance Training

Cardiovascular contraindications
    Unstable angina, untreated severe left main coronary artery disease
    Angina, hypotension, or arrhythmias provoked by resistance training
    Acute myocardial infarction
    End-stage congestive heart failure (New York Heart Association Class IV)
    Severe valvular heart disease
    Malignant or unstable arrhythmias[a]
    Large or expanding aortic aneurysm
    Known cerebral aneurysm
    Acute deep venous thrombosis
    Acute pulmonary embolism or infarction
    Recent intracerebral or subdural hemorrhage

Musculoskeletal contraindications
    Significant exacerbation of musculoskeletal pain with resistance training
    Unstable or acutely injured joints, tendons, or ligaments
    Fracture within last 6 months (delayed union)
    Acute inflammatory joint disease

Other contraindications
    Rapidly progressive or unstable neurological disease
    Failure to thrive, terminal illness
    Uncontrolled systemic disease[b]
    Symptomatic or large abdominal or inguinal hernias, hemorrhoids
    Severe dementia/behavioral disturbance
    Acute alcohol or drug intoxication
    Acute retinal bleeding or detachment or severe proliferative diabetic retinopathy
    Recent ophthalmic surgery[c]
    Severe cognitive impairment
    Uncontrolled COPD/CAL
    Prosthesis instability

COPD chronic obstructive pulmonary disease, *CLA* chronic airways limitations

[a]Ventricular tachycardia, complete heart block without pacemaker, atrial flutter, and junctional rhythms

[b]For example, uncontrolled diabetes (symptomatic hyper- or hypoglycemia; $HbA_{1c} >$ 10%), hypertension (untreated systolic BP > 170 mmHg), thyroid disease, congestive heart failure, sepsis, acute illness, and fevers

[c]Laser, cataract extraction, retinal surgery, glaucoma surgery, etc. (collated from Fiatarone Singh)

GUIDELINES FOR INCREASING DAILY PHYSICAL ACTIVITY

The process for motivating an inactive person with diabetes to become physically active is a challenging one. Nevertheless, increasing daily physical activity can be effectively incorporated into a patient's plan of therapy. Health care professionals are in a unique and influential position to motivate their sedentary patients to begin and maintain an effective program of regular physical activity. DiLoreto et al. *(48)* undertook a study to validate a counseling strategy that could be used by physicians

Table 9
Recommendations for Safe and Effective Progressive
Resistance Training in Type 2 Diabetes

Modality
  Machine and/or free weights training
  Large muscle groups of upper and lower body and trunk
  Dynamic lifting through full pain-free range of motion
  Slow velocity during eccentric phase (3–4 s)

Intensity
  Moderate-high (60–80% IRM)
  15–18 on Borg Scale of perceived exertion

Volume
  Two to three set of eight repetitions; 1–2 min rests between sets

Frequency
  Every 48–72 hours

Precautions
  Preactivity medical clearance
  Avoid excessive breath-holding
  Avoid sustained isometric contractions
  Take care with ankle cuffs because of risk of soft tissue injury
  Ensure good posture and technique to avoid back pain

in their daily outpatient practice to promote the adoption and maintenance of physical activity by T2DM patients. Patients were randomized to a behavioral approach to increase daily physical activity or to a usual care treatment group. Outcomes after 2 years included 69% of the patients in the intervention group and 18% of the patients in the control group achieving the target of >10 MET hours/week. In addition, the intervention group achieved significant improvements in body mass index and HbA_{1c} compared to the control group.

The 1996 Surgeon General's report by the US Department of Health and Human Services on Physical Activity and Health states: "Having confidence in one's ability to be active; enjoying physical activity; receiving support from family, friends or peers; and perceiving that the benefits of physical activity outweigh its barriers or costs appear to be central determining factors influencing activity levels across the life span" *(49)*. Health care professionals should use structured counseling in recommending physical activity to their patients with diabetes which includes motivation, self-efficacy, pleasure, support, comprehension, problem solving of barriers to increased physical activity, and recording daily physical activity. See Figs. 3 and 4 for counseling guidelines and establishing specific goals for lifestyle activity in patients with diabetes.

PHARMACOTHERAPY IN CONJUNCTION WITH PRESCRIBING EXERCISE

Treatment of persons with diabetes mellitus includes pharmacotherapy (oral drug therapy and/or insulin injections) as well as making changes in eating patterns, beginning an exercise regimen, and choosing effective ways to manage stress in their life. Patients with T2DM are most prone to experience hypoglycemia during the course of their exercise therapy. Signs of hypoglycemia include nausea, trembling, anxiety, extreme hunger, increased sweating, and rapid heartbeat. This brief review will focus on discussing drugs that *may* and drugs that *do not* contribute to hypoglycemia *(50)*.

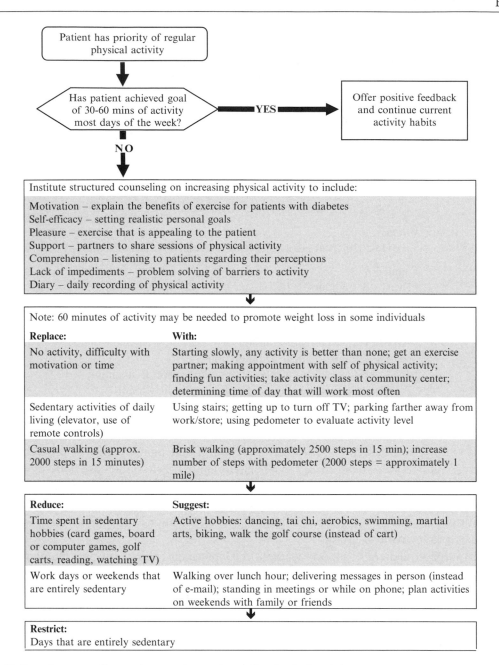

Fig. 3. Guidelines for counseling patients on increasing daily physical activity.

Drugs that may contribute to hypoglycemia:

Sulfonylureas: The sulfonylureas are a class of pharmacological agents that stimulate the release of insulin from β-cells in the pancreas. The possibility of medication-induced hypoglycemia should be a consideration in any patient taking a sulfonylurea. Patients who skip meals, engage in frequent strenuous exercise, and experience significant weight reduction will have an added risk. Sulfonylureas may also be combined with other antidiabetic medications with alternate mechanisms of action, such as metformin and thiazolidinediones. They can also be used in conjunction with insulin therapy, though that is not a first-line combination.

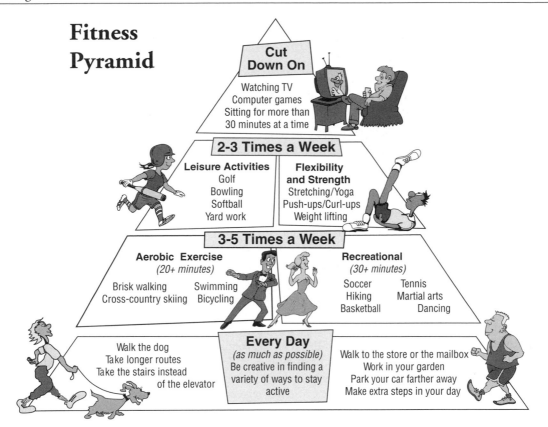

Fitness Pyramid

Cut Down On
Watching TV
Computer games
Sitting for more than
30 minutes at a time

2-3 Times a Week

Leisure Activities
Golf
Bowling
Softball
Yard work

Flexibility and Strength
Stretching/Yoga
Push-ups/Curl-ups
Weight lifting

3-5 Times a Week

Aerobic Exercise
(20+ minutes)
Brisk walking   Swimming
Cross-country skiing   Bicycling

Recreational
(30+ minutes)
Soccer   Tennis
Hiking   Martial arts
Basketball   Dancing

Walk the dog
Take longer routes
Take the stairs instead
of the elevator

Every Day
(as much as possible)
Be creative in finding a
variety of ways to stay
active

Walk to the store or the mailbox
Work in your garden
Park your car farther away
Make extra steps in your day

**Each week, try to increase your physical activity using this guide.
Here's how to start:**

**If you are <u>inactive</u>
(rarely do activity)**

Increase daily activities at the base of the
pyramid by:
- taking the stairs instead of the elevator
- hiding the TV remote control
- making extra trips around the home
  and yard
- stretching while standing in line
- walking when you can

**If you are <u>sporadic</u>
(active some of the time,
but not regularly)**

Become consistent with activity by
increasing activity in the middle of the
pyramid by:
- finding activities you enjoy
- planning activities in your day
- setting realistic goals

**If you are <u>consistent</u>
(active most of the time or
at least 4 days each week)**

Choose activities from the whole
pyramid by:
- changing your routine if you start
  to become bored
- exploring new activities

Above all...have fun!

Fig. 4. Fitness pyramid.

Meglitinides: Meglitinides are another class of hypoglycemics which work similarly to the sulfonylureas, but do not contain the sulfa structural element. They can also be combined with other hypoglycemics such as metformin, rosiglitazone, and pioglitazone, as well as insulin therapy. Similarly to the sulfonylureas, the meglitinides have the potential to cause hypoglycemia. They are of very short duration and may cause problems with hypoglycemia if a patient exercises within an hour of meal time. The risk of hypoglycemia is less with the meglitinides than with the sulfonylureas, as the insulin release is glucose-dependent, reducing the release of insulin when the blood glucose is low.

Insulin: T1DM patients, and many T2DM patients, may require exogenous insulin in addition to therapy with diet and exercise to maintain proper glucose control. The most common adverse effects associated with insulin therapy are hypoglycemia and lipodystrophies.

Newer products: Pramlintide is a synthetic analogue of amylin which lowers glucagon concentrations, slows gastric emptying, and increases satiety. It is indicated in insulin-requiring patients when insulin alone is insufficient. Pramlintide may cause hypoglycemia but does not induce weight gain.

Exenatide is a synthetic incretin which lowers glucagon concentrations, slows gastric emptying, and increases satiety plus stimulates the release of insulin. It is indicated in T2DM and is not approved to be given with insulin. Exenatide does not induce weight gain but may cause hypoglycemia.

See Table 10 for a summary of drugs that *may* contribute to hypoglycemia.

Drugs that do not contribute to hypoglycemia:

Biguanides: Metformin is the only hypoglycemic classified as a biguanide. The exact mechanism of action of metformin is not well understood. Therapeutic indications for metformin include monotherapy for T2DM combined with diet and exercise or in combination with a thiazolidinedione, sulfonylurea, or insulin therapy. Metformin has an advantage over sulfonylurea or insulin therapy in that it has not been shown to cause weight gain. Another advantage over the sulfonylureas is that it is not known to precipitate hypoglycemia.

Thiazolidinediones: Glitazones enhance insulin sensitivity by increasing the expression of glucose transporters (GLUT 1 and GLUT 4). There is a risk of weight gain in patients taking thiazolidinediones, especially if they are coadministered with a sulfonylurea or insulin therapy. Thiazolidinediones are indicated only in the treatment of T2DM and not T1DM. They are preferred to be used in conjunction with sulfonylurea, metformin, or insulin as use of glitazones as a monotherapy has been shown to be relatively ineffective, unless the patient is in the early stages of diabetes. These agents do not usually cause hypoglycemia at therapeutic doses.

α-Glucosidase inhibitors: By delaying the absorption of glucose after a meal, the α-glucosidase inhibitors can reduce postprandial hyperglycemia. However, these agents have relatively no effect on fasting glucose levels. It is essential that these agents be taken with the first bite of the patient's meal. With proper administration, hypoglycemia is not a common side effect of the α-glucosidase inhibitors, though it can occur if these agents are combined with other antidiabetic medication regimens.

Sitagliptin: It inhibits dipeptidyl peptidase-4 resulting in increased insulin release and decreased glucagon release. This drug can be used as monotherapy or in combination with metformin or a glitazone. It does not induce hypoglycemia or weight gain.

Table 10
Drugs that may Contribute to Hypoglycemia During Exercise

Drug	Brand name	Class
Repaglinide	Prandin	Meglitinides
Nateglinide	Starlix	Meglitinides
Glyberide + Metformin	Glucovance	Combination
Glipizide + Metformin	Metaglip	Combination
Pramlintide	Symlin	Synthetic amylin
Exenatide	Byetta	Synthetic incretin
Glimepiride	Amaryl	Sulfonylurea
Glipizide	Glucotrol	Sulfonylurea
Glyburide	Micronase, Diabeta, Glynase	Sulfonylurea
Insulin		

Muraglitazar: It has "glitazone" glucose-lowering effects plus fibrate-like lipid-lowering properties. This medication is more apt to include fluid retention and weight gain compared to glitazones and does not cause hypoglycemia.

See Table 11 for a summary of drugs that do not contribute to hypoglycemia.

β-Blockers can blunt the adrenergic symptoms of hypoglycemia, possibly increasing risk of hypoglycemia unawareness. ACE inhibitors may modestly increase insulin sensitivity, and both ACE inhibitors and aspirin may increase risk of hypoglycemia in some individuals *(2)*.

HYPERGLYCEMIA/HYPOGLYCEMIA: TO EXERCISE OR NOT TO EXERCISE? THAT IS THE QUESTION

The recommendation to avoid physical activity if plasma glucose is >300 mg/dl, even in the absence of ketosis *(51–53)*, is more cautious than necessary for a person with T2DM, especially in a postprandial state. Badenhop et al. *(54)* demonstrated that patients with T2DM who exercise in a cardiac rehabilitation program typically have systematic improvements in blood sugar levels after an exercise training session. Patients who presented with elevated pre-exercise blood sugars rarely exhibited symptomatic hypoglycemia or, in particular, symptomatic hyperglycemia or ketosis during the 24 hours postexercise. Therefore, provided the patient feels well and urine ketones are negative, it is not necessary to postpone exercise based simply on hyperglycemia *(3)*.

If the medication dose or carbohydrate ingestion is not altered, physical activity can cause hypoglycemia in individuals taking insulin and/or insulin secretagogues. Episodes of hypoglycemia are not likely in patients with diabetes who are not treated with insulin or insulin secretagogues. It was previously suggested by the ADA that added carbohydrate should be eaten if pre-exercise glucose levels are <100 mg/dl *(55)*. This recommendation stands for diabetic patients on insulin and/or insulin secretagogues. The revised ADA guidelines identify that supplementary carbohydrate is generally not needed for diabetic patients treated with diet, metformin, α-glucosidase inhibitors, and/or thiazolidinediones without insulin or insulin secretagogues *(2, 3)*.

Patients taking insulin or insulin secretagogues should check blood sugars before, after, and again several hours after completing physical activity. Those patients who show a tendency toward hypoglycemia in response to exercise can either reduce their dose of insulin or insulin secretagogues before activity, consume extra carbohydrates before or during physical activity, or both *(3, 56)*.

Table 11
Drugs that do not Contribute to Hypoglycemia During Exercise

Drug	Brand name	Class
Rosiglitazone	Avandia	Glitazones
Pioglitazone	Actos	Glitazones
Acarbose	Precose	α-Glucosidase inhibitors
Miglitol	Glyset	α-Glucosidase inhibitors
Metformin	Glucophage	Biguanides
Avandia + Metformin	Avandamet	Combination
Actos + Metformin	Actoplus	Combination
Sitagliptin	Januvia	
Muraglitazar	Pargluva	

Guidelines for monitoring diabetic control and patients' response to exercise:

When patients with diabetes begin an exercise program, blood glucose levels associated with exercise should be monitored systematically *(5, 14, 26, 27)*. Monitoring and recording a patient's blood glucose level before and after exercise is important for the following reasons:

- Many patients perceive and report that their diabetes is under good control when it is not!
- Checking blood sugars before and after exercise helps a patient identify when he or she is at immediate risk of becoming hypoglycemic or hyperglycemic.
- Checking blood sugars helps provide the basis for progressing their exercise prescription.
- Monitoring of blood sugars provides positive feedback regarding the effects of exercise.

Guidelines for monitoring patients with diabetes:

It is understood that clinical judgment should be used in conjunction with all finger-stick blood sugar numbers stated below. Clinical judgment should be considered along with:

- What type of insulin/oral medication will be taken?
- What time insulin/oral medication will be taken?
- Time patient last ate.
- Time of exercise session.
- Level of exercise to be performed.

Refer to Tables 12 and 13.

Unless ketosis, symptomatic hyperglycemia, symptomatic hypoglycemia, or diabetes-related symptoms are present, it is acceptable to allow a patient to continue his or her exercise program while at the same time developing a specific plan in conjunction with the patient's physician to optimize blood sugar control. Measures of HbA_{1c} provide a useful approximation of long-term glucose control, which helps in regulating dosing of medications, exercise, and weight-loss goals. A desirable HbA_{1c} reflecting good long-term glucose control and a low likelihood of complications is 7.0 mg/dl or lower.

Foot care is an important consideration for patients with diabetes who exercise. Problems most often develop when blood flow is poor or when there is nerve damage in the legs and feet. Such problems can include very dry skin that may peel or crack, the buildup of calluses that may ulcerate, and foot ulcers particularly at the ball of the foot or on the bottom of the big toe. Exercise staff should routinely inspect diabetic patient's feet, and encourage patients to examine their own feet daily. Patients should be strongly encouraged to bring any sores, infections, or inflammation to the immediate attention of the exercise staff or their physician or podiatrist. In addition, assessment for peripheral

Table 12
Recommended Procedures for Checking Blood Sugar Levels Associated with Exercise

Patients with diabetes taking an oral hypoglycemic agent or insulin for control of their diabetes will have finger-stick blood sugar performed pre- and postexercise for six exercise sessions in order to establish the patient's level of glucose control and subsequent response to exercise. Pre- and postexercise checks of finger-stick blood sugar will continue if values of ≤90 or ≥300 mg/dl are recorded.

A dietitian should be alerted when patients are in poor diabetic control to facilitate reinforcement of dietary aspects of self-care.

When patterns of diabetes control show change (improvement or worsening), a staff member will contact the patient's physician to provide data so that the primary care physician or endocrinologist can make medication adjustments as needed.

Table 13

Recommended Procedure for Managing Finger-Stick Blood Sugar Measures Pre- and Postexercise

If preexercise FSBS is ≥300 mg/dl, a urine sample will be checked for ketones.

No exercise if ketones are present. The patient's physician will be informed.

If FSBS is ≥300 mg/dl, but no ketones, patient may exercise unless:

Type 1 (insulin dependent)	
If FSBS ≥ 300 mg/dl	No exercise[a]
Type 2 (on oral agent/insulin requiring)	
If FSBS ≥ 300 mg/dl and symptomatic	No exercise[a]
Type 2 (on oral agent/insulin requiring)	
If FSBS ≥ 300 mg/dl and asymptomatic	Exercise[a]

Patients should be encouraged to test their blood sugar 1 h after exercise at home or work and be made aware of potential hypoglycemic responses for 24–48 hours after an exercise session.

Patients may need to bring their own glucose-measuring devices to ensure adequate technique and equipment operation and to cross-check with devices used in the health care setting.

Snacks appropriate for abnormal pre- or postexercise blood sugar measures should contain 15–30 g of carbohydrate:

- 4–8 ounces of fruit juice (not tomato juice)
- Four glucose tablets
- Half to one banana
- One cup skim milk

[a]In all of these cases, the patient's physician will be contacted.

neuropathies and pulses should be performed by a physician or podiatrist before a patient with diabetes undertakes a regular exercise program. Staff should instruct patients on the following procedures for care of their feet *(40)*. Refer to Table 14.

Please refer to Chapter (13) for further information on the subject of foot care and neuropathy.

SUMMARY

Regular physical activity provides improved glycemic control, reduces the risks and complications associated with CVD, and improves overall health with minimal risk. In addition to aerobic exercise, current guidelines also recommend resistance training as clinically important for managing glycemic control in older patients with T2DM. Exercise is not considered a primary component of treatment in Type 1 diabetics but patients with T1DM should exercise to reduce their risk for CVD and to enhance their sense of well-being.

Health care professionals should follow established guidelines for screening patients with diabetes before undergoing a moderate to vigorous exercise program. Exercise professionals should know under what conditions (i.e., hypoglycemia/hyperglycemia) it is safe for patients to proceed with exercise and know which medications may or may not cause problems with exercise. Special emphasis should be placed on proper foot care in the treatment of diabetics. Knowing the recommended guidelines related to mode, frequency, intensity, duration, and progression of an exercise prescription is essential. Counseling diabetic patients on strategies to increase their daily physical activity is challenging but is effective in achieving significant improvement in fasting blood glucose and body weight reduction.

Table 14
Instructions for Foot Care of Patients with Diabetes

Inspect feet daily for blisters, cuts, and scratches

Wash feet daily. Dry carefully, especially between the toes

Avoid bathing in extreme temperatures

If feet feel cold at night, wear socks

Do not walk on hot surfaces such as sandy beaches or pool decks

Do not walk barefoot

Do not use chemical agents for the removal of corns and calluses

Do not use adhesive tape on the feet

Inspect the insides of shoes daily for rough areas

Nails and calluses should be trimmed regularly by a podiatrist

Do not soak feet

Apply baby oil for dry feet after bathing and drying feet

Wear properly fitting stockings. Do not wear mended stockings. Avoid stockings
     with seams. Change stockings daily

Do not wear garters

Shoes should be comfortable at the time of purchase

Do not wear shoes without stockings

Do not wear sandals with thongs between the toes

Wear wool socks and protective footwear in the winter

Cut toenails straight across

Do not cut corns and calluses

Be sure that the feet are examined at each physician visit

Notify your physician at once should you develop a blister or sore on your foot

Alternate between two pairs of shoes for exercise in order to keep feet dry

The combination of structured exercise and increasing daily physical activity as therapy, appropriate adjustment of medications, and proper monitoring of finger-stick blood sugar pre- and postexercise in a health care setting may maximize the benefits and minimize the risks for patients with diabetes who make the lifelong commitment of habitual daily physical activity.

REFERENCES

1. American College of Sports Medicine. Guidelines for Exercise Testing and Prescription, 7th Edition. Philadelphia: Lippincott Williams & Wilkins, 2006.
2. Sigal RJ, Kenny GP, Wasserman DH, Castaneda-Sceppa C. Physical activity/exercise and T2DM: A technical review by the American Diabetes Association. *Diabetes Care* 2004;27:2518–2539.
3. Sigal RJ, Kenny GP, Wasserman DH, Castaneda-Sceppa C, White RD. Physical activity/exercise and T2DM; A consensus statement from the American Diabetes Association. Diabetes Care 2006;29:1433–1438.
4. DeFronzo RA, Ferrannmi E, Sato A, Yfelig P, Wahren J. Synergistic interaction between exercise and insulin on peripheral glucose metabolism. *J Clin Invest* 1981;68:1468–1474.
5. Koivisto VA, DeFronzo RA. Exercise in the treatment of Type II diabetes. *Acta Endocrinologica Suppl* 1984;262:107–111.
6. Reitman JS, Vasquez B, Klimes I, Nagulesparan M. Improvement of glucose homeostasis after exercise training in non-insulin dependent diabetics. Diabetes Care 1984;7:434–441.
7. Rogers MA, Yamamoto C, King DS, Hagberg JM, Ehsani AA, Holoszy JO. Improvement in glucose tolerance after 1 week of exercise in patients with mild NIDDM. Diabetes Care 1988;11:613–618.
8. Helmrich SP, Ragland DR, Leung RW, Paffenbarger RS. Physical activity and reduced occurrence of non-insulin-dependent diabetes mellitus. *N Engl J Med* 1991;325:147–152.

9. American College of Sports Medicine and American Diabetes Association Joint Position Statement. Diabetes mellitus and exercise. Med Sci Sports Exerc 1997;29(12):i–vi.

10. American Diabetes Association. Clinical practice recommendations: Diabetes mellitus and exercise (position statement). Diabetes Care 1999;22(Suppl 1):549–553.

11. Franz MJ. Exercise and the management of diabetes mellitus. *J Am Dietetic Assoc* 1987;87(7):872–880.

12. Walberg-Henriksson H. Exercise and diabetes mellitus. In: Hooloszy JO, eds. Exercise and Sport Sciences Reviews. Vol. 20. Baltimore, MD: Williams & Wilkins, 1992:339–368.

13. Kannel W, McGee D. Diabetes and cardiovascular disease: the Framingham Study. *JAMA* 1979;241:2035–2038.

14. Barrett-Connor E, Orchard T. Insulin-dependent diabetes mellitus and ischemic heart disease. Diabetes Care 1985;8:65–70.

15. Robertson W, Strong J. Atherosclerosis in persons with hypertension and diabetes mellitus. *Lab Invest* 1968;18:538–551.

16. Ruderman NB, Schneider SH. Diabetes, exercise and atherosclerosis. Diabetes Care 1992;15(Suppl 4):1787–1793.

17. Holloszy JO, Schultz J, Kusnierkiewic J, Hagberg JM, Ehsani AA. Effects of exercise on glucose tolerance and insulin resistance. *Acta Med Scand* 1986;711:55–65.

18. Myers J, Prakash M, Froelicher V, Do D, Partington S, Atwood JE. Exercise capacity and mortality among men referred for exercise testing. *N Engl J Med* 2002;346:793–801.

19. Thomas N, Alder E, Leese GP. Barriers to physical activity in patients with diabetes. *Postgrad Med J* 2004;80:287–291.

20. Ford ES, Herman WH. Leisure-time physical activity patterns in the U.S. diabetic population. Findings from the 1990 National Health Interview Survey-Health Promotion and Disease Prevention Supplement. Diabetes Care 1995;18:27–33.

21. Nelson KM, Reiber G, Boyko EJ. Diet and exercise among adults with Type 2 diabetes: Findings from NHANES III. Diabetes Care 2002;25:1722–1728.

22. Yamanouchi K, Shinozaki T, Chikada K, Nishikawa T, Ito K, Shimizu S, Ozawa N, Suzuki Y, Maeno H, Kato K, Oshida Y, Sato Y. Daily Walking combined with diet therapy is a useful means for obese NIDDM patients not only to reduce body weight but also to improve insulin sensitivity. Diabetes Care 1995;18:775–778.

23. Walker KZ, Piers LS, Putt RS, Jones JA, O'Dea K. Effects of regular walking on cardiovascular risk factors and body composition in normoglycemic women and women with T2DM. Diabetes Care 1999;22:555–561.

24. Braith RW, Stewart KJ. Resistance exercise training. Its role in the prevention of cardiovascular disease. *Circulation* 2006;113: 2642–2650.

25. Dunstan DW, Daly RM, Owen N, Jolley D, DeCourten M, Shaw J, Zimmet P. High-intensity resistance training improves glycemic control in older patients with T2DM. Diabetes Care 2002;25:1729–1736.

26. Castaneda C, Layne JE, Munoz-Orians L, Gordon PL, Walsmith J, Foldvari M, Roubenoff R, Tucker KL, Nelson ME. A randomized controlled trial of resistance exercise training to improve glycemic control in older adults with T2DM. Diabetes Care 2002;25:2335–2341.

27. Willey KA, Fiatarone Singh MA. Battling insulin resistance in elderly obese people with T2DM. Diabetes Care 2003;26:1580–1588.

28. Eriksson J, Taimela S, Eriksson K, Parviainen S, Peltonen J, Kujala U. Resistance training in the treatment of NIDDM. *Int J Sports Med* 1997;18:242–246.

29. Ishii T, Yamakita T, Sato T, Tanaka S, Fujii S. Resistance training improves insulin sensitivity in NIDDM subjects without altering maximal oxygen uptake. Diabetes Care 1998;21:1353–1355.

30. Honkola A, Forsen T, Eriksson J. Resistance training improves the metabolic profile in individuals with T2DM. *Acta Diabetol* 1997;34:245–248.

31. Dunstan DW, Puddey IB, Beilin LJ, Burke V, Morton AR, Stanton KG. Effects of a short-term circuit weight training program on glycaemic control in NIDDM. *Diabetes Res Clin Pract* 1998;40:53–61.

32. Benn SJ, McCartney N, McKelvie RS. Circulatory responses to weight lifting, walking, and stair climbing in older males. *J Am Geriatr Soc* 1996;44:121–125.

33. Hubinger A, Ridderskamp I, Lehmann E. Metabolic response to different forms of physical exercise in type I diabetics and the duration of the glucose lowering effect. *Eur J Clin Invest* 1985;15:197–205.

34. Wasserman DH, Zinman B, Exercise in individuals with IDDM. Diabetes Care 1994;17:924–937.

35. Zinman B, Zuniga-Guajardo S, Kelly D. Comparison of the acute and long-term effects of exercise on glucose control in Type I diabetes. Diabetes Care 1984;7:515–519.

36. Wallberg-Henriksson H, Gunnarsson R, Rossner S, Wahren J. Long-term physical training in female Type 1 diabetic patients: Absence of significant effect on glycaemic control and lipoprotein levels. *Diabetologia* 1986;29:53–57.

37. Albright AL. Diabetes. In: Durstine JL, ed. ACSM's Exercise Management for Persons with Chronic Diseases and Disabilities. Champaign, IL: Human Kinetics, 1997:94–100.
38. Gordon NF. The exercise prescription. In: Handbook of Exercise in Diabetes. Alexandria, VA: American Diabetes Association, 2002:269–288.
39. Vinik AI, Erbas T. Neuropathy. In: Ruderman N, Devlin JT, Schneider SH, Kriska A Handbook of Exercise in Diabetes. 2nd ed. Alexandria, VA, American Diabetes Association, 2002:463–496.
40. Levin ME. The Diabetic foot. In: Handbook of Exercise in Diabetes. Alexandria, VA: American Diabetes Association, 2002:385–399.
41. Aiello LP, Wong J, Cavallerano JD, Bursell S-E, Aiello LM. Retinopathy. In: Handbook of Exercise in Diabetes. Alexandria, VA: American Diabetes Association, 2002:401–413.
42. Castaneda C, Gordon PL, Uhlin KL, Levey AS, Kehayias JJ, Dwyer JT, Fielding RA, Roubenoff R, Singh MF. Resistance training to counteract the catabolism of a low-protein diet in patients with chronic renal insufficiency: A randomized, controlled trial. *Ann Intern Med* 2002;135:965–976.
43. Report of the Expert Committee on the Diagnosis and Classification of Diabetes Mellitus. Diabetes Care 1997;20:1183–1197.
44. Schneider SH, Khachadurian AK, Amorosa LF, Clemow L, Ruderman NB. Ten-year experience with an exercise-based outpatient life-style modification program in the treatment of diabetes mellitus. Diabetes Care 1992;15:1800–1810.
45. Zarich S, Waxman S, Freeman R, Mittleman M, Hegarty P, Nesto RW. Effect of autonomic nervous system dysfunction on the circadian pattern of myocardial ischemia in diabetes mellitus. *J Am Coll Cardiol* 1994;24:956–962.
46. Langer A, Freeman RM, Josse RG, Steiner G, Armstrong PW. Detection of silent myocardial ischemia in diabetes mellitus. *Am J Cardiol* 1991;67:1073–1078.
47. Gordon NF, Exercise guidelines for patients with NIDDM: An update. *J Cardiopulmonary Rehab* 1994;14:217–220.
48. DiLoreto C, Fanelli C, Lucidi P, Murdolo G, DeCicco A, Parlanti N, Santeusanio F, Brunetti P, DeFeo P. Validation of a counseling strategy to promote the adoption and the maintenance of physical activity by Type 2 diabetic subjects. Diabetes Care 2003;26:404–408.
49. US Department of Health and Human Services. Physical Activity and Health: Report of the Surgeon General. Executive Summary 1–14. Atlanta, Centers for Disease Control and Prevention, 1996.
50. Mauro VF, Taylor ML, Dawson KL, Tabb NC. A Review of Diabetes Mellitus and Its Therapeutic Options. The University of Toledo College of Pharmacy and College of Medicine, November 2006.
51. Jaspan JB. Monitoring and controlling the patient with non-insulin dependent diabetes mellitus. *Metabolism* 1987;36(2) (Suppl 1):22–27.
52. Staten MA. Managing diabetes in older adults. *Phys Sportsmed* 1991;19: 66–77.
53. Taunton JE, McCargar L. Managing activity in patients who have diabetes. *Phys Sportsmed* 1995;23: 41–52.
54. Badenhop DT, Dunn CB, Eldridge S, English SM, Hickey AP, Mayo CH, Gerardo JA, Pruitt TH, Smith R. Monitoring and management of cardiac rehabilitation patients with T2DM. *Clin Exerc Physiol* 2002;3(2):71–77.
55. Zinman B, Ruderman N, Campaigne BN, Devlin JT, Schneider SH. Physical activity/exercise and diabetes mellitus. Diabetes Care 2003;26(Suppl. 1):S73–S77.
56. Berger M. Adjustment of insulin and oral agent therapy. In: Handbook of Exercise in Diabetes. Alexandria, VA: American Diabetes Association, 2002:365–376.

10 Behavior Change Strategies for Increasing Exercise in Diabetes

Brent Van Dorsten

Contents

Abstract

Diabetes is associated with a variety of adverse health conditions including cardiovascular morbidity and mortality. Sedentary activity is a primary contributor to the rapidly escalating prevalence of prediabetes and diabetes in the United States, and a majority of US adults are not meeting recommended guidelines for exercise. This chapter reviews the available research regarding the influence of daily lifestyle activity and structured exercise on health improvement for persons with diabetes. A number of behavioral prescription recommendations are derived from this literature, and the benefit of utilizing behavioral modification techniques in the development and maintenance of increased exercise efforts is discussed. Examples for using specific behavioral techniques in exercise are provided and environmental challenges to creating large-scale behavioral interventions to promote increases in the public's activity level are reviewed.

Key words: Behavior change; Behavior modification; Readiness for change; Motivational interviewing; Exercise; Physical activity; Diabetes.

From: *Contemporary Diabetes: Diabetes and Exercise*
Edited by: J. G. Regensteiner et al. (eds.), DOI: 10.1007/978-1-59745-260-1_10
© Humana Press, a part of Springer Science+Business Media, LLC 2009

INTRODUCTION

A wealth of literature exists to document the increasing prevalence of overweight, obesity, prediabetes, and diabetes in all age groups world wide (1–5). Flegal et al. (3) reported that nearly 65% of the US population is overweight with the prevalence of obesity exceeding 30%, and overweight or obesity has been shown to constitute the strongest predictor for the development of diabetes (6). By 2000, approximately 8.6% of US adults or 16.7 million individuals had been diagnosed with diabetes, with the prediction that this number would more than double in the next 25 years (7, 8). Mokdad et al. (4) reported a 5.6% one-year increase in the prevalence of diabetes from 7.35% to 7.9% in 2000–2001, and a 61% increase in the prevalence of diabetes in USA between 1990 and 2001. Diabetes is associated with a variety of adverse health outcomes culminating in a highly increased prevalence of cardiovascular morbidity and mortality (9, 10). Perhaps none of these data are more ominous that those of Jemal et al. (5) who reported a 45% increase in diabetes-related deaths in US adults in the 15 years from 1987 to 2002.

Additional strong evidence exists to support the potential physiological health improvements that result from increased physical activity and exercise for those with diabetes and prediabetes. Physical activity has been shown to play a major role in the prevention of Type 2 diabetes in high-risk patients separate from its role on body weight (11). Often in combination with dietary changes and weight loss, physical exercise has been shown to actively contribute to the prevention of diabetes in persons with impaired glucose tolerance (1, 12, 13), and to improvements in cardiovascular fitness, improved insulin sensitivity, glycemic control, and hemoglobin A1c measures in patients with Type 2 diabetes (14–19) and reductions in all-cause mortality (20–25). Structured exercise programs have shown to be equally efficacious as pharmacotherapy for improving both glycemic control and cardiovascular risk (26, 27).

Sedentary behavior is a primary contributor to the increase in body weight and prevalence of diabetes in USA. Sedentary activity levels have been shown to associate with a doubled risk of all-cause cardiovascular mortality (28, 29), and the cardiovascular risks associated with sedentary activity may exceed the cardiac risk attributed to chronic disease processes such as diabetes (30). Unlike many of the lifestyle features that behavioral modification strategies have been used to address (e.g., eating, drinking, sleep, and sexual behaviors), there is no human biological drive to exercise (ref). In fact, intentional exertion for the explicit purpose of expending energy seems almost counter to the human physiological tendency to conserve. As such, one of the compelling behavioral challenges in increasing exercise is that an individual likely determines to attempt this change because they "should" or that "it will be good for them" rather than in response to a biological or physiological urge or sensation. For the purposes of this chapter, published definitions of physical activity and exercise will be used. *Physical activity* is typically defined as bodily movement produced via skeletal muscle requiring energy expenditure in excess of resting energy expenditure. *Exercise* is generally defined as intentional, structured, repetitive bodily movements performed with the goal of improving or maintaining physical fitness (7, 31, 32).

In a nationwide effort to combat the deleterious effects of sedentary behavior, it is now widely recommended that adults accumulate at least 30 min of moderate-intensity physical activity on most, preferably all, days of the week (33). However, the Institute of Medicine (34) suggested that this level of activity may be insufficient to maintain normal body weight in adults (e.g., BMI ≤ 25 kg/m^2) and to fully realize the health benefits of consistent exercise. The Institute of Medicine thus offered a recommendation for acquiring at least 60 min of moderate-intensity physical activity (e.g., walking or jogging at 4–5 mph pace) per day. Despite available data which support both recommendations, population surveys suggest that the average adult in USA remains far from meeting these objectives. National data has revealed that over 70% of US women and over 65% of US men fail to achieve the 30-min per day goal *(35)*. Approximately 60% of US adults report no regular or sustained leisure time activity and less than 15% regularly engage in vigorous physical activity *(32)*.

ENVIRONMENTAL INFLUENCES ON SEDENTARY BEHAVIORS

Rapid advances in urbanization and mechanization have contributed to the increasingly sedentary nature of humans. A variety of environmental and technological changes have contributed to the lack of required exercise for the population, with several authors now using the term "toxic environment" *(36–39)* to describe the deleterious impact of these changes on the public's health. In many ways, the increasingly sedentary population may be perceived as a direct by-product of technological advances that require less energy expenditure via physical labor in employment, transportation, increased leisure time, computers, internet, videogames, increased television viewing, decreased availability of and emphasis on physical education in schools, decreasing convenience of walking space, and increasing safety concerns which restrict access to walking, playgrounds, and other outdoor pursuits *(40–43)*. Not surprisingly, the convenience of local destinations and "walkability" of neighborhoods has been shown to associate with higher pedometer readings. King et al. (2003) reported that living within 20 min of a park, walking trail, or retail stores produced increases in walking in neighboring residents *(40)*. While the health benefits of consistent, moderate-intensity exercise are well known, the significant challenge to motivate and sustain long-term behavioral change against these obstacles remains *(44)*.

Watching television, sitting at one's work desk, and working on a computer comprise the majority of daily activities for many US adults. In fact, the average US male spends 29 h/week and the average US female 34 h/week watching television *(45)*. Time spent watching television has been reported to be independently and significantly associated with the risk of developing diabetes, with these estimated weekly viewing averages more than doubling Type 2 diabetes risk for both men and women *(6, 46)*. Hu et al. (2003) reported that each 2 h/day increment that females watch television poses a 23% increased risk for the development of obesity and a 14% risk for development of Type 2 diabetes *(6)*. This would grossly equate to a 56% increased risk of obesity and 34% increased risk of diabetes for women at the estimated average of 34 h of television viewing per week. These authors suggest that each additional 2 h daily increment of sedentary behaviors such as sitting at a desk may add an additional 5% risk of Type 2 diabetes for women. In contrast, even minimal activity change such as standing or walking in one's home can reduce this risk by more than 10%. One hour per day of brisk walking was shown to associate with a 24% reduction in risk for obesity and a 34% risk reduction for developing Type 2 diabetes. The authors conclude that 30% of new cases of obesity and 43% of new cases of Type 2 diabetes could be prevented by making modest lifestyle changes including <10 h of television per week and at least 30 min of brisk walking per day.

PHYSICIAN COUNSELING REGARDING EXERCISE

The average adult in US attends approximately two office visits per year with their primary physician *(47, 48)*, and prior studies suggest that patients desire information about physical activity from their doctors *(49)*. A variety of prominent organizations including the American Heart Association and the US Preventive Services Task Force *(50)* recommend that physicians advise and counsel their patients to increase or sustain physical activity. DiLoreto et al. *(51)* reported that a behavioral physician counseling strategy devised to increase motivation, self-efficacy, pleasure, behavior skills to problem-solving obstacles, and self-monitoring assisted patients in meeting exercise goals associated with improvements in BMI and HbA1c. Nonetheless, it is widely reported that primary care physicians do not regularly counsel patients regarding physical activity and a number of barriers to this counseling have been reported including time constraints, limited reimbursement for efforts, limited knowledge of specific behavioral skills, and lack of confidence in the efficacy of these counseling efforts *(52–55)*.

BEHAVIORAL CONCEPTUALIZATION OF EXERCISE RECOMMENDATIONS

In order to develop explicit behavioral recommendations to increase physical activity in the general public, many specifics of the proposed exercise guidelines must be elucidated including clarifying the most desirable type of activities to pursue, specifying both the amount of time and intensity required, and identifying acceptable derivations of exercise that will achieve the overall goal. As such, a brief review of exercise program specifics shown to be efficacious in improving cardiorespiratory health is provided.

Lifestyle Physical Activity vs. Structured Activity

Lifestyle physical activity is defined as "the daily accumulation of at least 30 minutes of self-selected activities, which includes all leisure, occupational, or household activities that are at least moderate to vigorous in their intensity and could be planned or unplanned activities that are part of everyday life" *(56,* p. 399). In a widely cited study called Project Active *(57)*, 235 sedentary men and women were randomized to either a lifestyle physical activity group ("Lifestyle") or a structured gym-based exercise program ("Structured") for 24 months of intervention (6 months intensive and 18 months maintenance). Lifestyle participants were advised to accumulate 30 min of moderate-intensity physical activity on most, preferably all days per week, and attended weekly group sessions focusing on cognitive and behavioral strategies related to exercise behavior. After 6 months, group meetings were decreased to twice per month. Structured exercise participants were requested to attend at least three supervised exercise sessions per week (50–85% of maximal aerobic capacity for 20–60 min) and to gradually increase participation to five sessions per week. This group received additional supervised instruction in behavioral strategies for 3 weeks then chose preferred activities for an individualized program. During months 7–24, this group attended quarterly meetings and received newsletters and monthly activity calendars to keep them abreast of benefits of exercise. Results indicated that both groups showed similar significant improvements in physical health and cardiorespiratory (VO_2 max) measures, yet neither group produced significant weight change. These results are supported by those of Anderson et al. *(58)* who reported that treatments involving diet plus lifestyle activities (e.g., encouragement to increase walking or using stairs) offered similar health benefits (e.g., weight, triglycerides, and cholesterol) to diet plus supervised structured activity consisting of step aerobics increased from 30 to 45 min three times per week.

Amount of Exercise: How Much is Enough?

The national recommendations for exercise accumulation previously cited suggest some lack of consensus as to the ideal amount of exercise per day to maximize health benefits. In fact, the simple conceptualization of "some is good and more may be better" appears to apply. Brill et al. *(59)* found that groups of individuals exercising either 30 or 60 min per day five times per week in combination with diet achieved similar health benefits despite no changes in body weight. Jakicic et al. (2003)

reported similar results in a study comparing varying degrees of walking intensity and duration *(60)*. In this study, 201 sedentary women were randomized to one of four exercise conditions with variable levels of intensity (high vs moderate) and duration (high duration equaling 2000 kcal/week expenditure vs moderate duration equaling 1,000 kcal/week expenditure) on a 5 day/week basis. A moderately reduced energy diet of 1,200–1,500 kcal/day was recommended. Results after 12 months of treatment indicated significant weight loss in all exercise groups with no between group differences. Cardiorespiratory fitness levels also showed significant improvement in all exercise conditions and no between group differences. Blair et al. *(61)* concluded that 30 min/day of moderate-intensity exercise can provide a substantial and broad range of health benefits for sedentary adults. They further suggested that for those individuals achieving and maintaining 30 min/day, a gradual increase to 60 min/day can offer additional health benefits. SoJung et al. *(62)* reported substantial decreases in visceral fat and skeletal muscle lipids in obese people with and without Type 2 diabetes following 13 weeks of supervised aerobic exercise (60 min/day on five occasions per week). DiLoreto et al. *(27)* similarly supported a gradual accumulation of 60 min of exercise per day by reporting that at least 30 min/day of aerobic leisure time activity (moderate-intensity walking) improved HbA1c and cardiorespiratory measures, but that a dose–response relationship was identified suggesting that additional health benefits could be achieved by increasing exercise accumulations to 60 min/day.

Type of Exercise Prescribed

Given the multitude of available types of exercise, several studies have been conducted to determine the optimal exercise regimens to achieve health improvements. As has been noted throughout this chapter, moderate-intensity exercise consisting of brisk-paced walking is the most commonly recommended physical activity, and walking has been shown to produce multiple health improvements which can lower mortality in persons with diabetes *(21, 43, 63–66)*. Blair et al. *(61)* again suggested that individuals maintaining 30 min/day of exercise may achieve additional health benefits with a gradual increase to 60 min/day utilizing a combination of aerobic, resistance training, and stretching exercises. This recommendation for combinations of different types of exercise was supported by Snowling and Hopkins *(64)* who found that aerobic, resistance, and combined exercise efforts each appeared beneficial in reducing HbA1c, with some evidence supporting combination exercise approaches. Sigal et al. *(31)* provided a comprehensive review of the beneficial effects of different types of physical exercise for individuals with prediabetes, Type 2 diabetes, and obesity. The results of several studies reported that persons with diabetes showed HbA1c improvement after participating in resistance exercise *(17, 31)*. In a meta-analysis of 14 controlled moderate-intensity aerobic and resistance training studies involving individuals with Type 2 diabetes, Boule et al. (2001) identified reductions in HbA1c by an average of 0.66%, an amount that should reduce risk of diabetes complications *(67)*. These results were again achieved despite no changes in body mass.

Long Exercise Bouts vs. Accumulated Short Bouts

While it may intuitively seem beneficial to accumulate exercise minutes in one continuous long-duration bout, available research has not supported this premise. DeBusk et al. *(68)* were among the first to report similar improvements in cardiorespiratory (e.g., VO_2 max) fitness in 18 healthy male subjects who performed either one 30-min exercise bout or accumulated three 10-min bouts on several occasions per week. Jakicic et al. *(69)* randomized 56 overweight adult females to diet plus short-bout exercise (total 40 min for 5 days per week cumulative of several 10-min exercise bouts) vs. long-bout exercise (one 40-min bout of moderate-intensity walking five times per week). Results demonstrated similar cardiorespiratory (VO$_2$ max) improvements in both groups, but with improved adherence (greater number of days, greater cumulative minutes per week) for participants in the short-bout condition. Jakicic et al. *(70)* then expanded upon these results by randomizing 148 sedentary, overweight females to diet plus long-bout exercise sessions, multiple short-bout sessions, or multiple short-bout sessions plus home exercise equipment (e.g., treadmill). All groups showed increased cardiorespiratory fitness from baseline and modest weight loss with no significant between group differences. Weight loss at 18 months was significantly greater in participants exercising more than 200 min/week as compared with those exercising less than 200 min/week, and the provision of home exercise equipment was associated with higher levels of long-term short-bout exercise adherence. In a modest adaptation of these research designs, Schmidt et al. *(71)* randomized a cohort of overweight females to one of three exercise conditions including one 30-min session, two 15-min sessions, or three 10-min sessions per day. Subjects in all groups demonstrated improved cardiorespiratory fitness (VO$_2$ max) and all demonstrated similar weight loss. No significant differences were noted between groups on any measure.

From a behavioral perspective, these results suggest that a minimum of 30 min of moderate-intensity exercise on five occasions per week formulates the basis of exercise goals. This frequency of exercise is supported for persons with diabetes by research suggesting improved insulin sensitivity in insulin-resistant individuals for 16–24 h after a single exercise training bout, and up to 48–72 h after exercise with extended physical training *(72–76)*. Increases to 60 min/day of moderate-intensity exercise may provide additional health improvement benefits for those able to achieve and sustain this exercise level. Structured exercise options have been proven to facilitate health improvement, but research suggests that encouraging increases in lifestyle physical activity can also produce valuable health improvements. As for the type of exercise to prescribe, moderate-intensity walking is the most readily available and cost-effective resource available to most people. Research supports health improvements with moderate-intensity walking for at least 30 min on most days per week *(21, 77)*. Adding additional resistance, aerobic, and stretching exercise components may produce additional health value and offer critical variety in exercise patterns to sustain motivation and pleasure. Multiple short bouts (e.g., at least 10 min duration) can be accumulated within an exercise day to meet the 30 min goal and produce health improvements. These short bouts may be easier to incorporate into busy schedules and may formulate the cornerstone of health behavior change strategies at the outset of attempting to develop and integrate exercise into a daily schedule for sedentary individuals. It appears to be of critical importance that efforts to increase physical activity in persons with obesity or diabetes must also incorporate specific plans to decrease sedentary activities in addition to strategically increasing physical activity to maximize long-term health improvement.

BEHAVIOR MODIFICATION AND EXERCISE

Behavior modification is a specialized area of psychology that utilizes specific theory-based strategies to analyze and modify behavior. The "functional analysis" of behavior involves specifying the relationship between environmental variables and specific behaviors, and "behavioral modification" occurs via the implementation of strategies to modify environmental, cognitive, or affective factors to facilitate the development of adaptive new behaviors *(78, 79)*. Behavioral modification techniques formulate the cornerstone of intentional lifestyle change and have been proven effective in improving exercise habits, dietary change, alcohol and drug misuse, and sleep problems. For decades, applying behavioral change tactics to increase exercise, change diets, and adhere to pharmacotherapy has composed the foundation of diabetes treatment *(64, 80)*.

The basic premise of health behavior change is that graded efforts to increase awareness of maladaptive behavioral patterns and to increase adaptive health behaviors can result in health improvement.

This premise has been widely supported by recent large-scale, multiyear, multicenter investigations of people with prediabetes (1, 13) and Type 2 diabetes (81, 82). The Diabetes Prevention Program (1) was a multiyear, multicenter investigation of the differential effectiveness of an intensive lifestyle intervention, medication, and placebo to delay or prevent the diabetes onset in at risk adults. Behaviorists were an integral part of the study in order to maximally effect the desired lifestyle changes. The goals of the lifestyle intervention were to achieve at least 7% total body weight reduction via dietary modification and at least 150 min/week of physical activity/exercise (e.g., moderate-intensity walking). Over 2.8-year follow-up, the incidence of diabetes was 11.0, 7.8, and 4.8 cases per 100 person years in the placebo, medication, and lifestyle arms, respectively. The lifestyle intervention was found to reduce the incidence of diabetes by 58%, which was significantly greater than all other arms. These impressive results were created by modest lifestyle changes over 2–3 years in which participants lost an approximate average of 10 pounds and increased walking (e.g., nearly three-quarters of lifestyle participants achieved the goal of 150 min or more). The results of the Diabetes Prevention Program study (1) are similar to those reported by Thomilehto et al. (13), who randomized 522 Finish adults with impaired glucose tolerance to either a similar intensive lifestyle intervention (e.g., supervised exercise and personalized dietary counseling) or a control group (e.g., oral and written information about dietary change and increasing exercise but with no personalized instruction). At an average follow-up of 3.2 years, participants in the intensive lifestyle intervention group showed significantly greater weight loss and improved metabolic measures, and a significantly greater number achieved the physical activity goal of more than 240 min/week. Amazingly, the risk of developing diabetes in intervention subjects was reduced by an identical 58% compared to control subjects as previously reported (1). Positive results supporting the protective and preventive effects of intensive and personalized lifestyle interventions including dietary change and activity increase have also been reported in Chinese and Japanese adults with impaired glucose tolerance (12, 83). The results of these large-scale trials are particularly important since they stand in direct contrast to the demoralizing perception that small-to-moderate lifestyle changes are insufficient to produce meaningful health improvement. Blair and Leemakers (84) offered the example that a 75-kg person would gain an average of 1–1.5 kg/year by consuming an extra 10–15 kcal/day, but that this same person could remain weight neutral by burning 15 kcal/day with 2.5 min of moderate-intensity walking. Gregg et al. (21) reported that adults with diabetes who walked at least 2 h/week had a 39% lower all-cause mortality rate and a 34% lower CVD mortality rate than inactive individuals who walked less than 2 h/week. These authors concluded that one death per year for every 61 people with diabetes might be prevented if they were to walk at least 2 h/week.

Brownell et al. (85) suggested three essential phases of behavior change including commitment and motivation for change, initiation of active change strategies, and relapse prevention strategies to maintain change. Behavior change techniques can be applied to overt or observable behaviors, cognitive, and mood factors influencing behavior. Behavioral modification strategies have been successfully applied to motivate exercise efforts, restructure environmental stimuli to promote increased exercise, develop and implement health behaviors, and modify thoughts and self-perceptions which influence physical activity (46, 86–91).

READINESS FOR EXERCISE ADOPTION

Utilization of behavioral modification strategies should be initiated well before a person begins walking or offers their first efforts at increasing exercise. Behavioral techniques can be used both to identify and influence factors affecting a person's decision to embark upon behavior change and to devise, implement, and evaluate specific strategies for producing desired changes. Determining readiness for behavioral change has been suggested as a useful factor in predicting participation with behavior change efforts *(92, 93)*, and the readiness for change construct has been specifically applied to exercise *(94, 95)*. Stage of change, also known as the transtheoretical model (TTM), suggests that individuals consider behavior change via a series of stages that take into account both current behavior and intention to change behavior in a specified time frame. For example, those in the first stage, Precontemplation, are not currently consistently engaging in exercise and have no plans to begin exercising in the next 6 months, while the next progressive stage, Contemplation, includes those who are not exercising but intend to do so regularly within the next 6 months. Those in the Preparation stage are not currently exercising but have begun making small changes in anticipation of beginning, while those in the Active stage have regularly exercised for a period less than 6 months. Those in the Maintenance phase have successfully sustained regular exercise for the last 6 months or longer. Available data suggest that individuals in the Precontemplation stage report the lowest levels of physical activity, while those in the Action and Maintenance stages reported the highest. This is supported by evidence suggesting a significant relationship between reported stage of readiness for change and measures of energy expenditure in women *(95)*. Cowan et al. *(96)* assessed 182 primary care patients and found 15% in the Precontemplation stage, 26% in Contemplation, 50% in Preparation, 7% in Action, and 13% in Maintenance, suggesting that only a small percentage of medical patients may be actively engaged in exercise at a given time.

The TTM further integrates the stage of change constructs of self-efficacy (perceived confidence in one's ability to consistently perform a desired behavior in challenging circumstances), decision balance (a systematic evaluation of the pros and cons of changing behavior), and the processes of behavior change (a series of five cognitive and five behavioral strategies that can assist one to progress through the stages of change). Review of the TTM literature supports that individuals with greater levels of perceived self-efficacy are more likely to adopt exercise behavior *(97, 98)*. An important reminder regarding the readiness for change stages is that an individual may cycle between stages and can relapse back to earlier stages of inactivity at various times. As such, literature assessing decision balance (personal perceptions of pros and cons of becoming increasingly active) has suggested that this assessment is significantly related to stage of change adoption *(99)*, and that increasing the ratio of perceived pros to cons predicted advancing stages of physical activity behaviors *(100)*.

MOTIVATIONAL INTERVIEWING

Introduced by Miller and Rollnick in 1991 *(101)*, motivational interviewing (MI) has been defined as a "client centered, directive method for enhancing intrinsic motivation to change by exploring and resolving ambivalence" *(102*, p. 25). An important part of this definition is the emphasis that motivation for change emanates from within the individual as opposed to requiring persuasion by a healthcare "expert." The historic use of dramatic clinical tactics to motivate change (e.g., the black lung picture, threats of mortality, and group confrontation about behavior) has suggested that external pressure to convince another into pursuing change is unlikely to be successful and potentially risks increasing resistance to change *(102, 103)*. In assessing readiness for change, healthcare providers are increasingly using MI techniques to assist patients in elucidating personal reasons that health behavior change may be desirable, and to acknowledge and validate feelings of ambivalence, one may feel about committing to behavior change. MI is designed to allow individuals to verbalize personal reasons to pursue lifestyle change, to anticipate obstacles that might be encountered, and to identify personal resources to navigate these barriers.

Hettema et al. *(104)* reported meta-analysis results of 72 clinical trials investigating various applications of MI across a range of problematic health behaviors. These authors reported promising initial results for various MI applications to promote increased exercise, dietary adherence, and success in eating disorder programs. Other research has suggested moderate effects sizes for diet and exercise behaviors with study results having been well maintained *(105)*. Motivational interview strategies used in combination with other behavioral interventions have shown promise in increasing reported physical exercise *(106–109)*, and studies utilizing MI techniques in obesity treatment with various diet and exercise strategies have demonstrated improved adherence with treatment *(110, 111)*. In a recent review of the applications of MI in weight loss, Van Dorsten *(112)* concluded that the current literature supports the use of MI adaptations in weight loss, weight loss maintenance, exercise behaviors, and regimen adherence.

Empirical isolation of specific MI effects has been difficult given that multiple adaptations of the MI interview approach have been published. Motivational interviews were originally designed as a pretreatment motivational strategy, but the MI effect may be enhanced or prolonged with additional repetitions or booster sessions *(104)*. Serial assessments of motivation for change can be conducted at specific time increments such as annually or even seasonally. MI interviews can be repeated every three months to identify specific motivations to sustain healthy behavior change efforts during different seasons when tangible obstacles or motivations may vary greatly. MI techniques were also initially designed to be used on an individual basis, yet many assessment and intervention strategies in health care may be best delivered on a group basis. Rollnick et al. *(113)* suggested that conducting MI in group settings may hold considerable promise in terms of time economy and clinical utility. Initial efforts to utilize MI techniques in clinical group settings have shown considerable promise *(114–116)* and a manual to incorporate MI principles into psychoeducational groups has been developed *(117)*.

COMMONLY USED BEHAVIORAL STRATEGIES IN EXERCISE ADOPTION

A body of evidence exists to support behavior modification interventions in improving glycemic control in diabetes *(86, 89, 90, 118)*. The research findings reviewed in aggregate suggest that even minimal increases in physical activity for sedentary individuals with diabetes may produce positive health improvements, and that the gradual development of a consistent exercise regimen may produce additional health benefits. Behavior modification techniques are readily applicable for assisting individuals to improve exercise behaviors. The fundamental goals of a behavioral approach are to increase awareness of current or deleterious health patterns, identify explicit behavior change goals, break individual behaviors into operational units, devise strategies to incrementally develop and master the desired behaviors, and plan relapse prevention strategies to sustain the long-term performance of the newly developed health behaviors. A brief discussion of several applicable behavioral techniques in establishing exercise behaviors follows, and a number of examples of applications of these principles in exercise adoption appear in Table 1.

Self-Monitoring

A mandatory first step in approaching health behavior change is increasing objective awareness of current behavioral patterns. Many individuals perceive themselves as being more active and much closer to meeting published exercise recommendations than they actually are. In fact, errors in unstructured estimates of energy expenditure have been reported to be as high as 50% *(119, 120)*. Others may perceive themselves as completely sedentary and overwhelmed with the prospective challenge of eventually achieving sufficient levels of exercise to improve their health. Self-monitoring is the term used to describe the systematic recording of behaviors selected for change. In exercise adoption, numbers of steps accumulated via pedometer recordings, minutes of intentional daily exercise, number of stairs walked, increases in lifestyle activities (e.g., minutes spent raking leaves, mowing the lawn), or amount of time spent watching television, sitting at a desk, or working on a computer may all be targeted for

Table 1
Examples of Behavioral Modification Strategies in Exercise Adoption and Maintenance

Behavioral technique	Purpose(s)	Target uses/Examples
Self-monitoring	Increase awareness of behavior patterns Increase accuracy of behavior estimates Reinforce changes in target behaviors	Daily activity minutes/steps Type of activity utilized each day Factors influencing activity pattern • mood, negative thoughts • weather, pain • medication adherence • television/computer time • glucose before/after exercise
Goal setting	Specify realistic, measurable, obtainable incremental goals for target behaviors Decreasing sedentary behaviors	Graded activity increases • achieving moderate-intensity • minutes per day/week • number of pedometer steps • number of days per week Reducing time spent watching television or working on a computer
Behavioral contracting	Specify criteria for increases in target behaviors, decreases in maladaptive behaviors Specify rewards for contract fulfillment	• activity amount/type/frequency • time management schedule • incremental goals • reinforcement/rewards
Reinforcement planning	Extrinsic Intrinsic	• positive comments from others • buying new shoes, clothes • entering walks, fun-runs • pleasurable activities, massage • self-perception ("a walker") • positive self-esteem changes • increased stamina • changes in body appearance • improved metabolic measures
Problem-solving	Stepwise algorithm to modify challenges to consistent efforts at behavior change	Obstacles to exercise adherence • adverse weather • mall walking • minor injuries • apathy • mood challenges • walking partners/social support
Stimulus control/cues	Prompt occurrence of target behaviors	Color dots to prompt awareness • exercise goals • taking stairs Increase visual cues to prompt activity • equipment, clothes, shoes Electronic calendar prompts to exercise

(*continued*)

Table 1
(continued)

Behavioral technique	Purpose(s)	Target uses/Examples
Changing the environment	Make changes in home/work environments to support performance of the target behavior	Keep walking shoes in sight at home/office Packing exercise clothing for work Preparing exercise equipment for easy use Changing one's social environment to increase exposure to others attempting positive activity change
Cognitive restructuring	Identify/modify self-defeating thoughts	Inaccurate self-perceptions • too out of shape to start • won't do any good • lazy, weak, failure • lack will-power
	Increase self-rewarding thoughts to motivate change efforts	Encouraging thoughts • I can do it this time • will succeed in the long run • little changes will help • a lapse is not a crisis • proud of myself for trying again
Social support	Identify positive resources Identify new/extended resources	• Enlist family/friends in efforts • Medical treatment providers • Community/public resources/clubs • Exercise groups • Professional organization exercise classes (e.g., Arthritis Foundation) • Online support groups for activity
Relapse prevention	Define lapse and relapse Develop plans to reengage Develop resources to contact to assist with reengaging	• Set explicit criteria to reengage • Identify multiple resources to assist re-engagement efforts • Multiple community resources for activity, continued contact, and support

self-monitoring to quantify current patterns. Daily monitoring of additional factors which influence exercise intention (e.g., mood states, perceived obstacles, weather, time availability) can also provide critical information in explicitly clarifying influences on exercise behavior. Self-monitoring of activity can provide an objective baseline level of activity and may frequently stimulate adaptive changes in the target behavior in response to the feedback acquired from recording. From the information acquired via self-monitoring, individually-tailored incremental goals for behavior change can be established. It is important to remember that self-monitoring should be used to increase awareness of positive behavioral patterns as well as maladaptive behaviors and to identify interpersonal strengths. Far too often, daily recording of behavior is used solely to identify problem areas and becomes perceived as a "weapon" rather than an assessment tool. Creatively using self-monitoring to episodically increase awareness of positives may increase long-term motivation and provide reward for initial change efforts.

Goal Setting

For many people, the chasm between current behavioral practices and the ultimate amount of behavior change they perceive as necessary to improve health can be immobilizing from both a motivational and a behavioral perspective. Using information obtained via the daily recording of behavior, the development of realistic, obtainable, and measurable goals for the graded increase in exercise performance is critical to long-term success. Overall goals must be divided into individual weekly goals, and these weekly goals can be sequentially increased over an extended time period. Initial behavior change goals may include setting a minimum number of minutes per day to walk or meeting a step goal, or reducing the amount of time watching television or working on a computer. The initial goal can be established as perhaps a 10% increase in the amount of time or number of steps monitored at baseline. In time, incremental goals can be linked together until a person might achieve three or more 10-min walking sessions per day and thereby meet their ultimate minute goal. For completely sedentary individuals, appropriate initial goals may include increasing the amounts of time or steps acquired via increasing leisure time or lifestyle activities (e.g., increasing number of steps in the home, decreased time reclining), with a goal to eventually work up to one 10-min exercise bout at moderate-intensity effort. Continued graded efforts might eventually allow the individual to achieve two or more 10-min walking or exercise bouts. Social support and reinforcement for persistent effort is critical as it realistically may take weeks or months to increase activity levels to achieve the desired number of minutes per day and/or the number of days per week.

Behavioral Contracts and Reinforcement Planning

Behavioral or *contingency* contracting is yet another tool which can be used to specify the "rules" and rewards for performance. Behavioral contracts are commonly an "effort agreement" between two parties (e.g., the person attempting behavior change and a family member, health care professional, or peers also attempting to be more active) in which the goal behavior is explicitly defined, the number of repetitions of the exercise behavior is specified, and the time frame for completion is defined. An initial contract for a sedentary person attempting to increase activity may include walking at moderate intensity (e.g., a more rapid pace than usual), for a given number of minutes, for a minimum number of days per week for the next one or two weeks. This contract should also include the identification of very specific rewards which will be provided when the contingencies in the contract are achieved. Self-reward is a necessary component of exercise contracts and is the basis of the premise of self-management of behavior. As it is unlikely that an external resource may always be available to provide support, peers can verify performance and offer rewards. Behavior change contracts, often signed by others witnessing the commitment, can be important strategies in motivating patients to maintain efforts over time *(121, 122)*. As an individual's performance gradually improves, contracts may be extended to longer time periods, with specified increases in exercise minutes or steps, or number of days per week of exercise to achieve an overall goal.

An associated and critical portion of contingency contracting is the specification of a reward or *reinforcer* that can be administered at the successful conclusion of an incremental contract. This reward is intended to increase the probability that the target behavior will increase in frequency. Reinforcers need to be individually determined and logically scrutinized for convenience, availability, and feasibility. Rewards may be primarily *extrinsic* or externally provided early in behavior change and may include pleasurable activities (e.g., camping, bowling), movies, clothing, a massage or spa day, motivating comments by others, or purchasing a desired but inexpensive item. Over time, rewards may become increasingly *intrinsic* or from within the individual. Intrinsic reinforcers might include changes in self-esteem (e.g., feeling better about oneself, looking more healthy, perceiving ease of activity, or daily movement) or improved self-perceptions (e.g., more confident in abilities, increased pride for efforts, positive self-statements). Long-term behavior change may be facilitated by a gradual change in the way an individual perceives and defines themselves (e.g., going from "trying to walk more" to someone who defines themselves as "a walker.")

Problem Solving

As was previously discussed, MI can precede behavior change to identify potential obstacles that might interfere with consistent change efforts. It is quite unlikely, however, that anyone might realistically anticipate the entire range of challenges which might be encountered when performing high-frequency behaviors over time. As such, formal training in the stepwise process of problem solving constitutes a valuable component of behavioral modification skill instruction in exercise. Problem-solving techniques generally include five steps which are: identifying and operationally defining specific obstacles to long-term behavioral performance, brainstorming a number of potential solutions to each challenge, considering the ease of applicability of each option, selecting and implementing a high-probability option to navigate a given obstacle, and evaluating the success of the chosen option. This problem-solving algorithm can be flexibly applied to both overt/environmental challenges (e.g., winter weather, transportation, financial issues, physical injuries, and schedule conflicts) and covert/intrapersonal obstacles (e.g., amotivation, depression, and negative self-statements). Both external and internal factors may challenge the successful integration of long-term behavior changes and must be addressed. Wanko et al. *(43)* reported a series of anticipated barriers to long-term exercise performance including painful injury, lacking "willpower" or feeling that one's health is not good enough to begin an exercise regimen, lack of specific insights about what to do, and a host of convenience and safety concerns (e.g., having no one to exercise with, lack of convenience of a place to exercise out of the home, and safety concerns). Any of these barriers to exercise may materialize at different time periods and instructing an adaptive problem-solving strategy which can be used to navigate these challenges can improve long-term outcomes.

Stimulus Control/Prompting

Stimulus control is the behavioral strategy designed to identify and modify environmental cues or prompts associated with increasing activity. Multiple environmental cues are present each day which may prompt inactivity (e.g., television remote controls and easy access transportation) and a commitment to increase activity comes with an inherent acknowledgement that behavior change is not initially convenient. Being sedentary is *convenient*, and identifying rival "convenient" resources to expedite changes in activity is a necessary prerequisite for successful behavior change. Multiple prompts can be strategically placed in one's home and work environment to cue activity increases. For example, placing exercise clothes in readily available carry bags for work, creating a convenient space for home exercise equipment to facilitate ease of use, keeping walking shoes in sight at both home and work, charting of walking days and times, using electronic schedule prompts to remind of exercise times, or placing simple adhesive color dots in high-traffic areas to prompt one to acquire walking minutes can all be successfully incorporated into home and work places to increase salient "reminders" of commitment and to fulfill each day's exercise goal.

Changing the Environment

Many of the behavioral tactics discussed can be utilized to modify the environment from one that tolerates or promotes inactivity to one that makes physical activity increasingly convenient and accessible. Jakicic et al. *(70)* reported that availability of home exercise equipment improved long-term adherence with exercise goals. Many people have exercise equipment that remains in a box, under a bed, in storage, in the garage, or tucked away in a seldom used part of the home. Placing exercise equipment in prominent sight near televisions or windows increases the availability and convenience and provides an important visual prompt to exercise. Keeping exercise clothing and shoes convenient and accessible further increases the ease of initiating exercise sessions. Rearranging home and work schedules to include exercise periods can raise the probability that exercise will occur. Surveying one's neighborhood for available parks, sidewalks, malls, or facilities that can be incorporated into an exercise regimen is critical. Using an automobile to gauge relative distances can be incorporated along with pedometer steps in measuring relative distances to establish incremental goals. Finally, changing one's environment might include modifying the social environment as well to increase exposure to others who are similarly attempting behavior change or to increase contact with those who support and encourage increased physical activity to improve health.

Cognitive Restructuring

Just as humans develop a variety of daily physical habits that become increasingly "automatic" determinants of behavior, we are equally prone to developing cognitive "habits" that influence our perceptions of ourselves, our world, and our daily behavior. Most people contemplating activity increases have made multiple prior unsuccessful attempts to exercise. The aggregate impact of prior attempts may be positive (e.g., person has gradually acquired skills that will help them eventually succeed) or profoundly negative (e.g., person has "learned" that they "lack willpower" or are "too weak" to succeed). As such, a review of cognitions and beliefs impacting previous attempts will very often identify negative and self-defeating thoughts and beliefs regarding one's ability to succeed in making future behavioral changes. Negative thoughts can become self-defeating as they may adversely impact a person's motivation to attempt future exercise and may serve as a strong prompt for abandoning activity efforts.

Cognitive-behavioral theory suggests that cognition and behavior are partially determined by one's self-perceptions and the amount of control one perceives to make changes in their world. Cognitive restructuring strategies can be used to make individuals more aware of maladaptive "distortions" or self-defeating perceptions *(123)*. Once these perceptual "tendencies" are identified, behavioral strategies can be used to actively challenge self-defeating self-perceptions (e.g., "will never succeed"). A number of behavioral techniques may be combined to modify these distortions including self-monitoring to increase awareness, problem-solving strategies to combat negative self-talk, and planning reinforcement to reward efforts to confront maladaptive perceptions. While it may be tempting to overlook cognitions related to exercise performance, clinical experience suggests that thoughts and beliefs may have considerable impact on the initial motivation for activity increase and the long-term consistency of change efforts.

Social Support

Involving influential others in behavior change efforts can have a significant effect on long-term motivation and productivity. Individuals attempting activity increases are encouraged to keep social support members aware of goals and to involve others whenever possible in exercise sessions *(124)*. Wallace et al. *(125)* reported that individuals who began a fitness program with their spouse had higher levels of adherence at 12 months than those who joined alone. In an interesting report of the potential influence of social others on exercise performance, Brekke et al. *(126)* reported that brief educational interventions with nondiabetic relatives of people with diabetes had a positive and statistically significant influence on producing increased physical activity in sedentary family members with diabetes. Consistent with previous discussions of barriers to exercise, having no one to exercise with has been reported as a primary barrier to exercise maintenance (43). Rather than relying exclusively on one walking partner (e.g., the buddy system) or one's spouse, individuals embarking on exercise behavior change should be encouraged to identify and enlist as many influential others as possible for the purpose of walking companionship, encouragement, and reviewing goal achievement. Online support resources, walking groups, and fitness facilities may provide consistent and positive exposure to others with similar goals to influence success.

Relapse Prevention

Available research supports that it is notoriously difficult to sustain participation with moderate or intensive activity regimens to achieve long-term effects. More than 50% of individuals who begin exercise regimens discontinue within 3–6 months (127, 128). Sallis et al. (129) reported that among women adopting either moderate or vigorous intensity activity, discontinuation rates were 30% and 50% for moderate and vigorous exercisers, respectively, between 6 and 12 months. Most individuals will cycle between the stages of readiness for exercise and episodically fall out of the active stage. Waning motivation, significant schedule changes, loss of exercise partners, or physical injury may all contribute to an episodic hiatus from activity.

Short-duration interruptions of exercise are referred to as a "lapse," while longer-term "relapses" are defined as a discontinuation of exercise behavior for a sufficient period so as to allow one's baseline status to return (85). A more concerning notion of "collapse" was suggested by Marlatt and Gordon (130) and cautioned that if a sufficient number of relapse episodes were experienced by an individual in repeated efforts to change behavior, motivation for future efforts could be diminished. As such, defining lapse threats and conceptualizing them as realistically inevitable in long-term behavioral change is recommended. Utilizing motivational strategies to reinvigorate efforts and enlisting problem-solving techniques to navigate obstacles and devise restart efforts can successfully shorten lapses away of action. Relapse may reasonably occur following more severe events (e.g., significant injury), but is often the product of failure to explicitly define relapse indicators (e.g., no exercise periods for seven days or exercising only once per week for four consecutive weeks). Once these criteria are developed, awareness of relapse threats is heightened, and a specific action plan (e.g., returning to structured exercise options, devising a reintroduction plan, and contacting social support or providers) can be established to facilitate prompt return to active performance. Failure to consider and specify relapse criteria may prolong inactivity until basal levels of sedentary activity return.

Among the factors shown to associate with behavior change adherence is maintaining long-term contact with treatment providers and/or peers (131, 132). Follow-up contacts can be efficiently accomplished via episodic individual or group meetings, telephone, or internet (56, 133, 134). The optimal frequency of maintenance contacts is largely unknown, but should be devised in response to attendance frequency and exercise performance. Improved results of structured exercise programs in the last two decades may be related to extending active program lengths from weeks to ten months or longer (131). For persons with access to structured exercise resources, restart programs offering the opportunity to reengage in an active intervention strategy during maintenance (e.g., exercise groups or supervised activity programs) should be considered to reestablish and strengthen beneficial behavioral patterns. Alternatively, provision of personal trainers and monetary incentives to sustain healthy lifestyle behaviors (135, 136) and group-contingent work site competitions (122, 137) have been successfully used to achieve ongoing participation with weight loss and exercise programs.

SUMMARY AND FUTURE WORK

Historically, it has proven difficult to isolate the effect of behavioral modification instruction on exercise outcomes or improving diabetes outcomes as most studies have employed varying combinations of exercise, diet, pharmacotherapy, and behavioral modification packages. Meta-analytic attempts to determine these specific effects have yielded small-to-moderate short-term effect sizes for behavioral self-management interventions in diabetes management (86, 87, 91). Continued efforts to elucidate the most efficacious behavioral and educational components of diabetes self-management approaches are needed. Given the lack of definition of the ultimate behavioral package or approach, clinicians and researchers must remain creative in combining behavioral techniques to promote exercise adoption and long-term maintenance.

A number of practical behavioral recommendations for increasing exercise can be derived from the data in this chapter. Improving health outcomes via exercise has become a combination task of reducing daily sedentary activity and increasing activities designed to intentionally expend energy. Making efforts to increase lifestyle, leisure, and recreational activities in addition to structured activity has been shown to produce health improvement. Daily exercise quotas can be accumulated via multiple short bouts as well as extended single sessions of activity. Individuals with diabetes seeking improved cardiorespiratory fitness should exercise as many times per week as possible but with a minimum goal of 4–5 days/week to maintain enhanced insulin sensitivity. Accumulating 30 min of exercise has shown to produce fitness improvements, and additional health benefits may be achieved by increasing exercise duration to 60 min/day. As it is known that more than half of people initiating behavior efforts to increase exercise discontinue within 6 months, longer-term and sustainable behavioral strategies must be emphasized in treatment planning. Implementing readiness for change and MI strategies have shown promise in maintaining efforts and must be consistently utilized in future programs. Rollnick et al. (138) have recently authored an MI text to facilitate specific applications with healthcare patients (138).

Profound environmental challenges exist to increasing the activity level of the general public. Dunn et al. (56) reported that studies employing intense and frequent behavioral skill instruction have shown success in increasing physical exercise with multiple populations, but that these results have not yet been far reaching as they have been largely confined to small group instruction in clinical settings. These authors recommended increasing the availability of behavioral skill instruction to larger numbers of individuals via their introduction in naturalistic work-site programs, computer-based programs, or web-based behavior change programs. Wing et al. (139) presented an excellent summary of environmental challenges that need be navigated to promote increases in physical activity and intentional exercise in USA. These authors encourage the development of large-scaled interventions including improved community development to increase activity convenience (e.g., sidewalks and improved lighting) and community program development (e.g., walking programs) to address the broad need to increase the general publics' participation in regular physical activity.

Significant behavioral challenges exist in improving the physical activity levels of adults, adolescents, and children in USA. Epidemiological data suggests that population rates of obesity and diabetes are rapidly increasing and that sedentary lifestyle is independently related to chances of developing diabetes. Fortunately, the data reviewed in this chapter supports the benefits of increasing physical activity even by a relatively small amount and holds promise that both small- and large-scale activity programs might improve the fitness levels of the general population and someday reverse the alarming health trends of the last two decades.

REFERENCES

1. Diabetes Prevention Program Research Group. Reduction in the incidence of Type 2 diabetes with lifestyle intervention or metformin. *N Engl J Med* 2002; 346:393–403.
2. Mokdad AH, Serdula MK, Dietz WH, Bowman BA, Marks JS, Koplan JP. The spread of the obesity epidemic in the United States, 1991–98. *JAMA* 1999; 282:1519–1522.
3. Flegal KM, Carroll MD, Ogden CL, Johnson CL. Prevalence and trends in obesity among US adults, 1999–2000. *JAMA* 2002; 288:1723–1727.
4. Mokdad AH, Ford ES, Bowman BA, Dietz WH, Vinicor F, Bales VS, Marks JS. Prevalence of obesity, diabetes, and obesity-related health risk factors, 2001. *JAMA* 2003; 282:76–79.
5. Jemel A, Ward E, Hao Y, Thun M. Trends in leading causes of death in the United States, 1970–2002. *JAMA* 2005; 294:1255–1259.
6. Hu FB, Leitzmann MF, Stampfler MJ, Colditz GA, Willett WC, Rimm EB. Physical activity and television watching in relation to risk of Type 2 diabetes in men. *Arch Int Med* 2001; 1612:1542–1548.
7. LaMonte MJ, Blair SN, Church TS. Physical activity and diabetes prevention. *J Appl Physiol* 2005; 99:1205–1213.
8. King H, Aubert RE, Herman WH. Global burden of diabetes 1995–2025: Prevalence, numerical estimates, and projections. *Diabetes Care* 1998; 21:1414–1431.
9. Grundy SM, Benjamin IJ, Burke GL, Chait A, Eckel RH, Howard BV, Mitch W, Smith SCJ, Sowers JR. Diabetes and cardiovascular disease: A statement for healthcare professionals for the American Heart Association. *Circulation* 1999; 100:1134–1146.
10. Howard BV, Rodriguez BL, Bennett PH, Harris MI, Hamman R, Kuller LH, Pearson TA, Wylie-Rosett J. Prevention Conference VI: Diabetes and Cardiovascular Disease; Writing Group 1: Epidemiology. *Circulation* 2002; 105:132–137.
11. Kriska AM, Saremi A, Hanson RL, Bennett PH, Kobes S, Williams DE, Knowler WC. Physical activity, obesity, and the incidence of Type 2 diabetes in a high risk population. *Am J Epidemiol* 2003; 158:669–675.
12. Pan XR, Li GW, Hu YH, Wang JX, Yang YW, An ZX, Hu ZX, Lin J, Xiao JZ, Cao HB, Liu PA, Jiang XG, Jiang YY, Wang JP, Zheng H, Zhang H, Bennett PH, Howard BV. Effects of diet and exercise in preventing NIDDM in people with impaired glucose tolerance. The Da Qing IGT and Diabetes Study. *Diabetes Care* 1997; 20:537–544.
13. Tuomilehto J, Linstrom J, Eriksson JG, Valle TT, Hamalainen H, Ilanne-Parikka P, Keinanen-Kiukaanniem S, Laakso M, Louheranta A, Rastas J, Salminen V, Uusitupa M. Prevention of Type 2 diabetes mellitus by changes in lifestyle among subjects with impaired glucose tolerance. *N Engl J Med* 2001; 344:1343–1350.
14. Bassuk SS, Manson JE. Epidemiological evidence for the role of physical activity in reducing risk of Type 2 diabetes and cardiovascular disease. *J Appl Physiol* 2005; 99:1193–1204.
15. Boule NG, Kenny GP, Haddad E, Wells GA, Sigal RJ. Meta-analysis of the effect of structured exercise training on cardiorespiratory fitness in Type 2 diabetes mellitus. *Diabetologia* 2003; 46:1071–1081.
16. Ellis SE, Elasy TA, Sigal RJ, Boule NG, Kenny G. Exercise and glycemic control in diabetes. *JAMA* 2001; 286:2941–2942.
17. Dunstan DW, Daly RM, Owen N, Jolley D, DeCourten M, Shaw J, Zimmet P. High-intensity resistance training improves glycemic control in older patients with Type 2 diabetes. *Diabetes Care* 2002; 25:1729–1736.
18. Fritz T, Rosenqvist U. Walking for exercise – Immediate effect on blood glucose levels in Type w diabetes. *Scand J Health Care* 2001; 19:31–33.
19. Weinstein AR, Sesso HD, Min Lee I, Rexrode RM, Cook NR, Manson JE, Buring JE, Gaziano M. The joint effects of physical activity and body mass index on coronary heart disease risk in women. *Arch Int Med* 2008; 168:884–890.
20. Jonker JT, DeLaet C, Franco OH, Peeters A, Mackenbach J, Nusselder WJ. Physical activity and life expectancy with and without diabetes. *Diabetes Care* 2006; 29:38–43.
21. Gregg EW, Gerzoff RB, Caspersen CJ, Williamson DF, Narayan KMV. Relationship of walking to mortality among US adults with diabetes. *Arch Int Med* 2003; 163:1441–1447.
22. Tanasescu M, Leitzmann MF, Rimm EB, Hu FB. Physical activity in relation to cardiovascular disease and total mortality among men with Type 2 diabetes. *Circulation* 2003; 107:2435–2439.
23. Warburton DER, Nicol CW, Bredin SSD. Health benefits of physical activity: The evidence. *Can Med Assoc J* 2006; 174:801–809.
24. Wei M, Gibbons LW, Kampert JB, Nichaman MZ, Blair SN. Low cardiorespiratory fitness and physical inactivity as predictors of mortality in men with Type 2 diabetes. *Ann Intern Med* 2000; 132:605–611.
25. Leitzmann MF, Park Y, Blair A, Ballard-Barbash R, Mouw T, Hollenbeck AR, Shatzkin A. Physical activity recommendations and decreased risk of mortality. *Arch Int Med* 2007; 167:2453–2460.
26. Conn VS, Hafdahl AR, Mehr DR, Lemaster JW, Brown SA, Nielsen PJ. Metabolic effects of interventions to increase exercise in adults with type 2 diabetes. *Diabetologia* 2007; 50:913–921.
27. DiLoreto C, Fanelli C, Lucidi P, Murdolo G, DeCicco A, Parlanti N, Ranchelli A, Fatone C, Taglioni C, Santeusanio F, DeFeo P. Make your diabetic patients walk: Long term impact of different amounts of physical activity on Type 2 diabetes. *Diabetes Care* 2005; 28:1295–1302.
28. Blair SN, Kohl HW, Paffenbarger RS, Clark DG, Cooper KH, Gibbons LW. Physical fitness and all-cause mortality: A prospective study of healthy men and women. *JAMA* 1989; 262:2395–2401.

29. Kujala UM, Kaprio J, Sarna S, Koskenvuo M. Relationship of leisure-time physical activity and mortality. *JAMA* 1998; 279:440–444.

30. Blair SN, Kampert JB, Kohl HW, Barlow CE, Macera CA, Paffenbarger RS, Gibbons LW. Influences of cardiorespiratory fitness and other precursors on cardiovascular disease and all-cause mortality in men and women. *JAMA* 1996; 276:205–210.

31. Sigal RJ, Kenny GP, Wasserman DH, Castaneda-Sceppa C. Physical activity/exercise and Type 2 diabetes. *Diabetes Care* 2004; 27:2518–2539.

32. Department of Health and Human Services, Centers for Disease Control and Prevention, National Center for Chronic Disease Prevention and Health Promotion. Physical activity and health: A report of the Surgeon General. Atlanta, GA, 1996.

33. Pate RR, Pratt M, Blair SN, Haskell WL, Macera CA, Bouchard C, Buchner D, Ettinger W, Heath GW, King AC. Physical activity and public health: A recommendation for the Centers for Disease Control and Prevention and the American College of Sports Medicine. *JAMA* 1995; 273:402–407.

34. Institute of Medicine of the National Academies of Science. Dietary reference intakes for energy, carbohydrate, fiber, fat, fatty acids, cholesterol, protein, and amino acids (micronutrients). Washington DC: National Academy Press, 2002.

35. Schoenborn CA, Barnes PM. Leisure-time physical activity among adults: United States, 1997–1998. Advance Data from Vital and Health Statistics; No. 325. Hyattsville, MD: National Center for Health Statistics; 2002.

36. Battle-Horgen K, Brownell KD. Confronting the toxic environment: Environmental and public health actions in a world crisis. In: Wadden TA & Stunkard AJ eds. Handbook of Obesity Treatment. New York: Guilford Press, 2002:95–107.

37. Hill JO, Peters JR. Environmental contributions to the obesity epidemic. *Science* 1998; 280:1371–1374.

38. Wadden TA, Brownell KD, Foster GD. Obesity: Responding to the global epidemic. *J Cons Clin Psych* 2002; 70:510–525.

39. Van Dorsten B. Behavioral modification in the treatment of obesity. In: Barnett AH & Kumar S eds. Obesity and diabetes. London: John Wiley & Sons, 2004.

40. King AC, Brach JS, Belle S, Killingsworth R, Fenton M, Kriska AM. The relationship between convenience of destinations and walking levels in older women. *Am J Public Health* 2003; 18:74–82.

41. Owen N, Leslile E, Salmon J, Fotheringham MJ. Environmental determinants of physical activity and sedentary behavior. *Exerc Sport Sci Rev* 2000; 28–153–158.

42. Humpel N, Owen N, Leslile E. Environmental factors associated with adults' participation in physical activity: A review. *Am J Prev Med* 2002; 22:188–199.

43. Wanko NS, Brazier CW, Young-Rogers D, Dunbar VG, Blyd B, George CD, Rhee MK, El-Kebbi IM, Cook CB. Exercise preferences and barriers in urban African Americans with Type 2 diabetes. *Diabetes Educ* 2004; 30:502–513.

44. Dubbert PM. Physical activity and exercise: Recent advances and current challenges. *J Consult Clin Psychol* 2002; 70:526–536.

45. Nielsen Report on Television. New York: Neilsen Media Research, 1998.

46. Hu FB, Li TY, Colditz GA, Willett WC, Manson JE. Television watching and other sedentary behaviors in relation to risk of obesity and Type 2 diabetes mellitus in women. *JAMA* 2003; 289:1785–1791.

47. Simons-Morton DG, Calfas KJ, Oldenburg B, Burton NW. Effects of interventions in health care settings on physical fitness or cardiorespiratory fitness. *Am J Prev Med* 1998; 14:413–430.

48. Shappert SM. National Ambulatory Medical Care Survey: 1991 Summary. 230th ed. Hyattsville, MD: National Center for Health Statistics, 1993.

49. Godin G, Shephard R. An evaluation of the potential role of the physician in influencing community exercise behavior. *Am J Health Promot* 1990; 4:225–229.

50. Preventive Services Task Force. The guide to clinical preventive services. (AHRQ Publication No. 06–0588). Rockville, MD: Agency for Healthcare Research and Quality, 2006.

51. DiLoreto C, Fanelli C, Lucidi P, Murdolo G, DeCicco A, Parlanti N, Santeusanio F, Brunetti P, DeFeo P. Validation of a counseling strategy to promote the adoption and the maintenance of physical activity by Type 2 diabetes subjects. *Diabetes Care* 2003; 26:404–408.

52. Kushner RF. Barriers to providing nutrition counseling by physicians: A survey of primary care practitioners. *Prev Med* 1995; 24:546–552.

53. Wells KB, Lewis CE, Leake B, Ware JE. Do physicians preach what they practice? A study of physicians' health habits and counseling practices. *JAMA* 1984; 252:2846–2848.

54. Lewis CE, Clancy C, Leake B, Schwartz JS. The counseling practices of internists. *Ann Intern Med* 1991; 114:54–58.

55. Wee CC. Physical activity counseling in primary care: The challenge of effecting behavioral change. *JAMA* 2001; 286:717–719.

56. Dunn AL, Anderson RE, Jakicic JM. Lifestyle physical activity interventions: History, short and long-term effects and recommendations. *Am J Prev Med* 1998; 15:398–412.

57. Dunn AL, Marcus BH, Kampert JB, Garcia ME, Kohl HW, Blair SN. Comparison of lifestyle and structured interventions to increase physical activity and cardiorespiratory fitness: A randomized trial. *JAMA* 1999; 281:327–334.

58. Anderson RE, Wadden TA, Bartlett SJ, Zemel B, Verde TJ, Franckowiak SC. Effects of lifestyle activity vs. structured aerobic exercise in obese women: A randomized trial. *JAMA* 1999; 281:335–340.

59. Brill JB, Perry AC, Parker L, Robinson A, Burnett K. Dose-response effect of walking exercise on weight loss. How much is enough? *Int J Obes* 2002; 26:1484–1493.

60. Jakicic JM, Marcus BH, Gallagher KI, Napolitano M, Lang W. Effect of exercise duration and intensity on weight loss in overweight, sedentary women. *JAMA* 2003; 290:1323–1330.

61. Blair SN, LaMonte MJ, Nichaman MZ. The evolution of physical activity recommendations: How much is enough? *Am J Clin Nutr* 2004; 79(Suppl):913S-920S.

62. SoJung L, Kuk, JL, Davidson LE, Hudson, R., Kilpatrick K, Graham TE, Ross R. Exercise without weight loss is an effective strategy for obesity reduction in obese individuals with and without type 2 diabetes. *J Appl Physiol* 2005; 99:1220–1225.

63. Jakicic JM. Exercise in the treatment of obesity. *Endocrinol Metab Clin North Am* 2003; 32:967–980.

64. Snowling NJ, Hopkins WG. Effects of different modes of exercise training on glucose control and risk factors for complications in Type 2 diabetic patients: A meta-analysis. *Diabetes Care* 2006; 29:2518–2527.

65. Praet SFE, van Loon LJC. Exercise: The brittle cornerstone of type 2 diabetes treatment. *Diabetologia* 2008; 51:398–401.

66. Simmons RK, Griffin LJ, Steele R, Wareham NJ, Ekelund U. Increasing overall physical activity and aerobic fitness is associated with improvements in metabolic risk: Cohort analysis of the ProActive trial. *Diabetologia* 2008; 51:787–794.

67. Boule NG, Haddad E, Kenny GP, Wells GA, Sigal RJ. Effects of exercise on glycemic control and body mass in Type 2 diabetes mellitus: A meta-analysis of controlled clinical trials. *JAMA* 2001; 286:1218–1227.

68. DeBusk RF, Stenestrand U, Sheehan M, Haskell WL. Training effects of long versus short bouts of exercise in healthy subjects. *Am J Cardiol* 1990; 15:1010–1013.

69. Jakicic JM, Wing RR, Butler BA, Robertson RJ. Prescribing exercise in multiple short bouts versus one continuous bout: Effects of adherence, cardiovascular fitness, and weight loss in overweight women. *Int J Obes Relat Metab Disord* 1995; 19:893–901.

70. Jakicic JM, Winters C, Lang W, Wing RR. Effects of intermittent exercise and use of home exercise equipment on adherence, weight loss and fitness in overweight women. *JAMA* 1999; 282:1554–1560.

71. Schmidt WD, Biwer CJ, Kalscheuer LK. Effects of long versus short bout exercise on fitness and weight loss in overweight females. *J Am Coll Nutr* 2001; 20:494–501.

72. American College of Sports Medicine. Exercise and type 2 diabetes. *Med Sci Sport Exer* 2000; 32:1345–1360.

73. Schneider SH, Amorosa LF, Khachadurian AK, Ruderman NB. Studies on the mechanism of improved glucose control during regular exercise in type 2 diabetes. *Diabetologia* 1984; 26:325–360.

74. Borghouts LB, Keizer HA. Exercise and insulin sensitivity: A review. *Int J Sports Med* 1999; 20:1–12.

75. Perseghin G, Price TB, Falk Petersen K, Roden M, Cline GW, Gerow K, Rothman DL, Shulman GI. Increased glucose transport-phosphorylation and muscle glycogen synthesis after exercise training in insulin-resistant subjects. *N Engl J Med* 1996; 335:1357–1362.

76. Mikines KJ, Sonne B, Farrell PA, Tronier B, Galbo H. Effect of physical exercise on sensitivity and responsiveness to insulin in humans. *Am J Physiol* 1988; 254:248–259.

77. Hu FB, Sigal RJ, Rich-Edwards JW, Colditz GA, Solomon CG, Willett WC, Speizer FE, Manson JE. Walking compared with vigorous physical activity and risk of type 2 diabetes in women. *JAMA* 1999; 282:1433–1439.

78. Kazdin AE. Behavioral Modification in Applied Settings. Pacific Grove, CA: Brooks/Cole Publishing Company, 1994.

79. Miltenberger RG. Behavior Modification: Principles and Procedures. Pacific Grove, CA: Brooks/Cole Publishing Company, 1997.

80. American Diabetes Association. Diabetes mellitus and exercise. *Diabetes Care* 1997; 20:1908–1912.

81. Ismail K, Winkley K, Rabe-Hesketh S. Systematic review and meta-analysis of randomized controlled trials of psychological interventions to improve glycaemic control in patients with type 2 diabetes. *Lancet* 2004; 363:1589–1597.

82. Ridgeway NA, Harvill DR, Harvill LM, Falin TM, Forester GM, Gose OD. Improved glycemic control of type 2 diabetes mellitus: A practical education/behavior modification program in a primary care clinic. *South Med J* 1999; 92:667–672.

83. Kosaka K, Noda M, Kuzuya T. Prevention of Type 2 diabetes by lifestyle intervention: A Japanese trial in IGT males. *Diabetes Res Clin Pract* 2005; 67:152–162.

84. Blair SN, Leermakers EA. Exercise and weight management. In: Wadden TA & Stunkard AJ eds. Handbook of Obesity Treatment. New York: Guilford Press, 2002:283–300.

85. Brownell KD, Marlatt GA, Lichtenstein E, Wilson GT. Understanding and preventing relapse. *Am Psychol* 1986; 41:765–782.

86. Brown S. Interventions to promote diabetes self-management: State of the science. *Diabetes Educ* 1999; 25:52–61.

87. Gary TL, Genkinger JM, Guallar E, Peyrot M, Brancatti FL. Meta-analysis of randomized educational and behavioral interventions in Type 2 diabetes. *Diabetes Educ* 2003; 29:488–501

88. Sherwood NE, Jeffery RW. The behavioral determinants of exercise: Implications for physical activity interventions. *Annu Rev Nutr* 2000; 20:21–44.

89. Steed L, Cooke D, Newman S. A systematic review of psychosocial outcomes following education, self-management and psychological interventions in diabetes mellitus. *Patient Educ Couns* 2003; 51:5–15.

90. Norris SL, Engelgau MM, Narayan KM. Effectiveness of self-management training in Type 2 diabetes: A systematic review of randomized clinical trials. *Diabetes Care* 2001; 24:561–587.

91. Norris SL, Zhang X, Avenell A., Gregg E, Bowman B, Serdula M, Brown TJ, Schmid CH, Lau J. Long-term effectiveness of lifestyle and behavioral weight loss interventions in adults with Type 2 diabetes: A meta-analysis. *Am J Med* 2004; 117:762–774.

92. Prochaska JL, DiClemente CC, Norcross JC. In search of how people change: Applications to addictive behaviors. *Am Psychol* 1992; 47:1102–1114.

93. Prochaska JL, Redding C, Evers K. The transtheoretical model of behavioral change. In: Glanz K, Lewis FM & Rimer BK eds. Health Behavior and Health Education: Theory, Research and Practice. 2nd ed. San Francisco: Jossey Bass, 1994:60–84.

94. Spencer L, Adams TB, Malone S, Roy L, Yost E. Applying the transtheoretical model to exercise: A systematic and comprehensive review of the literature. Health Promot Pract 2006; 7:428–433.

95. Fahrenwald NL, Walker SN. Application of the transtheoretical model of behavior change to the physical activity behavior of the WIC mothers. Publ Health Nurs 2003; 20:307–317.

96. Cowan R, Logue E, Milo L, Britton PJ, Smucker W. Exercise stage of change and self-efficacy in primary care: Implications for intervention. J Clin Psychol Med Settings 1997; 4:295–311.

97. McAuley E. The role of efficacy cognitions in the prediction of exercise behavior in middle-aged adults. J Behav Med 1992; 15:65–88.

98. McAuley E, Jacobson L. Self-efficacy and exercise participation in sedentary adult fremales. Am J Health Promot 1991; 5:185–191.

99. Marcus BH, Rakowski W, Rossi JS. Assessing motivational readiness and decision making for exercise. Health Psychol 1992; 11:257–261.

100. Marcus BH, Eaton CA, Rossi JS, Harlow LL. Self-efficacy, decision making, and stages of change: An integrative model of physical exercise. J Appl Soc Psychol 1994; 94:489–508.

101. Miller WR, Rollnick S. Motivational Interviewing: Preparing People for Change Addictive Behavior. New York: Guilford Press, 1991.

102. Miller WR, Rollnick S. Motivational Interviewing: Preparing People for Change. 2nd ed. New York: Guilford Press, 2002.

103. Stott NCH, Pill RM. "Advise yes, dictate no": Patient's views on health promotion in consultation. Fam Pract 1990; 7:125–131.

104. Hettema J, Steele J, Miller WR. Motivational interviewing. Annu Rev Clin Psychol 2005; 1:91–111.

105. Burke BL, Arkowitz H, Menchola M. The efficacy of motivational interviewing: A meta-analysis of controlled clinical trials. J Consult Clin Psychol 2003; 71:843–861.

106. Harland J, White M, Drinkwater C, Chinn D, Farr L, Howel D. The Newcastle exercise project: A randomized controlled trial of methods to promote physical activity in primary care. BMJ 1999; 319:828–832.

107. Brodie DA, Inoue A. Motivational interviewing to promote physical activity for people with chronic heart failure. J Adv Nurs 2005; 50:518–527.

108. Jones KD, Burchhardt CS, Bennett JA. Motivational interviewing may encourage exercise in persons with fibromyalgia by enhancing self efficacy. Arthritis Rheum 2004; 51:864–867.

109. Scales R, Miller JH. Motivational techniques for improving compliance with an exercise program: Skills for primary care physicians. Curr Sports Med Rep 2003; 2:166–172.

110. DiLillo V, Siegfried NJ, Smith-West D. Incorporating motivational interviewing into behavioral obesity treatment. Cogn Behav Pract 2003; 10:120–130.

111. Smith D, Heckemeyer C, Kratt P, Mason D. Motivational interviewing to improve adherence to a behavioral weight-control program for older obese women with NIDDM. Diabetes Care 1997; 20:52–58.

112. Van Dorsten B. The use of motivational interviewing in weight loss. Curr Diab Rep 2007; 7:386–390.

113. Rollnick S, Mason P, Butler C. Health behavior change: A guide for practitioners. London: Churchill Livingstone, 1999.

114. Lincour P, Kuettel TJ, Bombardier DH. Motivational interviewing in a group setting with mandated clients: A pilot study. Addict Behav 2002; 27:381–391.

115. Van Horn DHA, Bux D. A pilot test of motivational interviewing groups for dually diagnosed inpatients. J Subst Abuse Treat 2001; 20:191–195.

116. Santa Ana EJ, Wulfert E, Neitart PJ. Efficacy of group motivational interviewing (GMI) for psychiatric inpatients with chemical dependency. J Consult Clin Psychol 2008; 75:816–822.

117. Ingersoll KS, Wagner CC, Gharib S. Motivational groups for community substance abuse programs. Richmond VA: Mid-Atlantic Addiction Technology Transfer Center, Virginia Commonwealth University, 2000.

118. Padgett D, Mumford E, Hynes M, Carter R. Meta-analysis of the effects of educational and psychosocial interventions on management of diabetes mellitus. J Clin Epidemiol 1988; 41:1007–1030.

119. Irwin ML, Ainsworth BE, Conway JM. Estimation of energy expenditure from physical activity measures: Determinants of accuracy. Obes Res 2001; 9:517–525.

120. Lichtman SW, Pisarska K, Berman ER, Pestone M, Dowling H, Offenbacher E, Weisel H, Heshka S, Matthews DE, Heymsfield SB. Discrepancy between self-reported and actual caloric intake and exercise in obese subjects. N Engl J Med 1992; 327:1893–1898.

121. Ureda JR. The effect of contract witnessing on motivation and weight loss in a weight control program. Health Educ Quart 1980; 7:163–184.

122. Zandee GL, Oermann MH. Effectiveness of contingency contracting. Am Assoc Occup Health Nurs J 1996; 44:183–188.

123. Beck AT, Weishar M. Cognitive therapy. In: Freeman A, Simon KM, Beutler LE & Arkowitz H eds. Comprehensive Handbook of Cognitive Therapy. New York: Plenum Publishing Company, 1989.

124. Wing RR, Jeffrey RM. Benefits of recruiting participants with friends and increasing social support for weight loss maintenance. J Consult Clin Psychol 1999; 67:132–138.

125. Wallace JP, Raglin JS, Jastremski CA. Twelve month adherence of adults who joined a fitness program with a spouse vs without a spouse. *J Sports Med Phys Fitness* 1995; 35:206–213.

126. Brekke HK, Jansson PA, Mansson JE, Lenner RA. Lifestyle changes can be achieved through counseling and follow-up in first-degree relatives of patients with Type 2 diabetes. *J Am Diet Assoc* 2003; 103:835–843.

127. Dishman RK. Overview. In: Dishman R. ed. Exercise Adherence. City, IL: Human Kinetics, 1988.

128. Carmody TP, Senner JW, Manilow MR, Matarazzo, JD. Physical exercise rehabilitation: Long term dropout rate in cardiac patients. *J Behav Med* 1980; 3:163–168.

129. Sallis JF, Haskell WL, Fortmann SP, Vranizan KM, Taylor CB, Solomon DS. Predictors of adoption and maintenance of physical activity in a community sample. *Prev Med* 1986; 15:331–341.

130. Marlatt GA, Gordon JR. Relapse prevention: Maintenance strategies in the treatment of addictive behaviors. New York: Guilford Press, 1985.

131. Perri MG, McAdoo WG, McAllister DA, Lauer JB, Jordan RC, Yancey DZ, Nezu AM. Effects of peer support and therapist contact on long term weight loss. *J Consult Clin Psychol* 1987; 55:615–617.

132. Perri MG, McAdoo WG, McAllister DA, Lauer JB, Yancey DZ. Enhancing the efficacy of behavior therapy for obesity: Effects of aerobic exercise and a multi-component maintenance program. *J Consult Clin Psychol* 1986; 54:670–675.

133. Lindstrom LL, Balch P, Reese S. In person versus telephone treatment for obesity. *J Behav Ther Exp Psychiatry* 1976; 7:367–369.

134. Tate DF, Jackvony EH, Wing RR. Effects of internet behavioral counseling on weight loss in adults at risk for type 2 diabetes. *JAMA* 2003; 289:1833–1836.

135. Jeffrey RW, Bjornson-Benson WM, Rosenthal BS, Kurth CL, Dunn MM. Effectiveness of monetary contracts with two repayment schedules on weight reduction in men and women from self-referred and population samples. *Behav Ther* 1984; 15:273–279.

136. Jeffrey RW, Wing RR, Thorson C, Burton LR. Use of personal trainers and financial incentives to increase exercise in a behavioral weight loss program. *J Consult Clin Psychol* 1998; 66:777–783.

137. Brownell KD, Yopp-Cohen R, Stunkard AJ, Felix MRJ, Cooley NB. Weight loss competitions at the work site: Impact on weight, morale, and cost-effectiveness. *Am J Pub Health* 1984; 74:1283–1285.

138. Rollnick S, Miller WR, Butler CC. Motivational interviewing in health care: Helping patient's change behavior. New York: Guilford Press, 2008.

139. Wing RR, Goldstein MG, Action KJ, Birch LL, Jakicic JM, Sallis JF, Smith-West D, Jeffrey RW, Surwit RS. Behavioral science research in diabetes. *Diabetes Care* 2001; 24:117–123.

11 Nutritional Management of Diabetes

Norica Tomuta, Nichola Davis, Carmen Isasi, Vlad Tomuta, and Judith Wylie-Rosett

CONTENTS

ABSTRACT

Medical nutrition therapy (MNT) is a cornerstone of treatment for the estimated 20.8 million people with diabetes in the United States. MNT is a more intensive and focused comprehensive nutrition therapy service that relies heavily on follow-up and provides repeated reinforcement to help change behavior. The long-term goal of medical nutrition therapy in diabetes is to prevent and/or delay diabetes complications by restoring metabolism to as close-to-normal as possible. Strategies used in MNT differ depending on the type of diabetes. In type 1 diabetes, the focus may be coordinating insulin treatment to diet and physical activity, and in type 2 diabetes, the focus may be weight reduction. This chapter will review the goals of MNT in type 1, type 2, and gestational diabetes. We will review macronutrient composition including carbohydrate metabolism, micronutrient composition, and vitamin use in diabetes. We will clarify the terms used to describe carbohydrates and how they affect blood glucose (glycemic index, glycemic load, advanced glycosylation products, net carbohydrate, available carbohydrate, and glycemic glucose equivalent). Additionally, strategies for decreasing energy intake (lowering dietary energy density, reduced portion size, meal replacements, and structured meal plans) will be discussed. MNT is an integral component of diabetes prevention, management, and self-management education. All care providers involved in diabetes treatment need to be knowledgeable about nutrition therapy to help individuals with diabetes achieve recommendations for a healthy lifestyle.

Key words: Medical nutrition therapy; Physical activity; Diabetes; Weight loss diets; Macronutrient composition.

From: *Contemporary Diabetes: Diabetes and Exercise*
Edited by: J. G. Regensteiner et al. (eds.), DOI: 10.1007/978-1-59745-260-1_11
© Humana Press, a part of Springer Science+Business Media, LLC 2009

OVERVIEW OF NUTRITIONAL ISSUES

Obesity and a sedentary lifestyle are associated with a worldwide increase in the prevalence of diabetes. Governmental and voluntary agencies in the USA and elsewhere are focusing on obesity, diabetes, and sedentary lifestyle as public health problems. In addition to exercise, medical nutrition therapy (MNT) is a cornerstone of treatment for the estimated 20.8 million people in the USA who have diabetes (14.6 million undiagnosed and 6.2 million diagnosed) (1). The global prevalence of diabetes is expected to more than double between 2000 and 2030 from 171 to 366 million (2). Despite the strong link between diabetes (type 2) and obesity, paradoxically populations that have been exposed to famine and individuals exposed to early undernutrition appear to have disproportionately high rates of diabetes (3, 4). The estimated proportion of the US population between 40 and 74 years of age with diabetes increased by 49% (from 8.9 to 12.3%) between the first and second National Health and Nutrition Examination Surveys, which were conducted in 1971–1975 and 1988–1991, respectively (3). Ironically, both low-birth weight and high-birth weight infants can be at increased risk for developing diabetes later in life.

Age, race, ethnicity, and body weight greatly affect the prevalence of diabetes mellitus (DM) (5, 6). Compared with Caucasians, the risk for developing type 2 DM (T2DM) is twofold greater in African Americans, 2.5-fold greater in Hispanic Americans, and fivefold greater in native Americans (1, 2). Other population groups at high risk for developing T2DM include Asian Indians and Pacific Islanders.

The risk for developing diabetes is closely linked to lifestyle and obesity (5). Lifestyle changes are therefore important in achieving metabolic control and need to be addressed to reduce the growing global public health burden of diabetes (2, 3).

Four basic types of DM are recognized: type 1 (formerly known as insulin-dependent or juvenile DM), type 2 (formerly known as noninsulin-dependent DM or adult-onset diabetes), gestational DM (hyperglycemia identified during pregnancy), and secondary diabetes (due to pancreatic damage or insulin resistance caused by other diseases or treatments) (6). T2DM accounts for 90–95% of all cases of diabetes. Development of T2DM is associated with insulin resistance and inadequate pancreatic beta-cell compensatory insulin production. Because of the growing public health burden of diabetes in the USA and throughout the world, and in the light of recent scientific data, three approaches to reduce the burden of diabetes are considered to be of importance (7):

1. Primary prevention of diabetes in individuals at high risk for ultimately developing this condition (controlling weight);
2. Secondary prevention of diabetes complications (controlling the metabolic disorders associated with diabetes);
3. Tertiary prevention (controlling and medically managing diabetes complications to reduce morbidity and mortality).

The "ABCs of Diabetes" campaign is designed to increase awareness of the goals for metabolic control (8).

- A stands for HbA1c (<7%),
- B for blood pressure (<130/80 mmHg),
- C for low-density lipoprotein cholesterol (<100 mg/mL) (9).

This chapter focuses on the current evidence-based recommendations regarding the role of MNT in diabetes management to prevent diabetes complications, which is considered secondary prevention.

Historical Perspective

Nutrition has been considered important in diabetes management, but specific dietary recommendations have been debated for over 3,500 years. The first diabetes dietary recommendation from Papyrus Ebers in 1550 BC focused on eating carbohydrate-containing foods, but restriction of carbohydrate containing foods emerged in the sixth century AD. During the seventeenth and eighteenth centuries recommendations varied from replacing sugar loss with a high carbohydrate diet to eating meat and fat and "avoiding" carbohydrate. During the nineteenth and early twentieth centuries, fasting and measured diabetic diets that limited carbohydrate were widely used, but some patients were treated with higher carbohydrate diets that focused on potatoes or oatmeal. High carbohydrates became the preparatory diet for glucose tolerance tests during the 1930s *(15, 16)*.

Since the 1950s, the American Diabetes Association (ADA) has utilized expert groups to develop recommendations and educational materials for the nutritional management of diabetes *(9, 10)*. Initially, the focus was on an "exchange system" for meal planning with precalculated meal plans to achieve a macronutrient distribution of 20% protein, 40% fat, and 40% carbohydrate. Recommendations focused on achieving ideal body weight, avoiding simple sugars, and individualizing programs within an exchange system approach. Gradually, as cardiovascular disease (CVD) complications became a larger part of diabetes, recommendations focused on decreasing dietary fat and increasing carbohydrate up to 60% of calories with a focus on the differing needs of patients with type 1 and type 2 diabetes. By 1994, the ADA focused on individualization based on dietitian assessment, with no specific recommendations for the balance between total fat and carbohydrate intake *(9, 10)*. The ADA's overall goal of nutrition recommendations is to achieve and maintain improvement in metabolic control to reduce the risk of acute and long-term diabetes complications. Standards of care and recommendations are reviewed by a multidisciplinary panel and published annually (clinical practice recommendations are found in www.diabetes.org). Periodically, an expert nutrition panel conducts a more comprehensive literature review as a technical review or scientific statement to assure that nutrition recommendations address relevant advances in nutrition knowledge related to diabetes and its complications *(10–15)* [Table 1; *(16)*].

Rationale for MNT Distinct from Diabetes Self-Management Training

MNT for persons with diabetes may need to be distinguished from overall diabetes self-management training (DSMT) when addressing services with policymakers and third-party payer organizations *(17, 18)*. The intent of DSMT is to provide overall guidance and is related to all aspects of diabetes self-management and glycemic control. MNT is a more intensive and focused comprehensive nutrition therapy service that relies heavily on follow-up and provides repeated reinforcement to help

Table 1
Medical Nutrition Therapy Implementation Strategies for Type 2 Diabetes Mellitus

If overweight, reduce calorie intake to achieve 5–10% weight loss.
Increase physical activity.
Monitor blood glucose approximately 4 times per day to assess pattern of glycemic control.
If postprandial glucose level is high, spread food intake throughout the day (using 5 or 6 small meals/snacks rather than having fewer larger ones).
Reduce and/or modify type of fat to achieve weight and lipid goals.

change behavior. Issues of who decides on the content of MNT, what the scientific review process is, who delivers this important therapeutic approach, and how economic considerations should affect decisions vary greatly by health system, culture, and country *(17, 18)*.

MEDICAL NUTRITION THERAPY IN DM

For persons with either type 1 or type 2 diabetes, management may necessitate several modalities. These include a variety of pharmacological agents, close personal and laboratory monitoring, for example, self-blood glucose testing, A1C and renal function testing, etc., and careful assessment by a variety of health professionals.

The long-term goal of MNT in diabetes is to prevent and/or delay diabetes complications by restoring metabolism to as close-to-normal as possible. The focus is on adjusting energy intake and expenditure to achieve a modest weight loss of ~10% and reducing the impact of CVD risk factors such as hypertension and dyslipidemia. The distribution of macronutrient intake may vary based on a number of factors including matching insulin to lifestyle in type 1 DM (T1DM) and reducing cardiovascular risk factor in T2DM. MNT should begin with an assessment of how lifestyle relates to metabolic measures associated with diabetes and its comorbidities *(10, 11)*. The assessment also addresses the interrelationship of lifestyle and medications as they impact on the metabolic parameters. The concept of instructing patients to follow the diabetic diet is outdated and grossly oversimplifies the issues that need to be addressed in MNT. Medicaid, Medicare, and other third-party payers cover MNT provided by registered dietitians *(17)*. Wide varieties of educational tools are used in conjunction with MNT. The diabetes exchange system was the primary tool used in teaching patient for many years, but carbohydrate counting and other tools are widely used in MNT.

MNT Approach in T1DM

The main role of MNT is to assist in trying to achieve and maintain metabolic normality in persons with T1DM. This means coordinating nutrition approaches with insulin treatment and physical activity, as well as strict monitoring of blood glucose levels throughout the day with self-blood glucose measurement. The process of intensifying T1DM management to improve glycemic control involves several stages as well as an individualized approach to insulin therapy, increasing physical activity, blood glucose monitoring, and nutrition therapy. The initial stage, usually lasting three to four visits, focuses on teaching basic skills needed by newly diagnosed patients, especially those with little or no previous nutrition or a history of poor glycemic control. Nutrition counseling emphasizes the consistency of carbohydrate intake and eating times. Blood glucose monitoring provides information about the patterns of response. Patients need to master a basic understanding of the relationship between insulin action and lifestyle before moving on to learn more complex planning in order to achieve both better glycemic control, and a more flexible lifestyle. An initial bolus dose of insulin for covering meals or snack is often estimated based on carbohydrate intake (e.g., 1 unit per 15 g of carbohydrate). Gradually algorithms are developed to adjust insulin for changes in carbohydrate intake or physical activity. After mastering insulin adjustment and supplementation, patients learn to adjust insulin for changes in food or activity using a ratio of carbohydrate intake to insulin dosage *(13)*.

MNT Approach in T2DM

Diet and exercise are cornerstones for diabetes management with emphasis on improving diabetes-related health risk associated with overweight and obesity. Reducing cardiovascular risk is another primary goal for MNT in T2DM *(10, 14)*. Current research is examining how much lifestyle intervention and weight loss add to cardiovascular risk reduction in patients with T2DM, whose treatment also include control of cardiovascular risk factors *(20)*. An earlier meta-analysis of lifestyle intervention weight loss studies in T2DM indicated that dietary intervention (often using very low calorie diets) achieves weight loss and improves glycemic control *(21)*. Data from randomized, controlled clinical trials further indicate that combining physical activity, dietary change, and behavioral strategies achieves the best long-term weight loss. A modest weight loss of 5–10% body weight has been associated with improvements in glycemic control and cardiovascular risk factors *(5, 10)*.

A multinational observational study, which did not evaluate lifestyle, found no improvement in morbidity or mortality associated with weight loss in individuals with T2DM *(22)*. It is not known if undetected illness or unhealthy dietary habits may have affected the study results. An evidence-based review concluded that undertaking lifestyle changes to lose a modest amount of weight could improve health outcomes *(5)*.

There is considerable interest in how dietary composition affects weight loss and health outcomes. One study evaluating the effects of a 381 J (1,600 kcal) isocaloric diet utilizing a 12-week parallel study found that energy restriction independent of dietary composition caused weight loss and improved glycemic control *(23)*. Increasing monounsaturated fatty acids and carbohydrate were both effective as substitutes for saturated fat in lowering LDL cholesterol levels. The high carbohydrate diet reduced HDL cholesterol levels at weeks 4 and 8, but it returned to the baseline level by week 12. A recent study by Samaha et al., compared a very low carbohydrate diet with a ketosis induction phase to a low fat diet, and included a subset of patients with T2DM. After 6 and 12 months on the diet, the diabetic patients in the low carbohydrate arm required less medication for diabetes and tended to have better HbA1c levels than those in the low fat arm *(24, 25)*. Additional studies with a larger sample of patients with diabetes and a longer follow-up period are needed to assess the long-term efficacy and safety of very low carbohydrates in diabetes management.

Much of the emphasis in T2DM is on controlling dyslipidemia and hypertension, which are exceedingly common comorbidities that are linked to cardiovascular complications. Various combinations of antihyperglycemic agents are used to improve blood glucose levels because monotherapy is usually inadequate *(26)*. Thus, patients with diabetes are likely to be on multiple medications and MNT is implemented within the context of overall diabetes management. Diabetes MNT can help achieve weight loss and improve metabolic parameters including glucose, blood pressure, and lipids levels. Potentially medication dosages and their side effects could be reduced by diabetes MNT.

MNT and Other Types of Diabetes

GESTATIONAL DM

The goal of diabetes therapy in gestational DM is to achieve and maintain euglycemia to improve pregnancy outcomes; reduce risks to the fetus/baby, such as macrosomia and perinatal complications; and perhaps reduce chances of fetal malnutrition, with subsequent increased risk for adult chronic diseases *(27–29)*. Women with gestational DM actually have nutrition requirements similar to those of other pregnant women but are much more likely to also be overweight.

SECONDARY DIABETES

Secondary diabetes is the result of direct pancreatic injury (by trauma, pancreatitis, etc.) or of various endocrine disorders (e.g., Cushing's disease, acromegaly) leading to increased production of counterregulatory hormones. Some pharmacologic agents, such as, steroids and antipsychotic medications can also cause secondary diabetes by increasing insulin resistance or insulin requirements.

Managing secondary diabetes is very challenging, since it involves balancing the need for glycemic control with the treatment of the underlying disease.

When possible, medications that treat the underlying disease should be modified to reduce the adverse effects on blood sugar levels (e.g., in treatment of severe asthma replace oral steroids, that have systemic effects, with inhaled steroids, that are only locally active) [Table 2; *(10)*].

MACRONUTRIENT ISSUES FOR THE MANAGEMENT OF DIABETES

Carbohydrate in Diabetes Management

Simple carbohydrate (sugar) refers often to mono- and disaccharides and complex disaccharides refer to polysaccharides. The most common natural monosaccharide is fructose, found in fruits and vegetables.

The term dextrose is used to refer to glucose. The most common disaccharides are sucrose (glucose + fructose), lactose (glucose + galactose), and maltose (glucose + glucose).

Table 2
Evidence for MNT for Type 2 Diabetes Compared with Other Forms of Diabetes

Nutrition interventions for type 2 diabetes

Individuals with type 2 diabetes are encouraged to implement lifestyle modifications such as reduced intakes of energy, saturated and trans-fatty acids, cholesterol, and sodium and increase physical activity in an effort to improve glycemia, dyslipidemia, and blood pressure. (E)

Plasma glucose monitoring can be used to determine whether adjustments in foods and meals will be sufficient to achieve blood glucose goals or if medication(s) need to be combined with MNT. (E)

Nutrition interventions for type 1 diabetes

For individuals with type 1 diabetes, insulin therapy should be integrated into an individual's food and physical activity pattern. (E)

Individuals using a rapid-acting insulin by injection or an insulin pump should adjust the meal and snack insulin doses based on the carbohydrate content of meals or snacks. (A)

For individuals using fixed daily insulin doses, carbohydrate intake on a day-to-day basis should be kept consistent with respect to time and amount. (C)

For planned exercise, insulin doses can be adjusted. For unplanned exercise, extra carbohydrate may be needed. (E)

Nutrition interventions for pregnancy and lactation with diabetes

Adequate energy intake that provides for appropriate weight gain is recommended. Weight loss is not recommended; however, for overweight and obese women with gestational diabetes, modest energy and carbohydrate restriction may be appropriate. (E)

Ketonemia from ketoacidosis or starvation ketosis should be avoided. (C)

Medical nutrition therapy for gestational diabetes focuses on food choices for appropriate weight gain, normoglycemia, and absence of ketones. (E)

Because gestational diabetes is a risk factor for subsequent development of type 2 diabetes, lifestyle modifications after delivery aimed at reducing weight and increasing physical activity are recommended. (A)

Special issues for older adults with diabetes

Obese older adults with diabetes may benefit from a modest energy restriction and an increase in physical activity; energy requirement may be less than for a younger individual of a similar weight. (E)

A daily multivitamin supplement may be appropriate, especially for those older adults with reduced energy intake. (C)

A large well-designed multicenter or multiple randomized clinical trials or well done meta-analyses, *B* examination of cohort follow-up studies or limited from one or more randomized trials, *C* more limited evidence from intervention studies, which may lack rigor with respect to the control group comparison, or more limited observation data, *E* expert consensus (but no evidence from clinical trial)

Sucrose can be found in sugar cane, sugar beets, honey, and corn syrup; lactose can be found in milk products; and maltose in malt.

The control of blood glucose levels is a primary goal of diabetes management. Food and nutrition interventions that reduce postprandial blood glucose excursions are important in this regard since dietary carbohydrate is the major determinant of postprandial glucose levels. Low carbohydrate diets might seem to be a logical approach to lower postprandial glucose. However, carbohydrate containing foods can be important sources of energy, fiber, vitamins, and minerals *(10)*. Issues related to dietary carbohydrate and glycemia have previously been extensively reviewed in ADA reports, and nutrition recommendations for the general public have been made. These recommendations can be summarized as eating a minimum of 130 g of carbohydrate per day, eating a variety of vegetables and fruit, consuming half of grains eaten as whole grains, and selecting fiber-rich options containing more than 5 g of fiber per serving, for example, beans, peas, and high-fiber cereals *(10, 15, 30, 31)*.

Blood glucose concentration in the postprandial state can vary based on the rate of appearance of glucose in the blood stream (digestion and absorption) and its clearance from the circulation *(11)*. Insulin secretion normally maintains blood glucose in a narrow range. For people with diabetes, defects in insulin action, insulin secretion, or both impair regulation of postprandial glucose in response to dietary carbohydrate. Both the quantity and the type or source of carbohydrates found in foods can influence postprandial glucose levels *(10)*.

Dietary Carbohydrate in Diabetes Management

A (2008) ADA statement addresses the effects of the amount and type of carbohydrate in diabetes management *(10)*. As noted previously, the recommended daily allowance (RDA) for carbohydrate is a minimum of 130 g/day *(30)*. Although there are no data specifically in patients with diabetes, the ADA considered the RDA in its decision to not recommend diets that restrict total carbohydrate to <130 g/day in the management of diabetes. The amount of carbohydrate ingested is usually the primary determinant of postprandial response. However, the type of carbohydrate can also affect this response. Intrinsic variables that influence the effect of carbohydrate-containing foods on blood glucose response include the specific type of food ingested, type of starch (amylose vs amylopectin), and style of preparation (cooking method and time, amount of heat or moisture used), and degree of processing. Extrinsic variables that may influence glucose response include fasting or preprandial blood glucose level, macronutrient distribution of the meal in which the food is consumed, available insulin and degree of insulin resistance *(10)*.

A variety of terminologies is used to further describe carbohydrates and how they affect blood glucose. Glycemic index, glycemic load, formation of advanced glycosylation end products, net carbohydrate, available carbohydrate, and glycemic glucose equivalent are different terms reflecting ways in which the effects of carbohydrate on blood glucose can be classified.

GLYCEMIC INDEX

The glycemic index (GI) of foods was developed in 1981 as a method to compare the postprandial responses to constant amounts of different carbohydrate-containing foods while controlling for the amount of carbohydrate eaten *(32)*. The GI of a food is the increase above fasting in the blood glucose area under the curve over 2 h after ingestion of a constant amount of that food (usually a 50-g carbohydrate portion) divided by the response to a reference food (usually glucose or white bread) *(10)*. The Food and Agriculture Organization of the United Nations and the World Health Organization issued an extensive report on various aspects of carbohydrate in the diet concluding that eating legumes and potentially other foods with a lower GI may be helpful in preventing obesity *(33)*. Slowly absorbed foods could be beneficial because they trigger less of a rise and fall in blood glucose, and thus less of a rise and fall in insulin and other hormones involved in energy regulation. Numerous difficulties with using the GI as a basis for clinical advice have arisen. For instance, the GI values for a specific food can vary considerably. Published GI for boiled white rice, for instance, varied from 45 to 112 (glucose = 100). Bananas ranged from 30 to 70, partially depending on their degree of ripeness. White durum-wheat semolina spaghetti varied from 46 to 65, depending on length of cooking time. The GI for different types of spaghetti (different brands, different types of wheat) varied even more widely. Prepared foods, which might be assumed to have manufacturing control of content, fared no better. Kellogg's All-Bran Cereal ranged from 30 in Australia to 51 in Canada, and Doritos corn chips varied from 72 in 1985 to 42 in 1998 *(34)*. Pi-Sunyer has pointed out that simple preparation (mashing a potato) can change the GI by 25%. Other types of processing and cooking can further vary the GI value by adding fiber, sugar, or acids such as vinegar *(35)*.

The role of insulin in regulating the postprandial glucose level needs to be considered, and the insulin response to a given food is not predictable as a dose response. Wolever et al. *(36)* demonstrated varied postprandial insulin responses among four different patient populations (lean, obese, impaired glucose tolerance, and overt diabetes) following meals with a relatively constant GI. Therefore GI is not a reliable predictor of insulin response.

Raben reviewed 31 studies that compared low-GI versus high-GI intake with respect to appetite or food intake. Approximately half the studies reported decreased hunger (or increased satiety) and decreased food intake with low-GI diets *(37)*. Of the 28 studies where the energy, macronutrient, and fiber compositions of the diets were similar, it was an even split. Of three long-term studies of low-versus high-GI isoenergetic weight maintenance diets, two studies have shown a decrease in body weight and one an increase in body weight with a low-GI diet *(37)*. Overall, many of these studies did not demonstrate a clear pattern of difference between low- and high-GI diets in terms of decreased food intake or weight loss. On the other hand, Pawlak et al. *(38)* noted that several single-meal studies demonstrated that GI is directly related to postprandial hunger and food intake. They have also pointed out that low-GI diets may have other benefits such as lowering triglycerides and raising high-density lipoprotein cholesterol. Contrary to the complaint that a low-GI diet is too complex for clinical use, in several studies of low-GI diets involving patient self-selection of food, patients described the diets as "simple and practical" *(38)*.

The effects of dietary fiber on glycemic response and appetite may be important when considering the role of glycemic indexing. The addition of dietary fiber, which lowers GI and slows absorption of carbohydrate, has been shown to decrease hunger, and promote a negative energy balance *(38)*. It has also been suggested that the classic studies showing the effectiveness of high-carbohydrate diets for glycemic control in people with diabetes were high in fiber, and therefore, "probably de facto low-GI diets" *(39)*.

Studies evaluating effects of GI on weight are inconsistent, as are the studies of GI effects on glycemic control. Several randomized clinical trials have reported that low-GI diets reduce glycemia in diabetic subjects, but other clinical trials have not confirmed this effect *(11)*. Moreover, the variability in GI responses to specific carbohydrate-containing food is a concern. Nevertheless, a recent meta-analysis of trials using a low-GI diet in diabetic subjects demonstrated that such diets produced a 0.4% decrement in hemoglobin A1c when compared to high-GI diets *(39)*.

GLYCEMIC LOAD

The glycemic load of foods, meals, and diets are calculated by multiplying the GI of the constituent foods by the amounts of carbohydrate in each food and then totaling the values for all foods *(10)*. Foods with low GIs include oats, barley, bulgur, beans, lentils, legumes, pasta, pumpernickel (coarse rye) bread, apples, oranges, milk, yogurt, and ice cream. Fiber, fructose, lactose, and fat are dietary constituents that tend to lower glycemic response. Carrots illustrate the leveling effect of using glycemic load. Carrots have a high GI but contain relatively little carbohydrate, and thereby have modest glycemic load. In theory because a low-glycemic-load diet slows glucose absorption and lessens hyperinsulinemia, a low-glycemic-load diet may promote appropriate weight loss, improve cardiovascular health, and reduce diabetes. Along these lines, Ludwig has developed an alternative food pyramid based on the GI, which promotes intake of vegetables and fruits with secondary emphasis on reduced-fat dairy, lean protein, nuts, and legumes (40).

ADVANCED GLYCOXIDATION END PRODUCTS

Advanced glycoxidation end products (AGEs) are formed when sugars become nonenzymatically attached to proteins (41). When heat is applied to foods containing sugar, protein cross-linking of the glycated proteins can reduce tissue elasticity and impede cellular function. The AGEs are associated with microvascular and macrovascular diabetic complications. Diet is an underappreciated source of AGE toxicity and food preparation impacts AGE content. High temperature cooking (broiling, grilling, frying, roasting) increases significantly the AGE content, while lower temperature cooking for shorter times and with more water (boiling, steaming) is responsible for smaller increases in AGE. An estimated 10% of AGEs ingested enter the circulation, and two-thirds of those absorbed are retained. Normal renal function is important to AGE clearance, since renal impairment decreases the clearance of AGEs in both diabetic and nondiabetic populations. Diet changes aimed at reducing the AGE content of food are effective, feasible, and in concordance with the current recommendations of American Diet Association and American Heart Association (41).

"NET" CARBOHYDRATE AND "AVAILABLE" CARBOHYDRATE

"Net" and "available" carbohydrates are terms used to describe the metabolically available carbohydrate in food products. Net carbohydrate for food labels is not a standardized calculation. For some food products, net carbohydrate is being calculated by subtracting the grams of fiber from the total carbohydrate content (46). However, for many other products the sugar alcohol content is also subtracted. Subtracting the fiber content appears to be reasonable because it does not appreciably affect energy intake. However, the sugar in alcohol can substantially increase energy intake.

By definition, available carbohydrate is that "absorbed via the small intestine and used in metabolism," and it was originally seen as that component of carbohydrate that should be considered in regulating blood glucose control in diabetes (55). Theoretically, carbohydrate would be classified as "unavailable," as it would not affect blood glucose response because it is not absorbed. More recently, it has been suggested that unavailable carbohydrates be subdivided based on whether the carbohydrate is subject to fermentation (55). Classifying food based on glycemic response (32, 39) is not consistent with the original purpose of classifying carbohydrates as available or unavailable as described by the Food and Agriculture Organization in 1998. Available carbohydrate (approx. 4 cal/g) has gross energy that is used fully to fuel metabolism. Unavailable carbohydrate such as sugar alcohol (approx. 2 cal/g) contributes 50% of its gross energy to fuel metabolism. Nonfermentable carbohydrate such as fiber is excreted unchanged and makes no appreciable contribution to caloric intake (42, 43).

GLYCEMIC GLUCOSE EQUIVALENT

Glycemic glucose equivalent is the glycemic load per 100-g fresh weight or per serving (44–46). The glycemic glucose equivalent can be determined directly based on the glycemic response without the need to analyze the available carbohydrate (or other component) in the food.

Prior research has included the use of total carbohydrate, total carbohydrate less dietary fiber, and directly available carbohydrate to define the type of carbohydrates that influence the glycemic response. Among these representations of available carbohydrate, several methods are available for the dietary fiber analysis required, and analysts may or may not include nondigestible oligosaccharides with dietary fiber. Direct determinations of available carbohydrate may or may not capture digestible oligosaccharides. The mode of expression of available carbohydrate is a source of variation between authors; some authors use available carbohydrate by difference (the actual weight of the available carbohydrate plus the sum of errors in all other components), some authors use the sum weight of sugars, dextrins, and starches determined directly and some authors use adjustment or more direct determination as "monosaccharide equivalents." There can also be a 20% difference in the levels (mol/g carbohydrate) of waters of hydration and condensation (excluding moisture) (47). While the glycemic glucose equivalent has many potentially attractive features, food classification using this approach is not available for use in the clinical management of diabetes or in diabetes MNT. Nonetheless, testing postmeal glucose response is useful in helping compare foods for which the amount of carbohydrate and its glycemic effects are difficult to separate.

In diabetes management, it is important to match doses of insulin and insulin secretagogues to the carbohydrate content of meals. A variety of methods can be used to estimate the nutrient content of meals including carbohydrate counting, the exchange system, and experience-based estimation. By testing pre- and postprandial glucose, many individuals use experience to evaluate and achieve postprandial glucose goals with a variety of foods.

FIBER

People with diabetes are encouraged to include in there daily intake foods such as legumes, fiber-rich cereals (>5 g of fiber per serving), fruits, vegetables, and whole grain products because they provide vitamins, minerals, and other substances important for good health. Additionally, there are data suggesting that consuming a high fiber diet (~50-g fiber per day) reduces glycemia in subjects with T1DM and glycemia, hyperinsulinemia, and lipemia in subjects with T2DM (15). Palatability, limited food choices and gastrointestinal side effects are potential barriers to achieving such high fiber intakes. However, increased fiber intake appears to be desirable for people with diabetes and a first priority might be to encourage these individuals to achieve the fiber intake goals set for the general population of 14 g/1,000 kcal (30).

SWEETENERS

Substantial evidence from clinical studies demonstrates that dietary sucrose does not increase glycemia more than isocaloric amounts of starch (15). Thus, intake of sucrose and sucrose-containing foods by people with diabetes does not need to be restricted because of concern about aggravating hyperglycemia. Sucrose can be substituted for other carbohydrate sources in the meal plan or, if added to the meal plan, adequately covered by taking insulin or another glucose-lowering medication. Additionally, intake of other nutrients ingested with sucrose, such as fat, needs to be taken into account to avoid excess energy intake.

In individuals with diabetes, fructose produces a lower postprandial glucose response when it replaces sucrose or starch in the diet; however, this benefit is tempered by concern that fructose may adversely affect plasma lipids (15, 30).

Much of the carbohydrate consumed today is in the form of high-fructose corn syrup, which usually contains 55% fructose. Sucrose or common table sugar is 50% fructose. Overall, the hormonal pattern seen with ingestion of fructose is the opposite of that seen with glucose. Fructose does not require insulin for cell uptake and many aspects of its metabolism. Thus, insulin secretion is not increased, and leptin (a hormone known to suppress appetite) appears to be reduced. Additionally, hormones such as ghrelin that stimulates appetite and are reduced postprandially do not appear to be suppressed with fructose ingestion *(48)*.

The increase in fructose consumption and the pattern of hormonal response to fructose intake has led Bray to suggest that fructose, especially as high-fructose corn syrup in beverages, contributes to the epidemic of obesity in the USA *(49)*. Compared with eucaloric glucose ingestion, fructose ingestion favors de novo lipogenesis, which could increase adiposity. Theoretically, fructose intake could increase overall food intake because of decreased satiety, resulting from its effects on ghrelin, leptin, and insulin *(48, 49)*.

Fructose is also associated with other negative metabolic states. Animal studies have shown a relationship between fructose intake and insulin resistance, possibly through decreases in adiponectin – a protein released by adipocytes that improves insulin sensitivity *(50)*.

Although it has not been shown in humans *(51)*, high-fructose diets can cause hypertension in dogs and rodents *(52)*. Additionally, when fructose has been added to a high-fiber, high-carbohydrate, low-fat diet used by people with T2DM, glucose levels improved, but they gained weight *(53)*.

The use of added fructose as a sweetening agent in the diabetic diet is not recommended *(10)*. There is however, no reason to recommend that people with diabetes avoid naturally occurring fructose in fruits, vegetables, and other foods. Fructose from these sources usually accounts for only 3–4% of energy intake *(10)*.

Reduced calorie sweeteners approved by the FDA include sugar alcohols (polyols) such as erythritol, isomalt, lactitol, maltitol, mannitol, sorbitol, xylitol, tagatose, and hydrogenated starch hydrolysates. Studies of subjects with and without diabetes have shown that sugar alcohols produce a lower postprandial glucose response than sucrose or glucose and have lower available energy *(15)*. Sugar alcohols contain, on average, about 2 cal/g (1/2 the calories of other sweeteners such as sucrose). When calculating carbohydrate content of foods containing sugar alcohols, subtraction of one-half of sugar alcohol grams from total carbohydrate grams is appropriate. Use of sugar alcohols as sweeteners reduces the risk of dental caries. However, there is no evidence that the amounts of sugar alcohols likely to be consumed will reduce glycemia, energy intake, or weight. The use of sugar alcohols appears to be safe; however, they may cause diarrhea, especially in children.

FDA approved nonnutritive sweeteners include acesulfame potassium, aspartame, neotame, saccharin, and sucralose. Before being allowed on the market, all underwent rigorous scrutiny and were shown to be safe when consumed by the public, including people with diabetes and women during pregnancy. Clinical studies involving subjects without diabetes provide no indication that nonnutritive sweeteners in foods will cause weight loss or weight gain *(54)*.

RESISTANT STARCH/HIGH AMYLOSE FOODS

Although there are no published long-term studies in subjects with diabetes to prove benefit from the use of resistant starch, it has been proposed that foods containing resistant starch (starch physically enclosed within intact cell structures as in some legumes, starch granules as in raw potato, and retrograde amylose from plants modified by plant breeding to increase amylose content) or high amylose foods such as especially formulated cornstarch may modify postprandial glycemic response, prevent hypoglycemia, and reduce hyperglycemia *(10)*.

The challenge of translating the carbohydrate-related recommendations into practical clinical advice involves prioritizing intervention steps to focus on metabolic goals. Therefore, for patients whose HbA1C is greater than 7% or who have the goal of normal postmeal glucose, the steps could include:

1. Monitor blood glucose 1–2 h after eating (normal values are <140 mg/dL 2 h after the meal, but goals need to be individualized based on the risk of hypoglycemia)

2. Determine if the amount of carbohydrates eaten is contributing to any post meal elevation (keeping the amount of carbohydrate consistent will make assessing the effects on postprandial glucose easier)

3. Examine the portion size, especially accounting for potential errors in estimating how many grams of carbohydrate may be in foods with variable portion size (e.g., pasta, bagels, muffin)

4. Examine components of carbohydrate such as fiber in legumes that may affect the postprandial response and the glycemic load of food intake.

These steps are designed to help guide decision making with respect to the amount and type of carbohydrate eaten *(55)*.

Dietary Fat and Cholesterol in Diabetes Management

The primary goal with respect to dietary fat in individuals with diabetes is to limit saturated fatty acids, trans-fatty acids and cholesterol intakes to reduce risk for CVD. Saturated and trans-fatty acids are the principal dietary determinants of plasma LDL cholesterol. In nondiabetic individuals, reducing saturated and trans-fatty acids and cholesterol intakes decreases plasma total and LDL cholesterol. Reducing saturated fatty acids may also reduce HDL cholesterol. Importantly, the ratio of LDL cholesterol to HDL cholesterol is not adversely affected. Studies in individuals with diabetes demonstrating the effects of specific percentages of dietary saturated and trans-fatty acids and specific amounts of dietary cholesterol on plasma lipids are not available. Therefore, because of a lack of specific information, it is recommended that the dietary goals for individuals with diabetes be the same as for individuals with preexisting CVD, since the two groups appear to have equivalent cardiovascular risk. Thus, saturated fatty acids <7% of total energy, minimal intake of trans-fatty acids, and cholesterol intake <200 mg daily are recommended *(10)*.

In metabolic studies in which energy intake and weight are held constant, diets low in saturated fatty acids and high in either carbohydrate or *cis*-monounsaturated fatty acids lowered plasma LDL cholesterol equivalently *(50, 54)*. The high carbohydrate diets (~55% of total energy from carbohydrate) increased postprandial plasma glucose, insulin, and triglycerides when compared to high monounsaturated fat diets. However, high monounsaturated fat diets have not been shown to improve fasting plasma glucose or hemoglobin A1c values. In other studies when energy intake was reduced, the adverse effects of high carbohydrate diets were not observed *(23, 57)*. Individual variability in response to high carbohydrate diets suggest plasma triglyceride response to dietary modification should be monitored carefully, particularly in the absence of weight loss.

Diets high in polyunsaturated fatty acids appear to have effects similar to monounsaturated fatty acids on plasma lipid concentrations *(58–61)*. A modified Mediterranean diet, in which polyunsaturated fatty acids were substituted for monounsaturated fatty acids, reduced overall mortality in elderly Europeans by 7% *(62)*. Very long chain n-3 polyunsaturated fatty acid supplements have been shown to lower plasma triglyceride levels in individuals with T2DM who are hypertriglyceridemic. Although the accompanying small rise in plasma LDL cholesterol is of concern, an increase in HDL cholesterol may offset this concern *(63)*. Glucose metabolism is not likely to be adversely affected. Very long chain n-3 polyunsaturated fatty acid studies in individuals with diabetes have primarily used fish oil supplements. Consumption of omega-3 fatty acids from fish or from supplements had been shown to reduce adverse CVD outcomes, but the evidence for alpha-linolenic acid is sparse and inconclusive *(64)*. In addition to providing n-3 fatty acids, fish frequently displace high saturated fat containing foods from the diet *(65)*. Two or more servings of fish per week (with the exception of commercially fried fish filets) *(66, 67)* is recommended.

Plant sterol and stanol esters block the intestinal absorption of dietary and biliary cholesterol. In the general public and in individuals with T2DM *(68)*, plant sterols and stanols in amounts of approximately 2 g/day have been shown to lower plasma total and LDL cholesterol. A wide range of foods and beverages are now available, which contain plant sterols. If these products are used, they should displace, rather than be added to the diet to avoid weight gain. Soft gel capsules containing plant sterols are also available.

Protein in Diabetes Management

The Dietary Reference Intakes' (DRI) acceptable macronutrient distribution range for protein is 10–35% of energy intake with 15% being the average adult intake in the USA and Canada. The RDA is 0.8 g of good quality protein/kg body weight per day (on average, about 10% of calories) *(30)*. Good quality protein sources are defined as having high PDCAAS (protein digestibility corrected amino acid scoring) scores and provide all nine indispensable amino acids. Examples are meat, poultry, fish, eggs, milk, cheese, and soy. Excluded from the "good" category are cereals, grains, nuts, and vegetables. In meal planning, protein intake should be greater than 0.8 g/kg/day to account for mixed protein quality in foods.

Dietary intake of protein should be similar in individuals with diabetes compared to that of the general public and usually does not exceed 20% of energy intake. A number of studies in healthy individuals and in individuals with T2DM have demonstrated that glucose produced from ingested protein does not increase plasma glucose concentration but does produce increases in serum insulin responses *(50, 69)*. Abnormalities in protein metabolism may be caused by insulin deficiency and insulin resistance; however, these are usually corrected with good blood glucose control *(70)*. There is increasing interest in the role of protein in weight loss, which is vitally important in diabetes management. Utilizing protein as energy is less efficient than carbohydrate and fat because of the energy requirements for breakdown and utilization of protein and amino acids. Therefore, increasing protein could theoretically be beneficial in a weight loss program *(57)*.

Small, short-term studies in diabetes suggest that diets with protein content greater than 20% of total energy reduce glucose and insulin concentrations, reduce appetite, and increase satiety *(71, 72)*. However, the effects of high protein diets on long-term regulation of energy intake, satiety, weight, and the ability of individuals to follow such diets long term have not been adequately studied.

Optimal Mix of Macronutrients

Although numerous studies have attempted to identify the optimal mix of macronutrients for the diabetic diet, it is unlikely that one such combination of macronutrients exists *(10)*. The daily balance of carbohydrate, protein, and fat varies based on individual circumstances. For those individuals seeking guidance as to macronutrient distribution in healthy adults, the DRIs may be helpful *(30)*. The DRI report recommends that, to meet the body's daily nutritional needs while minimizing risk for chronic diseases, healthy adults should consume 45–65% of total energy from carbohydrate, 20–35% from fat, and 10–35% from protein. It must be clearly recognized that regardless of the macronutrient mix, total caloric intake must be appropriate to weight management goals. Additionally the above ranges should be modified, as needed, based on the previously stated considerations for each macronutrient group.

Alcohol in Diabetes Management

For people with a history of alcohol abuse or dependence, women during pregnancy, and people with medical problems (pancreatitis, liver disease advanced neuropathy, severe hypertriglyceridemia) abstention from alcohol should be advised *(10)*. If individuals choose to consume alcohol, intake should be limited to a moderate amount (less than one drink per day for adult women and less than two drinks per day for adult men). One alcohol-containing beverage is defined as 12-oz beer, 5-oz wine, or 1.5-oz distilled spirits. Each contains ~15-g alcohol.

Moderate amounts of alcohol when ingested with food have a minimal but acute effect on plasma glucose and serum insulin concentrations. However, carbohydrate ingested together with alcohol may raise blood glucose. Caution is needed to reduce the risk of hypoglycemia in patients whose treatment includes insulin or insulin secretagogues. Evening consumption of alcohol may increase the risk of nocturnal and fasting hypoglycemia. When an alcoholic beverage is consumed, no decrease in calories from other sources should be made. Excessive amounts of alcohol (three or more drinks per day) on a consistent basis, contribute to hyperglycemia (73).

In individuals with diabetes, as with the general population, light to moderate alcohol intake (1–2 drinks per day; 15–30 g of alcohol) is associated with a decreased risk of coronary heart disease (CHD) (73). The reduction in CHD does not appear to be due to an increase in plasma HDL cholesterol. The type of alcohol-containing beverage consumed does not appear to make a difference. The ADA and other health organizations recommend limiting alcoholic beverages to two drinks per day for men and one per day for women (10).

Micronutrients in Diabetes Management

Uncontrolled diabetes is often associated with micronutrient deficiencies (74). Individuals with diabetes should be aware of the importance of acquiring daily vitamin and mineral requirements from natural food sources and a balanced diet. In select groups such as the elderly, pregnant or lactating women, strict vegetarians, or those on calorie-restricted diets, a multivitamin supplement may be needed (15).

ANTIOXIDANTS IN DIABETES MANAGEMENT

Since diabetes is a state of increased oxidative stress, there has been great interest in antioxidant therapy. Unfortunately, there are no studies examining the effects of dietary intervention on circulating levels of antioxidants and inflammatory biomarkers in diabetic volunteers. The few small clinical studies involving diabetes and functional foods thought to have high antioxidant potential (tea, cocoa, and coffee) are inconclusive. Clinical trial data not only indicate the lack of benefit with respect to glycemic control and progression of complications but also provide evidence of the potential harm of vitamin E, carotene, and other antioxidant supplements (8, 75, 76). In addition, available data do not support the use of antioxidant supplements for CVD risk reduction (77).

Chromium, Other Minerals, and Herbs in Diabetes Management

Chromium, potassium, magnesium, and possibly zinc deficiency may aggravate carbohydrate intolerance. Serum levels can readily detect the need for potassium or magnesium replacement, but detecting deficiency of zinc or chromium is more difficult (78).

Chromium is found in tissues throughout the body. A chromium-containing compound commonly known as glucose tolerance factor is involved in glucose homeostasis. Severe chromium deficiency is associated with glucose intolerance. In the late 1990s, a randomized, placebo-controlled, clinical trial conducted on 180 patients with T2DM in China studied the effect of chromium supplementation on cholesterol levels and glycemic control. In this study, supplemental chromium had significant beneficial effects on HbA1c, glucose, insulin, and cholesterol variables in subjects with type 2 diabetes. The beneficial effects of chromium in individuals with diabetes, however, were observed at levels higher than the upper limit of the Estimated Safe and Adequate Daily Dietary Intake (79). Additionally, the chromium status of the study populations was not evaluated either at baseline or following supplementation. In an uncontrolled study of 13 patients treated with corticosteroids, chromium picolinate supplementation reduced the rise in fasting glucose and the need for antihyperglycemic medication *(80)*.

Data from recent small studies indicate that chromium supplementation may have a role in the management of glucose intolerance, gestational diabetes, and corticosteroid-induced diabetes *(81–83)*. However, other well-designed studies have failed to demonstrate any significant benefit of chromium supplementation in individuals with impaired glucose intolerance or T2DM *(84, 85)*. Similarly, a meta-analysis of randomized controlled trials failed to demonstrate any benefit of chromium picolinate supplementation in reducing body weight *(86)*. The FDA concluded that although a small study suggested that chromium picolinate may reduce insulin resistance, the existence of such a relationship between chromium picolinate and either insulin resistance or T2DM was uncertain. However, most patients with diabetes do not appear to be chromium deficient, and further studies are needed to determine for whom chromium supplementation could improve carbohydrate metabolism *(79)*.

Magnesium is a cofactor in various enzyme pathways involved in glucose oxidation, and it modulates glucose transport across cell membranes. It may increase insulin secretion and/or improve insulin sensitivity and peripheral glucose uptake. It has not been shown to have an effect on hepatic glucose output and nonoxidative glucose disposal *(78, 87)*.

Poorly controlled diabetes can induce hypomagnesemia by increasing urinary excretion, and hypomagnesemia can increase insulin resistance *(89)*. The clinical usefulness of supplementation, which is usually by intake of magnesium-based antacids, for patients with T2DM and insulin resistance, is not established. Studies have examined magnesium's potential role in the evolution of such complications as neuropathy, retinopathy, thrombosis, and hypertension. However, its role in glycemic control is unknown.

Because magnesium is an intracellular cation, it is difficult to measure it accurately, and total body stores are seldom measured. Of the seven RCTs examining magnesium supplementation for glycemic control in diabetes, only two small trials from one investigator group ($n = 8$ and $n = 9$) reported a decrease in fasting plasma glucose and increase in postprandial insulin *(87, 88)*. Several trials did not observe a change in blood glucose or HbA1c *(89–91)*. One trial ($n = 128$) did find a decrease in serum fructosamine, a short-term marker of glycemic control *(89)*. Another study ($n = 40$) reported one subject with an exanthema and one who had transient gastrointestinal pain with magnesium supplementation *(90)*. The available data for magnesium are mixed, and thus the evidence for efficacy in diabetes is inconclusive.

Other inorganic trace elements such as vanadium, copper, iron, potassium, sodium, and nickel may play an important role in the maintenance of normoglycemia by activating the beta cells of the pancreas, and sources of these elements are often contained in various alternative/complementary medications. For example, analysis of the mineral content of the leaves from four Asian traditional medicinal plants (*Murraya koenigii*, *Mentha piperitae*, *Ocimum sanctum*, and *Aegle marmelos*) yielded moderate levels of copper nickel, zinc, potassium and sodium, which may account for the therapeutic benefit if the basic food supply is inadequate *(91)*. The seven most promising supplements at present include *Coccinia indica*, *American ginseng*, *Momordica charantia*, nopal, l-carnitine, *Gymnema sylvestre*, *Aloe vera*, and vanadium.

Until more definitive studies help to clarify our questions, clinicians should remain cautious, yet open-minded, regarding adjunctive use of these supplements. One clinical study that evaluated the effects of a multivitamin supplement on quality of life and missed days of activity found some benefit for the subgroup with diabetes and those over 65 years of age *(92)*. A survey of providers of alternative therapies used in diabetes found that the 10 most commonly recommended supplements were biotin, vanadium, chromium, vitamin B6, vitamin C, vitamin E, zinc, selenium, alpha-lipoic acid, and fructooligosaccharides, and the most commonly recommended herbal supplements uses were gymnema, psyllium, fenugreek, bilberry, garlic, Chinese ginseng, dandelion, burdock, prickly pear cactus, and bitter melon *(93)*. While antioxidant nutrients appear to play a role in reducing oxidative stress and possibly in increasing insulin sensitivity, there is insufficient evidence at present to warrant making any specific recommendation about use of these substances in diabetes management *(9, 10)*. Having an open dialogue about the use of alternative therapies provides the opportunity to explore how they may interact with prescribed medications beneficially or harmfully *(93)*.

VITAMINS IN DIABETES MANAGEMENT

Vitamin C. In a trial conducted by Eriksson and Kohvakka, high doses of vitamin C (2 g/day) showed a beneficial effect for type 2 diabetic patients, improving the glycemic control (decreasing both fasting glucose and HbA1c) and the lipid profile, while magnesium supplements did not influence the glycemic control or the lipid profile in the same group of subjects *(94)*.

The B Vitamin Group represents a final category to consider, particularly thiamin, riboflavin, niacin, and vitamin B6 – all of which are involved in glucose metabolism. Among persons with poorly controlled diabetes and polyuria associated with hyperglycemia, requirements may be altered by excess excretion. Nicotinic acid (niacin) + independently can worsen glycemic control when it is used to treat hyperlipidemia, but uncontrolled studies suggest it may also potentially help protect beta cell function from autoimmune destruction *(95, 96)*. Folate and vitamin B12 levels play a role in homocysteine metabolism, and plasma levels of these nutrients are inversely related to homocysteine levels. In patients with T2DM, plasma homocysteine concentration is a significant predictor of cardiovascular events and death, perhaps due to worsening of endothelial dysfunction and/or structural vessel properties induced by oxidative stress *(95)*. Of interest, elevated fasting homocysteine levels appear to be a biomarker for subsequent development of T2DM in women *(96)*. However, to confirm that a particular measurement is actually a risk factor (vs a risk marker), it is desirable that a randomized controlled trial be conducted to show that the alteration in the compound being measured is associated with benefits to patients. Such clinical trials are still pending, so that evidence-based advice can be developed in the future.

There is insufficient evidence to demonstrate efficacy of individual herbs and supplements in diabetes management *(97)*. In addition, commercially available products are not standardized and vary in the content of active ingredients. Herbal preparations also have the potential to interact with other medications *(98)*. Therefore, it is important that health care providers be knowledgeable about the use of these products by their patients and be on alert for possible side effects [Table 3 ; Nutrition Recommendations *(10)]*.

OBESITY AND WEIGHT LOSS ISSUES

People with T2DM experience more difficulty losing weight than their overweight spouses *(99)*. However, a weight loss of as little as 10 lb or 5% of body weight has resulted in improved metabolic control *(99)*. In addition, modest weight losses of at least 15 lb have been associated with significant improvements in glycemic control, fasting blood glucose, insulin levels, HDL cholesterol, and triglyceride levels within the first year in people with T2DM, whereas those who gained weight had significant worsening of glycemic control *(100)*. The treatment goal is to achieve a 5–10% weight loss in 6 months with a comprehensive approach that combines dietary, physical activity, and behavior intervention [Table 4; *(10)]*.

Table 3
Nutrients Recommendations for Managing Diabetes

Carbohydrate	A dietary pattern that includes carbohydrate from fruits, vegetables, whole grains, legumes, and low-fat milk is encouraged for good health. (B)
	Monitoring carbohydrate, whether by carbohydrate counting, exchanges, or experienced-based estimation remains a key strategy in achieving glycemic control. (A)
	The use of glycemic index and load may provide a modest additional benefit over that observed when total carbohydrate is considered alone. (B)
	Sucrose-containing foods can be substituted for other carbohydrates in the meal plan or, if added to the meal plan, covered with insulin or other glucose-lowering medications. Care should be taken to avoid excess energy intake. (A)
	As for the general population, people with diabetes are encouraged to consume a variety of fiber-containing foods. However, evidence is lacking to recommend a higher fiber intake for people with diabetes than for the population as a whole. (B)
	Sugar alcohols and non-nutritive sweeteners are safe when consumed within the daily intake levels established by the Food and Drug Administration. (A)
Fat and cholesterol	Limit saturated fat to <7% of total calories. (A)
	Intake of trans-fat should be minimized. (E)
	In individuals with diabetes, low dietary cholesterol to <200 mg/day. (E)
	Two or more servings of fish per week (with the exception of commercially fried fish filets) provide n-3 polyunsaturated fatty acids and are recommended. (B)
Protein	For individuals with diabetes and normal renal function, there is insufficient evidence to suggest that usual protein intake (15–20% of energy) should be modified. (E)
	In individuals with type 2 diabetes, ingested protein can increase insulin responses without increasing plasma glucose concentrations. Therefore, protein should not be used to treat acute or prevent night-time hypoglycemia. (A)
	High-protein diets are not recommended as a method for weight loss at this time. The long-term effects of protein intake >20% of calories on diabetes management and its complications are unknown. Although such diets may produce short-term weight loss and improved glycemia, it has not been established that these benefits are maintained long-term. (E)
Alcohol	If adults with diabetes choose to use alcohol, daily intake should be limited to a moderate amount (one drink per day or less for women and two drinks per day or less for men). (E)
	To reduce risk of nocturnal hypoglycemia in individuals using insulin or insulin secretagogues, alcohol should be consumed with food. (E)
	In individuals with diabetes, moderate alcohol consumption (when ingested alone) has no acute effect on glucose and insulin concentrations but carbohydrate co-ingested with alcohol (as in a mixed drink) may raise blood glucose. (B)
Micronutrients	There is no clear evidence of benefit from vitamin or mineral supplementation in people with diabetes (compared to the general population) who do not have underlying deficiencies. (A)
	Routine supplementation with antioxidants, such as vitamins E and C and carotene, is not advised because of lack of evidence of efficacy and concern related to long-term safety. (A)
	Benefit from chromium supplementation in persons with diabetes or obesity has not been clearly demonstrated and therefore cannot be recommended. (E)

A large well-designed multicenter or multiple randomized clinical trials or well done meta-analyses, *B* examination of cohort follow up studies or limited from one or more randomized trials, *C* more limited evidence from intervention studies, which may lack rigor with respect to the control group comparison, or more limited observation data, *E* expert consensus (but no evidence from clinical trials)

Energy Intake and Nutrient Composition

Weight loss occurs when energy expenditure exceeds energy intake. An energy deficit of 500–1,000 kcal/day will result in a loss of ~1–2 pounds/week and an average total weight loss of about 8% after 6 months. A variety of diets have been proposed to treat obesity. Although many different dietary approaches may result in short-term weight loss, the limitation of most diets is poor long-term compliance and weight regain. The optimal dietary macronutrient composition that facilitates lasting and safe weight loss is not known *(101)*.

A low-fat (e.g., 25–30% of calories from fat) diet is considered the conventional therapy for treating obesity. Data obtained from obese persons who were successful at maintaining long-term weight loss *(102)*, diet intervention trials designed to decrease the risk of CVD *(103)*, and randomized controlled trials that evaluated diet therapy for obesity indicate that decreasing dietary fat intake (to 25–30% of total calories) results in decreased total energy intake and weight loss. Data regarding the long-term effect of a very-low-fat diet (~15% of total calories from fat) on weight loss are limited because few studies have successfully achieved this level of intake *(104)*.

Additionally, in some diabetic patients, the concomitant increase in carbohydrate intake can exacerbate the dyslipidemia (elevated triglyceride, low HDL cholesterol levels) frequently associated with insulin resistance/T2DM *(105–108)*.

There has been an increasing interest in the use of low-carbohydrate diets as therapy for obesity. The results of five randomized controlled trials in adults *(24, 25, 109–111)* found that subjects randomized to a low-carbohydrate, high-protein/high-fat diet (~25–40% carbohydrate) achieved greater short-term (6 months) *(24, 109, 110)*, and similar long-term (12 months) *(24, 25)*, weight loss compared to a low-fat diet (~25–30% fat, 55–60% carbohydrate). The data from these studies also found greater improvements in serum triglycerides and HDL cholesterol concentrations, but not in serum LDL-cholesterol concentration, in the low-carbohydrate compared to the low-fat group. In addition, glycemic control was better with low-carbohydrate than low-fat diet therapy in subjects who had T2DM *(24, 25)*. Data from a 1-year study by Stern et al. *(25)* indicate, among the subset with diabetes,

Table 4
Evidence for Importance of Energy Balance, Overweight, and Obesity

In overweight and obese insulin-resistant individuals, modest weight loss has been shown to improve insulin resistance. Thus, weight loss is recommended for all such individuals who have or are at risk for diabetes. (A)

For weight loss, either low-carbohydrate or low-fat calorie-restricted diets may be effective in the short term (up to 1 year). (A)

For patients on low-carbohydrate diets, monitor lipid profiles, renal function, and protein intake (in those with nephropathy), and adjust hypoglycemic therapy as needed. (E)

Physical activity and behavior modification are important components of weight loss programs and are most helpful in maintenance of weight loss. (B)

Weight loss medications may be considered in the treatment of overweight and obese individuals with type 2 diabetes and can help achieve a 5–10% weight loss when combined with lifestyle modification. (B)

Bariatric surgery may be considered for some individuals with type 2 diabetes and BMI 35 kg/m^2 and can result in marked improvements in glycemia. The long-term benefits and risks of bariatric surgery in individuals with pre-diabetes or diabetes continue to be studied. (B)

A large well-designed multicenter or multiple randomized clinical trials or well done meta-analyses, *B* examination of cohort follow up studies or limited from one or more randomized trials, *C* more limited evidence from intervention studies, which may lack rigor with respect to the control group comparison, or more limited observation data that the reduction in fasting glucose was 21 and 28 mg/dL for the low carbohydrate and low fat diets, respectively (adjusted $p = 0.019$ with no significant difference for change in HbA1c levels). Data from a study conducted in overweight adolescents found that altering dietary glycemic load by reducing both total carbohydrate content (45–50% of energy intake) and consuming low-GI foods resulted in more weight loss when compared with a conventional low-fat (25–30%) diet *(112)*. Additional research is needed to clarify the long-term efficacy and safety of low-carbohydrate diets, particularly in patients with diabetes.

Tailoring Weight Loss Guidance

It is unlikely that one diet is optimal for all overweight/obese persons. Dietary guidance should be individualized to allow for specific food preferences and individual approaches to reducing energy intake *(15, 113)*. A variety of strategies are available for decreasing energy intake. For example, lowering dietary energy density (e.g., by increasing fruit and vegetable intake and limiting foods that are high in fat) can reduce energy intake while maintaining a volume of food that might help control hunger *(114)*. Achieving portion control by reducing portion sizes *(114)*, using meal replacement products *(115–117)*, and following structured meal plans *(118, 119)* can also enhance compliance with energy-deficit diets.

The MNT process involves selecting an appropriate meal-planning approach and educational materials based on an individual assessment of a person's ability or willingness to learn, motivation to make changes in eating habits, clinical and nutrition goals, diabetes medications, activity level, and lifestyle. The selection of a meal-planning approach considers type of diabetes, literacy, and the degree of emphasis desired on weight loss, metabolic control, structure, and complexity *(120, 121)*.

Table 5 provides an overview of methods used to help achieve the dietary goals in diabetes management that include: guidelines and food pyramids, meal planning and monitoring tools, and lifestyle-change books.

There is an interactive web page to help consumers tailor their goals using the USDA's Food Guide Pyramid, which now emphasizes weight management. Similarly, the ADA's website has the Interactive Diabetes Learning Center, which includes a plate tool for teaching consumer to choose meals that are half vegetable in order to limit meat (protein foods) and starch to one-fourth of the meal each.

Meal-planning approaches have traditionally included menus, such as individualized menus or Month of Meals, exchange lists, and counting methods, each of which can have an emphasis on weight loss. Individualized menus are based on a person's food preferences and treatment goals and specify the portions and types of foods to be consumed at meals and snacks. The five Month of Meals books each contain 28 days of complete menus for breakfast, lunch, dinner, and snacks providing 1,200, 1,500, or 1,800 cal/day. Exchange lists include the Exchange Lists for Meal Planning, which divides foods into three food groups—carbohydrate, meat and meat substitutes, and fat—and can be used as a basis for teaching the calorie and fat content of foods *(121)*. Counting methods include calorie counting, fat-gram counting, carbohydrate counting, or a combination of fat-gram and calorie counting. These approaches teach flexibility and control over food choices, but do not guarantee carbohydrate consistency.

Another type of meal planning approach that should be considered and added to the meal-planning options is the meal-replacement approach. This involves using formula shakes or bars, or prepackaged meals to control portions and simplify food decisions. Typically, formula drinks or bars are used to replace two meals and one snack per day to achieve weight loss and to replace one meal per day for weight maintenance. The relative effectiveness of each of the different meal-planning approaches that can be used to achieve a low calorie diet has not been adequately studied. Evidence has been

Table 5
Meal-Planning Approaches for Weight Loss in Type 2 Diabetes

Approach	Examples
Guidelines and food pyramids: Materials are free from website links and focus on the principles of a balanced approach to eating. Some websites offer interactive tools that can be used for tailoring goals.	Interactive Diabetes Learning Center[a] Rate Your Plate Virtual Grocery Store Diabetes Food Pyramid USDA Food Guide Pyramid[b]
Meal plans and Meal planning tools: Materials include daily menus with recipes, exchange food grouping to be used to teach meal planning, and nutrient counting approaches to be used in self-monitoring. Menus	Month of Meals book series (menus with nutrient information and exchanges at several calorie levels)[a]
Exchanges Counting (carbohydrate, fat, calories)	Exchange Lists for Meal Planning[a] Wide range of carbohydrate counting material ranging from stickers to advanced books[a]
Meal Replacements: This approach simplifies decision making, but some individuals compensate by eating between meals.	Formula drinks or bars Prepared entrée (Supermarket and catered home delivery options)
Lifestyle change: These self-help workbooks include information on behavioral change, nutrition, and physical activity.	The Complete Weight Loss Workbook[a] *(123)* The Learn Program for Weight Control *(124)*

[a] http://www.diabetes.org/home.jsp
[b] http:www.mypyramid.gov

accumulating regarding the role of meal replacements as a viable meal-planning approach for the treatment of obesity.

There is greater emphasis on lifestyle issues in books such as Facilitating Lifestyle Change: A Resource Manual *(121, 122)*, which focuses on using self-monitoring problem solving and goal setting to promote lifestyle change and improve eating habits and activity levels. Other types of manuals that use the lifestyle-change approach are The Complete Weight Loss Workbook *(123)* and The Learn Program for Weight Control *(124)*, both of which have been used in weight reduction programs to achieve successful weight loss outcomes *(125, 126)* (Table 5).

Research Issues in the Area of Weight Loss

Little research has focused on comparing educational approaches to weight control in diabetes management. The Look-AHEAD (Action for Health in Diabetes) trial is a multicenter, randomized controlled clinical trial, designed to determine whether intentional weight loss reduces cardiovascular morbidity and mortality in overweight individuals with T2DM *(119)*. This 16-center trial, which has enrolled 5,145 overweight individuals with T2DM, is examining cardiovascular morbidity and mortality for up to 12 years in persons randomly assigned to one of two study arms. Participants in a diabetes support and education group receive their usual medical care, provided by their own primary care physicians, plus three group educational sessions per year for the first 4 years. Participants in a lifestyle intervention group receive usual medical care, combined with an intensive 4-year program designed to increase physical activity and reduce initial weight by 7% or more *(20)*. All individuals are encouraged to use meal replacement for two meals, typically breakfast and lunch *(116)*. Participants are to consume an evening meal of conventional foods (which includes the option of frozen food entrees) and to add fruits and vegetables to their diet until they reach their daily calorie goal. Participants could choose from meal replacements in the form of a liquid shake or as a bar from four companies, which include Slim-Fast (Slim-Fast Foods Company, Englewood, NJ), Glucerna (Ross Laboratories, Columbus, OH), OPTIFAST (Novartis Nutrition, Fremont, MI), and HMR (Health Management Resources, Boston, MA).

We anticipate that results from the Look-Ahead study will help to determine the role of meal replacement as a weight loss strategy in patients with diabetes, and effects of weight loss achieved with this method on cardiovascular risk *(20)*.

A small randomized trial that utilized meal replacement in T2DM found that greater weight loss resulted from using a liquid formula meal replacement approach than an individualized meal planning. Further, a meta-analysis of six RCTs showed that liquid meal replacements induced a loss approximately 3 kg greater than that produced by a conventional diet *(127)*. However, previous research suggests that providing menus may be as effective as providing food to promote weight loss *(119)*. Therefore, more research is needed to determine the value of providing a guideline for food intake in achieving energy intake goals and weight loss. The short- and long-term effects of these formulas on metabolic parameters are also of interest.

To date, research on metabolic effects has largely focused on ill patients. Results indicated that, compared to standard formulas, diabetes-specific formulas significantly reduced postprandial rise in blood glucose, peak blood glucose concentration, and the glucose area under curve. Individual studies reported a reduced requirement for insulin (26–71% lower) and fewer acute complications with diabetes-specific formulas than with those for standard nutrition. However, there were no significant differences in HDL, total cholesterol, or triglyceride concentrations *(128)*.

Portion-controlled servings of conventional foods similarly facilitate weight loss, as shown by Jeffery and Wing *(119)*, among other investigators *(129, 130)*. Ultimately, the simple act of providing patients detailed menu plans, with accompanying shopping lists, offers sufficient structure to significantly increase weight loss.

Evaluation of the patient's impetus to lose weight is also an integral part of the assessment. The treatment goal in general is to achieve a 10% weight loss in 6 months with a comprehensive approach that combines dietary, physical activity, and behavioral interventions *(5, 9, 10)*.

Obesity Medications and Surgery

Weight loss medication can help achieve weight loss when combined with lifestyle change, but their use is generally restricted *(131)*. Medication approved for long-term weight loss such as orlistat (Xenical) and sibutramine (Meridia) have been demonstrated to achieve a 5–10% weight loss when accompanied by diet and exercise. Orlistat is also available at a lower dosage as an over the counter medication (Alli). There are side effects to such medications *(132)*.

For Orlistat, these include the following:

Oily spotting/discharge, fatty stools
Gas with discharge
Urgent need to have a bowel movement, increased number of bowel movements, and inability to control bowel
    movements.

In case of Sibutramine there were reported serious side effects, such as the following:

Allergic reactions
Irregular heartbeat
High blood pressure
Seizures

Other, less serious, side effects may occur while on treatment with Sibutramine:

Restlessness or tremor
Nervousness or anxiety
Mild headache or dizziness
Insomnia
Dry mouth
Constipation

Weight loss through these medications may have a role in management of diabetes, but additional studies will need to be done to determine their long-term efficacy.

Bariatric surgery is increasingly utilized as a method of weight loss. Long-term risk and benefits of bariatric surgery need further study, but a meta-analysis of studies of bariatric surgery reported improvement or normalization of fasting blood glucose levels in 86% of patients with diabetes *(133, 134)*. However, for the subset with HbA1C measurements the mean change was 0.31% after controlling for potential confounders *(131)*. Therefore, while fasting glucose appears to dramatically decrease, the overall improvement in glycemic control measured by the HbA1c was modest. In the Swedish Obese Subjects Study (SOS), a 10-year follow-up of individuals undergoing bariatric surgery who achieve a mean body weight loss of 23.4%, roughly one-third of the subjects with diabetes had remission of diabetes, compared to 13% of matched controls who did not receive surgery *(133, 134)*. All cardiovascular risk factors except hypercholesterolemia improved in the surgical patients (Table 6).

NUTRITION AND THE ROLE OF PHYSICAL ACTIVITY

In MNT, physical activity is a key component of the lifestyle intervention for patients with diabetes or at risk for developing diabetes. As such, the effects of physical activity on glycemia and weight need to be understood. Making sure that any physical activity program is safe and enjoyable for the patient is as important as the activity itself.

For young patients treated with insulin or medications that enhance insulin secretion, safety issues usually focus on the risks of hypoglycemia. Special care should also be given to older patients and those with long-standing diabetes with regard to cardiovascular risk status. These persons should have thorough screening for any other underlying complications prior to beginning an exercise program *(135)*.

Exercise and T1DM

People with T1DM can perform all levels of physical activity, including leisure activities, recreational sports, and competitive professional sports. This last assumes that they do not have complications and have good blood glucose control. The ability to adjust the therapeutic regimen (insulin and MNT) to allow safe participation and high performance is recognized as an important management strategy in these individuals. In particular, the importance of glucose self-monitoring to improve overall athletic performance and enhance safety is now fully accepted by the medical community.

Table 6
Treating and Controlling Diabetes Complications (Tertiary Prevention)

Microvascular complications

Reduction of protein intake to 0.8–1.0 g/kg body weight per day in individuals with diabetes and the earlier stages of chronic kidney disease (CKD) and to 0.8 g/kg body weight per day in the later stages of CKD may improve measures of renal function (e.g., urine albumin excretion rate, glomerular filtration rate). (B)

Medical nutrition therapy that favorably affects cardiovascular risk factors may also have a favorable effect on microvascular complications such as retinopathy and nephropathy. (C)

Treatment and management of CVD risk

Target A1C is as close to normal as possible without significant hypoglycemia. (B)

For patients with diabetes as risk for CVD, diets high in fruits, vegetables, whole grains, and nuts may reduce the risk. (C)

For patients with diabetes and symptomatic heart failure, dietary sodium intake of <2,000 mg/day may reduce symptoms. (C)

In normotensive and hypertensive individuals, a reduced sodium intake (e.g., 2,300 mg/day) with a diet high in fruits, vegetables, and low fat dairy products lowers blood pressure.

In most individuals, a modest amount of weight loss beneficially affects blood pressure. (C)

Hypoglycemia

Ingestion of 15–20 g of glucose is the preferred treatment for hypoglycemia, although any form of carbohydrate that contains glucose may be used. (A)

The response to treatment of hypoglycemia should be apparent in 10–20 min; however, plasma glucose should be tested again in ~60 min as additional treatment may be necessary. (B)

Acute illness

During acute illnesses, insulin and oral glucose lowering medications should be continued. (A)

During acute illnesses, testing of plasma glucose and ketones, drinking adequate amounts of fluids, and ingesting carbohydrate are all important. (B)

Acute health care facilities

Establishing an interdisciplinary team, implementation of MNT, and timely diabetes-specific discharge planning improves the care of patients with diabetes during and after hospitalizations. (E)

Hospitals should consider implementing a diabetes meal planning system that provides consistency in the carbohydrate content of specific meals. (E)

Long-term care facilities

The imposition of dietary restrictions on elderly patients with diabetes in long-term care facilities is not warranted. Residents with diabetes should be served a regular menu, with consistency in the amount and timing of carbohydrate. (C)

An interdisciplinary team approach is necessary to integrate nutrition therapy for patients with diabetes into overall management. (E)

There is no evidence to support the prescribing of diets such as "no concentrated sweets" or "no sugar added." (E) In the institutionalized elderly, undernutrition is likely and caution should be exercised when prescribing weight loss diets. (B)

A large well-designed multicenter or multiple randomized clinical trials or well done meta-analyses, *B* examination of cohort follow-up studies or limited from one or more randomized trials, *C* more limited evidence from intervention studies, which may lack rigor with respect to the control group comparison, or more limited observation data, *E* expert consensus (but no evidence from clinical trials)

The risk of hypoglycemia, which can occur during, immediately after, or many hours after physical activity, can be minimized or avoided. Minimizing risk requires that the patient has both an adequate knowledge of the metabolic and hormonal responses to physical activity and well-tuned self-management skills. The increasing use of intensive insulin therapy has provided patients with the flexibility to make appropriate insulin dose adjustments for various activities.

Physical activity can improve the lipid profile, reduce blood pressure and improve cardiovascular parameters of patients with T1DM. The ADA has concluded that research has failed to show an independent effect of exercise on glycemic control, as measured by HbA1C levels. Such information is critical in the paradigm shift from focusing only on glycemic control to focusing on lifestyle changes with multiple benefits *(135)*.

RECOMMENDATIONS REGARDING PHYSICAL ACTIVITY IN T1DM *(135, 136)*

1. Achieving metabolic control before beginning a program of increased physical activity

   (a) Avoid physical activity if fasting glucose levels are >250 mg/dl and ketosis is present, and use caution if glucose levels are >300 mg/dl and no ketosis is present.
   (b) Ingest added carbohydrate if glucose levels are <100 mg/dl.

2. Blood glucose monitoring before and after physical activity

   (a) Identify when changes in insulin or food intake are necessary.
   (b) Learn the glycemic response to different physical activity conditions.

3. Adjusting (or monitoring) food intake as needed

   (a) Consume added carbohydrate as needed to avoid hypoglycemia.
   (b) Carbohydrate-based foods should be readily available during and after physical activity.

With vigorous activity, dehydration can negatively affect blood glucose levels and heart function. Therefore, special attention to maintaining hydration is important, especially when heat is also a factor. Adequate hydration prior to physical activity is recommended (e.g., 17 oz of fluid consumed 2 h before physical activity). During physical activity, fluids should be taken early and frequently in an amount sufficient to compensate for losses in sweat reflected in body weight loss. Precautions should be taken when exercising in extremely hot or cold environments.

Exercise and T2DM

There are important benefits of physical activity for the patient with T2DM. Poor aerobic fitness is associated with many of the cardiovascular risk factors, and reducing levels of these parameters has been linked to a decrease in plasma insulin levels *(134)*. Therefore, beneficial effects of physical activity on cardiovascular risk are likely to be related to improvements in insulin sensitivity. In addition, regular exercise appears to have a direct benefit with regard to decreasing the levels of triglyceride-rich VLDL and blood pressure levels. An ADA and AHA common statement has addressed the role of physical activity in preventing CVD in for people with diabetes *(137)*. To improve glycemic control, assist with weight loss or maintenance, and reduce risk of CVD, at least 150 min of moderate-intensity aerobic physical activity or at least 90 min of vigorous aerobic exercise per week is recommended. The physical activity should be distributed over at least 3 days per week, with no more than two consecutive days without physical activity. For long-term maintenance of major weight loss, a larger amount of exercise (7 h of moderate or vigorous aerobic physical activity per week) may be helpful *(136)*.

In T2DM exercise can be a strategy for improving blood glucose as well as for losing weight. Exercise may need dietary adjustment to prevent hypoglycemia in patients treated with insulin or other medications that enhance insulin secretion.

Exercise and Diabetes Prevention

The greatest benefit from physical activity may occur early in the progression from insulin resistance to impaired glucose tolerance to overt hyperglycemia. The Diabetes Prevention Program (DPP), in which patients participated in an intensive lifestyle intervention, recorded a 58% reduction in incidence of diabetes over 3.2 years for patients who averaged a 7% weight loss. This level of weight loss was achieved by 49% of participants *(137)*. After accounting for weight loss, self-reported changes in physical activity or fat intake did not lead to additional reductions in diabetes risk. However, if participants did meet the activity goals of 150 min per week achieved a 44% reduction in diabetes incidence, despite not achieving the weight loss goal *(138)*. Overall the 150 min/week activity goal was achieved by three quarters of DPP lifestyle participants at the end of the core curriculum and by two-thirds at the end of the study *(119)*. In the context of worldwide T2DM epidemics, the importance of promoting physical activity as a vital component of the prevention as well as management of T2DM must be viewed as a high priority.

CONCLUSIONS

MNT is an integral component of diabetes prevention, management, and self-management education. Achieving nutrition-related goals require a coordinated team effort that includes the active involvement of the patient with prediabetes or diabetes. Because of the complexity of nutrition issues, Medicare and several other third-party payers cover MNT provided by a registered dietitian. However, all care providers involved in diabetes treatment need to be knowledgeable about nutrition therapy and help individuals with diabetes to achieve recommendations for a healthy lifestyle *(135)*.

RESOURCES FOR NUTRITION INFORMATION ABOUT DIABETES

American Association of Diabetes Educators
  1-800-TEAM-UP4 (800-832-6874)
  www.diabeteseducator.org
  American Diabetes Association
  1-800-DIABETES (800-342-2383)
  www.diabetes.org
  American Dietetic Association
  1-800-366-1655 (in English and Spanish)
  www.eatright.org
  Centers for Disease Control and Prevention
  1-877-232-3422
  www.cdc.gov/diabetes
  Centers for Medicare & Medicaid Services
  1-800-MEDICARE or (800-633-4227)
  www.cms.hhs.gov/MLNProducts/downloads/expanded_benefits_06-08-05.pdf.

REFERENCES

1. Centers for Disease Control. National Diabetes Fact Sheet. 2005. Available at: http://www.cdc.gov/diabetes/pubs/factsheet05.htm. Accessed Nov. 27, 2005.
2. Wild S, Roglic F, Green A, et al. Global prevalence of diabetes: estimated for the year 2000 and projections for 2030. *Diabetes Care* 2004;27:1047–1053.
3. Vinicor F. The public health burden of diabetes and the reality of the limits. *Diabetes Care* 1998;21 (Suppl 3):C15–C18.

4. Laaksonen DE, Niskanen L, Lakka HM, Lakka TA, Uusitupa M. Epidemiology and treatment of the metabolic syndrome. *Ann Med* 2004;36:332–346.

5. Obesity Education Initiative Expert Panel Clinical guidelines on the identification evaluation, and treatment of overweight and obesity in adults: the evidence report. U.S. Department of Health and Human Services, Public Health Service, National Institutes of Health, National Heart Lung and Blood Institute. http://www.nhlbi.nih.gov/guidelines/obesity/ob_home.htm. Accessed January 14, 2005).

6. American Diabetes Association Position Statement (2006). Diagnosis and Classification of DM. Diabetes Care 2006 29:S43–49. Available at: http://care.diabetesjournals.org/cgi/reprint/29/suppl–1/s43.

7. U.S. Department of Health and Human Services. Diabetes Prevention and Control: A Public Health Imperative. Available at: http://www.healthierus.gov/steps/summit/prevportfolio/strategies/reducing/diabetes/contents–diabetes.htm.

8. National Diabetes Education Program (NDEP) Four Steps to Diabetes Control: Know Your Diabetes ABCs. Available at: http://www.ndep.nih.gov/diabetes/control/4Steps.htm_Step2.

9. American Diabetes Association. Position Statement: Standards of medical care in diabetes-2007. *Diabetes Care* 2007;30 (Suppl 1):S4–S41.

10. American Diabetes Association. Position Statement: Nutrition recommendations and Interventions for Diabetes-2008. *Diabetes Care*. 2008;30 (Suppl 1):S61–S78.

11. Sheard NF, Clark NG, Brand-Miller JC, et al. Dietary carbohydrate (amount and type) in the prevention and management of diabetes: statement by the American Diabetes Association. *Diabetes Care* 2004;27:2266–2271.

12. American Diabetes Association, North American Association for the Study of Obesity, American Society for Clinical Nutrition. Weight management through lifestyle modification for the prevention and management of type 2 diabetes: rationale and strategies. *Diabetes Care* 2004;27:2067–2073.

13. Nutrition Practice Guidelines for Type 1 and Type 2 Diabetes Mellitus [CD-ROM]. Chicago: American Dietetic Association, 2002.

14. American Diabetes Association. Frequently asked Questions about Diabetes Self-Management and Medical Nutrition Therapy. Available at: http://www.diabetes.org/for-health-professionals-and-scientists/recognition/dsmt-mntfaqs.jsp.

15. Franz MJ, Bantle JP, Beebe CA, Brunzell JD, Chiasson JL, Garg A, Holzmeister LA, Hoogwerf B, Mayer-Davis E, Mooradian AD, Purnell JS, Wheeler M. Evidence-based nutrition principles and recommendations for the treatment and prevention of diabetes and related complications (technical review). *Diabetes Care* 2002;25:148–198.

16. Wylie-Rosett J, Vinicor F. Diabetes mellitus. In: Present Knowledge in Nutrition, 9th ed., Section IX: Nutrition and Chronic Disease, Chapter 50, 2006.

17. American Dietetic Association and the American Association of Diabetes Educators. Medicare, Part B: Referral Forms for Diabetes Self-Management Training and Medical Nutrition Therapy. Available at: http://www.eatright.org/cps/rde/xchg/ada/hs.xsl/nutrition_accessmnt_ENU_HTML.htm.

18. American Diabetes Association. Therapy for Diabetes Mellitus and Related Disorders, 4th ed. AlexandriaVA: American Diabetes Association, 2004.

19. Grundy SM, Benjamin IJ, Burke GL, Chait A, Eckel RH, Howard BV, Mitch W, Smith SC Jr, Sowers JR. Diabetes and Cardiovascular Disease. A statement for healthcare professionals from the American Heart Association. *Circulation* 1999;100:1134–1146.

20. Ryan DH, Espeland MA, Foster GD, Haffner SM, Hubbard VS, Johnson KC, Kahn SE, Knowler WC, Yanovski SZ; Look AHEAD Research Group. Look AHEAD (Action for Health in Diabetes): design and methods for a clinical trial of weight loss for the prevention of cardiovascular disease in type 2 diabetes. *Control Clin Trials*. 2003;24:610–628.

21. Brown AS, Upchurch S, Anding R, Winter M, Rameriz G. Promoting weight loss in type II diabetes. *Diabetes Care* 1996;19:613–624.

22. Chaturvedi N, Fuller JH. Mortality risk by body weight and weight change in people with NIDDM. The WHO Multinational Study of Vascular Disease in Diabetes. *Diabetes Care* 1995;18(6):766–774.

23. Heibronn LK, Noakes M, Clifton PM. Effects of energy restriction, weight loss, and dietary composition on plasma lipids and glucose in patients with type 2 diabetes. *Diabetes Care* 1999;22:889–895.

24. Samaha FF, Iqbal N, Seshadri P, Chicano KL, Daily DA, McGrory J, Williams T, Williams M, Gracely EJ, Stern L. Low-carbohydrate as compared with a low-fat diet in severe obesity. *N Engl J Med*. 2003;348:2074–2081.

25. Stern L, Iqbal N, Seshadri P, Chicano KL, Daily DA, McGrory J, Williams M, Gracely EJ, Samaha FF. The effects of low-carbohydrate versus conventional weight loss diets in severely obese adults: one-year follow-up of a randomized trial. *Ann Intern Med* 2004;140:778–785.

26. Campbell RK, White J, White J Jr. Medications for the Treatment of Diabetes. Alexandria, VA: American Diabetes Association, 2003.

27. Jovanovic L, Pettit D. Gestational diabetes mellitus. *JAMA* 2004;286:2516–2518.

28. Nutrition Practice Guidelines for Gestational Diabetes Mellitus. Chicago, IL: American Dietetic Association, 2002.

29. Gunderson EP. Gestational diabetes and nutritional recommendations. *Curr Diab Rep* 2004;4:377–386.

30. Institute of Medicine: Dietary Reference Intakes: Energy, Carbohydrate, Fiber, Fat, Fatty Acids, Cholesterol, Protein, and Amino Acids. Washington, DC: National Academies Press, 2002.

31. The Department of Health and Human Services, the Department of Agriculture: Dietary Guidelines for Americans. Washington, DC: U.S. Govt. Printing Office, 2005.

32. Jenkins DJ, Wolever TM, Taylor RH, Barker H, Fielden H, Baldwin JM, Bowling AC, Newman HC, Jenkins AL, Goff DV. Glycemic index of foods: a physiological basis for carbohydrate exchange. *Am J Clin Nutr* 1981;34:362–366.

33. Joint FAO/WHO Expert Consultation. Carbohydrates in human nutrition (FAO Food and Nutrition Paper 66). Rome: FAO, 1998.

34. Foster-Powell K, Holt SHA, Brand-Miller JC. International table of glycemic index and glycemic load values. *Am J Clin Nutr* 2002;76:5–56.

35. Pi-Sunyer FX. Glycemic index and disease. *Am J Clin Nutr* 2002;76(S):290–298.

36. Wolever TMS, Chiasson J-L, Hunt JA, Palmason C, Ross SA, Ryan EA. Similarity of relative glycaemic but not relative insulinaemic responses in normal IGT, and diabetic subjects. *Nutr Res* 1998;18:1667–1676.

37. Raben A. Should obese patients be counseled to follow a low-glycaemic index diet? No. *Obes Rev* 2002;3:245–256.

38. Pawlak DB, Ebbeling CB, Ludwig DS. Should obese patients be counseled to follow a low-glycaemic index diet? Yes. *Obes Rev* 2002;3:235–243.

39. Brand-Miller J, Hayne S, Petocz P, Colagiuri S. Low glycemic index diets in the management of diabetes: a meta analysis of randomized controlled trials. *Diabetes Care* 2003;25:2261–2267.

40. Ludwig DS. Dietary glycemic index and obesity. *J Nutr* 2000;130(S):280–283.

41. Huebschmann AG, Regensteiner J, Vlassara H, Reusch JEB. Diabetes and advanced glycoxidation end products. *Diabetes Care* 2006;29:1420–1432.

42. Livesey G. A perspective on food energy standards for nutrition labeling. *Br J Nutr* 2001;85:271–287.

43. Livesey G. Thermogenesis associated with fermentable carbohydrate in humans, validity of indirect calorimetry, and implications of dietary thermogenesis for energy requirements, food energy and body weight. *Int J Obes Relat Metab Disord* 2002;26(12):1553–1569.

44. Liu P, Perry T, Monro JA. Glycaemic glucose equivalent: validation as a predictor of the relative glycaemic effect of foods. *Eur J Clin Nutr* 2003;57(9):1141–1149.

45. Monro J. Redefining the glycemic index for dietary management of postprandial glycemia. *J Nutr* 2003;133(12):4256–4258.

46. Monro JA. Glycaemic glucose equivalent: combining carbohydrate content, quantity and glycaemic index of foods for precision in glycaemia management. *Asia Pac J Clin Nutr* 2002;11(3):217–224.

47. Livesey G. Low-glycaemic diets and health: implications for obesity. *Proc Nutr Soc* 2005;64(1):105–113.

48. Teff KL, Elliott SS, Tschop M, et al. Dietary fructose reduces circulating insulin and leptin, attenuates postprandial suppression of ghrelin, and increases triglycerides in women. *J Clin Endocrinol Metab* 2004;89:2963–2972.

49. Bray GA, Nielsen SJ, Popkin BM. Consumption of high fructose corn syrup in beverages may play a role in the epidemic of obesity. *Am J Clin Nutr* 2004;79:537–543.

50. Elliott SS, Keim NL, Stern JS, Teff K, Havel PJ. Fructose, weight gain, and the insulin resistance syndrome. *Am J Clin Nutr* 2002;76:911–922.

51. Daly M. Sugars, insulin sensitivity, and the postprandial state. *Am J Clin Nutr* 2003;78(S):865–872.

52. Hwang IS, Ho H, Hoffman BB, Reaven GM. Fructose induced insulin resistance and hypertension in rats. *Hypertension* 1987;10:512–516.

53. Ha TKK, Lean MEJ. Technical review: recommendations for the nutritional management of patients with diabetes mellitus. *Eur J Clin Nutr* 1998;52:467–481.

54. Raben A, Vasilaras TH, Moller AC, Astrup A. Sucrose compared with artificial sweeteners: different effects on ad libitum food intake and body weight after 10 wk of supplementation in overweight subjects. *Am J Clin Nutr* 2002;76:721–729.

55. Wylie-Rosett J, Segal-Isaacson CJ, Segal-Isaacson A. *Carbohydrates and increases in obesity: does the type of carbohydrate make a difference? Obes Res* 2004;12 (S2):124–129.

56. Garg A, Bantle JP, Henry RR, Coulston AM, Griver KA, Raatz SK, Brinkley L, Chen YD, Grundy SM, Huet BA, et al. Effects of varying carbohydrate content of diet in patients with non-insulin-dependent diabetes mellitus. *JAMA* 1994;271:1421–1428.

57. Parker B, Noakes M, Luscombe N, Clifton P. Effect of a high-protein, high-monounsaturated fat weight loss diet on glycemic control and lipid levels in type 2 diabetes. *Diabetes Care* 2002;25:425–430.

58. Hu FB, van Dam RM, Liu S. Diet and risk of type II diabetes: the role of types of fat and carbohydrate. *Diabetologia* 2001;44:805–817.

59. Summers LK, Fielding BA, Bradshaw HA, Ilic V, Beysen C, Clark ML, Moore NR, Frayn KN. Substituting dietary saturated fat with polyunsaturated fat changes abdominal fat distribution and improves insulin sensitivity. *Diabetologia* 2002;45:369–377.

60. Salmeron J, Hu FB, Manson JE, Stampfer MJ, Colditz GA, Rimm EB, Willett WC. Dietary fat intake and risk of type 2 diabetes in women. *Am J Clin Nutr* 2001;73:1019–1026.

61. Tapsell LC, Gillen LJ, Patch CS, Batterham M, Owen A, Bare M, Kennedy M. Including walnuts in a low-fat/modified fat diet improves HDL cholesterol–to total cholesterol ratios in patients with type 2 diabetes. *Diabetes Care* 2004;27:2777–2783.

62. Trichopoulou A, Orfanos P, Norat T, et al. Modified Mediterranean diet and survival: EPIC-elderly prospective cohort study. *BMJ* 2005;330:991.

63. West SG, Hecker KD, Mustad VA, Nicholson S, Schoemer SL, Wagner P, Hinderliter AL, Ulbrecht J, Ruey P, Kris-Etherton PM. Acute effects of monounsaturated fatty acids with and without omega-3 fatty acids on vascular reactivity in individuals with type 2 diabetes. *Diabetologia* 2005;48:113–122.

64. Wang C, Harris WS, Chung M, Lichtenstein AH, Balk EM, Kupelnick B, Jordan HS. n-3 Fatty acids from fish or fish-oil supplements, but not alpha-linolenic acid, benefit cardiovascular outcomes in primary- and secondary-prevention studies: a systematic review. *Am J Clin Nutr* 2006;84:5–17.

65. Kris-Etherton PM, Harris WS, Appel LJ. Fish consumption, fish oil, omega-3 fatty acids, and cardiovascular disease. *Circulation* 2002;106:2747–2757.

66. Mozaffarian D, Bryson CL, Lemaitre RN, Burke GL, Siscovick DS. Fish intake and risk of incident heart failure. *J Am Coll Cardiol* 2005;45:2015–2021.

67. Erkkila AT, Lichtenstein AH, Mozaffarian D, Herrington DM. Fish intake is associated with a reduced progression of coronary artery atherosclerosis in postmenopausal women with coronary artery disease. *Am J Clin Nutr* 2004;80:626–632.

68. Lee YM, Haastert B, Scherbaum W, Hauner H. A phytosterol-enriched spread improves the lipid profile of subjects with type 2 diabetes mellitus: a randomized controlled trial under free-living conditions. *Eur J Nutr* 2003;42:111–117.

69. Gannon MC, Nuttall JA, Damberg G, Gupta V, Nuttall FQ. Effect of protein ingestion on the glucose appearance rate in people with type 2 diabetes. *J Clin Endocrinol Metab* 2001;86:1040–1047.

70. Gougeon R, Styhler K, Morais JA, Jones PJ, Marliss EB. Effects of oral hypoglycemic agents and diet on protein metabolism in type 2 diabetes. *Diabetes Care* 2000;23:1–8.

71. Gannon MC, Nuttall FQ. Effect of a high-protein, low-carbohydrate diet on blood glucose control in people with type 2 diabetes. *Diabetes* 2004;53:2375–2382.

72. Gannon MC, Nuttall FQ, Saeed A, Jordan K, Hoover H. An increase in dietary protein improves the blood glucose response in persons with type 2 diabetes. *Am J Clin Nutr* 2003;78:734–741.

73. Howard AA, Arnsten JH, Gourevitch MN. Effect of alcohol consumption on diabetes mellitus: a systematic review. *Ann Intern Med* 2004;140:211–219.

74. Mooradian AD. Micronutrients in diabetes mellitus. *Drugs, Diet and Disease* 1999;2:183–200.

75. Hasanain B, Mooradian AD. Antioxidant vitamins and their influence in diabetes mellitus. Curr Diab Rep 2002;448–456.

76. Lonn E, Yusuf S, Hoogwerf B, Pogue J, Yi Q, Zinman B, Bosch J, Dagenais G, Mann JF, Gerstein HC. Effects of vitamin E on cardiovascular and microvascular outcomes in high-risk patients with diabetes: results of the HOPE study and MICRO-HOPE substudy. *Diabetes Care* 2002;25:1919–1927.

77. Kris-Etherton PM, Lichtenstein AH, Howard BV, Steinberg D, Witztum JL. Antioxidant vitamin supplements and cardiovascular disease. *Circulation* 2004;110:637–641.

78. Mooradian AD, Failla M, Hoogwerf B, Maryniuk M, Wylie-Rosett J. Selected vitamins and minerals in diabetes. *Diabetes Care* 1994;17:464–479.

79. Anderson RA, Cheng N, Bryden NA Polansky MM, Cheng N, Chi J, Feng J. Elevated intakes of supplemental chromium improves glucose and insulin variables in individuals with type 2 diabetes. *Diabetes* 1997;46:1786–1791.

80. Ravina A, Slezak L, Mirsky N, Bryden NA, Anderson RA. Reversal of corticosteroid-induced diabetes with supplemental chromium. *Diabet Med* 1999;16:164–167.

81. Cefalu WT, Hu FB. Role of chromium in human health and in diabetes. *Diabetes Care* 2004;27:2741–2751.

82. Ryan GJ, Wanko NS, Redman AR, Cook CB. Chromium as adjunctive treatment for type 2 diabetes. *Ann Pharmacother* 2003;37:876–885

83. Althuis MD, Jordan NE, Ludington EA, Wittes JT. Glucose and insulin responses to dietary chromium supplements: a meta-analysis. *Am J Clin Nutr* 2002;76:148–155

84. Gunton JE, Cheung NW, Hitchman R, Hams G, O'Sullivan C, Foster-Powell K, McElduff A: Chromium supplementation does not improve glucose tolerance, insulin sensitivity, or lipid profile: a randomized, placebo-controlled, double-blind trial of supplementation in subjects with impaired glucose tolerance. Diabetes Care 2005;28:712–713.

85. Kleefstra N, Houweling ST, Jansman FG, Groenier KH, Gans RO, Meyboom-de Jong B, Bakker SJ, Bilo HJ. Chromium treatment has no effect in patients with poorly controlled, insulin-treated type 2 diabetes in an obese Western population: a randomized, double-blind, placebo-controlled trial. *Diabetes Care* 2006;29:521–525.

86. Pittler MH, Stevinson C, Ernst E. Chromium picolinate for reducing body weight: meta-analysis of randomized trials. *Int J Obes Relat Metab Disord* 2003;27:522–529.

87. Paolisso G, Sgambato S, Gambardella A, Pizza G, Tesauro P, Varricchio M, D'Onofrio F. Daily magnesium supplements improve glucose handling in elderly subjects. *Am J Clin Nutr* 1992;55:1161–1167.

88. Paolisso G, Sgambato S, Pizza G, Passariello N, Varricchio M, D'Onofrio F. Improved insulin response and action by chronic magnesium administration in aged NIDDM subjects. *Diabetes Care* 1989;12:265–269.

89. de Lourdes LM, Crua T, Pousada JC, Rodrigues LE, Barbosa K, Cangucu V. The effect of magnesium supplementation in increasing doses on the control of type 2 diabetes. *Diabetes Care* 1998;21:682–686.

90. Eibl NL, Kopp HP, Nowak HR, Schnack CJ, Hopmeier PG, Schernthaner G. Hypomagnesemia in type 2 diabetes: effect of a 3-month replacement therapy. *Diabetes Care* 1995;18:188–192.

91. Eriksson J, Kohvakka A. Magnesium and ascorbic acid supplementation in diabetes mellitus. *Ann Nutr Metab* 1995;39:217–223.

92. Barringer TA, Kirk JK, Santaniello AC, Foley KL, Michielutte R. Effect of a multivitamin and mineral supplement on infection and quality of life. A randomized, double-blind, placebo-controlled trial. *Ann Intern Med* 2003;138: 365–371.

93. Cicero AF, Derosa G, Gaddi A. What do herbalists suggest to diabetic patients in order to improve glycemic control? Evaluation of scientific evidence and potential risks. *Acta Diabetol* 2004;41:91–98.

94. Eriksson J, Kohvakka A. Magnesium and ascorbic acid supplementation in diabetes mellitus. *Ann Nutr Metab* 1995;39:217–223.

95. Huijberts MS, Becker A, Stehouwer CD. *Homocysteine and vascular disease in diabetes: a double hit? Clin Chem Lab Med* 2005;43:993–1000.

96. Cho NH, Lim S, Jang HC, Park HK, Metzger BE. Elevated homocysteine as a risk factor for the development of diabetes in women with a previous history of gestational diabetes mellitus: a 4-year prospective study. *Diabetes Care* 2005;28: 2750–2755.

97. Yeh GY, Eisenberg DM, Kaptchuk TJ, Phillips RS. Systematic review of herbs and dietary supplements for glycemic control in diabetes. *Diabetes Care* 2003;26:1277–1294.

98. Tariq SH. Herbal therapies. *Clin Geriatr Med* 2004;20:237–257.

99. Wing RR, Marcus MD, Epstein LH, Salata R Type II diabetic subjects lose less weight than their overweight non-diabetic spouses. *Diabetes Care* 1987;10:563–566.

100. Wing RR, Koeske R, Epstein LH, Nowalk MP, Gooding W, Becker D. Long-term effects of modest weight loss in type 2 diabetic patients. *Arch Intern Med* 1987;147:1749–1753.

101. National Institutes of Health, National Heart, Lung and Blood Institute, National Institute of Diabetes and Digestive and Kidney Diseases: Clinical Guidelines on the Identification, Evaluation, and Treatment of Overweight and Obesity in Adults. Bethesda, MD, National Institutes of Health, 1998

102. Klem ML, Wing RR, McGuire MT, Seagle HM, Hill JO. A descriptive study of individuals successful at long-term maintenance of substantial weight loss. *Am J Clin Nutr* 1998;66:239–246.

103. Yu-Poth S, Zhao G, Etherton T, Naglak M, Jonnalagadda S, Kris-Etherton PM. Effects of the National Cholesterol Education Program's Step I and Step II dietary intervention programs on cardiovascular disease risk factors: a meta-analysis. *Am J Clin Nutr* 1999;69:632–646.

104. Lichtenstein AH, Van Horn L. Very low fat diets. *Circulation* 1998;98:935–939.

105. Grundy SM: Hypertriglyceridemia, insulin resistance, and the metabolic syndrome. *Am J Cardiol* 1999;83:25F–29F.

106. Garg A, Bonanome A, Grundy SM, Zhang ZJ, Unger RH. Comparison of a high-carbohydrate diet with a high-mono-unsaturated-fat diet in patients with non-insulin-dependent diabetes mellitus. *N Engl J Med* 1988;319:829–834.

107. Garg A, Grundy SM, Unger RH. Comparison of effects of high and low carbohydrate diets on plasma lipoproteins and insulin sensitivity in patients with mild NIDDM. *Diabetes* 1992;41:1278–1285.

108. Garg A, Bantle JP, Henry RR, Coulston AM, Griver KA, Raatz SK, Brinkley L, Chen YD, Grundy SM, Huet BA. Effects of varying carbohydrate content of diet in patients with non-insulin-dependent diabetes mellitus. *JAMA* 1994;271:1421–1428.

109. Foster GD, Wyatt HR, Hill JO, McGuckin BG, Brill C, Mohammed BS, Szapary PO, Rader DJ, Edman JS, Klein S: A randomized trial of a low-carbohydrate diet for obesity. *N Engl J Med* 2003;48:2082–2090.

110. Brehm BJ, Seeley RJ, Daniels SR, D'Alessio DA. A randomized trial comparing a very low carbohydrate diet and a calorie-restricted low fat diet on body weight and cardiovascular risk factors in healthy women. J Clin Endocrinol Metab 203;88:1617–1623.

111. Yancy WS Jr, Olsen MK, Guyton JR, Bakst RP, Westman EC. A low-carbohydrate, ketogenic diet versus a low-fat diet to treat obesity and hyperlipidemia: a randomized, controlled trial. Ann Intern Med 2004;140:769–777.

112. Ebbeling CB, Leidig MM, Sinclair KB, Hangen JP, Ludwig DS. A reduced-glycemic load diet in the treatment of adolescent obesity. Arch Pediatr Adolesc Med 2003;157:773–779.

113. National Institutes of Health, National Heart, Lung and Blood Institute, North American Association for the Study of Obesity: The Practical Guide: Identification, Evaluation, and Treatment of Overweight and Obesity in Adults. Bethesda, MD: National Institutes of Health, 2000.

114. Rolls BJ, Bell EA. Dietary approaches to the treatment of obesity (Review). Med Clin North Am 2000;84:401–418.

115. McGuire MT, Wing RR, Klem ML, Seagle HM, Hill JO. Long-term maintenance of weight loss: do people who lose weight through various weight loss methods use different behaviors to maintain their weight? Int J Obes Relat Metab Disord 1998;22:572–577.

116. Ditschuneit HH, Flechtner-Mors M, Johnson TD, Adler G. Metabolic and weight-loss effects of a long-term dietary intervention in obese patients. Am J Clin Nutr 1999;69:198–204.

117. Heber D, Ashley JM, Wang HJ, Elashoff RM. Clinical evaluation of a minimal intervention meal replacement regimen for weight reduction. J Am Coll Nutr 1994;13:608–614.

118. Jeffery RW, Wing RR, Thorson C, Burton LR, Raether C, Harvey J, Mullen M. Strengthening behavioral interventions for weight loss: a randomized trial of food provision and monetary incentives. J Consult Clin Psychol 1993;61:1038–1045.

119. Wing RR, Jeffery RW: Food provision as a strategy to promote weight loss. Obes Res 2001;9(S):271–275.

120. Monk A, Barry B, McClain K, Weaver T, Cooper N, Franz MH. Practice guidelines for medical nutrition therapy provided by dietitians for persons with non-insulin dependent diabetes mellitus. J Am Diet Assoc 1995;95:999–1006.

121. Green Pastors J. Expanding meal-planning approaches. In Handbook of Diabetes Medical Nutrition Therapy. Powers MA, Ed.Gaithersburg, Md., Aspen Publishers, Inc., 1996:207–224.

122. Green Pastors J, Barrier P, Rich M, Gallagher S, Galligos C, Wheeler M. Facilitating Lifestyle Change: A Resource Manual. Alexandria, VA., and Chicago, Ill. American Diabetes Association and American Dietetic Association, 1996.

123. Wylie-Rosett J, Swencionis C, Caban A, Friedler A, Schaffer N. The Complete Weight Loss Workbook: Proven Techniques for Controlling Weight-Related Health Problems. Alexandria, VA., American Diabetes Association, 1997.

124. Brownell KD. The Learn Program for Weight Control. Dallas, TX: American Health Publishing Co., 1998.

125. Wylie-Rosett J, Swencionis C, Ginsberg M, Cimino C, Wassertheil-Smoller S, Caban A, Segal-Isaacson CJ, Martin T, Lewis J. Computerized weight loss intervention optimizes staff time: the clinical and cost results of a controlled clinical trial conducted in a managed care setting. J Am Diet Assoc 2001;101:1155–1162.

126. Ashley JM, St. Jeor ST, Schrage JP, Perumean-Chaney SE, Gilbertson MC, McCall NL, Bovee V. Weight control in the physician's office. Arch Intern Med 2001;161:1599–1604.

127. Heymsfield SB, van Mierlo CA, van der Knaap HC, Heo M, Frier HI. Weight management using a meal replacement strategy: meta and pooling analysis from six studies. Int J Obes 2003;27:537–549.

128. Elia M, Ceriello A, Laube H, Sinclair AJ, Engfer M Stratton RJ. Enteral nutritional support and use of diabetes-specific formulas for patients with diabetes: a systematic review and meta-analysis. Diabetes Care 2005;28:2267–227979.

129. Metz JA, Stern JS, Kris-Etherton P, et al. A randomized trial of improved weight loss with a prepared meal plan in overweight and obese patients: impact of cardiovascular risk reduction. Arch Intern Med 2000;160:2150–2158.

130. Haynes RB, Kris-Etherton P, McCarron DA, et al. Nutritionally complete prepared meal plan to reduce cardiovascular risk factors: a randomized clinical trial. J Am Diet Assoc 1999;99:1077–1083.

131. Wadden TA SWD, Delahanty LM, Jakicic JM, Rejeski J, Berkowotz RI, Williamson DA, Kelley DE, Kumanika SK, Hill JO, Tomachee CM and the Look AHEAD Research Group. The Look AHEAD study: A description of the lifestyle intervention and the evidence supporting it. Obesity 2006;14:737–752.

132. Perrio MJ, Wilton LV, Shakir SA. The safety profiles of orlistat and sibutramine: results of prescription-event monitoring studies in England. Obesity 2007, 15(11): 2712–2722.

133. Buchwald H, Avidor Y, Braunwald E, Jensen MD, Pories W, Fahrbach K, Schoelles K. Bariatric surgery: a systemic review and meta-analysis. JAMA 2004;292:1724–1737.

134. Sjostrom L, Lindroos AK, Peltonen M, Torgerson J, Buchard C, Carlsson B, Dahlgren S, Larsson B, Narbro K, Sjostrom CD, Sullivan M, Wedwl H. Lifestyle diabetes, and cardiovascular risk factors 10 years after bariatric surgery. N Engl J Med 2004;351:2683–2693.

135. American Diabetes Association-Position Statement. Physical Activity/Exercise and Diabetes. *Diabetes Care* 2004; 27(S1):58–62.

136. American Diabetes Association and American Heart Association Statement-Primary Prevention of Cardiovascular Diseases in People With Diabetes Mellitus. *Diabetes Care* 2007;30:162–172.

137. DPP Research Group-Reduction in the incidence of Type 2 Diabetes with lifestyle intervention or Metformin. *N Engl J Med* 2002;346(6):393–403.

138. Hamman RF, Wing RR, Edelstein SL, Lachin JM, Bray GA, Delahanty L, Hoskin M, Kriska AM, Mayer-Davis EJ, Pi-Sunyer X, Regensteiner J, Venditti B, Wylie Rosett J. Effect of weight loss with lifestyle intervention on risk of Diabetes. *Diabetes Care* 2006;29:2102–2107.

12

Guidelines for Exercise Testing in Diabetics Starting an Exercise Program

Barry A. Franklin, Wendy M. Miller, Katherine Nori, and Peter A. McCullough

CONTENTS

ABSTRACT

Because diabetes mellitus is considered a major risk factor for cardiovascular disease, the clinical evaluation of the patient with diabetes is an assessment performed by primary care and specialty physicians on a daily basis. A careful history, medical record review, current treatment (oral agents, insulin), related comorbidities (hypertension, obesity, metabolic syndrome, coronary artery disease), electrocardiogram (ECG), laboratory studies (blood glucose, hemoglobin A1c, serum creatinine, estimated glomerular filtration rate, urine albumin/creatinine ratio), ankle/brachial systolic pressure index, and exercise stress test may be important components of this evaluation. In addition to the indications and contraindications and appropriate methodology (protocols) for exercise testing, key diagnostic and prognostic variables include: the resting and exercise ECG, especially the provocation of significant ST-segment displacement and/ or arrhythmias during or after exercise testing; anginal symptoms; dyspnea; chronotropic incompetence; abnormal heart rate recovery; exertional hyper or hypotension; exercise capacity, expressed as metabolic equivalents (METs; 1 MET = 3.5 mL/kg/min); and combined information (e.g., treadmill scores [Duke Treadmill Score]). Echocardiographic studies may also reveal impaired left ventricular diastolic function, a condition that is common in diabetes, which often precedes systolic dysfunction. Collectively, these data should prove helpful in prescribing exercise and identifying treatment targets to prevent end-organ complications and major cardiovascular events in this escalating patient population.

Key words: Diabetes; Exercise testing; Exercise capacity; Evaluation of patients with diabetes mellitus.

Exercise testing and training are vital components in the evaluation and medical treatment of patients with diabetes mellitus. Nevertheless, there are associated risks of exercise training, specific exercise precautions, and contemporary guidelines for the medical evaluation and exercise testing of

From: *Contemporary Diabetes: Diabetes and Exercise*
Edited by: J. G. Regensteiner et al. (eds.), DOI: 10.1007/978-1-59745-260-1_12
© Humana Press, a part of Springer Science+Business Media, LLC 2009

diabetics prior to initiating an exercise program. This chapter addresses these issues, with specific reference to the conduct and interpretation of exercise testing in assessing patients with known or suspected diabetes mellitus.

MEDICAL EVALUATION AND ASSESSMENT OF THE DIABETIC PATIENT

Diabetes mellitus (DM) has two major forms, types 1 and 2, with two very different etiologies and clinical courses. Most patients with type 1 diabetes develop this form during childhood and develop complications during middle age. In contrast, most patients with type 2 diabetes present during adulthood, and this form is largely due to being overweight or obese, and being physically inactive. Because type 2 diabetes represents >90% of prevalent cases, the following text concerning the evaluation of the diabetic patient before exercise pertains to type 2 DM.

Diabetes mellitus is considered a major cardiovascular disease (CVD) risk factor and is independently related to an approximate twofold increased risk of myocardial infarction, stroke, heart failure, and cardiovascular death across all age and gender groups. The rates of cardiovascular events are similar for DM with and without known CVD. Thus, DM is considered a "cardiovascular risk equivalent." Major medical complications to be avoided or prevented in a patient with DM include cardiovascular events, blindness due to retinopathy, end-stage renal disease requiring dialysis, peripheral arterial disease (PAD), and amputation due to extremity ulcers, infection, and osteomyelitis.

Components of the initial clinical evaluation of DM include historical information such as the duration of known DM, current treatment (oral agents, insulin, others), and related comorbidities (hypertension, coronary artery disease [CAD], etc.). In addition, evidence for end-organ complications secondary to DM should be obtained. Diabetic nephropathy occurs in approximately 50% of patients; thus, the serum creatinine, estimated glomerular filtration rate (eGFR), and urine albumin:creatinine ratio should be noted in the medical records. In general, if the eGFR < 60 mL/min/1.73 m^2 or if the spot urine albumin:creatinine ratio is >30 mg/g, then diabetic nephropathy is present. It is important to realize that a patient with diabetic nephropathy is more likely to die of CVD than progress to end-stage renal disease requiring dialysis in the next five to ten years. Another important end-organ complication is diabetic retinopathy, which is a leading cause of blindness. This condition requires a comprehensive examination by an ophthalmologist on an annual basis.

One of the most important aspects of the physical examination in a patient with DM is measurement of the resting blood pressure in the brachial artery. Hypertension is a major determinant of end-organ complications, as discussed earlier. When the blood pressure consistently exceeds >140/90 mmHg, hypertension is present (1). Currently, there is a greater emphasis on the systolic blood pressure as the treatment target. In general, an uncomplicated patient with DM should have the systolic blood pressure treated to <130 mmHg. Patients with DM and kidney disease with proteinuria should be treated to an even lower target, that is, <120 mmHg.

A careful general physical examination of the extremities should be made for evidence of skin breakdown or discoloration. Reduced macro- and microvascular flow to the skin increases the risk of minor cuts and abrasions developing into penetrating diabetic ulcers, which can lead to deep tissue infections including osteomyelitis. Proper socks and shoes should be recommended for a patient about to embark on an exercise program to reduce the likelihood of diabetic foot lesions.

A focused evaluation for the manifestations of underlying CVD should be conducted. Any self-reported history of myocardial infarction, stroke, or heart failure should be corroborated by medical records and additional diagnostic testing, if indicated. The presence of angina should be quantified according the Canadian Cardiovascular Society (Classes 1–4) (2). An electrocardiogram (ECG) is essential on the initial visit with attention to the presence of Q-waves, left ventricular hypertrophy, and abnormalities of the conduction system. The physical examination should attempt to identify normal versus reduced systolic function. A normally placed point of maximal impulse, normal S1 and S2, and an unremarkable ECG in the same patient strongly suggest the left ventricular ejection fraction is preserved. Other findings, including soft heart tones, an S3, and electrocardiographic evidence of Q-waves or bundle branch patterns, make it more likely that the ejection fraction is reduced. Echocardiographic studies may also reveal impaired left ventricular diastolic function, a condition that is common in diabetes, and will often precede systolic dysfunction. Finally, the examination should attempt to identify the presence of PAD. A history of stroke, leg claudication, or carotid or peripheral revascularization suggests PAD. The presence of bruits in the neck, the abdomen, or over the femoral arteries may represent other signs of PAD. In addition, if the posterior tibial artery pulse is reduced, PAD at some level in the lower extremity circulation is present. The dorsalis pedis pulse is less reliable in its anatomic position in the dorsum of the foot; thus, its absence on examination is not especially helpful. The ankle/brachial systolic pressure index (or ABI) is derived by measuring the brachial artery cuff systolic pressure, and dividing it by the systolic pressure measured in the posterior tibial artery using a cuff and a continuous wave Doppler probe. Of note, the ABI should be measured in each leg by dividing the ankle blood pressure from each leg by the highest blood pressure from either arm. Because of peripheral amplification of the arterial pulse wave, the ABI should normally be ≥1.00. When this value becomes <0.90, PAD is present and a comprehensive lower extremity vascular examination may be recommended, using a dedicated vascular laboratory with ultrasound and plethysmography. Discovering and documenting PAD, with or without intermittent claudication, is important since it is a common limiting factor in aerobic exercise and can be a treatment target. Moreover, exercise therapy improves PAD symptoms and quality of life for the patient (3).

The laboratory evaluation for the DM patient should include a biochemistry profile with serum creatinine, hemoglobin A1c (glycohemoglobin), urine albumin:creatinine ratio, and lipid profile. The glycohemoglobin, which reflects the prior 90 days of glycemic control, should normally be <6.0%. In DM, the treatment goal for A1c should be <7.0%. In general, when this value exceeds 8.0%, there is poor chronic control of blood glucose and medication changes are indicated. As discussed earlier, the treatment goal for the urine albumin:creatinine ratio is <30 mg/g. This is usually accomplished with strict blood pressure control, including drugs which block the renin–angiotensin system. For most patients with DM, the current low density lipoprotein cholesterol goal should be <70 mg/dL, requiring use of a statin medication (4).

All patients with DM are considered to be at a similar risk to those with CAD; thus, baseline exercise stress testing is often advised prior to initiating an exercise program. If any of the examination features suggest the presence of coronary or peripheral atherosclerosis, a stress test with cardiac imaging (nuclear scintigraphy or echocardiography) may serve to further improve risk stratification of these patients (5). Evidence of large reversible myocardial perfusion abnormalities, left ventricular dysfunction, or both, should signal the need for additional cardiology evaluation and treatment and approval before initiating an exercise program.

In summary, the clinical evaluation of the patient with DM is an important activity performed by primary care and speciality physicians on a daily basis. A careful history, medical record review, ECG, laboratory evaluation, and stress test are important components of this evaluation. The spirit of the evaluation is to discover treatment targets to prevent end-organ complications and major cardiovascular events.

CONDUCTING AND INTERPRETING THE EXERCISE STRESS TEST

Exercise testing permits evaluation of the following variables: aerobic capacity (the estimated or actual peak or maximal oxygen consumption [VO$_2$ max]); hemodynamic responses including the heart rate and systolic/diastolic blood pressure responses during and after exercise; adverse clinical signs or symptoms (e.g., exertional angina and/or dyspnea); and, associated changes in electrical functions of the heart, especially supraventricular and ventricular arrhythmias and ST-segment displacement. When an exercise test that includes metabolic testing is performed, valuable cardiopulmonary data obtained include the ventilatory-derived anaerobic threshold (V-AT; the break point in linearity when carbon dioxide production [VCO_2] is plotted as a function of oxygen consumption [VO_2]), expressed as a percentage of the VO_2 max, may be determined. This method has been reported to provide a valid and reliable noninvasive technique for the detection of the onset of metabolic acidosis *(6)*. Variables other than VO_2 max or VO_2-AT, such as the minute ventilation (VE)/ VO_2 slope or VE/VCO_2 slope, have also been used to classify functional limitations, breathing economy, and, more recently, to risk stratify patients *(7)*. Accordingly, exercise tests with metabolic assessment have immediate value in directly assessing cardiopulmonary capacity and the safety of physical exertion as well as diagnostic and prognostic significance in regard to CAD and its associated morbidity and mortality.

This section addresses the physiological basis and rationale for exercise testing in assessing asymptomatic and symptomatic patients, especially those with DM and known or suspected CAD, with specific reference to indications and contraindications, end points, test modalities/protocols, and test interpretation, including ECG, symptomatic, and hemodynamic responses, exercise capacity, and treadmill scores.

Rationale for Stress Testing in Patients with Diabetes Mellitus: Contemporary Guidelines

CVD is the leading cause of morbidity and mortality in patients with DM *(8)*; an estimated 80% die from CVD, and 75% of these fatalities are attributed to CAD *(9)*. Nearly two decades ago, the Framingham Study *(10)* demonstrated that diabetic individuals had a two- to fivefold risk of developing the manifestations of coronary disease (e.g., angina pectoris, acute myocardial infarction, congestive heart failure). When individuals younger than 45 years of age are examined, the risk of CVD escalates to >11-fold that of the general population *(11)*. Although early detection of occult CAD in diabetics is important, the role of routine exercise testing in this patient population is controversial, since outcome data from randomized controlled trials are lacking *(12)*.

In 1998, consensus guidelines issued by the American Diabetes Association (ADA) indicated that screening by stress testing was appropriate in diabetics with two or more additional risk factors *(9)*. Subsequently, the ADA expanded this recommendation by suggesting that an exercise stress test should be conducted in virtually all diabetic individuals who were beginning a moderate or vigorous exercise program *(13)*. However, the earlier recommendation has been challenged in two recent studies *(14, 15)* that have identified silent myocardial ischemia and/or angiographically documented CAD in asymptomatic patients with type 2 diabetes, independent of the risk factor profile.

Writing groups from the American College of Cardiology/American Heart Association Guidelines on Exercise Testing *(5)* and the American College of Sports Medicine (ACSM) *(16)* have addressed the role of exercise testing before exercise training for patients with DM. The former group classified routine exercise testing in asymptomatic persons with DM who plan to start vigorous exercise (≥60% VO_2 reserve) as a Class IIa recommendation (i.e., weight of evidence/opinion is in favor of usefulness/ efficacy). Similarly, the ACSM recommended exercise testing for diabetics who plan to start a moderate (40–59% VO_2 reserve) to vigorous exercise program. In contrast, the US Preventive Services Task Force *(17, 18)* came to the conclusion that insufficient evidence exists to determine the benefits and limitations of exercise stress testing before exercise programs or, for that matter, in the routine screening of asymptomatic individuals at low CAD risk (<10% risk of a cardiac event over 10 years). Recently, the latter recommendation was echoed by the ADA *(19)*.

A major limitation of exercise testing is that a truly positive exercise test requires a hemodynamically significant coronary lesion (e.g., >75% stenosis; Fig. 1), whereas nearly 90% of acute myocardial infarctions occur at the site of previously nonobstructive atherosclerotic plaques *(20)*. These findings, coupled with the extremely low rate of cardiovascular complications in asymptomatic persons who exercise *(21)*, suggest that it is impractical and cost prohibitive to use exercise testing to forestall serious cardiovascular events in all asymptomatic exercisers. Accordingly, physicians and health care providers should evaluate the entire atherosclerotic risk profile in diabetic patients, as well as the anticipated exercise intensity, degree of competition, and potential for superimposed cognitive and/or environmental stressors, before recommending exercise stress testing as a prelude to exercise training.

Indications and Contraindications

Exercise stress testing is generally recommended for the following reasons: to aid in the diagnosis of occult or suspected CAD in asymptomatic or symptomatic individuals; to evaluate cardiorespiratory fitness, expressed as mL/kg/min or metabolic equivalents (METs; 1 MET = 3.5 mL/kg/min); to assess the efficacy of interventions such as pacemaker implantation, coronary revascularization, anti-ischemic medications, or physical training; to establish the safety of vigorous physical exertion; to formulate a safe and effective exercise prescription; and, to assess work-related capabilities after an acute coronary event or intervention *(22)*.

Common contraindications to peak or symptom-limited exercise testing include a recent significant change in the resting ECG suggesting cardiac ischemia (e.g., ST-T wave abnormalities), recent myocardial infarction (within 2 days), unstable angina, uncontrolled symptomatic heart failure and/or atrial or ventricular arrhythmias that may compromise cardiac function, severe aortic stenosis, acute infection, third-degree heart block (without pacemaker), and active myocarditis or pericarditis *(23)*. Patients with relative contraindications such as electrolyte abnormalities (e.g., hypokalemia, hypomagnesemia), severe arterial hypertension (i.e., resting systolic and/or diastolic blood pressure >

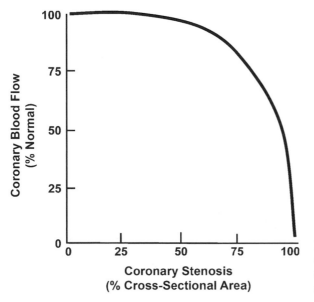

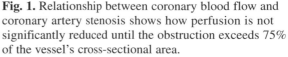

Fig. 1. Relationship between coronary blood flow and coronary artery stenosis shows how perfusion is not significantly reduced until the obstruction exceeds 75% of the vessel's cross-sectional area.

200 or >110 mmHg, respectively), hypertrophic cardiomyopathy and other forms of outflow obstruction, ventricular aneurysm, or uncontrolled metabolic disease (e.g., DM) may be tested after careful medical evaluation of the risk/benefit ratio (23). Oftentimes, individuals with relative contraindications can be exercised with caution using modified protocols (e.g., initial work rates ~2–3 METs) and/or low-level end points, especially if they are asymptomatic at rest.

Test Modalities/Protocols

Both treadmill exercise and cycle ergometry have advantages and disadvantages in evaluating patients with and without documented CAD. Alternatively, dynamic arm exercise testing provides a reproducible method to evaluate cardiovascular function in individuals with neurologic, vascular, or orthopedic impairment of the lower extremities (24).

The cycle ergometer has the advantage of requiring less space, making less noise, and generally costing less than the treadmill. It also minimizes movement of the torso and arms, which facilitates better quality ECG recordings and more audible blood pressure measurements. Table 1 shows the approximate energy expenditure in mL/kg/min during progressive leg cycle ergometry, expressed as kilogram meters per minute (kg/m/min), which at a given power output or work rate is inversely related to body weight (16).

Conversely, treadmill testing provides a more common form of physiologic stress (i.e., walking) in which subjects are more likely to attain a slightly higher VO_2 max and peak heart rate. The test should generally last 8–12 min for patients limited by fatigue, highlighting the importance of appropriate protocol selection. Figure 2 shows three commonly used multistage treadmill exercise protocols, involving a constant walking speed (range, 2.0–3.4 mph) and standardized increases in grade or incline and aerobic requirements (1 MET/stage). The conventional Bruce treadmill protocol is perhaps the most widely used because it offers a rapid and safe exercise progression for which aerobic capacity can be estimated from the treadmill time in men, women, and patients with CAD (Table 2)

Table 1
Approximate Energy Expenditure (mL/kg/min) During Leg Cycle Ergometry

Body weight		Power output or work rate (kg/m/min)[a]						
Kg	lb	300	450	600	750	900	1,050	1,200
50	110	17.9	23.1	28.7	34.0	39.6	44.8	50.1
60	132	16.1	20.7	24.9	29.4	34.0	38.5	43.1
70	154	14.7	18.6	22.4	26.3	30.1	34.0	37.8
80	176	13.7	17.2	20.7	23.8	27.3	30.8	34.0
90	198	13.0	16.1	18.9	22.1	24.9	28.0	31.2
100	220	12.3	15.1	17.9	20.7	23.1	25.9	28.7

Estimated values of approximate energy expenditure are based on completion of each 3-min stage. To convert to METs, divide the estimated value (mL/kg/min) by 3.5.

[a] The work rate or power output is expressed as kilogram meters per minute (kg/m/min) and is determined by the designated internal resistance (kg), pedal speed (in revolutions per minute), and the distance in meters (m) the flywheel travels for one pedal revolution. This distance is 6 m for Monarch leg ergometers, and 3 m for Tunturi and Body Guard ergometers.

Balke		**3.4 mph**														
			2	4	6	8	10	12	14	16	18	20	22	26	26
Balke		**3.0 mph**														
			0	2.5	5	7.5	10	12.5	15	17.5	20	22.5			
Naughton	1.0	**2.0 mph**														
	0	0	3.5	7	10.5	14	17.5									
METs	**1.6**	**2**	**3**	**4**	**5**	**6**	**7**	**8**	**9**	**10**	**11**	**12**	**13**	**14**	**15**	**16**
mL/kg/min	5.6	7		14		21		28		35		42		49		56
Clinical Status		Symptomatic Patients														
		Diseased, Recovered														
			Sedentary/Healthy													
				Physically Active Subjects												
Functional Class	IV	III		II		I and Normal										

Fig. 2. Metabolic cost of three common treadmill protocols. One MET signifies resting energy expenditure, equivalent to approximately 3.5 mL/kg/min. Unlabeled numbers refer to the treadmill grade, expressed as percent. The patient's clinical status and functional class (I–IV) for the peak-attained workload are also shown.

(25). Alternatively, newer ramp protocols can overcome many of the limitations of some multistage exercise tests, which may impose excessive initial workloads and/or simultaneous increases in speed and grade. In contrast, ramp protocols provide a nearly continuous and uniform increase in aerobic requirements *(26).*

End Points for Testing

Commonly used criteria for discontinuing an exercise test include attaining a predetermined end point of submaximal performance (e.g., ≥70% or 85% of age-predicted maximal heart rate, perceived exertion ≥ 13 ["somewhat hard"] or ≥ ["hard"] on the category scale [6–20]), volitional fatigue, or emergence of abnormal signs or symptoms. Absolute and relative end points for terminating an exercise test are listed in Table 3 *(23).*

Electrocardiographic, Symptomatic, Hemodynamic, and Cardiorespiratory Responses to Exercise Testing and Their Prognostic Significance

Risk or prognostic evaluation is a critical activity in contemporary medical practice on which many patient management decisions are based (e.g., prescription of cardioprotective medications, need for coronary revascularization and/or an implantable cardioverter defibrillator). Data derived from a resting ECG and from exercise testing are most helpful in this regard, especially when considered in

Table 2
The Conventional Bruce Treadmill Protocol with MET Values for Each
Minute Interval Completed

Stage	MPH	Grade	Min	MET requirement[a]		
				Men	Women	Cardiac
			1	3.2	3.1	3.6
I	1.7	10%	2	4.0	3.9	4.3
			3	4.9	4.7	4.9
			4	5.7	5.4	5.6
II	2.5	12%	5	6.6	6.2	6.2
			6	7.4	7.0	7.0
			7	8.3	8.0	7.6
III	3.4	14%	8	9.1	8.6	8.3
			9	10.0	9.4	9.0
			10	10.7	10.1	9.7
IV	4.2	16%	11	11.6	10.9	10.4
			12	12.5	11.7	11.0
			13	13.3	12.5	11.7
V	5.0	18%	14	14.1	13.2	12.3
			15	15.0	14.1	13.0

Adapted from *(25)*.

[a]MET values are for each minute *completed*. Note that women and cardiac patients achieve *lower* VO_2 for equivalent workload. Holding on to front rail will *increase* the apparent MET capacity.

the context of other clinical information. Important prognostic variables that can be derived from the exercise test include electrocardiographic, symptomatic, and hemodynamic responses, as well as functional capacity (mL/kg/min or METs). In fact, by incorporating several of these measurements and/or related clinical data into a mathematical formula or treadmill score, conventional exercise testing can often outperform the newer, more costly, noninvasive studies.

BUNDLE BRANCH BLOCK

The prognostic significance of left and right bundle branch block was determined from the baseline or resting ECG in 7,073 adults who were referred for symptom-limited nuclear exercise testing *(27)*. Over a 6.7-year follow-up, all-cause mortality was greater in those patients who demonstrated either anomaly (24% for complete right or left bundle branch block) than in those without these findings (11%). After adjustment for exercise capacity, nuclear perfusion defects, and other risk factors, right bundle branch block was as strong an independent predictor of mortality as left bundle branch block, yielding identical hazard ratios (1.5). In contrast, incomplete right bundle branch block was not associated with an increased risk of mortality. Although the mechanisms underlying this relationship remain unclear, it has been suggested that complete bundle branch block (right or left) may reflect a greater likelihood of underlying CAD, manifested as left ventricular dysfunction, threatening ventricular arrhythmias, or both.

Table 3
Common End Points for Terminating Exercise Testing

Absolute Indications

Exertional hypotension (drop in systolic blood pressure ≥10 mmHg from baseline blood pressure despite an increase in workload, when accompanied by signs and/or symptoms of myocardial ischemia)

Moderate to severe angina pectoris (≥2/4 chest pain)

Signs of poor perfusion or central nervous system dysfunction (ataxia, cyanosis or pallor, staggering, failure to respond to questions)

Onset of ventricular tachycardia (≥3 consecutive premature ventricular contractions [PVCs])

ST-segment elevation (≥1.0 mm) in ECG leads without diagnostic Q waves (other than V_1 or aVR)

Technical difficulties monitoring the ECG or systolic blood pressure (i.e., equipment malfunction)

Subject's desire to stop[a]

Relative Indications

Excessive horizontal or downsloping ST-segment depression (≥2 mm)

Selected supraventricular or ventricular arrhythmias (e.g., increasing multifocal PVCs and/or ventricular couplets, supraventricular tachycardia, bradyarrhythmias)

Development of bundle branch block or intraventricular conduction delay that cannot be distinguished from ventricular tachycardia

Exertional hypotension in the absence of other evidence of myocardial ischemia

Hypertensive blood pressure response (systolic and/or diastolic pressure > 250 mmHg or 115 mmHg, respectively)

Marked fatigue, shortness of breath, or limiting claudication

Adapted from *(23)*.

[a]Ratings of perceived exertion ≥17 (very hard) on the Borg category scale, signifying near-maximal to maximal exertion, or a peak heart rate ~100% of the predicted maximal heart rate, can be especially helpful in this regard.

ST-SEGMENT DISPLACEMENT

The increased cardiac demands during progressive physical exertion may serve as the basis by which exercise testing may uncover occult obstructive CAD. By progressively challenging the coronary circulation with a higher rate-pressure product and contractile state, exercise raises myocardial oxygen demand. Stenotic arteries are unable to adequately respond to the requirements for increased blood flow, especially when the obstruction exceeds 75% of the vessel's cross-sectional area (Fig. 1). As a result, myocardial territories in jeopardy are rendered ischemic, and this may be manifested on the surface ECG as alterations in electrical repolarization currents (e.g., ST-segment displacement).

The interpretation of exercise-induced myocardial ischemia has historically relied on the presence of three types of ST-segment depression: horizontal, downsloping, and slow upsloping *(22)*. However, negative tests are often considered "inconclusive" when the peak heart rate achieved is <85% of the predicted maximum, because of inadequate cardiac stress. In contrast, exercise-induced ST-segment elevation in leads displaying a previous Q wave infarction almost always reflects an aneurysm or a wall motion abnormality, manifested as left ventricular dysfunction *(28)*. Furthermore, the development of ST-segment elevation during exercise in the absence of a previous myocardial infarction suggests a high-grade coronary stenosis and transmural rather than subendocardial ischemia, and is highly arrhythmogenic *(28)*.

Limitations of the Conventional Exercise ECG. Although useful in many patients, the conventional exercise ECG lacks specificity and sensitivity when screening for CAD in low- and high-risk populations, respectively *(12)*. Consequently, this diagnostic study is most useful in patients at moderate risk for CAD. Moreover, some patients may not be able to achieve adequate cardiac demands during treadmill exercise testing because of underlying obesity, deconditioning, PAD, or sensory or motor neuropathy. Others may be taking medications (i.e., beta blockers) or have preexisting anomalies on the resting ECG (e.g., substantial ST-segment depression at rest, left ventricular hypertrophy, left bundle branch block) that make ST-segment abnormalities that develop during exercise uninterpretable with respect to evidence of myocardial ischemia. Because many of these concerns apply to the diabetic patient, and early detection of CAD and intervention may prevent progression of disease and decrease the risk of clinical events, several recent reports have highlighted the diagnostic value of stress echocardiography and stress myocardial perfusion imaging with or without gated single-photon emission computed tomography in this escalating patient population *(12, 29–32)*.

SUPRAVENTRICULAR ARRHYTHMIAS

Isolated atrial beats and short runs of supraventricular tachycardia commonly occur during exercise testing and do not seem to have any diagnostic or prognostic significance for CAD *(22)*. Patients who regularly experience paroxysmal atrial tachycardia, especially if symptomatic, may be effectively treated with selected beta or calcium channel blockers or, in some cases, catheter ablation.

EXERCISE-INDUCED PREMATURE VENTRICULAR CONTRACTIONS (PVCs)

To clarify the long-term prognosis in persons with exercise-induced PVCs, researchers evaluated the risk of death from cardiovascular causes in 6,101 French men aged 42–53 years without known or suspected CAD who underwent conventional graded exercise testing and were followed for an average of 23 years *(33)*. Both signs/symptoms of myocardial ischemia and the occurrence of frequent PVCs during exercise were independently associated with an increased cardiovascular mortality, with similar relative risks (2.63 and 2.53, respectively). More recently, researchers at the Cleveland Clinic Foundation reported that frequent PVCs during exercise predicted an increased risk of death (9% vs. 5% among patients without frequent ventricular ectopy during exercise), but frequent ventricular ectopy during recovery was a stronger predictor (11% vs. 5%) *(34)*. Collectively, these studies suggest that frequent ventricular ectopy during and especially after symptom-limited exercise testing provides an important, independent predictor of an increased risk of death.

ANGINAL SYMPTOMS

It is critical for the clinician to note all symptoms that occur during and after the exercise test. Especially important are symptoms that may represent classic angina pectoris, such as substernal pressure radiating across the chest and/or down the left arm, back, or jaw, or lower neck pain or discomfort. Such symptoms can be subjectively rated by the patient on a 4-point scale: 1 = perceptible but mild; 2 = moderate; 3 = moderately severe; and, 4 = severe. Ratings of ≥2 should be used as end points for exercise testing *(22, 23)*.

Although asymptomatic patients may demonstrate marked exercise-induced ST-segment abnormalities, when angina pectoris occurs in conjunction with ST-segment displacement the likelihood of ECG changes being due to CAD is significantly increased. Moreover, exercise-induced angina pectoris per se is now considered an independent variable that identifies a subset of patients at increased risk for subsequent coronary events *(35)*.

DYSPNEA AND CARDIAC PROGNOSIS

Although dyspnea is a common symptom, few data are available regarding its prognostic significance among patients referred for cardiac stress testing. Recently, investigators reported on 17,991 patients who underwent resting and stress myocardial-perfusion single-photon-emission computed tomography using symptom-limited stress induced by either a treadmill exercise (66%) or a vasodilator (34%) *(36)*. Patients were divided into five categories according to their self-reported symptoms of chest pain and dyspnea at the time of testing: none; nonanginal chest pain; atypical angina; typical angina; and, dyspnea. After a mean ± SD follow-up of 2.7 ± 1.7 years, patients with dyspnea, both those with and without known CAD, had increased cardiovascular and all-cause mortality rates. Among patients with no known history of CAD, those with dyspnea had 4.6 times the annualized rate (%/years) of sudden cardiac death of asymptomatic patients and 2.6 times the risk of patients with typical angina. It was concluded that dyspnea may represent myocardial ischemia (an anginal equivalent) and underlying CVD, and that this response should be documented and included in the clinical assessment of patients referred for cardiac stress testing.

HEMODYNAMIC RESPONSES

Although exercise-induced ST-segment displacement and angina pectoris have been the primary, and often sole diagnostic and prognostic criteria to identify occult or progressive CAD, the evaluation of hemodynamic responses (i.e., heart rate and blood pressure) before, during and immediately after exercise enhance the predictive value of exercise testing. Chronotropic incompetence, a delayed decrease in the recovery heart rate immediately after peak or symptom-limited exercise testing, and exertional hypotension are associated with underlying CAD and increased mortality.

Chronotropic Incompetence.   Sustained relative bradycardia (subsequently termed chronotropic incompetence), that is, the inability to achieve an expected peak or maximal heart rate on exercise testing, has been shown to independently predict significant CAD, even in the absence of other abnormal signs or symptoms *(37)*. For patients who are not taking beta-blockers (or other heart rate blunting drugs) and whose tests are terminated due to volitional fatigue, chronotropic incompetence is apparent if the heart rate reserve – calculated as follows: (peak heart rate – resting heart rate)/ ([220 – age] – resting heart rate) – is less than 80% during exercise-induced stress *(38)*. For example, a 60-year-old male, with a resting heart rate of 75 beats/min in the upright position, attains a maximal exercise heart rate of 138 beats/min at which point the test is terminated due to volitional fatigue. His heart rate reserve would be calculated as 220 – 60 – 75 = 85 beats/min. A normal maximal heart rate would be 80% or more of 85 beats/min, added to the resting heart rate of 75 beats/min, that is, ≥143 beats/min. Thus, this man would be classified as demonstrating chronotropic incompetence.

Recovery Heart Rate.   The decrement in heart rate after peak or symptom-limited exercise testing has also been suggested as an important predictor of mortality, even after accounting for ST-segment depression and/or angina pectoris, angiographic severity of CAD, left ventricular function, cardiorespiratory fitness, chronotropic incompetence, and the Duke treadmill score *(39)*. Previously, after adjusting for potential confounding variables, researchers reported that a delayed decrease in heart rate, defined as a reduction of 12 beats/min or less from the heart rate at peak exercise, was associated with a relative risk of 2.0 (CI = 1.5–2.7) *(40)*. It was concluded that this response, which may be a reflection of decreased vagal activity, is a powerful predictor of overall mortality. Another study of a large cohort of asymptomatic men with diabetes found that heart rate recovery measured even as long as 5 min following maximal exercise was independently associated with higher cardiovascular and all-cause mortality *(41)*.

Heart Rate Profile.   Recently, the heart rate profile before, during, and after maximal exercise testing was assessed in a cohort of 5,713 asymptomatic working men (between the ages of 42 and 53 years), none of whom had documented CAD *(42)*. During a 23-year follow-up, the relative risk (RR) of sudden cardiac death was increased in subjects with a resting heart rate that was greater than 75 beats/min (RR = 3.9), in subjects with an increase in heart rate during exercise that was less than 89 beats/min (RR = 6.2), and in subjects with a decrease in heart rate of less than 25 beats/min at one minute after the termination of exercise (RR = 2.2). After adjusting for potential confounding variables, these three responses remained strongly associated with an increased risk of sudden death. It was concluded that abnormalities in autonomic function, that is, impairment of the ability to increase both sympathetic and vagal activity rapidly, may precede manifestations of CAD and contribute to the early identification of persons at high risk for sudden cardiac death.

Prognostic Blood Pressure Responses.   The "normal" hemodynamic response to exercise is a progressive increase in systolic blood pressure, typically 8–12 mmHg per MET, with a possible plateau at peak exercise *(16, 22)*. Exertional hypotension (systolic blood pressure that fails to rise or falls [>10 mmHg]) with incremental exercise may signify myocardial ischemia, left ventricular dysfunction, or both. Men with a maximal exercise systolic blood pressure < 140 mmHg had a 3.8- and 14.7-fold increase in the annual rate of sudden cardiac death as compared with those whose pressures reached 140–200 mmHg and exceeded 200 mmHg, respectively *(43)*.

The normal response to exercise is no change or a slight decrease in diastolic blood pressure. An exercise-induced increase of more than 15 mmHg in diastolic pressure may signify severe CAD, even in the absence of ischemic signs and symptoms *(44)*.

EXERCISE CAPACITY

Large cohort and clinical studies have identified a low level of aerobic fitness as an independent risk factor for all-cause and cardiovascular mortality *(22, 45, 46)*, as well as varied comorbid conditions, including diabetes. Previously, researchers at the Cooper Institute/Clinic studied >8,600 nondiabetic men who were followed for approximately 6 years *(47)*. After adjusting for confounding variables, men in the low-fitness group (the least 20% of the cohort) at baseline had a 1.9- and 3.7-fold risk of developing impaired fasting glucose and diabetes, respectively, as compared with those in the high-fitness group (the most fit 40% of the cohort). A more recent report by several of these investigators found that diabetic men in the lowest, second, and third quartiles of cardiorespiratory fitness had 4.5-, 2.8-, and 1.6-fold greater risk for overall mortality than men in the highest quartile of cardiorespiratory fitness, even after adjusting for age, risk factors, and other potential modulating factors *(48)*.

Numerous studies in men and women suggest that each 1-MET increase in exercise capacity appears to convey an 8–17% reduction in mortality risk *(22)*. The Aerobic Center Longitudinal Study represents a unique database regarding fitness and mortality. Tables 4 and 5 illustrate low, moderate,

Table 4
Fitness and Mortality in Men, ACLS, Fitness Categories

Fitness group	*Age groups (years)*			
	20–39	*40–49*	*50–59*	*60+*
Low	≤10.5	≤9.9	≤8.8	≤7.5
Moderate	10.6–12.7	10.0–12.1	8.9–10.9	7.6–9.7
High	>12.7	>12.1	>10.9	>9.7

Courtesy of the Cooper Institute for Aerobics Research, Dallas, TX, with permission.

Table values are maximal METs attained during treadmill exercise testing.

Table 5
Fitness and Mortality in Women, ACLS, Fitness Categories

Fitness group	*Age groups (years)*			
	20–39	*40–49*	*50–59*	*60+*
Low	≤8.1	≤7.5	≤6.5	≤5.7
Moderate	8.2–10.5	7.6–9.5	6.6–8.3	5.7–7.5
High	>10.5	>9.5	>8.3	>7.5

Courtesy of the Cooper Institute for Aerobics Research, Dallas, TX, with permission.

Table values are maximal METs attained during treadmill exercise testing.

and high fitness levels (in METs), expressed as a function of age and gender. The low-fitness groups are at increased mortality risk, whereas the high-fitness groups generally have an excellent prognosis, regardless of existing comorbidities or underlying CAD. These data should be helpful in counseling patients regarding their current exercise capacity and long-term fitness goals. For example, a 55-year-old man who achieves 7 min on the conventional Bruce treadmill protocol, corresponding to an estimated aerobic capacity of 8.3 METs (Table 2), would be classified in the low fitness category (Table 4), which is associated with an increased mortality rate. An initial goal would be to increase his fitness to the moderate category (8.9–10.9 METs) and higher (>10.9 METs), if possible, in the future. Conversely, a 65-year-old woman who achieves 6 min on the conventional Bruce treadmill protocol, would have an estimated aerobic capacity of 7.0 METs (Table 2), corresponding to the moderate or average fitness category (Table 5). A goal for her would be to achieve high fitness, or >7.5 METs.

THE DUKE TREADMILL SCORE

Researchers at Duke University have incorporated three treadmill test variables into a mathematical formula or treadmill score, which has proven to be extremely valuable in assessing prognosis and the severity of underlying CAD. Initially, the Duke treadmill score was validated on a population of inpatients with chest pain who underwent both cardiac catheterization and treadmill testing *(49)*, and subsequently on outpatients (men and women) referred for noninvasive evaluation of CAD, but without recent myocardial infarction or coronary revascularization *(50)*. The score has also been shown to predict significant (≥75% coronary obstruction) and severe (three-vessel or left main) CAD *(51)*. Accordingly, treadmill scores can help to determine the type and advisability of further diagnostic testing.

The Duke Treadmill Score uses exercise time (minutes), based on the conventional Bruce treadmill protocol (Table 2), ST-segment displacement (millimeters), and an anginal index (0, none; 1, occurring during the treadmill test; 2, reason for terminating the test):

$$\text{Treadmill Score} = \text{Exercise time} - (5 \times \text{ST displacement}) - (4 \times \text{Angina index})$$

Using these calculations, treadmill scores identified patients at low (≤+5 points), moderate (−10 to +4), and high (≤−11) risk of subsequent cardiac events. Low-risk patients could be spared from additional diagnostic studies, whereas high-risk patients would be referred for cardiac catheterization. Thus, for these patient subsets, treadmill scores render additional noninvasive testing unnecessary. To provide a simpler method of determining prognosis, the earlier referenced responses were plotted as a nomogram that provides an estimate of 5-year survival and average annual mortality *(52)*.

To determine the predictive accuracy of exercise testing in diabetics, researchers studied 100 diabetics and 202 age- and sex-matched nondiabetic controls without known CAD stratified by the Duke Treadmill Score and followed for an average duration of 6.6 years *(53)*. Although diabetics had higher rates of major adverse cardiac events than nondiabetics, the Duke Treadmill Score was a strong independent predictor of composite events in both diabetics and nondiabetics, highlighting its value in this patient cohort who carry a high risk for CAD.

REFERENCES

1. Chobanian AV, Bakris GL, Black HR, et al. The Seventh Report of the Joint National Committee on Prevention, Detection, Evaluation, and Treatment of High Blood Pressure: the JNC 7 report. *JAMA* 2003;289:2560–2572.
2. Gibbons RJ, Abrams J, Chatterjee K, et al. ACC/AHA 2002 guideline update for the management of patients with chronic stable angina – summary article: a report of the American College of Cardiology/American Heart Association Task Force on Practice Guidelines (Committee on the Management of Patients with Chronic Stable Angina). *Circulation* 2003;107:149–158.
3. Stewart KJ. Exercise training for claudication. *N Engl J Med* 2002;347:1941–1951.
4. Grundy SM, Cleeman JI, Merz CN, et al. Implications of recent clinical trials for the National Cholesterol Education Program Adult Treatment Panel III guidelines. *Circulation* 2004;13;110:227–239.
5. Gibbons RJ, Balady GJ, Bricker JT, et al. ACC/AHA 2002 guideline update for exercise testing: Summary article. A report of the American College of Cardiology/American Heart Association Task Force on Practice Guidelines (Committee to Update the 1997 Exercise Testing Guidelines). *Circulation* 2002;106:1883–1892.
6. Beaver WL, Wasserman K, Whipp BJ. A new method for detecting the anaerobic threshold by gas exchange. *J Appl Physiol* 1986;60:2020–2027.
7. Corrà U, Mezzani A, Bosimini E, Scapellato F, Imparato A, Giannuzzi P. Ventilatory response to exercise improves risk stratification in patients with chronic heart failure and intermediate functional capacity. *Am Heart J* 2002;143:18–26.
8. American Diabetes Association. Standards of medical care for patients with diabetes mellitus. *Diabetes Care* 2002;25:S33–S49.
9. Barrett EJ, Ginsberg HN, Pauker SG, et al. Consensus Development Conference on the Diagnosis of Coronary Heart Disease in People with Diabetes: 10–11 February 1998, Miami, Florida. *Diabetes Care* 1998;21:1551–1559.
10. Kannel WB, D'Agostino RB, Wilson PW, Belanger AJ, Gagnon DR. Diabetes, fibrinogen, and risk of cardiovascular disease: the Framingham experience. *Am Heart J* 1990;120:672–676.
11. American Diabetes Association. Economic consequences of diabetes mellitus in the U.S. in 1997. *Diabetes Care* 1998; 21:296–309.
12. Inzucchi SE. Noninvasive assessment of the diabetic patient for coronary artery disease. *Diabetes Care* 2001;24:1519–1521.
13. Zinman B, Ruderman N, Campaigne BN, Devlin JT, Schneider SH. American Diabetes Association. Physical activity/exercise and diabetes mellitus (position statement). *Diabetes Care* 2003;26 (Suppl 1):S73–S77.
14. Wackers FJTh, Young LH, Inzucchi SE, et al. Detection of silent myocardial ischemia in asymptomatic diabetic subjects. The DIAD study. *Diabetes Care* 2004;27:2954–2961.
15. Scognamiglio R, Negut C, Ramondo A, Tiengo A, Avogaro A. Detection of coronary artery disease in asymptomatic patients with type 2 diabetes mellitus. *J Am Coll Cardiol* 2006;47:65–71.
16. American College of Sports Medicine. Guidelines for Exercise Testing and Prescription, 7th ed. Baltimore, MD: Lippincott Williams & Wilkins, 2005.
17. Fowler-Brown A, Pignone M, Pletcher M, Tice JA, Sutton SF, Lohr KN. Exercise tolerance testing to screen for coronary heart disease: a systematic review for the technical support for the U.S. Preventive Services Task Force. *Ann Intern Med* 2004;140:W9–W24.
18. U.S. Preventive Services Task Force. Screening for coronary heart disease: recommendation statement. *Ann Intern Med* 2004;140:569–572.
19. Sigal RJ, Kenny GP, Wasserman DH, Castaneda-Sceppa C. Physical activity/exercise and type 2 diabetes. *Diabetes Care* 2004;27:2518–2539.
20. Falk E, Shah PK, Fuster V. Coronary plaque disruption. *Circulation* 1995;92:657–671.
21. Malinow MR, McGarry DL, Kuehl KS. Is exercise testing indicated for asymptomatic active people? *J Cardiac Rehabil* 1984;4:376–380.
22. Franklin BA, Gordon NF. Contemporary Diagnosis and Management in Cardiovascular Exercise. Newtown, PA: Handbooks in Health Care, 2005.
23. Gibbons RA, Balady GJ, Beasely JW, et al. ACC/AHA guidelines for exercise testing: a report of the American College of Cardiology/American Heart Association Task Force on Practice Guidelines (Committee on Exercise Testing). *J Am Coll Cardiol* 1997;30:260–315.
24. Franklin BA. Exercise testing, training and arm ergometry. *Sports Med* 1985;2:100–119.

25. American College of Sports Medicine. Guidelines for Exercise Testing and Prescription, 4th ed. Philadelphia, PA: Lea & Febiger, 1991:61.
26. Myers J, Buchanan N, Walsh D, et al. Comparison of the ramp versus standard exercise protocols. *J Am Coll Cardiol* 1991;17:1334–1342.
27. Hesse B, Diaz LA, Snader CE, Blackstone EH, Lauer MS. Complete bundle branch block as an independent predictor of all-cause mortality: report of 7073 patients referred for nuclear exercise testing. *Am J Med* 2001;110:253–259.
28. Nostratian F, Froelicher VF. ST elevation during exercise testing. *Am J Cardiol* 1989;63:986–988.
29. Wackers FJTh, Zaret BL. Detection of myocardial ischemia in patients with diabetes mellitus. *Circulation* 2002;105:5–7.
30. Kamalesh M, Feigenbaum H, Sawada S. Challenge of identifying patients with diabetes mellitus who are at low risk for coronary events by use of cardiac stress imaging. *Am Heart J* 2004;147:561–563.
31. Wackers FJTh. Diabetes and coronary artery disease: The role of stress myocardial perfusion imaging. *Cleve Clin J Med* 2005;72:21–33.
32. Lauer MS. Coronary artery disease in diabetes: which (if any) test is best. *Cleve Clin J Med* 2005;72:6–9.
33. Jouven X, Zuriek M, Desnos M, Courbon D, Ducimetière P. Long-term outcome in asymptomatic men with exercise-induced premature ventricular depolarizations. *N Engl J Med* 2000;343:826–833.
34. Frolkis JP, Pothier CE, Blackstone EH, Lauer MS. Frequent ventricular ectopy after exercise as a predictor of death. *N Engl J Med* 2003;348:781–790.
35. Cole JP, Ellestad MH. Significance of chest pain during treadmill exercise: correlation with coronary events. *Am J Cardiol* 1978;41:227–232.
36. Abidov A, Rozanski A, Hachamovitch R, et al. Prognostic significance of dyspnea in patients referred for cardiac stress testing. *N Engl J Med* 2005;353:1889–1898.
37. Brener SJ, Pashkow FJ, Harvey SA, Marwick TH, Thomas JD, Lauer MS. Chronotropic response to exercise predicts angiographic severity in patients with suspected or stable coronary artery disease. *Am J Cardiol* 1995;76:1228–1232.
38. Lauer MS, Francis GS, Okin PM, Pashkow FJ, Snader CE, Marwick TH. Impaired chronotropic response to exercise stress testing as a predictor of mortality. *JAMA* 1999;281:524–529.
39. Vivekananthan DP, Blackstone EH, Pothier CE, Lauer MS. Heart rate recovery after exercise is a predictor of mortality, independent of the angiographic severity of coronary disease. *J Am Coll Cardiol* 2003;42:831–838.
40. Cole CR, Blackstone EH, Pashkow FJ, Snader CE, Lauer MS. Heart-rate recovery immediately after exercise as a predictor of mortality. *N Engl J Med* 1999;341:1351–1357.
41. Cheng YJ, Lauer MS, Earnest CP, et al. Heart rate recovery following maximal exercise testing as a predictor of cardiovascular disease and all-cause mortality in men with diabetes. *Diabetes Care* 2003;26:2052–2057.
42. Jouven X, Empana J-P, Schwartz PJ, Desnos M, Courbon D, Ducimetière P. Heart-rate profile during exercise as a predictor of sudden death. *N Engl J Med* 2005;352:1951–1958.
43. Irving JB, Bruce RA, DeRouen TA. Variations in and significance of systolic pressure during maximal exercise (treadmill) testing: relation to severity of coronary artery disease and cardiac mortality. *Am J Cardiol* 1977;39:841–848.
44. Sheps DS, Ernst JC, Briese FW, Myerburg RJ. Exercise-induced increase in diastolic pressure: indicator of severe coronary artery disease. *Am J Cardiol* 1979;43:708–712.
45. Snader CE, Marwick TH, Pashkow FJ, Harvey SA, Thomas JD, Lauer MS. Importance of estimated functional capacity as a predictor of all-cause mortality among patients referred for exercise thallium single-photon emission computed tomography: Report of 3,400 patients from a single center. *J Am Coll Cardiol* 1997;30:641–648.
46. Dutcher JR, Kahn J, Grines C, Franklin B. Comparison of left ventricular ejection fraction and exercise capacity as predictors of two- and five-year mortality following acute myocardial infarction. *Am J Cardiol* 2007;99:436–441.
47. Wei M, Gibbons LW, Mitchell TL, Kampert JB, Lee CD, Blair SN. The association between cardiorespiratory fitness and impaired fasting glucose and type 2 diabetes mellitus in men. *Ann Intern Med* 1999;130:89–96.
48. Church TS, Cheng YJ, Earnest CP, et al. Exercise capacity and body composition as predictors of mortality among men with diabetes. *Diabetes Care* 2004;27:83–88.
49. Mark DB, Hlatky MA, Harrell FE, Lee KL, Califf RM, Pryor DB. Exercise treadmill score for predicting prognosis in coronary artery disease. *Ann Intern Med* 1987;106:793–800.
50. Mark DB, Shaw L, Harrell FE, et al. Prognostic value of a treadmill exercise score in outpatients with suspected coronary artery disease. *N Engl J Med* 1991;325:849–853.
51. Shaw LJ, Peterson ED, Shaw LK, et al. Use of prognostic treadmill score in identifying diagnostic coronary disease subgroups. *Circulation* 1998;98:1622–1630.
52. Fletcher GF, Balady GJ, Amsterdam EA, et al. Exercise standards for testing and training. A statement for Healthcare Professionals from the American Heart Association. *Circulation* 2001;104:1694–1740.
53. Lakkireddy DR, Bhakkad J, Korlakunta HL, et al. Prognostic value of the Duke treadmill score in diabetic patients. *Am Heart J* 2005;150:516–521.

IV

SPECIAL CONSIDERATIONS FOR EXERCISE IN PERSONS WITH DIABETES

13 Conditions That May Interfere with Exercise

Susan Herzlinger Botein, Aristidis Veves, and Edward Horton

CONTENTS

ABSTRACT

Exercise often has many positive effects on diabetes management, including improved glycemic control, assistance with weight maintenance, increases cardiorespiratory fitness, and general sense of well-being. However, as diabetic patients can also have other conditions that can be negatively affected by exercise, such as cardiovascular disease and neuropathy that makes them vulnerable to foot problems and retinopathy, exercise should be carefully monitored by the health provider, especially during the initiation period. Therefore, careful evaluation of patients for complications that may present incremental risks or interfere with the capacity for exercise is an important first step in planning an appropriate exercise program. This chapter will review the currently available guidelines and will provide practical information regarding the implementation of exercise programs in diabetic patients with conditions that may interfere with exercise and will need additional attention.

Key words: Retinopathy; Neuropathy; Cardiovascular disease; Exercise.

Diabetes affects nearly 21 million children and adults in the USA or 7% of the population *(1)*. Diabetes is a chronic, often debilitating, and disabling illness due to the complications that accompany the disease. These complications, including coronary artery disease, peripheral neuropathy, nephropathy, and retinopathy, can largely be prevented through proper medical therapy and lifestyle measures, such as eating a healthy diet, maintaining a normal weight, and participating in regular exercise. However, only a minority of people with diabetes achieve adequate glycemic control (HcA1C < 7.0%)

From: *Contemporary Diabetes: Diabetes and Exercise*
Edited by: J. G. Regensteiner et al. (eds.), DOI: 10.1007/978-1-59745-260-1_13
© Humana Press, a part of Springer Science+Business Media, LLC 2009

and even fewer also reach established targets for blood pressure and lipids *(2)*. Consequently, long-term complications of diabetes are still prevalent and may even be present at the time of diagnosis in people with type 2 diabetes. Careful evaluation of patients for complications that may present incremental risks or interfere with the capacity for exercise is an important first step in planning an appropriate exercise program.

ROLE OF EXERCISE IN DIABETES MANAGEMENT

Exercise often has many positive effects on diabetes management. These include improved glycemic control, assistance with weight maintenance, increased cardiorespiratory fitness, and general sense of well-being. In type I diabetes, the primary exercise-related goal is to make it possible for patients to participate in recreational exercise and sports and to capture the general health benefits afforded by exercise. In type 2 diabetes, a regular program of physical exercise should be an integral part of the treatment program. The American Diabetes Association (ADA) recommends 150 min per week of moderate intensity exercise (50–70% of maximum heart rate) or 90 min per week of vigorous (>70% of maximum heart rate) exercise per week to maintain weight, improve glycemic control, and reduce cardiac risk *(3)*. In the absence of contraindications, the ADA and the American College of Sports Medicine also recommend resistance exercise three times per week to patients with type 2 diabetes.

Certainly, imparting the aforementioned recommendations to patients is quite facile. "Advised exercise regimen? Check." But diabetes complications plague many patients with diabetes before they undertake an exercise program and may affect ability to safely exercise. What advice is appropriate for the 25-year-old woman with type 1 diabetes and diabetic retinopathy who wants to start horseback riding? Or the 50-year-old man with peripheral neuropathy who wants to start exercising on a treadmill? This chapter outlines an approach to exercise in patients with preexisting complications of diabetes - neuropathy, nephropathy, and retinopathy. Patients with established coronary artery disease often require the monitored environment of cardiac rehabilitation, which is reviewed in the following chapter.

GLUCOSE CONTROL AND EXERCISE

All people with diabetes, particularly those with type 1 diabetes or people with type 2 diabetes, who require insulin therapy, may have problems with glucose control with exercise (see Table 1). There may be a decreased need for insulin during exercise, as well as increased risk of hypoglycemia. High-intensity, short-term exercise may also cause an acute rise in blood glucose in people, even with well-controlled diabetes *(5)*. Clearly glucose regulation, particularly in diabetes type I, is critical. Problems include hypoglycemia during and following exercise, as well as hyperglycemia and ketosis as a response to strenuous exercise. The details of glucose management and alterations in insulin and glucose physiology with exercise are covered elsewhere.

CARDIOVASCULAR DISEASE

Exercise has beneficial effects as well in patients with coronary artery disease. Exercise training as part of a cardiac rehabilitation program after myocardial infarction, for example, has been shown to decrease mortality *(6)*. Exercise also improves insulin sensitivity, lipid metabolism and expends calories, all of which may have a positive impact on the development of cardiovascular disease (CVD). As remarked elsewhere, however, patients with diabetes have high prevalence of CVD - both overt and

Table 1
Limiting Factors and Risks of Exercise for Patients
with Diabetic Complications (4)

Precipitating or exacerbating cardiovascular disease
Angina pectoris
Myocardial infarction
Arrhythmia
Sudden cardiac death
Proliferative retinopathy
Vitreous hemorrhage
Retinal detachment
Retinal hemorrhage
Nephropathy
Increased proteinuria
Peripheral neuropathy
Soft-tissue and joint injury
Autonomic neuropathy
Blunted cardiovascular response to exercise
Decreased maximal aerobic capacity
Impaired response to dehydration
Postural hypotension

undiagnosed. Hypercholesterolemia, hypertension, and associated cardiac disease frequently accompany diabetes. Some consider the diagnosis of diabetes akin to a coronary heart disease equivalent (7). For example, a large study in Finland found that the risk of first major coronary event in high-risk patients with diabetes was approximately equal to that of nondiabetic patients with prior myocardial infarcts (8). Complications of diabetes confer additional risks to patients. Autonomic neuropathy, for example, is associated with "silent" ischemia as well as increased risk of sudden death. People with diabetes have a lower survival rate after myocardial infarction and a poorer prognosis after diagnosis of coronary artery disease (9). Therefore, appropriate screening is necessary before initiating an exercise program. Procedures and limits related to testing are covered in Chap. 10.

Retinopathy

The confluence of diabetes and retinopathy poses an additional layer of concern for risks of exercise to the patient. As covered in other chapters, exercise may help to delay or prevent complications in diabetes. The concern is that exercise may exacerbate several diabetes-related complications. Among these, one of the most potentially serious is proliferative retinopathy, which predisposes to vitreous hemorrhage and traction retinal detachment. Exercises that increase blood pressure, particularly high-intensity exercise that involves Valsalva maneuvers, as well as jarring head motions, can precipitate these devastating complications. Patients with proliferative retinopathy have significant restrictions on the type and intensity of activity that they can safely engage in due to this risk of severe ocular damage.

The underlying mechanisms hypothesized to incite these devastating events include increasing systolic blood pressure causing vessel rupture and hemorrhage, trauma causing retinal detachment or hemorrhage. The loss of circulatory autoregulation in the eye of individuals with proliferative diabetic retinopathy may allow the retinal arteriole perfusion pressure to surpass the hemorrhagic threshold in the abnormal retinal vessels during exercise-induced blood pressure rise *(10)*. Such increases in systolic blood pressure could precipitate retinal or vitreous hemorrhage. Activities that include rapid head motion may also precipitate retinal detachment or vitreous hemorrhage *(4)*. There is no such concern in nonproliferative retinal disease or macular edema.

Systolic blood pressure increases linearly with work intensity, reaching peak values between 200 and 240 mm of mercury in normotensive persons in intense exercise, while diastolic pressure remains near resting levels *(4)*. This phenomenon is present both in resistance and aerobic exercise *(11)*. In a study of healthy older men, blood pressure and heart rate were measured during a variety of activities. Peak systolic blood pressure occurred with aerobic exercise and the military press (271 and 261 mmHg, respectively) *(12)*. Interestingly, in another study, exaggerated blood pressure increase with exercise (>60 mmHg) was associated with increased risk of developing hypertension at follow-up (4–15 years later) and may be a predictive tool *(13)*. Vigorous aerobic or resistance activity may be contraindicated in patients with proliferative retinopathy due to risk of inciting retinal detachment or retinal or vitreous hemorrhage due to blood pressure increases *(14)*. Preexercise testing to determine the heart rate at which blood pressure exceeds a predetermined limit may be helpful for patients to self-monitor during exercise *(15)*.

The general recommendation to patients with proliferative diabetic retinopathy is thus to avoid any activity that is jarring, traumatic, or involves excessive strain. The latter include maximal isometric contractions and Valsalva maneuvers, such as weight training. Practical general advice to the patient with proliferative retinopathy may include recommending avoidance of bending at the waist, lifting (particularly overhead), and near-maximal isometric contraction, which might be useful for the patient who exercises in classes at gyms or with a personal trainer and may or may not plan their own routines. Low-impact exercise, such as stationary biking (not maximal efforts as in spinning), walking, and swimming are recommended (see Table 2 for more details).

Despite these recommendations - or perhaps because of them -most retinal and vitreous hemorrhages do not occur with activity. In one retrospective report of diabetic patients with episodes of vitreous hemorrhage, the most common antecedent activity was sleep (36%) followed closely by sitting or lying (26%) *(16)*. Only one of six hemorrhages was associated with strenuous activity in this report. Finally, physical activity does not appear to be associated with progression or development of proliferative retinopathy. One large study followed subjects with diabetes diagnosed before the age of 30 for 6 years. There was no association between physical activity and development or progression of retinopathy, even with strenuous activity *(17)*.

In the early stages of retinopathy, however, exercise may be beneficial. Because exercise can lower blood pressure and increase high-density lipoprotein (HDL), exercise may reduce risk of developing proliferative diabetic retinopathy and diabetic macular edema. Regular ophthalmology follow-up, with or without diabetic retinopathy is essential as well. With proliferative diabetic retinopathy, follow-up should be every 1–2 months, and without evidence of eye complications, a minimum of annually *(14)*.

Nephropathy

There are no explicit limitations to exercise in patients with diabetic nephropathy. The pathophysiology underlying development of microalbuminuria has not been determined, but is generally considered to be associated with endothelial dysfunction and changes in renal blood flow. Increased blood pressure is related to albuminuria progression and, therefore, hemodynamic factors play a role. Numerous studies have noted that in patients with diabetes-related nephropathy, exercise can acutely increase urinary

Table 2
Recommendations to Patients with Proliferative Diabetic Retinopathy

Exercise	Recommendation	Exercise	Recommendation
Walking	Recommended	Yoga	Use extreme caution; avoid bending as in downward facing dog and shoulder stands
Running	Not recommended due to jarring	Pilates	Avoid due to Valsalva
Aerobics	Not recommended due to jarring	Dance	Use caution with rapid spinning
Rowing machine	Recommended at low intensity	Cycling/ spinning	Avoid highest intensity Valsalva in spinning; avoid trauma in mountain biking
Soccer	Not recommended due to heading	Tennis	Avoid *only if* significant Valsalva and active proliferative retinopathy and vitreous hemorrhage
Basketball	Use caution, avoid contact	Swimming	Use caution with kick-turns
Weightlifting	Not recommended due to Valsalva; 5–10 lb free weight okay	Downhill skiing	No jumps
Horseback riding	Avoid due to risk of trauma	Snowboarding	Not recommended
		Alpine skiing	Use caution

protein excretion. For example, one study examined children and adolescents with and without type 1 diabetes. While baseline albumin excretion rates were similar between the groups, albumin excretion rates after exercise were significantly higher in the subjects with diabetes type 1 *(18)*.

In another study of children and adolescents with diabetes type 1, postexercise albuminuria was not correlated with the development of microalbuminuria at 6-year follow-up *(19)*. In contrast, a study of adults with insulin-dependent diabetes who were initially normoalbuminuric for 10 years found that the postexercise urine albumin to creatinine ratio at baseline was predictive of rest microalbuminuria in 80% of affected subjects at 10-year follow-up *(20)*. Another study examined postexercise albuminuria in children with differing durations with diabetes. While children who had diabetes for less than 5 years did not have significant albuminuria with exercise, those with disease for longer than 5 years did have significant albuminuria with exercise, and 43% had accompanying immunoglobulin G (IgG) and transferrin, indicating glomerular damage *(21)*. In a similar study, participants exercised at a fixed workload; exercise-induced increases in systolic blood pressure were exaggerated in subjects with diabetes-related microalbuminuria as compared to patients with uncomplicated diabetes and control subjects *(22)*.

Angiotensin-converting enzyme (ACE) inhibitors may decrease the amount of exercise-induced albumin excretion in type 1 diabetes *(23, 24)*, perhaps through reduction in renal intracapillary pressure by inhibiting angiotensin-induced vasoconstriction on the efferent glomerular artery *(22)*. ACE inhibitors are currently standard care for rest microalbuminuria.

Efforts to link exercise-induced proteinuria to a precursor stage of microalbuminuria have been inconclusive *(22)*. One study of fixed workload demonstrated that exercise-induced albuminuria was not a useful predictor of microalbuminuria at 6 years of follow-up *(25)*. Alternatively, another fixed-workload study found that exercise-induced albuminuria improved with lowering hemoglobin A1C, and that a "window" exists during which an elevated exercise-related albumin excretion may be reversed by improved glucose control *(26)*. Regardless of whether postexercise microalbuminuria is a harbinger of overt nephropathy, there is no evidence that exercise accelerates the course of diabetic nephropathy.

In chronic kidney disease, the rationale for including exercise as a part of therapy is targeted at reversing the catabolism and reduced exercise capacity that often accompanies end-stage renal disease *(27)*. There are few rigorous trials looking at the effect of exercise in chronic kidney disease. One small study of dialysis patients in Greece showed that an exercise rehabilitation program improved muscle atrophy and overall exercise performance *(28)*. In another study of participants with moderate renal insufficiency, resistance training improved muscle mass and nutritional status in the context of the challenges presented by a low-protein diet and uremia that accompany renal disease *(29)*.

Limited randomized-control trials have been performed; there is no evidence that exercise improves or decreases glomerular filtration rate over time *(30)*. There is, however, evidence that the presence of diabetic nephropathy is associated with diminished exercise capacity (peak VO_2max) *(31)*. Anemia contributes to this relationship. In addition, exercise capacity may be used as a predictor of risk for cardiovascular events; presence of nephropathy may be associated with increased risk of CVD. The risk factors for nephropathy are similar to those for coronary artery disease, so appropriate preexercise screening should be performed as covered in Chap. 10.

In summary, as there is no evidence that exercise accelerates the course of diabetic nephropathy, there are no recommended limits on participation in exercise in these patients. However, the fatigue and anemia that often accompany chronic kidney disease may hamper patients' desire and ability to exercise.

Neuropathy

Peripheral neuropathy, along with peripheral arterial disease, is a main underlying cause of foot pathology in patients with diabetes. Neuropathy can predispose to muscular atrophy resulting of clawing of the toes, and collagen glycation can lead to limited joint mobility, changing foot pressures, and ulceration *(32)*. Peripheral neuropathy results in decreased pain sensation in the extremities, which can lead to injury unawareness and, ultimately, Charcot joint morphology *(33)*.

Because peripheral neuropathy results in impaired proprioception, the patient needs to rely on vision. Mirrors can help the patient orient without having to look at their feet. Equilibrium training and use of external supports may also be helpful. Range of motion exercises is also important for preventing and minimizing contractures *(32)*.

Some clinicians recommend complete avoidance of weight-bearing exercise in these patients, although education and proper footwear may help to prevent these complications. Certainly, limiting weight-bearing exercise and focusing instead on bicycling, swimming, and arm exercises is prudent. Daily inspection of feet, limiting wearing shoes to 5 h at a time are essential for patients with peripheral neuropathy and/or Charcot feet. Corrective footwear can also redistribute pressures to limit pressure on deformities.

Autonomic neuropathy presents both metabolic and hormonal derangements, both of which alter normal response to exercise. The adrenergic response of norepinephrine, epinephrine, growth hormone, cortisol, and pancreatic polypeptide is impaired in autonomic neuropathy *(34)*, although plasma metabolite concentration does not differ between diabetes patients with and without neuropathy *(35)*. Hypoglycemia is more common during exercise in patients with autonomic neuropathy as

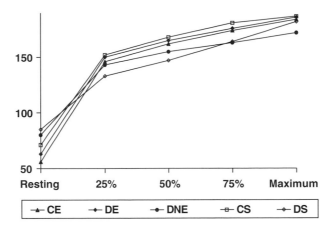

Fig. 1. The mean heart rate in healthy, nondiabetic subjects who exercised regularly (*CE*), diabetic patients – regular exercisers (*DE*), diabetic neuropathic regular exercisers (*DNE*), healthy nondiabetic subjects who did not exercise regularly (*CS*), and diabetic patients who did not exercise regularly (*DS*). All exercisers exercised regularly primarily in the form of endurance training (running) more than three times per week and at least 45 min per session. At resting conditions, heart rate was lowest in CE and highest in DS ($p < 0.0001$). No difference existed at the 25 and 50% of the total exercise time but at the 75% and maximal effort points the heart rate was lower in DNE compared with all other groups ($p < 0.05$) (*39*, 45).

the blunted adrenergic response to hypoglycemia limits counterregulatory activity on the liver. Neuropathic patients may also be more apt to be unaware of this hypoglycemia due to blunted autonomic activity. Diminished catecholamine-derived symptoms (including classic symptoms of tremor, sweating, and anxiety) may then result in progression to neuroglycopenia without antecedent warning (*4*). Gastroparesis - concomitant with autonomic neuropathy - may also result in variable delivery of calories, contributing to both hyper and hypoglycemia.

Autonomic neuropathy can also present increased risk of injury to the patient due to decreased cardiac response to exercise, postural hypotension, impaired thermoregulation, impaired thirst sensation, and gastroparesis (*36*). Most inhibiting to exercise is perhaps the impairments to heart rate and blood pressure adaptations to exercise. In terms of heart rate, autonomic neuropathy is associated with changes in resting work and impaired work capacity during exercise (*37, 38*). Patients with autonomic neuropathy often have an increased resting heart rate, likely secondary to a cardiac vagal defect (*10*). The increase in heart rate during exercise at low intensity is in part mediated by reduction in vagal tone, and increased heart rate in more intense exercise is related to sympathetic outflow. Patients with autonomic neuropathy do not exhibit the same increases in heart rate that unaffected people do, as autonomic neuropathy impairs both vagal tone and sympathetic outflow. In addition, maximal aerobic capacity is impaired in autonomic neuropathy, which may be related to the above detailed blunting of heart rate increase and cardiac output (*10*). For example, one study of young type 1 diabetic patients found that the exercise capacity of active subjects with both peripheral and autonomic neuropathy was reduced compared to active controls and diabetic patients without neuropathy (Fig. 1) (*39*). The exercise capacity of the physically active diabetic patients with neuropathy was similar to that of sedentary nondiabetic and diabetic subjects without neuropathy (*39*). Impaired lung function as well as reduction in oxidative capacity of muscle fibers may also contribute (*32*).

Patients with autonomic neuropathy also have lower-resting blood pressure and blunted blood pressure response to exercise compared to patients without diabetes and diabetic patients without neuropathy (*40–42*). The autonomic nervous system normally regulates increases in blood pressure with exercise. In autonomic neuropathy, blood pressure falls with exercise, due to decreased stimulus of the heart and vasculature from epinephrine and norepinephrine (12). Impaired exercise-induced increase in norepinephrine is associated with a fall in systemic vascular resistance (43), which reduces systemic blood pressure.

Because patients with autonomic neuropathy may not experience the same responses to vigorous exercise - such as heart rate and blood pressure - alternative measures of exertion need to be employed. A commonly used scale is the Borg Scale of Perceived Exertion. Sitting or recumbent exercise is beneficial for maintaining blood pressure during exercise; water therapy may also help maintain blood pressure during exercise (32). Autonomic neuropathy is also strongly associated with CVD and affected patients should undergo a cardiac work-up before initiating exercise.

SUMMARY

- Diabetes is an increasingly prevalent and debilitating disease. Exercise is an important part of general health for people with diabetes type 1 and essential to care for patients with diabetes type 2.
- Complications of diabetes — particularly coronary artery disease, retinopathy, nephropathy, and both peripheral and autonomic neuropathy — increase the risks associated with and can limit types of exercise.
- Exercise can precipitate angina and ischemia in patients with coronary artery disease, both known and unknown. Preexercise evaluation, including a graded exercise stress test, is advised.
- Patients with proliferative retinopathy need guidelines for activity; jarring and strenuous activities can predispose to traction retinal detachment and vitreous hemorrhage and should be avoided.
- After an acute retinal detachment or hemorrhage, exercise is limited and must be cleared by an ophthalmologist.
- Exercise may cause exercise-related microalbuminuria due to increases in blood pressure, but there is no evidence that exercise lead to progression of renal disease.
- Peripheral neuropathy can predispose to ulcers and Charcot foot morphology with exercise due to lack of sensation. Nonweight-bearing exercise is recommended.
- Autonomic neuropathy impairs cardiac reactivity to exercise and can lead to orthostasis. Gastroparesis and impaired sweating can further interfere with ability to exercise. Relative perceived level of exertion may be needed as a proxy for heart rate with exercise. Preexercise cardiac evaluation is essential.

REFERENCES

1. http://www.diabetes.org/about-diabetes.jsp.
2. Saydah SH, Fradkin J and Cowie CC. Poor control of risk factors for vascular disease among adults with previously diagnosed diabetes. *JAMA* 2004; 291: 335–342.
3. American Diabetes Association. Clinical practice recommendations 2007. Diabetes Care 2007; 30S1: S12–S14.
4. Steppel JH and Horton ES. Exercise. In: Therapy for Diabetes Mellitus and Related Disorders, 4th edition. American Diabetes Association, Alexandria, VA, 2003: 149–156.
5. Marliss EB and Vranic M. Intense exercise has unique effects on both insulin release and its roles in glucoregulation. *Diabetes* 2002; 51(S1): S271–S283.
6. O'Connor GT, Buring JE, Yusuf S, et al. An overview of randomized trials of rehabilitation with exercise after myocardial infarction. *Circulation* 1989; 80: 234–244.
7. National Cholesterol Education Program (NCEP) Expert Panel on Detection, Evaluation, and Treatment of High Blood Cholesterol in Adults (Adult Treatment Panel III). Third Report of the National Cholesterol Education Program (NCEP) Expert Panel on Detection, Evaluation, and Treatment of High Blood Cholesterol in Adults (Adult Treatment Panel III) Final Report. Circulation 2002; 106: 3143–3421.
8. Haffner SM, Lehto S, Ronnmaaa T, Pyorala K and Laakso M. Mortality from coronaty heart disease in subjects with diabetes type 2 and in nondiabetic subjects with and without prior myocardial infarction. *N Engl J Med* 1998; 339: 229–234.
9. Miettinen H, Lehto S, Salomaa V, Mahonen M, Niemela M, Haffner SM, Pyorala K and Tuomilehto J. Impact of diabetes on mortality after the first myocardial infarction. The FINMONICA Myocardial Infarction Register Study Group. *Diabetes Care* 1998; 21: 69–75.

10. Aiello LP, Cahill MT and Wong JS. Systemic considerations in the management of diabetic retinopathy. *Am J Opthalmol* 2001; 132: 760–776.

11. Sigal RJ, Kenny GP, Wasserman DH and Castaneda-Sceppa C. Physical activity/exercise and type 2 diabetes. *Diabetes Care* 2004; 27: 2518–2539.

12. Benn SJ, McCartney N and McKelvie RS. Circulatory responses to weight lifting, walking and stair climbing in older males. *J Am Geriatr Soc* 1996; 44: 121–125.

13. Matthews CE, Pate RR, Jackson KL, Ward DS, Macera CA, Kohl HW and Blair SN. Exaggerated blood pressure response to dynamic exercise and risk of future hypertension. *J Clin Epidemiol* 1998; 51: 29–35.

14. Aiello LP, Wong J, Cavallerano J, Bursell FE and Aielle LM. Retinopathy. In: Handbook of Diabetes in Exercise, 2nd edition. American Diabetes Association, Alexandria, VA, 2002: 401–413.

15. Graham C and Lasko-McCarthy P. Exercise options for persons with diabetic complications. *Diabetes Educ* 1990; 16: 212–220.

16. Anderson B. Activity and diabetic vitreous hemorrhages. *Ophthalmology* 1980; 87: 173–175.

17. Cruickshanks KJ, Moss SE, Klein R and Klein EK. Physical activity and the risk if progression of retinopathy or the development of proliferative retinopathy. *Ophthalmology* 1995; 102: 1177–1182.

18. Huttunen NP, Kaar M, Puukka R and Akerblom HK. Exercise-induced proteinuria in children and adolescents with type 1 diabetes. *Diabetologia* 1981; 21: 495–497.

19. Bognetti E, Meschi F, Pattarini A, Zoja A and Chiumello G. Postexercise Albuminuria does not predict microalbuminuria in type 1 diabetic patients. *Diabetes Med* 1994; 11: 850–855.

20. O'Brien SF, Watts GF, Powrie JK and Shaw KM. Exercise testing as a long-term predictor of the development of microalbuminuria in normoalbuminuric IDDM patients. *Diabetes Care* 1995; 18: 1602–1605.

21. Kruger M, Gordjani N and Rainer B. Postexercise albuminuria in children with different durations of diabetes mellius. *Pediatr Nephrol* 1996; 10: 594–597.

22. Dash R and Torffvit O. How to predict nephropathy in type 1 diabetic patients. Routine data or provocation by exercise testing. *Scand J Urol Nephrol* 2003; 37: 437–442.

23. Inserra F, Daccordi H, Ippolito J, Romano L, Zelechower H and Ferder L. Decrease of exercise-induced microalbuminuria in patients with type 1 diabetes by means of an angiotensin-converting enzyme inhibitor. *Am J Kidney Dis* 1996; 27: 26–33.

24. Poulson PL, Ebbelhoj E and Mogensen CE. Lisinopril rescues albuminuria during exercise in low grade microalbuminuric type 1 diabetic patients: a double-blind randomized study. *J Intern Med* 2001; 249: 433.

25. Bognetti E, Meschi F, Pattarini A, Zoja A and Chiumello G. Postexercise albuminuria does not predict microalbuminuria in type 1 diabetic patients. *Diabet Med* 1994; 11: 850–855.

26. Garg S, Chase P, Harris S, Marshall G, Hoops S and Osberg I. Glycemic control and longitudinal testing for exercise microalbuminuria in subjects with type 1 diabetes. *J Diabetes Complicat* 1990; 4: 154–158.

27. Cheema BSB, O'Sullivan AJ, Chan M, Patwardhan A, Kelly J, Gillin A and Singh MAF. Progressive resistance training during hemodialysis: rationale and method of a randomized-controlled trial. *Hemodial Int* 2006; 10: 303–310.

28. Kouidi E, Albani M, Natsis K, et al. The effects of exercise training on muscle atrophy in haemodialysis patients. *Nephrol Dial Transplant* 1998; 13: 685–689.

29. Castaneda C, Gordon P, Uhlin K, Levey A, Kehayias J, Dwyer J, Fielding RA, Roubenoff R and Singh MF. Resistance training to counteract the catabolism of a low-protein diet in patients with chronic kidney disease. *Ann Intern Med* 2001; 135: 965–976.

30. Harris D, Thomas M, Johnson D, Nicholls K and Gillin A. Caring for Australians with renal impairment (CARI). *Neprhology* 2006; 11 (Suppl. 1): S30.

31. Estacio RO, Regenstein JGM, Wolfel EE, Jeffers B, Dickenson M and Schrier RW. The association between diabetic complications and exercise capacity in NIDDM patients. *Diabetes Care* 1998; 21: 291–295.

32. LeBrasseur NK and Fielding RA. Exercise and diabetic neuropathy. Implications for exercise participation and prescription for patients with insulin-dependent and non-insulin-dependent diabetes mellitus. In: Veves A (ed), The Clinical Management of Diabetic Neuropathy. Humana Press, Totowa, NJ, 1998: 257–271.

33. Vinik A and Erbas T. Neuropathy. In: Handbook of Diabetes in Exercise, 2nd edition. American Diabetes Association, Alexandria, VA, 2002: 463–496.

34. Hilsted J, Galbo H and Christensen N. Impaired responses of catecholamines, growth hormone, and cortisol to graded exercise in diabetic autonomic neuropathy. *Diabetes* 1980; 29: 257–262.

35. Hilsted J. Cardiovascular, hormonal and metabolic studies. *Diabetes* 1982; 31: 730–737.

36. Levin ME. The diabetic foot. In: Handbook of Diabetes in Exercise, 2nd edition. American Diabetes Association, Alexandria, VA, 2002: 385–399.

37. Barkai L, Peja M and Varmosi I. Physical work capacity in diabetic children and adolescent with and without cardiovascular autonomic dysfunction. *Diabet Med* 1996; 13: 254–258.

38. Hilsted J, Galbo H and Christensen N. Impaired cardiovascular responses to graded exercise in diabetic autonomic neuropathy. *Diabetes* 1979; 28: 313–319.

39. Veves A, Saouaf R, Donaghue VM, Mullooly CA, Kistler JA, Giurini JM, Horton ES and Fielding RA. Aerobic exercise capacity remains normal despite impaired endothelial function in the micro- and macro-circulation in physically active IDDM patients. *Diabetes* 1997; 46: 1846–1852.

40. Hilsted J, Galbo N, et al.. Haemodynamic changes during graded exercise in patients with diabetic autonomic neuropathy. *Diabetologia* 1982; 22: 318–323.

41. Hornung RS, Mahler RF and Raftery EB. Ambulatory blood pressure and heart rate in diabetic patients: an assessment of autonomic function. *Diabet Med* 1989; 6: 579–585.

42. Radice MA, Rocca A, Bendon E, Musacchio N, Morabito A and Segalini G. Abnormal response to exercise in middle-aged NIDDM patients with and without autonomic neuropathy. *Diabet Med* 1996; 13: 259–265.

43. Smith GDP, Watson LP and Mathias CJ. Cardiovascular and catecholamine changes induced by supine exercise and upright posture in vasovagal syncope. *Eur Heart J* 1996; 17: 1882–1890.

14

Type 1 Diabetes Mellitus and Exercise

David Maahs, Craig E. Taplin, and Rosanna Fiallo-Scharer

CONTENTS

ABSTRACT

Exercise is an important aspect of the care of persons with type 1 diabetes and presents different challenges than in type 2 diabetes. In this chapter, American Diabetes Association recommendations for exercise will be reviewed as well as pathophysiologic differences in type 1 diabetes including counter-regulatory hormones with an emphasis on exercise-related hypoglycemia and exercise in youth with type 1 diabetes. The risks and benefits of exercise, practical considerations, and new technologies will also be discussed.

Key Words: Type 1 diabetes mellitus; Exercise; Hypoglycemia; Counterregulatory hormones; Self-monitoring blood glucose; Insulin pump.

INTRODUCTION

Exercise, in addition to diet and insulin, has been one of the essentials of diabetes management since early last century *(1)*. However, the specific pathophysiology of type 1 diabetes mellitus (T1DM) - in contrast to type 2 diabetes mellitus (T2DM) - requires treatment with exogenous insulin, which impairs the body's ability to maintain glycemic homeostasis during exercise and presents both the patient with T1DM and their health-care provider with challenges.

From: *Contemporary Diabetes: Diabetes and Exercise*
Edited by: J. G. Regensteiner et al. (eds.), DOI: 10.1007/978-1-59745-260-1_14
© Humana Press, a part of Springer Science+Business Media, LLC 2009

T1DM is characterized by autoimmune destruction of beta cells in the pancreas leading to absolute insulin deficiency and the need for daily insulin injections to control blood glucose concentrations *(2)*. A number of advances have been made in the past few decades in the care of persons with T1DM, which include home glucose monitoring *(3)*, development of insulin analogues *(4)*, demonstration of the benefit of intensive diabetes management on the prevention of microvascular *(5, 6)* and macrovascular disease *(7, 8)*, insulin pump therapy *(9)*, and, more recently, the advent of continuous glucose monitoring *(10)*. These advances have provided improved tools for daily management for persons with T1DM, but are labor intensive and require a sophisticated understanding of diet, exercise, and insulin actions. Despite these therapeutic advances, exercise for persons with T1DM requires thoughtful adaptations of daily dietary and insulin management and continues to be a challenge to patients and their health-care providers.

Early references stressed the importance of exercise for both control of glycemia and for general health *(1)*. A number of fundamental differences exist concerning the pathophysiology of T1DM as compared to T2DM that have important implications for both the study of exercise in T1DM and for practical guidelines for exercise for persons with T1DM. In addition to both exogenous insulin and carbohydrate intake, disregulated counterregulatory hormone and autonomic responses are of great importance in exercise for people with T1DM and will be discussed. In this chapter we will review the pathophysiology of T1DM in regard to exercise as well as practice guidelines and expert opinion on management of exercise, particularly in youth with T1DM, and the risks and benefits of exercise.

ADA RECOMMENDATIONS

The American Diabetes Association (ADA) recognizes both the importance and challenges of exercise in T1DM and specifically addresses these issues in a recent position statement *(11)*: "For people with type 1 diabetes, the emphasis must be on adjusting the therapeutic regimen to allow safe participation in all forms of physical activity consistent with an individual's desires and goals." While exercise is considered an important part of routine T1DM management, evaluation of the patient with T1DM prior to initiating exercise is recommended with a graded exercise test for anyone, >35 years (or if >25 years with >15 years T1DM duration) or in the presence of any one of the following: any additional risk factor for coronary artery disease (CAD), microvascular disease, peripheral vascular disease, or autonomic neuropathy*(12, 13)*. Other recommendations for preparation for exercise include proper warm-up and cool-down periods and adequate hydration. Specific precautions for feet are necessary in many older individuals with T1DM. Certain activities are discouraged in the presence of diabetic complications (e.g., micro- or macrovascular disease), such as activities that increase blood pressure (e.g., weight lifting), may cause eye injuries (e.g., boxing), foot injury (e.g., in persons with Charcot joint), or hypoglycemia (e.g., in those persons with hypoglycemic unawareness).

General metabolic guidelines include adequate glycemic control prior to physical activity; avoid if fasting glucose is >250 mg/dl and elevated blood or urine ketones and use caution if >300 mg/dl and no ketonuria/ketonemia, ingest carbohydrates if glucose <100 mg/dl, monitor blood glucose before, during, and after physical activity, and consume food during extensive exercise to avoid hypoglycemia.

PATHOPHYSIOLOGY

Physiologic Differences in T1DM

A brief description of metabolic adaptations to exercise in nondiabetic individuals will be reviewed both as an introduction and for comparison with the physiologic changes that occur in T1DM. The normal physiologic adaptation to exercise in persons without T1DM involves complex neurohormonal regulation to maintain euglycemia. With exercise, muscles utilize circulating free fatty acids, muscle triglycerides and glycogen, and liver glycogen, with the proportion of fuel derived from muscle and liver glycogen increasing as the intensity of exercise increases. Concomitantly, insulin secretion is reduced while the counterregulatory hormones glucagon, growth hormone, cortisol, and cathecholamines are increased to maintain euglycemia as exercise continues (2, 13–15).

In T1DM, the inability of the pancreas to produce and regulate insulin concentrations impairs the normal metabolic adaptation to exercise. Compared to the normal physiologic response to decrease insulin concentrations with exercise, exogenous insulin delivery lacks the dynamic adaptability and precise control found in nondiabetics and can result in either too much or too little insulin for a given physiologic state. Excessive exogenous insulin during exercise can lead to hypoglycemia. Mechanistic explanations for this include inappropriate inhibition of hepatic glucose production and lipolysis, suppression of counterregulatory glucagon secretion with hypoglycemia, and decreased growth hormone and cortisol release [reviewed in (15, 16)]. Catecholamine response in T1DM has also been demonstrated to be impaired in youth during exercise (17) and this may be accentuated with strict glycemic control (18). Counterregulatory hormone responses have been found to be impaired in strictly controlled (hemoglobin A1 = 7.6 ± 0.7%) as compared to poorly controlled (hemoglobin A1 = 11.5 ± 1.7%) subjects with T1DM or nondiabetic controls (18). The subjects with T1DM also had a lower threshold of glucose required to trigger epinephrine release and an enhanced suppressive effect of insulin on hepatic glucose output. Exercise has been shown to significantly reduce glucagon, catecholamine, growth hormone, pancreatic polypeptide, and endogenous glucose production to subsequent hypoglycemia (19) and, likewise, hypoglycemia prior to exercise has been shown to blunt counterregulatory responses during exercise (20). The issue of gender differences in the responses to hypoglycemia after exercise (21) or to exercise after hypoglycemia (22) have been investigated with a better counterregulatory response described in women as compared to men.

Additional factors associated with exercise-induced hypoglycemia in T1DM include improved insulin sensitivity, increase in insulin-independent glucose transport, and the possible increase in subcutaneous insulin absorption secondary to increased blood flow to the area of the insulin injection. This can occur after injection into subcutaneous tissue in the leg prior to running, for example, and can lead to increasing, not decreasing insulin concentrations with exercise and consequent hypoglycemia (23).

In contrast, insufficient insulin during exercise can lead to hyperglycemia secondary to excessive hepatic glucose output as well as impaired muscle utilization of glucose. Insulin insufficiency can also lead to lipolysis with increased free fatty acid release and ketonemia. Dehydration resulting from hyperglycemia and resultant osmotic diuresis may further exacerbate the severity of ketonemia. High-intensity exercise can accentuate these pathophysiologic changes (24). Therefore, recommendations published by the ADA in 2004 are to avoid physical activity if preexercise blood glucose levels are >250 mg/dl with ketonuria/ketonemia and to use caution if >300 mg/dl (11). The recommendation to avoid strenuous exercise if preexercise glucose levels are >250 mg/dl with ketones was recently reinforced in guidelines published by the International Society of Pediatric and Adolescent Diabetes (25). They recommend a bolus dose of 0.05 U/kg (or 5% of total daily insulin dose) to be given and exercise be postponed until ketones have cleared.

Risks and Benefits

While exercise is encouraged for all people, including persons with T1DM, studies have been variable in demonstrating that exercise independently improves diabetic glycemic control (as measured by HbA1c levels) *(13)*. However, multiple benefits on cardiovascular disease (CVD) risk profile exist for exercise such as improved lipoprotein profile, blood pressure, cardiovascular fitness, quality of life, and insulin sensitivity and reduced insulin requirement and body weight *(11, 13, 26)*.

Epidemiologic data from people with T1DM followed long term in Pittsburgh suggest a beneficial association between physical activity and CVD and mortality *(27)*. Another report found that children and adolescents with T1DM spent more time in sporting activities than their nondiabetic siblings *(28)*. Activity correlated only with a reduced insulin dose, but not with HbA1c levels.

Exercise has been shown to improve insulin sensitivity in nondiabetic persons. Similarly, a recent study involving 50 children with T1DM who were randomized to 1 h of afternoon exercise on one study visit, or no exercise on another study visit, found significantly lower glucose levels until breakfast the next day following the exercise *(29)*. One mechanism explaining this might be an increase in translocation of the GLUT4 transport protein to muscle membrane upon insulin stimulation, which has been shown to occur for at least 3.5 h after exercise *(30)* and may contribute to the increase in insulin sensitivity which may be seen for up to 16 h *(31)*.

Previous studies utilizing the hyperinsulinemic-euglycemic clamp studies in adolescents suggested that youth with T1DM had similar physical fitness as assessed by VO_2max, but lower total-body insulin-mediated glucose metabolism as compared to controls ($p = 0.0002$) *(32)*. Insulin-mediated glucose metabolism correlated with VO_2max in both subjects with T1DM and controls, but for similar levels of physical fitness, subjects with T1DM had more insulin resistance than controls. Much of the insulin resistance was attributable to glycemic control as assessed by glycated hemoglobin *(32)*.

Increased insulin resistance has long been known to occur in persons with T1DM as compared to non-diabetes mellitus (DM) controls with studies using the euglycemic clamp technique *(33–38)*. Recent data has demonstrated that adult patients with T1DM show decreased insulin-mediated suppression of free fatty acid levels compared to controls *(39)*. Insulin sensitivity has also been shown to be decreased in T1DM youth, when compared to lean controls, with glycemia as the major contributor *(40)*. Importantly, and very recently, the assertion that exercise function, as assessed by VO_2max, is not different in adolescents with T1DM compared with controls has been challenged. Nadeau and colleagues have shown that, in fact, a reduction in exercise function (VO_2max) is found early in the pathophysiology of diabetes, regardless of diabetes type, and is directly related to insulin resistance *(41)*. Therefore, increasing exercise to reduce insulin resistance in persons with T1DM could have numerous health benefits that are self-potentiating, including reduction of CVD risk which is the leading cause of mortality in persons with T1DM *(42)*, as in persons with T2DM.

HYPOGLYCEMIA

The Diabetes Control and Complications Trial demonstrated the benefit of intensive glycemic control on both microvascular *(5, 6)* and macrovascular *(7, 8)* outcomes in persons with T1DM. Accompanying the improved glycemic control however was a two to sixfold increase in severe hypoglycemia in intensive as compared to conventionally treated subjects *(43)*. While hypoglycemia continues to be the most important barrier to tight glycemic control, the increased use of insulin pumps or nonpeaking basal insulin have decreased this risk *(44)* and continuous glucose monitoring has the potential for further reductions in hypoglycemic events.

Not only is hypoglycemia a concern in persons with T1DM, in general, but more so during exercise for the reasons outlined in the pathophysiology section. Furthermore, delayed hypoglycemia postexercise has been a well-described complication occurring most frequently 6–15 h after strenuous exercise or play *(45)*. When exercise takes place in the afternoon or early evening, as is often the case for school-aged children, this window of susceptibility to delayed hypoglycemia corresponds to the middle of the night. In fact, up to 75% of severe hypoglycemic events in children are nocturnal *(46)*. It has been shown that the glucose infusion rate (GIR) required to maintain euglycemia increases between 7 and 11 h after 45 min of bicycle exercise at 55% of VO_2max *(47)*. In these youth, who exercised in the after-school period, this corresponded to a maximal GIR between 11 p.m. and 3 a.m., a time when it might be expected that a child or adolescent and their parents are asleep and not monitoring blood sugars as one might during the waking hours.

Furthermore, in an experiment utilizing hyperinsulinemic-stepped hypoglycemic clamps, subjects with T1DM had reduced awakening from sleep during hypoglycemia as compared to nondiabetic subjects, likely due to impaired sympathoadrenal responses *(48)*. They concluded that impaired sleep-related autonomic responses to low blood glucose levels coupled with imperfect insulin replacement explained the high frequency of nocturnal hypoglycemia. Hypoglycemia-associated autonomic failure in diabetes has been reviewed recently, including syndromes of defective glucose counterregulation and hypoglycemic unawareness (and that antecedent hypoglycemia - described as a unifying concept of hypoglycemia-associated autonomic failure - can cause both) *(49, 50)*.

A series of experiments to further investigate the effects of exercise on youth with T1DM has been undertaken by the Diabetes Research in Children Network (DirecNet) Study Group. Youth ages 11–17 years were more likely to experience nocturnal hypoglycemia (<60 mg/dl) after an afternoon aerobic exercise session than on a "sedentary" day (48% vs. 28%, $p = 0.009$) when insulin doses and bedtime snacks were not adjusted. The authors identified that hypoglycemia was unusual on the "sedentary" night if the prebedtime glucose level was ≥ 130 mg/dl *(29)*. Furthermore, hypoglycemia was frequent (86% of subjects) during or within 45 min postexercise when preexercise glucose was <120 mg/dl as compared to 120–180 mg/dl (13%) or >180 mg/dl (6%) ($p < 0.001$). Regarding treatment of hypoglycemia, the authors reported that 15 g of oral glucose only increased glucose concentrations by approximately 20 mg/dl and suggested that 30–45 g of carbohydrate may be a more appropriate amount for treatment of exercise-induced hypoglycemia *(17)*. Of note, the counterregulatory hormones epinephrine and growth hormone levels (but not of cortisol or glucagon) were marginally higher in subjects whose glucose dropped below 70 mg/dl, but were clearly insufficient to prevent hypoglycemia. Further investigation of counterregulatory hormone responses to hypoglycemia found no difference in norepinephrine, cortisol, or glucagon responses to nocturnal hypoglycemia with only small increases in epinephrine and growth hormone *(17)*. The DirecNet study group subsequently performed an experiment in which pump basal insulin was suspended for 2 h during a 75-min exercise session. Suspension of pump basal insulin compared to continued basal insulin resulted in significantly reduced hypoglycemia during the exercise (16% vs. 43%; $p = 0.003$). After the exercise hyperglycemia ($\geq 20\%$ rise in blood glucose to ≥ 200 mg/dl) was more frequent in the group with suspended basal insulin (27% vs. 4%; $p = 0.002$), although there was no detection of elevated blood ketones *(51)*. This finding points out a potential benefit of insulin pump therapy in being able to make rapid changes in insulin treatment to adjust for exercise.

PRACTICAL CONSIDERATIONS FOR YOUTH WITH T1DM

Current recommendations are for school-age youth to receive 60 min of moderate to vigorous exercise daily for health benefits including cardiovascular and musculoskeletal health, maintaining a healthy weight, as well as beneficial psychosocial effects *(52)*. Although there is varied data on the beneficial effects of exercise specifically on glycemic control in youth with diabetes, expert opinion recommends exercise in youth with T1DM for the same reasons as in nondiabetic youth *(53, 54)*.

Practical strategies to prevent hypo- and hyperglycemia during exercise are numerous *(2)*. Self-monitoring blood glucose (SMBG) concentrations prior to, during, and after exercise are of the utmost importance. The ADA recommends delaying exercise if blood glucose is <100 mg/dl until additional carbohydrate can be ingested to raise blood glucose *(11)*. The DirecNet data suggests that a preexercise blood glucose of at least 120 mg/dl may be ideal *(17)*. Prolonged exercise can lower blood glucose and requires additional monitoring and ingestion of carbohydrate after each additional 30–60 min of continued exercise. Delayed hypoglycemia can occur for up to 12 h or more after exercise and additional glucose monitoring is essential. Frequent SMBG and each individual's past experience with exercise and ability to recognize hypoglycemia are extremely important. Snacks prior to and during exercise are often necessary to maintain euglycemia with rapidly absorbed carbohydrates required for treating hypoglycemia, whereas combining fat and protein with carbohydrate will have a more prolonged and blunted effect on glycemia. Reduction of preexercise insulin doses is often needed. Conversely, hyperglycemia can occur with under insulinization, excessive snacking, high-intensity exercise, or excitement (e.g., during a match vs practice) causing increased catecholamine release. However, exercise, especially in children, is often spontaneous. This can pose a challenge as reductions in insulin doses are often not possible and additional glucose monitoring and snacks as needed to maintain euglycemia and safety are required. If exercise is planned within 2 h of a rapid-acting insulin injection then a reduced dose (often by 50%) is recommended. Exercise later after an injection may also require reductions in longer-acting injected insulin or reductions in pump basal insulin infusion rates. Insulin pump therapy provides the flexibility to either disconnect from insulin infusion for up to 2 h or to set a reduced temporary basal rate of 50% or 75% of the usual basal for 30–60 min prior to and during exercise. This temporary reduction in basal rate can be continued postexercise if delayed hypoglycemia is a concern. An additional issue is to avoid injecting insulin into a part of the body that will be heavily used during exercise as exercise increases blood flow into the parts of the body that are moving and this increases insulin uptake. A final practical consideration is to make coaches, teammates, and exercise partners aware of the diabetes and provide hypoglycemia education as appropriate with easy availability of snacks, insulin, and glucose monitoring equipment. When hypoglycemia does occur, it is important to make certain that blood glucose levels rise prior to resuming the exercise.

Of note, despite the practical daily challenges presented by T1DM, highly accomplished athletes with T1DM include Adam Morrison (NBA), Gary Hall Jr. (multiple Olympic gold-medal winning swimmer), as well as past and present male and female professional athletes in baseball, football, golf, and other sports *(55)*. Although T1DM has presented an additional challenge to these highly performing athletes, they have succeeded in managing their diabetes care regimen and training to achieve outstanding accomplishments in their sports.

Types of Exercise

The type of exercise in addition to duration may play a role in maintaining euglycemia *(56)*. Specifically, the decline in glucose with intermittent high-intensity exercise was less than that of moderate-intensity exercise ($p < 0.05$) and likewise remained more stable postexercise ($p < 0.05$) *(57)*. A short maximal sprint of 10 s duration was explored as a possible counter to exercise-induced decreases in glucose levels and in comparison to control subjects was associated with stabilization of glycemia and increased levels of catecholamines, growth hormone, and cortisol *(58)*.

A recent review from Ridell and colleagues *(59)* provides very useful information for patients and providers, detailing the duration of common types of exercise equivalent to one carbohydrate exchange (15 g). For example, for a child with body weight of 40 kg, for every 15 min of soccer or 25 min of tennis, an extra 15 g of carbohydrate is required to maintain blood sugar levels, assuming no reduction in insulin is made. Tables and charts such as these may be extremely useful to help patients plan for known activities.

NEW TECHNOLOGIES

Newer insulin analogues have provided persons with T1DM an improved ability to more closely match exogenous insulin to metabolic requirements, both with rapid-acting insulins (Lispro, Aspart, Glulisine) to correct hyperglycemia and to match carbohydrate intake and longer duration basal insulins (Glargine, Detemir) with minimal peaks that have reduced the risk of nocturnal hypoglycemia *(60)*. Continuous subcutaneous insulin infusion delivered with insulin pumps has a theoretic advantage in allowing greater flexibility to adjust insulin delivery including temporary detachment (or temporary cessation of insulin delivery), temporary reduction of basal insulin delivery, and incremental dosage (delivery of rapid acting insulin as tenths of units) *(61)*.

More recent developments have included continuous glucose monitoring devices with real-time display that have been approved by the Food and Drug Administration. These devices, while not yet sufficiently accurate to completely replace SMBG, provide temporal blood glucose trends which can alert patients that blood glucose is falling (or rising) and that action should be taken (i.e., confirming with a SMBG, with appropriate bolusing with insulin or conversely suspending insulin infusion and ingesting carbohydrates). One obvious research goal is to improve on the technologic capabilities of both continuous insulin infusion systems and continuous glucose monitoring with the ultimate goal of a "closed-loop" system" in which insulin infusion would be automatically responsive to changes in glucose concentrations *(10, 62, 63)*. While advancements in this field have occurred, a number of challenges remain and the timeline for nonresearch availability of a "closed-loop" pancreas is still far off. Indeed, the challenges presented by exercise will provide a formidable safety trial for this technology. In the meantime, exercise remains and likely will always be an important component of care of persons with T1DM.

CONCLUSIONS

Exercise for persons with T1DM will continue to require close attention to SMBG with adjustment of insulin doses and food prior to, during, and after exercise. The benefits of exercise for persons with T1DM include a better CVD risk profile, body composition, insulin sensitivity, reduced insulin requirements, and quality of life. Numerous clinical and research challenges remain in handling exercise in youth with T1DM. These include data to direct clinical care to maintain euglycemia (and prevent hypoglycemia) during, and after, exercise as well as technologic advances that will better adapt insulin and counterregulatory hormone concentration response during exercise to more closely mimic the normal neuroendocrine milieu. With the proper precautions, including consultation with a qualified health care professional, exercise should be an important part of the daily life and the care of people with T1DM. The number of highly accomplished athletes and millions of people worldwide with T1DM who exercise routinely attest to this fact.

REFERENCES

1. Feudtner C. *Bittersweet: Diabetes, insulin, and the transformation of illness*. Chapel Hill: University of North Carolina Press. 2003.
2. Chase HP. *Understanding Diabetes: A Handbook for People Who Are Living with Diabetes*. 11th ed. 2006, Paros Press, Denvev, Co
3. Saudek CD, Derr RL, Kalyani RR. Assessing glycemia in diabetes using self-monitoring blood glucose and hemoglobin A1c. *JAMA* 2006 April 12;295(14):1688–97.
4. Hirsch IB. Insulin analogues. *N Engl J Med* 2005 January 13;352(2):174–83.
5. The effect of intensive treatment of diabetes on the development and progression of long-term complications in insulin-dependent diabetes mellitus. The Diabetes Control and Complications Trial Research Group. *N Engl J Med* 1993 September 30;329(14):977–86.
6. Effect of intensive diabetes treatment on the development and progression of long-term complications Trial. Diabetes Control and Complications Trial Research Group. *J Pediatr* 1994 August;125(2):177–88.
7. Nathan DM, Lachin J, Cleary P, Orchard T, Brillon DJ, Backlund JY, O'Leary DH, Genuth S. Intensive diabetes therapy and carotid intima-media thickness in type 1 diabetes mellitus. *N Engl J Med* 2003 June 5;348(23):2294–303.

8. Nathan DM, Cleary PA, Backlund JY, Genuth SM, Lachin JM, Orchard TJ, Raskin P, Zinman B. Intensive diabetes treatment and cardiovascular disease in patients with type 1 diabetes. *N Engl J Med* 2005 December 22;353(25):2643–53.

9. Tamborlane WV. Fulfilling the promise of insulin pump therapy in childhood diabetes. *Pediatr Diabetes* 2006 August;7(Suppl. 4): 4–10.

10. Klonoff DC. Continuous glucose monitoring: roadmap for 21st century diabetes therapy. *Diabetes Care* 2005 May; 28(5):1231–9.

11. Zinman B, Ruderman N, Campaigne BN, Devlin JT, Schneider SH. Physical activity/exercise and diabetes. *Diabetes Care* 2004 January;27(Suppl. 1):S58–62.

12. Gerstein HC, Bosch J, Pogue J, Taylor DW, Zinman B, Yusuf S. Rationale and design of a large study to evaluate the renal and cardiovascular effects of an ACE inhibitor and vitamin E in high- risk patients with diabetes. The MICRO-HOPE Study. Microalbuminuria, cardiovascular, and renal outcomes. Heart Outcomes Prevention Evaluation. *Diabetes Care* 1996;19(11):1225–8.

13. Wasserman DH, Zinman B. Exercise in individuals with IDDM. *Diabetes Care* 1994 August;17(8):924–37.

14. Camacho RC, Galassetti P, Davis SN, Wasserman DH. Glucoregulation during and after exercise in health and insulin-dependent diabetes. *Exerc Sport Sci Rev* 2005 January;33(1):17–23.

15. Jeanne H. Steppel, Edward S. Horton. Exercise for the patient with type 1 diabetes mellitus. In Diabetes mellitus: a fundamental and clinical text. Derek Leroith (ed.), Lippincott Williams & Wilkins 2006.p.671–81

16. Riddell MC, Iscoe KE. Physical activity, sport, and pediatric diabetes. *Pediatr Diabetes* 2006 February;7(1):60–70.

17. Tansey MJ, Tsalikian E, Beck RW, Mauras N, Buckingham BA, Weinzimer SA, Janz KF, Kollman C, Xing D, Ruedy KJ, Steffes MW, Borland TM, Singh RJ, Tamborlane WV. The effects of aerobic exercise on glucose and counterregulatory hormone concentrations in children with type 1 diabetes. *Diabetes Care* 2006 January;29(1):20–5.

18. Amiel SA, Tamborlane WV, Simonson DC, Sherwin RS. Defective glucose counterregulation after strict glycemic control of insulin-dependent diabetes mellitus. *N Engl J Med* 1987 May 28;316(22):1376–83.

19. Galassetti P, Mann S, Tate D, Neill RA, Costa F, Wasserman DH, Davis SN. Effects of antecedent prolonged exercise on subsequent counterregulatory responses to hypoglycemia. *Am J Physiol Endocrinol Metab* 2001 June;280(6):E908–17.

20. Galassetti P, Tate D, Neill RA, Morrey S, Wasserman DH, Davis SN. Effect of antecedent hypoglycemia on counterregulatory responses to subsequent euglycemic exercise in type 1 diabetes. *Diabetes* 2003 July;52(7):1761–9.

21. Galassetti P, Neill AR, Tate D, Ertl AC, Wasserman DH, Davis SN. Sexual dimorphism in counterregulatory responses to hypoglycemia after antecedent exercise. *J Clin Endocrinol Metab* 2001 August;86(8):3516–24.

22. Galassetti P, Tate D, Neill RA, Morrey S, Wasserman DH, Davis SN. Effect of sex on counterregulatory responses to exercise after antecedent hypoglycemia in type 1 diabetes. *Am J Physiol Endocrinol Metab* 2004 July;287(1):E16–24.

23. Koivisto VA, Felig P. Effects of leg exercise on insulin absorption in diabetic patients. *N Engl J Med* 1978 January 12;298(2):79–83.

24. Marliss EB, Vranic M. Intense exercise has unique effects on both insulin release and its roles in glucoregulation: implications for diabetes. *Diabetes* 2002 February;51(Suppl. 1):S271–83.

25. Robertson K, Adolfsson P, Riddell MC, Scheiner G, Hanas R. Exercise in children and adolescents with diabetes. ISPAD Clinical Practice Consensus Guidelines 2006–07. *Pediatr Diabetes* 2008 February;9(1):65–77.

26. Austin A, Warty V, Janosky J, Arslanian S. The relationship of physical fitness to lipid and lipoprotein(a) levels in adolescents with IDDM. *Diabetes Care* 1993 February;16(2):421–5.

27. LaPorte RE, Dorman JS, Tajima N, Cruickshanks KJ, Orchard TJ, Cavender DE, Becker DJ, Drash AL. Pittsburgh Insulin-Dependent Diabetes Mellitus Morbidity and Mortality Study: physical activity and diabetic complications. *Pediatrics* 1986;78:1027–33.

28. Raile K, Kapellen T, Schweiger A, Hunkert F, Nietzschmann U, Dost A, Kiess W. Physical activity and competitive sports in children and adolescents with type 1 diabetes. *Diabetes Care* 1999 November;22(11):1904–5.

29. Tsalikian E, Mauras N, Beck RW, Tamborlane WV, Janz KF, Chase HP, Wysocki T, Weinzimer SA, Buckingham BA, Kollman C, Xing D, Ruedy KJ. Impact of exercise on overnight glycemic control in children with type 1 diabetes mellitus. *J Pediatr* 2005 October;147(4):528–34.

30. Hansen PA, Nolte LA, Chen MM, Holloszy JO. Increased GKUT-4 translocation mediates enhanced insulin sensitivity of muscle glucose transport after exercise. *J Appl Physiol* 1998 Oct;85(4):1218–22.

31. Borghouts LB, Keizer HA. Exercise and insulin sensitivity: a review. *Int J Sports Med* 2000 January;21(1):1–12.

32. Arslanian S, Nixon PA, Becker D, Drash AL. Impact of physical fitness and glycemic control on in vivo insulin action in adolescents with IDDM. *Diabetes Care* 1990 January;13(1):9–15.

33. Perseghin G, Lattuada G, Danna M, Sereni LP, Maffi P, De Cobelli F, Battezzati A, Secchi A, Del Maschio A, Luzi L. Insulin resistance, intramyocellular lipid content and plasma adiponectin in patients with type 1 diabetes. *Am.J Physiol Endocrinol Metab* 2003; 285(6):E1174–81.

34. Williams KV, Erbey JR, Becker D, Arslanian S, Orchard TJ. Can clinical factors estimate insulin resistance in type 1 diabetes? *Diabetes* 2000 April;49(4):626–32.

35. Ekstrand AV, Groop PH, Gronhagen-Riska C. Insulin resistance precedes microalbuminuria in patients with insulin-dependent diabetes mellitus. *Nephrol Dial Transplant* 1998 December;13(12):3079–83.

36. Greenbaum CJ. Insulin resistance in type 1 diabetes. *Diabetes Metab Res Rev* 2002 May;18(3):192–200.

37. Nijs HG, Radder JK, Frolich M, Krans HM. The course and determinants of insulin action in type 1 (insulin-dependent) diabetes mellitus. *Diabetologia* 1989 January;32(1):20–7.
38. Reinehr T, Holl RW, Roth CL, Wiesel T, Stachow R, Wabitsch M, Andler W. Insulin resistance in children and adolescents with type 1 diabetes mellitus: relation to obesity. *Pediatr Diabetes* 2005 March;6(1):5–12.
39. Schauer IE, Bergman B, Snell-Bergeon J, Maahs DM, Kretowski A, Eckel RH, Rewers MJ, Insulin Sensitivity and free fatty acid suppression differ in person with type 1 diabetic compared to non-diabetic controls: the CACTI Study. Abstract 1300-P68th Scientific Sessions ADA 2008.
40 Nadeau KJ, West N, Sorenson E, Vehik K, Maahs DM, Zeitler PS, Liese A, Draznin B, Mayer-Davis EJ, Hamman RF, Dabelea D. Reduced insulin sensitivity in youth with type 1 and type 2 diabetes. Abstract 1804-P 68th Scientific Sessions ADA, 2008.
41. Nadeau KJ, Sorenson E, Brown M, Zeitler PS, Draznin B, Reusch J, Regensteiner JG. Exercise function is abnormal in adolescents with type 1 and type 2 diabetes. Oral Presentation 327-OR 68th Scientific Sessions ADA, 2008.
42. Libby P, Nathan DM, Abraham K, Brunzell JD, Fradkin JE, Haffner SM, Hsueh W, Rewers M, Roberts BT, Savage PJ, Skarlatos S, Wassef M, Rabadan-Diehl C. Report of the National Heart, Lung, and Blood Institute-National Institute of Diabetes and Digestive and Kidney Diseases Working Group on Cardiovascular Complications of Type 1 Diabetes Mellitus. *Circulation* 2005 June 28;111(25):3489–93.
43. Epidemiology of severe hypoglycemia in the diates control and complications trial. The DCCT Research Group. *Am J Med* 1991 April; 90(4):450–9.
44. Chase HP, Dixon B, Pearson J, Fiallo-Scharer R, Walravens P, Klingensmith G, Rewers M, Garg SK. Reduced hypoglycemic episodes and improved glycemic control in children with type 1 diabetes using insulin glargine and neutral protamine Hagedorn insulin. *J Pediatr* 2003 December;143(6):737–40.
45. MacDonald MJ. Postexercise late-onset hypoglycemia in insulin-dependent diabetic patients. *Diabetes Care* 1987 September;10(5):584–8.
46. Davis EA, Keating B, Byrne GC, Russell M, Jones TW. Hypoglycemia: incidence and clinical predictors in a large population-based sample of children and adolescents with IDDM. *Diabetes Care* 1997 January;20(1):22–5.
47. McMahon SK, Ferreira LD, Ratnam N, Davey RJ, Youngs LM, Davis EA, Fournier PA, Jones TW. Glucose requirements to maintain euglycemia after moderate-intensity afternoon exercise in adolescents with type 1 diabetes are increased in a biphasic manner. *J Clin Endocrinol Metab.* 2007 March;92(3):963–8.
48. Banarer S, Cryer PE. Sleep-related hypoglycemia-associated autonomic failure in type 1 diabetes: reduced awakening from sleep during hypoglycemia. *Diabetes* 2003 May;52(5):1195–203.
49. Cryer PE. Diverse causes of hypoglycemia-associated autonomic failure in diabetes. *N Engl J Med* 2004 May 27;350(22):2272–9.
50. Cryer PE. Mechanisms of hypoglycemia-associated autonomic failure and its component syndromes in diabetes. *Diabetes* 2005 December;54(12):3592–601.
51. Tsalikian E, Kollman C, Tamborlane WB, Beck RW, Fiallo-Scharer R, Fox L, Janz KF, Ruedy KJ, Wilson D, Xing D, Weinzimer SA. Prevention of hypoglycemia during exercise in children with type 1 diabetes by suspending basal insulin. *Diabetes Care* 2006 October;29(10):2200–4.
52. Strong WB, Malina RM, Blimkie CJ, Daniels SR, Dishman RK, Gutin B, Hergenroeder AC, Must A, Nixon PA, Pivarnik JM, Rowland T, Trost S, Trudeau F. Evidence based physical activity for school-age youth. *J Pediatr* 2005 June;146(6):732–7.
53. Silverstein J, Klingensmith G, Copeland K, Plotnick L, Kaufman F, Laffel L, Deeb L, Grey M, Anderson B, Holzmeister LA, Clark N. Care of children and adolescents with type 1 diabetes: a statement of the American Diabetes Association. *Diabetes Care* 2005 January;28(1):186–212.
54. Wolfsdorf JI. Children with diabetes benefit from exercise. *Arch Dis Child* 2005 December;90(12):1215–7.
55. Internet Communication 2007. Accessed January 1, 2007. http://www.diabetes.org
56. Guelfi KJ, Jones TW, Fournier PA. Intermittent high-intensity exercise does not increase the risk of early postexercise hypoglycemia in individuals with type 1 diabetes. *Diabetes Care* 2005 February;28(2):416–8.
57. Guelfi KJ, Jones TW, Fournier PA. The decline in blood glucose levels is less with intermittent high-intensity compared with moderate exercise in individuals with type 1 diabetes. *Diabetes Care* 2005 June;28(6):1289–94.
58. Bussau VA, Ferreira LD, Jones TW, Fournier PA. The 10-s maximal sprint: a novel approach to counter an exercise-mediated fall in glycemia in individuals with type 1 diabetes. *Diabetes Care* 2006 March;29(3):601–6.
59. Riddell M, Iscoe K. Physical activity, sport, and pedaitric diabetes. *Pediatr Diabetes* 2006;7:60–70.
60. Chase HP, Dixon B, Pearson J, Fiallo-Scharer R, Walravens P, Klingensmith G, Rewers M, Garg SK. Reduced hypoglycemic episodes and improved glycemic control in children with type 1 diabetes using insulin glargine and neutral protamine Hagedorn insulin. J Pediatr 2003 December;143(6):737–40.
61. Admon G, Weinstein Y, Falk B, Weintrob N, Benzaquen H, Ofan R, Fayman G, Zigel L, Constantini N, Phillip M. Exercise with and without an insulin pump among children and adolescents with type 1 diabetes mellitus. Pediatrics 2005 September;116(3):e348–55.
62. Hovorka R. Continuous glucose monitoring and closed-loop systems. Diabet Med 2006 January;23(1):1–12.
63. Shalitin S, Phillip M. Closing the loop: combining insulin pumps and glucose sensors in children with type 1 diabetes mellitus. *Pediatr Diabetes* 2006 August;7(Suppl. 4):45–9.

15

Exercise and Type 2 Diabetes in Youth

Kristen Nadeau, Jane E.B. Reusch,
and Judith G. Regensteiner

ABSTRACT

The antecedents of adult cardiovascular disease begin in childhood. Accompanying the dramatic increase in childhood obesity and decline in physical activity, the prevalence of type 2 diabetes mellitus (T2DM) in pediatrics is also rising, forecasting earlier macrovascular and microvascular complications. Poor physical fitness is associated with increased cardiovascular morbidity and mortality. The presence of T2DM appears to confer a specific exercise defect, as adults with T2DM have reduced VO_2max, slower $VO_{2kinetics}$, and slower heart rate kinetics when compared with age, pubertal stage, weight, and activity-matched controls. As little exercise data exists in youth with T2DM, our group assessed VO_2max in adolescents with T2DM, compared with nondiabetic, obese, and lean controls. We found significant impairments in maximal and submaximal exercise, not explainable by weight or activity level alone. VO_2max/kg was strongly related to insulin resistance, as well as inflammation, impaired endothelial function, and ectopic lipid deposition. Notably, these defects are already happening in very young patients, with no other comorbidities or reasons for exercise dysfunction. Therefore, since exercise capacity predicts cardiovascular and all cause mortality, it is critical to further assess the mechanisms of exercise dysfunction in T2DM youth, as well as the impact of diabetes treatments in adolescents. On the basis of studies in adults and in adolescents with obesity and insulin resistance, exercise interventions appear helpful, but further study in pediatric T2DM is required.

Key words: Exercise; Type 2 diabetes; Pediatrics; Insulin resistance.

The antecedents of adult cardiovascular disease (CVD) begin in childhood, as factors such as lipid levels and obesity track from childhood to adulthood *(1, 2)*. Acute cardiovascular deaths have been reported in adolescents with type 2 diabetes mellitus (T2DM), despite their young age *(3)*. Accompanying the dramatic increase in childhood obesity *(4)*, the prevalence of T2DM in pediatrics is also rising *(5)*. In 1992, pediatric T2DM was rare, but by 1994, it characterized up to 16% of new onset diabetes in urban areas, and by 1999, between 8 and 45%, depending on location, gender, and ethnicity *(5)*. Recent data demonstrate that the lifetime risk of developing T2DM for all children born in 2000 is 32.8% for males and 38.5% for females *(6)*. Therefore, a large and growing segment of the US population is likely to be affected with T2DM.

From: *Contemporary Diabetes: Diabetes and Exercise*
Edited by: J. G. Regensteiner et al. (eds.), DOI: 10.1007/978-1-59745-260-1_15
© Humana Press, a part of Springer Science+Business Media, LLC 2009

Importantly, the macrovascular and microvascular complications of T2DM are much more aggressive in patients diagnosed as young adults relative to those diagnosed at an older age *(7, 8)*. For example, young adults with early-onset T2DM have a much higher relative risk of developing CVD compared with age-matched control subjects than adults with later onset T2DM *(7)*. This increased relative risk is most striking with MI, in which young adults had a 14-fold increased risk compared with matched-control subjects *(7)*. Essentially, all of this increased risk occurred in young women with T2DM *(7)*. One potential explanation for the markedly increased risk of CVD detected in this study is that most young adults are heavier and have more metabolic syndrome components at diabetes diagnosis than adults, both important contributors to risk of CVD *(9)*.

In addition, the prevalence of CVD increases with increasing duration of diabetes *(10)*. Among the Pima Indians, T2DM raises the risk of death from all causes by 1.4 times if the age of onset is after age 20, but raises the risk of death by three times if the age of onset is less than 20 years *(8)*. Of great concern is that deaths among a significant number of Pimas with early onset diabetes are occurring in middle age, significantly shortening the lifespan *(8)*. Therefore, it is vital to address the metabolic effects of this disease in young people and devise effective treatment strategies for children with T2DM, as the development of comorbidities may differ between children and adults.

In adolescents, T2DM is more common in females *(11, 12)*. The development of diabetes in young females before the age of childbearing translates to more pregnancies complicated by diabetes. This is especially concerning because gestational diabetes greatly increases the risk of offspring developing diabetes *(12)*. Thus, T2DM increases the risk of CVD not just in an individual woman, but also in future generations. Although data to guide optimal care of CVD in adults with diabetes are limited, even less data exist in youth. Thus, it is vital to address the metabolic effects of T2DM in youth.

Poor physical fitness is associated with poor health and increased cardiovascular morbidity and mortality. For example, low cardiorespiratory fitness predicts mortality in normal weight and obese men and women *(13, 14)* and predicts cardiovascular events *(15)* and mortality in adults with diabetes *(16)*. Poor fitness is also associated with an unfavorable cardiovascular risk profile in children and adolescents *(17–20)*. Being physically fit increases the overall chance of survival *(21–23)*, decreases the incidence of T2DM *(24–26)*, and improves cardiovascular function in persons who already have T2DM *(25, 27)*. Exercise also helps improve metabolic control in adult and pediatric subjects with type 1 diabetes mellitus *(28–32)*. Thus, exercise is a cornerstone of the prevention and treatment of diabetes *(28, 33)*. In addition, higher levels of activity and fitness are associated with reduced risk of metabolic syndrome *(34–41)*.

However, despite the extensive data indicating the importance of exercise, 60–80% of adults with T2DM do not get the recommended amount of exercise, and adherence to exercise programs is lower than in nondiabetics *(29, 42)*. Unfortunately, this is not a phenomenon limited to adults. Physical activity and fitness in general have progressively declined among children in the USA, especially girls *(43)*, and this decrease is associated with increased body mass index (BMI) *(44)*. Black girls are even less active than white girls, having virtually no physical activity by the end of adolescence, and are also at higher risk for T2DM *(45)*. In a large study in 2003, measuring fitness by estimating VO_2max from the heart rate response to reference levels of submaximal work, low fitness was identified in 33.6% of 3,110 adolescents and 13.9% of 2,205 adults *(46)*. The prevalence of low fitness was similar in adolescent females (34.4%) and males (32.9%) but was higher in adult females (16.2%) than in males (11.8%) *(46)*. Non-Hispanic blacks and Mexican Americans were also less fit than non-Hispanic whites *(46)*. Low activity levels are not limited to youth in the United States. For example, in a Norwegian study in 2003, only 86.2% of the 9-year olds and 55.4% of the 15-year olds met physical activity recommendations for youth *(47)*. Similarly, the activity level of youth throughout Europe decreases throughout adolescence and is, significantly, lower among girls than among boys *(47, 48)*.

Physical activity among children has declined over the past several decades for multiple reasons *(49, 50)*. One reason is related to the lack of safe outdoor play areas in many cities. Outdoor play has been replaced by video games, television, listening to music, and computers. Budgetary limitations and curriculum changes have also resulted in a deemphasis on regular physical education programs in many schools. In addition, the increasing number of homes with two working parents or a single parent limits the ability of parents to provide access to regular physical activity.

Although activity has declined recently among all Americans *(51)*, people with T2DM are particularly inactive *(29)*. Recent research has focused on understanding why people with T2DM are not exercising. Regensteiner et al. found that adults with uncomplicated T2DM have reduced VO_2max, slower $VO_{2kinetics}$, and slower heart rate kinetics when compared with age, weight, and activity-matched controls *(30, 31, 52)*, despite similar respiratory exchange ratio (RER), indicating similar effort. Therefore, neither low habitual physical activity level, poor effort nor weight alone were sufficient to explain the exercise defects seen in subjects with T2DM *(52)*. Thus, the presence of T2DM appears to confer a specific exercise defect. Explanations for this may include a higher perceived level of exertion at any given workload in people with T2DM compared with that in controls. For example, adults with T2DM have a higher perceived exertion when compared with obese, nondiabetic, or lean controls at both 20 W, even when corrected for relative exercise capacity (unpublished, 2007). Therefore, subjects with T2DM may feel uncomfortable even during exercise at the level of activities of daily life.

The $VO_{2kinetic}$ data are perhaps the most concerning, as they demonstrate abnormalities at the level of activities of daily life, which certainly impacts quality of life and the likelihood that any exercise can be performed. In addition, in a study of young (34 ± 10 years), healthy, and normal glucose-tolerant subjects with either a first-degree relative (FDR) with T2DM (*n*= 183), or no family history of T2DM (*n*= 147), FDR's had significantly lower VO_2max/kg lean body mass than controls, even after adjusting for sex, age, BMI, habitual physical activity, and insulin sensitivity *(53)*. Therefore, exercise impairment may precede glucose abnormalities in subjects at risk for diabetes, making young patients a critical group to study. If therapies can be identified to target these early defects, our treatment of diabetes and its precursors will improve, hopefully preventing the morbidity and mortality seen in adults with T2DM.

If the response to exercise is already abnormal in adolescents, it may forecast potentially serious cardiac complications at young ages. While little exercise data exist in youth with T2D, exercise function has been studied in youth with obesity and with markers of insulin resistance. Previous studies of exercise capacity in obese children show no differences when compared to lean children if controlled for weight *(54)*, or lean body mass *(55)*. However, obese children report a higher level of perceived exertion at equal levels of work, and, therefore, either exercise for shorter duration *(56)* or perform more poorly during sustained exercise than lean controls *(57)*. This higher perceived level of exertion may result in avoidance of exercise. Studies in severely obese adolescents also show higher resting heart rates but lower maximal heart rates during exercise than lean controls *(57)*. This may indicate autonomic dysfunction, which could also contribute to decreased exercise ability.

Several exercise studies have also examined pediatric subjects with insulin resistance, with variable results. For example, treadmill physical work capacity (absolute or corrected for weight and lean body mass) was decreased in 11 children with fasting hyperinsulinemia, compared to 14 obese controls in a Hungarian study *(58)*. Similarly, treadmill exercise duration, VO_2max, and lactate threshold were all abnormal in 22 obese adolescent boys with the metabolic syndrome, when compared to 17 obese controls *(59)*. Furthermore, in a large study of 349 children (11–14 years), predicted bicycle VO_2max was significantly correlated to fasting insulin levels (Pearson correlation males = −0.418, females = −0.290, $p < 0.006$) *(60)*. After an exercise intervention, improvement in predicted VO_2max correlated with reductions in fasting insulin levels *(60)*. In combination, these studies implicate insulin resistance rather than just obesity per se, in causing exercise defects, as subjects with markers of insulin resistance performed more poorly than equally obese controls. In contrast, in a study of 163 obese Hispanic children (8–13 years) with a family history of T2DM, no significant differences were found in treadmill absolute VO_2max, VO_2max adjusted for gender, age, and body composition, or recreational physical activity levels between youth with or without the metabolic syndrome *(61)* or between youth with normal glucose tolerance and those with impaired glucose tolerance *(62)*. Shaibi et al. also reported that VO_2max was not independently related to insulin sensitivity or secretion, as measured by frequently sampled intravenous glucose tolerance test in a subset of 95 of the same subjects *(63)*. One possible explanation for these discrepancies is that subjects in the Shaibi et al. study were younger, and, therefore, may not yet have developed comorbidities associated with insulin resistance. In addition, other confounders may include differences in baseline activity level, pubertal stage, or dietary intake that were not controlled for. Finally, all of these studies use surrogate markers of insulin sensitivity, which may inaccurately classify the subject's actual insulin sensitivity.

There is evidence that physical activity improves insulin sensitivity in obese youth *(64–66)*, but longitudinal data are limited, as are data on the effects of exercise on cardiovascular risk factors in youth. Several intervention studies focused on lifestyle changes including increased physical activity *(67)*, or a physical activity-only component *(68, 69)* do provide encouraging overall findings. Sallis et al. and Pangrazi et al. showed that school-based programs promoting increased physical activity were effective at increasing the physical activity level or cardiorespiratory endurance (although not in reducing BMI) of youth, particularly in girls. However, there are not yet randomized-controlled trials showing that physical activity or exercise prevents T2DM in youth. Current limited intervention and observation studies suggest that to prevent and manage T2DM, daily goals for youth should include less than 60 min of daily screen (television, computer, or video game) time and 60–90 min of daily physical activity *(70–72)*. We are also currently involved with a large multicenter trial (the TODAY study) to assess the role of physical activity in treating T2DM in youth *(73)*.

Very little data are available regarding exercise function in adolescents with T2DM. In a study including adolescents with T2DM, measures of exercise beliefs, self-reported physical activity, bicycle VO_{2peak}, and heart rate variability were all significantly lower in a study of 27 adolescents with T2DM in comparison to 105 adolescents with type 1 diabetes *(74)*. Hba-1c was not reported in this study; therefore, the effect of glycemic control cannot be teased apart. In addition, insulin sensitivity itself was not measured. However, the poor performance in the T2DM subjects, who were likely more insulin resistant, suggests insulin resistance and its manifestations may be the culprit.

To further investigate exercise function in adolescents with T2DM, our group assessed VO_2max by bicycle ergometer in a group of adolescents with T2DM, compared to nondiabetic, obese and lean controls. Importantly, subjects were chosen to be similar for activity level, Tanner stage, and age, and received a study diet for 3 days prior to exercise to control for differences in dietary intake. Preliminary results show a significantly lower VO_2max in T2DM versus obese subjects despite similar BMI, and, significantly, lower VO_2max in T2DM and obese groups than lean subjects, despite similar RER (indicating similar effort) in all three groups (unpublished data, 2006, 2007). Similarly, T2DM subjects performed significantly less work at maximal effort than the obese or lean groups (unpublished data, 2006, 2007), and had slowed oxygen uptake kinetics during submaximal exercise compared with controls (unpublished data, 2008). Thus, adolescents with T2DM appear to have significant impairments in maximal and submaximal exercise, not explainable by their weight or activity level alone. Unique aspects of this study include control groups that were well matched for BMI, habitual physical activity level, Tanner stage, and age, all of which affect VO_2max. In addition, providing a study diet prior to exercise testing also controlled for differences in dietary composition, which also impacts VO_2max.

VO_2max reflects respiration, cardiac output, autonomic function, endothelial function, skeletal muscle blood flow, and O_2 extraction by skeletal muscle *(75)* among other factors. Therefore, abnormalities in any of these areas could lead to a decrease in VO_2max. Data from our lab and others in adult T2DM subjects suggest abnormalities in the cardiac and vascular system, which may limit nutrient delivery to skeletal muscle. For example, we found that pulmonary capillary wedge pressure rose more steeply and to a greater level with exercise in T2DM than in nondiabetic control subjects, suggesting abnormalities in cardiac output with T2DM *(76)*. Additional cardiac defects include diastolic dysfunction, as shown by reduced early diastolic relaxation and abnormal left ventricular filling pressure in subjects with T2DM, independent of age and body composition *(77)*. Multiple studies also implicate endothelial dysfunction in subjects with T2DM *(78–80)*. Finally, microvascular disease, as evidenced by diabetic nephropathy and diabetic neuropathy, also correlate with reductions in VO_2max *(81)*.

In addition to the heart and vasculature, intrinsic skeletal muscle properties also contribute importantly to VO_2max. Subjects with T2DM have abnormalities in skeletal muscle blood flow and glucose transport into muscle *(82)*. In addition, skeletal muscle oxidative enzyme activity is reduced in subjects with T2DM *(83)*. Moreover, capillary density is decreased in T2DM, which would specifically limit perfusion of skeletal muscle *(84)*. Finally, subjects with T2DM have an increased ratio of type IIb-to-type I muscle fibers *(84)*, which could cause dysfunction in muscle metabolism. All of these skeletal muscle abnormalities may compromise muscle performance during exercise and contribute to a reduced VO_2max.

Insulin resistance itself is a likely culprit in the link between T2DM and exercise dysfunction. We and others have now shown a clear relationship between insulin resistance and VO_2max in adults *(85–87)*. Based on all of the reported abnormalities in adults with T2DM, our group is now examining such potential causes of exercise defects in adolescents with T2DM.

In a preliminary analysis of our data in adolescents, resting echocardiograms showed no significant abnormalities in diastolic function in lean, obese, or T2DM youth but youth with T2DM did have evidence of left ventricular hypertrophy. There were also no differences in resting heart rate, peak heart rate, or recovery heart rate 2 min after exercise in any of the three study groups. Therefore, diastolic function and autonomic function appear to be normal in our adolescent population, and are not explanations for the reduced exercise capacity we observed. In contrast, both adolescents with T2DM and obese adolescents had significantly less blood flow in response to occlusion during plethysmography than lean subjects, indicating potential endothelial dysfunction. In addition, blood flow measured by plethysmography correlated negatively with VO_2max/kg ($r = -0.59$, $p < 0.0001$) (unpublished data, 2008), suggesting that endothelial dysfunction contributes to exercise dysfunction.

VO_2max/kg was also strongly negatively correlated with insulin sensitivity as measured by a hyperinsulinemic euglycemic clamp ($r = -0.83$, $p < 0.0001$) (unpublished data, 2008), suggesting that insulin sensitivity is also an important component of exercise function in adolescents. Other preliminary negative correlations with VO_2max/kg include highly sensitive C-reactive protein (CRP) ($r = -0.578$, $p < 0.0001$), implicating inflammation, and soleus intramyocellular lipid deposition ($r = -0.63$, $p < 0.0001$), suggesting that ectopic fat deposition also effects exercise function in youth (unpublished data, 2006).

Thus, preliminary data suggest that adolescents with T2DM have decreased exercise performance, which is potentially explained by insulin resistance, inflammation, impaired endothelial function, and ectopic lipid deposition. Importantly, these abnormalities are beyond what might be contributed by inactivity or obesity alone. Notably, this is already happening in very young patients, with no other comorbidities or reasons for exercise dysfunction. Therefore, since exercise capacity predicts cardiovascular and all cause mortality, it is critical to further assess baseline exercise capacity and its correlates, as well as the impact of diabetes treatments in adolescents.

Recent encouraging data from our group shows the possibility of improving exercise defects in adults with T2DM. As in subjects without diabetes, an exercise training intervention can improve VO_2max in subjects with T2DM (88). Even more intriguingly, we also found that use of the insulin sensitizer rosiglitazone improved VO_2max in subjects with T2DM, even in the absence of an exercise component (85). Rosiglitazone's effect may act directly through improvements in insulin sensitivity or via its ability to improve endothelial function (89). While we are hopeful that such interventions would help improve exercise capacity in the adolescent population, adolescents are different from adults in many aspects. They are growing, and going through puberty, and have not reached peak muscle or bone strength, therefore their nutritional and hormonal milieu is quite different from an adult. For example, insulin resistance increases during puberty (90, 91), and, therefore, adolescents have differences in insulin secretion and insulin requirements when compared to adults. In addition, teenagers live in families, attend school, are not cognitively mature, and exist amongst the social and psychological issues of adolescence, all affecting their response to potential interventions. Therefore, intervention studies need to be performed in the adolescent population rather that relying on extrapolations from the adult literature.

Although the effects of such interventions have not been tested in pediatric subjects with T2DM, exercise interventions have been studied in obese pediatric subjects. For example, 8 weeks of stationary cycling in 20 overweight children and adolescents, resulted in significant improvements in VO_{2peak}, high-density lipoprotein (HDL) and endothelial function versus controls (92). In another study, a middle school-based exercise intervention tested lifestyle-focused gym classes versus control standard gym classes for 9 months, and found a greater improvement in percent body fat, fasting insulin, and VO_2max in the treatment group versus controls (93). Therefore, VO_2 can be improved in youth by both traditional and school-based exercise interventions.

In addition, pediatric exercise interventions have other positive effects on metabolic health. For example, both lifestyle interventions including overall fitness (94) and resistance training (62) improved insulin sensitivity in youth from ethnic groups at risk for diabetes. Furthermore, a lifestyle intervention in 43 overweight youth (8–16 years) resulted in significant improvements in markers of the metabolic syndrome (BMI, systolic blood pressure, total, low-density lipoprotein, LDL, cholesterol triglycerides, and postprandial glucose) (95). Similarly, in a study of 80 obese adolescents randomly assigned to lifestyle education alone or in addition to moderate or high-intensity physical training, cardiovascular fitness, fasting triglycerides, TC/HDLC, and diastolic blood pressure were significantly improved by exercise training, especially high intensity. The exercise training also reduced visceral and total-body adiposity and increased LDL particle size, regardless of intensity (96, 97). In addition, a modest lifestyle intervention study in 15 obese adolescents improved insulin sensitivity, CRP, fibrinogen, IL-6, fat mass, and adiponectin, even in the absence of weight loss (98, 99). Finally, 100 obese 7–11-year olds were randomized to 13 weeks of no exercise, mild exercise (20-min aerobic activity), or moderate exercise (40-min aerobic activity) (100). Both exercise groups had less snoring and improved sleep quality as assessed by questionnaires, despite no changes in BMI z-score (100). Therefore, exercise can improve VO_2 and multiple markers of health in pediatric subjects, despite the absence of weight loss.

As T2DM is a relatively new phenomenon in the field of pediatrics, there are few data on diabetes prevention or therapy in this age group, and many diabetes therapies considered standard in adults have not been studied in young patients. There are also little data on exercise function in adolescents with T2DM, or response to interventions that work in adults with T2DM. In addition, there are no data on how the diabetes treatments currently used in youth with T2DM affect exercise function or its correlates. However, our recent data show that youth with T2DM have exercise defects. Based on studies in adults and in adolescents with obesity and insulin resistance, exercise interventions appear helpful in pediatric subjects. In summary, due to the current epidemic of obesity and T2DM in pediatrics, and its potential to end lives at an early age, we are in desperate need of data on why adolescents with T2DM are unable to exercise, and how we can improve this situation. If we are able to accomplish this goal, we can hopefully help such adolescents to exercise more, potentially reverse their diabetes, and prevent our country's youth from experiencing cardiovascular morbidity and mortality at young ages.

REFERENCES

1. Berenson, G.S., et al., Association between multiple cardiovascular risk factors and atherosclerosis in children and young adults. *N Engl J Med*, 1998. 338: p. 1650–56.
2. Raitakari, O.T., et al., Cardiovascular risk factors in childhood and carotid artery intima-media thickness in adulthood: the Cardiovascular Risk in Young Finns Study. *JAMA*, 2003. 290: p. 2277–83.
3. Pinhas-Hamiel, O. and P. Zeitler, Advances in the epidemiology and treatment of type 2 diabetes in children. *Adv Pediatr*, 2005. 52: p. 223–59.
4. Dietz, W.H., A.L. Franks, and J.S. Marks, The obesity problem [comment]. *N Engl J Med*, 1998. 338(16): p. 1157; author reply 1158.
5. Kaufman, F.R., Type 2 diabetes mellitus in children and youth: a new epidemic. *J Pediatr Endocrinol Metab*, 2002. 15 (Suppl. 2): p. 737–44.
6. Narayan, K.M., et al., Lifetime risk for diabetes mellitus in the United States. *JAMA*, 2003. 290(14): p. 1884–90.
7. Hillier, T. and K. Pedula, Complications in young adults with early-onset type 2 diabetes. *Diab Care*, 2003. 26: p. 2999–3005.
8. Pavkov, M.E., et al., Effect of youth-onset type 2 diabetes mellitus on incidence of end-stage renal disease and mortality in young and middle-aged Pima Indians. *JAMA*, 2006. 296: p. 421–6.
9. Hillier, T.A. and K.L. Pedula, Characteristics of an adult population with newly diagnosed type 2 diabetes: the relation of obesity and age of onset. *Diabetes Care*, 2001. 24(9): p. 1522–7.
10. Hu, F.B., et al., The impact of diabetes mellitus on mortality from all causes and coronary heart disease in women. *Arch Intern Med*, 2001. 161: p. 1717–23.
11. Fagot-Campagna, A., et al., Type 2 diabetes among North American children and adolescents: an epidemiologic review and a public health perspective. *J Pediatr*, 2000. 136(5): p. 664–72.
12. Kaufman, F.R., Type 2 diabetes mellitus in children and youth: a new epidemic. *J Pediatr Endocrinol Metab*, 2002. 15 (Suppl. 2): p. 737–44.
13. Wei, M., et al., Relationship between low cardiorespiratory fitness and mortality in normal-weight, overweight, and obese men. *JAMA*, 1999. 282(16): p. 1547–53.
14. Blair, S.N. and M. Wei, Sedentary habits, health, and function in older women and men. *Am J Health Promot*, 2000. 15(1): p. 1–8.
15. Seyoum, B., et al., Exercise capacity is a predictor of cardiovascular events in patients with type 2 diabetes mellitus. *Diab Vasc Dis Res*, 2006. 3(3): p. 197–201.
16. Wei, M., et al., Low cardiorespiratory fitness and physical inactivity as predictors of mortality in men with type 2 diabetes. *Ann Intern Med*, 2000. 132(8): p. 605–11.
17. Ribeiro, J., et al., Overweight and obesity in children and adolescents: relationship with blood pressure, and physical activity. *Ann Hum Biol*, 2003. 30(2): p. 203–13.
18. Koga, T., A. Kawaguchi, and H. Aizawa, Physical activity and cardiovascular risk in children. *Lancet*, 2006. 368(9544): p. 1326; author reply 1326–7.
19. Klasson-Heggebo, L., et al., Graded associations between cardiorespiratory fitness, fatness, and blood pressure in children and adolescents. *Br J Sports Med*, 2006. 40(1): p. 25–9; discussion 25–9.
20. Andersen, L.B., et al., Physical activity and clustered cardiovascular risk in children: a cross-sectional study (The European Youth Heart Study). *Lancet*, 2006. 368(9532): p. 299–304.
21. Vuori, I.M., Health benefits of physical activity with special reference to interaction with diet. *Public Health Nutr*, 2001. 4(2B): p. 517–28.
22. Erlichman, J., A.L. Kerbey, and W.P. James, Physical activity and its impact on health outcomes. Paper 1: The impact of physical activity on cardiovascular disease and all-cause mortality: an historical perspective. *Obes Rev*, 2002. 3(4): p. 257–71.
23. Smith, T.C., et al., Walking decreased risk of cardiovascular disease mortality in older adults with diabetes. *J Clin Epidemiol*, 2007. 60(3): p. 309–17.
24. Fulton-Kehoe, D., et al., A case-control study of physical activity and non-insulin dependent diabetes mellitus (NIDDM). The San Luis Valley Diabetes Study. *Ann Epidemiol*, 2001. 11(5): p. 320–7.
25. Li, S., B. Culver, and J. Ren, Benefit and risk of exercise on myocardial function in diabetes. *Pharmacol Res*, 2003. 48(2): p. 127–32.
26. Knowler, W.C., et al., Reduction in the incidence of type 2 diabetes with lifestyle intervention or metformin. *N Engl J Med*, 2002. 346(6): p. 393–403.
27. Krook, A., et al., Reduction of risk factors following lifestyle modification programme in subjects with type 2 (non-insulin dependent) diabetes mellitus. *Clin Physiol Funct Imaging*, 2003. 23(1): p. 21–30.

28. Anonyomous, American Diabetes Association: clinical practice recommendations. *Diabetes Care*, 2002. 25(1) p. S1–S147.

29. Krug, L.M., D. Haire-Joshu, and S.A. Heady, Exercise habits and exercise relapse in persons with non-insulin-dependent diabetes mellitus. *Diabetes Educ*, 1991. 17(3): p. 185–8.

30. Regensteiner, J.G., et al., Effects of non-insulin-dependent diabetes on oxygen consumption during treadmill exercise. *Med Sci Sports Exerc*, 1995. 27(6): p. 875–81.

31. Regensteiner, J.G., et al., Relationship between habitual physical activity and insulin area among individuals with impaired glucose tolerance. The San Luis Valley Diabetes Study. *Diabetes Care*, 1995. 18(4): p. 490–7.

32. Campaigne, B.N., et al., Effects of a physical activity program on metabolic control and cardiovascular fitness in children with insulin-dependent diabetes mellitus. *Diabetes Care*, 1984. 7(1): p. 57–62.

33. Sigal, R.J., et al., Physical activity/exercise and type 2 diabetes: a consensus statement from the American Diabetes Association. *Diabetes Care*, 2006. 29(6): p. 1433–8.

34. Brage, S., et al., Features of the metabolic syndrome are associated with objectively measured physical activity and fitness in Danish children: the European Youth Heart Study (EYHS). *Diabetes Care*, 2004. 27(9): p. 2141–8.

35. Ferreira, I., et al., Development of fatness, fitness, and lifestyle from adolescence to the age of 36 years: determinants of the metabolic syndrome in young adults: the Amsterdam growth and health longitudinal study. *Arch Intern Med*, 2005. 165(1): p. 42–8.

36. Platat, C., et al., Relationships of physical activity with metabolic syndrome features and low-grade inflammation in adolescents. *Diabetologia*, 2006. 49(9): p. 2078–85.

37. DuBose, K.D., J.C. Eisenmann, and J.E. Donnelly, Aerobic fitness attenuates the metabolic syndrome score in normal-weight, at-risk-for-overweight, and overweight children. *Pediatrics*, 2007. 120(5): p. e1262–e1268.

38. Kelishadi R., et al., Association of physical activity and the metabolic syndrome in children and adolescents: CASPIAN Study. *Horm Res*, 2007. 67(1): p. 46–52.

39. Eisenmann, J.C., et al., Fatness, fitness, and cardiovascular disease risk factors in children and adolescents. *Med Sci Sports Exerc*, 2007. 39(8): p. 1251–6.

40. Eisenmann, J.C., et al., Aerobic fitness, body mass index, and CVD risk factors among adolescents: the Quebec family study. *Int J Obes*, 2005. 29(9): p. 1077–83.

41. Eisenmann, J.C., et al., Relationship between adolescent fitness and fatness and cardiovascular disease risk factors in adulthood: the Aerobics Center Longitudinal Study (ACLS). *Am Heart J*, 2005. 149(1): p. 46–53.

42. Morrato, E.H., et al., Physical activity in U.S. adults with diabetes and at risk for developing diabetes, 2003. *Diabetes Care*, 2007. 30(2): p. 203–9.

43. Kimm, S.Y., et al., Longitudinal changes in physical activity in a biracial cohort during adolescence. *Med Sci Sports Exerc*, 2000. 32(8): p. 1445–54.

44. Chatrath, R., et al., Physical fitness of urban American children. *Pediatr Cardiol*, 2002. 23(6): p. 608–12.

45. Kim, Y., T.P. Ciaraldi, A. Kong, D. Kim, N. Chu, P. Mohideen, S. Mudaliar, R.R. Henry and , B.B. Kahn, Troglitazone but not metformin restores insulin-stimulated phosphoinositide 3-kinase activity and increased p110B protein levels in skeletal muscle of type 2 diabetic subjects. *Diabetes*, 2002. 51: p. 443–8.

46. Carnethon, M.R., M. Gulati, and P. Greenland, Prevalence and cardiovascular disease correlates of low cardiorespiratory fitness in adolescents and adults. *JAMA*, 2005. 294(23): p. 2981–8.

47. Klasson-Heggebo, L. and S.A. Anderssen, Gender and age differences in relation to the recommendations of physical activity among Norwegian children and youth. *Scand J Med Sci Sports*, 2003. 13(5): p. 293–8.

48. Riddoch, C.J., et al., Physical activity levels and patterns of 9- and 15-yr-old European children. *Med Sci Sports Exerc*, 2004. 36(1): p. 86–92.

49. Luepker, R.V., How physically active are American children and what can we do about it? *Int J Obes Relat Metab Disord*, 1999. 23 (Suppl. 2): p. S12–S17.

50. Flynn, M.A., et al., Reducing obesity and related chronic disease risk in children and youth: a synthesis of evidence with 'best practice' recommendations. *Obes Rev*, 2006. 7 (Suppl. 1): p. 7–66.

51. Steffen, L.M., et al., Population trends in leisure-time physical activity: Minnesota Heart Survey, 1980–2000. *Med Sci Sports Exerc*, 2006. 38(10): p. 1716–23.

52. Regensteiner, J.G., et al., Abnormal oxygen uptake kinetic responses in women with type II diabetes mellitus. *J Appl Physiol*, 1998. 85(1): p. 310–17.

53. Thamer, C., et al., Reduced skeletal muscle oxygen uptake and reduced beta-cell function: two early abnormalities in normal glucose-tolerant offspring of patients with type 2 diabetes. *Diabetes Care*, 2003. 26(7): p. 2126–32.

54. Maffeis, C., Maximal aerobic power during running and cycling in obese and non-obese children. *Acta Paediatr*, 1994. 83(1): p. 113–16.

55. Watanabe, K., Relationship between body composition and cardiorespiratory fitnmess in Japanese junior high school boys and girls. *Ann Physiol Anthropol*, 1994. 13(4): p. 167–74.

56. Marinov, B., S. Kostianev, and T. Turnovska, Ventilatory efficiency and rate of perceived exertion in obese and non-obese children performing standard exercise. *Clin Physiol Funct Imaging*, 2002. 22(4): p. 254–60.

57. Norman, A.C., et al., Influence of excess adiposity on exercise fitness and performance in overweight children and adolescents. *Pediatrics*, 2005. 115(6): p. e690–e696.

58. Molnar, D. and J. Porszasz, The effect of fasting hyperinsulinaemia on physical fitness in obese children. *Eur J Pediatr*, 1990. 149: p. 570–3.

59. Torok, K., Z. Szelenyi, J. Porszasz, and D. Molnar, Low physical performance in obese adolescent boys with metabolic syndrome. *Int J Obes*, 2001. 25: p. 966–70.

60. McMurray, R.G., et al., Effects of improvement in aerobic power on resting insulin and glucose concentrations in children. *Eur J Appl Physiol*, 2000. 81(1–2): p. 132–9.

61. Shaibi, G.Q., et al., Cardiovascular fitness and the metabolic syndrome in overweight latino youths. *Med Sci Sports Exerc*, 2005. 37(6): p. 922–8.

62. Shaibi, G.Q., et al., Effects of resistance training on insulin sensitivity in overweight Latino adolescent males. *Med Sci Sports Exerc*, 2006. 38(7): p. 1208–15.

63. Ball, G.D., et al., Insulin sensitivity, cardiorespiratory fitness, and physical activity in overweight Hispanic youth. *Obes Res*, 2004. 12(1): p. 77–85.

64. Ribeiro, M.M., et al., Diet and exercise training restore blood pressure and vasodilatory responses during physiological maneuvers in obese children. *Circulation*, 2005. 111(15): p. 1915–23.

65. Nassis, G.P., et al., Aerobic exercise training improves insulin sensitivity without changes in body weight, body fat, adiponectin, and inflammatory markers in overweight and obese girls. *Metabolism*, 2005. 54(11): p. 1472–9.

66. Carrel, A.L., et al., Improvement of fitness, body composition, and insulin sensitivity in overweight children in a school-based exercise program: a randomized, controlled study. *Arch Pediatr Adolesc Med*, 2005. 159(10): p. 963–8.

67. Nwobu, C.O. and C.C. Johnson, Targeting obesity to reduce the risk for type 2 diabetes and other co-morbidities in African American youth: a review of the literature and recommendations for prevention. *Diab Vasc Dis Res*, 2007. 4(4): p. 311–19.

68. Sallis, J.F., et al., The effects of a 2-year physical education program (SPARK) on physical activity and fitness in elementary school students. Sports, play and active recreation for kids. *Am J Public Health*, 1997. 87(8): p. 1328–34.

69. Pangrazi, R.P., et al., Impact of Promoting Lifestyle Activity for Youth (PLAY) on children's physical activity. *J Sch Health*, 2003. 73(8): p. 317–21.

70. McGavock, J., E. Sellers, and H. Dean, Physical activity for the prevention and management of youth-onset type 2 diabetes mellitus: focus on cardiovascular complications. *Diab Vasc Dis Res*, 2007. 4(4): p. 305–10.

71. Crespo, C.J., et al., Television watching, energy intake, and obesity in US children: results from the third National Health and Nutrition Examination Survey, 1988–1994. *Arch Pediatr Adolesc Med*, 2001. 155(3): p. 360–5.

72. Berkey, C.S., et al., One-year changes in activity and in inactivity among 10- to 15-year-old boys and girls: relationship to change in body mass index. *Pediatrics*, 2003. 111(4, Part 1): p. 836–43.

73. Zeitler, P., et al., Treatment options for type 2 diabetes in adolescents and youth: a study of the comparative efficacy of metformin alone or in combination with rosiglitazone or lifestyle intervention in adolescents with type 2 diabetes. *Pediatr Diabetes*, 2007. 8(2): p. 74–87.

74. Faulkner, M.S., et al., Cardiovascular endurance and heart rate variability in adolescents with type 1 or type 2 diabetes. *Biol Res Nurs*, 2005. 7(1): p. 16–29.

75. Rowell, L., Human circulation regulation during physical stress. New York: Oxford University Press, 1986.

76. Regensteiner, J.G., et al., Recently diagnosed type 2 diabetes mellitus adversely affects cardiac function during exercise. *Diabetes*, 2002. 51 (Suppl. 2): p. A59.

77. Baldi, J.C., et al., The effect of type 2 diabetes on diastolic function. *Med Sci Sports Exerc*, 2006. 38(8): p. 1384–8.

78. Regensteiner, J.G., et al., Oral L-arginine and vitamins E and C improve endothelial function in women with type 2 diabetes. *Vasc Med*, 2003. 8(3): p. 169–75.

79. Williams, S., J.A. Cusco, M.A. Roddy, M.T. Johnstone, and M.A. Creager, Impaired nitric oxide-mediated vasodilation in patients with non-insulin-dependent diabetes mellitus. *J Am Coll Cardiol*, 1996. 27: p. 567–74.

80. Kingwell, B., M. Formosa, M. Muhlmann, S.J. Bradley, and G.K. McConell, Type 2 diabetic individuals have impaired leg blood flow responses to exercise: role of endothelium-dependent vasodilation. *Diabetes Care*, 2003. 26(3): p. 899–904.

81. Estacio, R., J.G. Regensteiner, E.E. Wolfel, B. Jeffers, M. Dickenson and, R.W. Schrier, The association between diabetic complications and exercise capacity in NIDDM patients. *Diabetes Care*, 1998. 21: p. 291–5.

82. Steinberg, H.O. and A.D. Baron, Vascular function, insulin resistance and fatty acids. *Diabetologia*, 2002. 45: p. 623–34.

83. Simoneau, J.-A. and D.E. Kelley, Altered glycolytic and oxidative capacities of skeletal muscle contribute to insulin resistance in NIDDM. *J Appl Physiol*, 1997. 83: p. 166–71.

84. Marin, P., M. Krotkiewski, B. Anderson, and P. Bjorntorp, Muscle fiber composition and capillary density in women and men with NIDDM. *Diabetes Care*, 1994. 17: p. 382–6.

85. Regensteiner, J.G., T.A. Bauer, and J.E. Reusch, Rosiglitazone improves exercise capacity in individuals with type 2 diabetes. *Diabetes Care*, 2005. 28(12): p. 2877–83.

86. Mikines, K.J., et al., Effect of training on the dose-response relationship for insulin action in men. *J Appl Physiol*, 1989. 66(2): p. 695–703.

87. Ferrara, C.M., et al., Effects of aerobic and resistive exercise training on glucose disposal and skeletal muscle metabolism in older men. *J Gerontol A Biol Sci Med Sci*, 2006. 61(5): p. 480–7.

88. Brandenburg, S., J. Reusch, T.A. Bauer, B.W. Jeffers, W.R. Hiatt, and J.G. Regensteiner, Effects of exercise training on oxygen uptake kinetic responses in women with type 2 diabetes. *Diabetes Care*, 1999. 22(10): p. 1640–6.

89. Albertini, J.P., et al., Effect of rosiglitazone on factors related to endothelial dysfunction in patients with type 2 diabetes mellitus. *Atherosclerosis*, 2007. 195: p. e159–e166.

90. Travers, S.H., et al., Gender and Tanner stage differences in body composition and insulin sensitivity in early pubertal children. *J Clin Endocrinol Metab*, 1995. 80(1): p. 172–8.

91. Moran, A., et al., Insulin resistance during puberty: results from clamp studies in 357 children. *Diabetes*, 1999. 48(10): p. 2039–44.

92. Kelly, A.S., et al., Inflammation, insulin, and endothelial function in overweight children and adolescents: the role of exercise. *J Pediatr*, 2004. 145(6): p. 731–6.

93. Carrell, A., R.R. Clark, S.E. Peterson, B.A. Nemeth, J. Sullivan, and D.B. Allen, Improvement of fitness, body composition, and insulin sensitivity in overweight children in a school-based exercise program. *Arch Pediatr Adolesc Med*, 2005. 159: p. 963–8.

94. Ritenbaugh, C., et al., A lifestyle intervention improves plasma insulin levels among Native American high school youth. *Prev Med*, 2003. 36(3): p. 309–19.

95. Monzavi, R., et al., Improvement in risk factors for metabolic syndrome and insulin resistance in overweight youth who are treated with lifestyle intervention. *Pediatrics*, 2006. 117(6): p. e1111–e1118.

96. Gutin, B., et al., Effects of exercise intensity on cardiovascular fitness, total body composition, and visceral adiposity of obese adolescents. *Am J Clin Nutr*, 2002. 75(5): p. 818–26.

97. Kang, H.S., et al., Physical training improves insulin resistance syndrome markers in obese adolescents. *Med Sci Sports Exerc*, 2002. 34(12): p. 1920–7.

98. Balagopal, P., et al., Lifestyle-only intervention attenuates the inflammatory state associated with obesity: a randomized controlled study in adolescents. *J Pediatr*, 2005. 146(3): p. 342–8.

99. Balagopal, P., et al., Reversal of obesity-related hypoadiponectinemia by lifestyle intervention: a controlled, randomized study in obese adolescents. *J Clin Endocrinol Metab*, 2005. 90(11): p. 6192–7.

100. Davis, C.L., et al., Aerobic exercise and snoring in overweight children: a randomized controlled trial. *Obesity*, 2006. 14(11): p. 1985–91.

Index